Essential Obstetrics and Gynaecology

Essential Obstetrics and Gynaecology

Sixth Edition

Edited by

Ian Symonds
MB BS MMedSci DM FRCOG FRANZCOG

Dean of Medicine – University of Adelaide;
Head of School, Adelaide Medical School;
Visiting Medical Specialist in Obstetrics,
Women's and Children's Hospital,
Adelaide, South Australia

Sir Sabaratnam Arulkumaran
PhD DSc FRCSE FRCOG FRANZCOG(Hon)

Professor Emeritus,
Division of Obstetrics and Gynaecology,
St George's University of London,
London, UK

ELSEVIER Edinburgh London New York Oxford Philadelphia St Louis Sydney 2020

First edition 1987
Second edition 1992
Third edition 1998
Fourth edition 2004
Fifth edition 2013
Sixth edition 2020

Notices

Practitioners and researchers must always rely on their own experience and knowledge in evaluating and using any information, methods, compounds or experiments described herein. Because of rapid advances in the medical sciences, in particular, independent verification of diagnoses and drug dosages should be made. To the fullest extent of the law, no responsibility is assumed by Elsevier, authors, editors or contributors for any injury and/or damage to persons or property as a matter of products liability, negligence or otherwise, or from any use or operation of any methods, products, instructions, or ideas contained in the material herein.

ISBN: 978-0-7020-7638-1
International ISBN: 978-0-7020-7639-8

Content Strategist: Pauline Graham
Content Development Specialist: Sally Davies, Kirsty Guest
Project Manager: Karthikeyan Murthy
Design: Bridget Hoette
Illustration Manager: Paula Catalano
Marketing Manager: Deborah Watkins

Printed in China

Last digit is the print number: 9 8 7 6 5 4 3 2 1

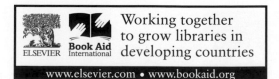

Contents

Contributors

Petra Agoston MD
Clinical Fellow in Obstetrics and Gynaecology
St George's University Hospitals NHS Foundation Trust
London, UK

Sir Sabaratnam Arulkumaran PhD DSc FRCSE FRCOG FRANZCOG(Hon)
Professor Emeritus
Division of Obstetrics and Gynaecology
St George's University of London
London, UK

Shankari Arulkumaran BSc MSc MRCOG MD
Consultant Obstetrician and Gynaecologist
St Mary's Hospital, Imperial College Healthcare NHS Trust
London, UK

Jo Black MB BS MRCPsych
Consultant Perinatal Psychiatrist
Devon Partnership NHS Trust
Exeter, Devon, UK
Associate National Clinical Director for Perinatal Mental Health
NHS England

Fiona Broughton Pipkin MA DPhil FRCOG *ad eundem*
Emeritus Professor of Perinatal Physiology
School of Medicine
University of Nottingham
Nottingham, UK

Karen K.L. Chan MBBChir FRCOG FHKCOG FHKAM (O&G) Cert RCOG (Gyn Onc)
Clinical Associate Professor
Department of Obstetrics and Gynaecology
The University of Hong Kong
Hong Kong, China

Edwin Chandraharan MBBS MS(Obs & Gyn) DFFP DCRM FSLCOG FRCOG
Lead Consultant, Labour Ward
Consultant Obstetrician and Gynaecologist
St George's University Hospitals NHS Foundation Trust
London, UK

Caroline de Costa AM PhD MPH FRANZCOG FRCOG
Professor of Obstetrics and Gynaecology
James Cook University College of Medicine and Dentistry
Cairns, Queensland, Australia

Stergios K. Doumouchtsis MSc MPH PhD MRCOG
Consultant Obstetrician, Gynaecologist, and Urogynaecologist
Epsom and St Helier University Hospitals NHS Trust
Epsom, Surrey
Honorary Senior Lecturer
St George's University of London
London, UK,
Visiting Professor, University of Athens
Athens, Greece

Paul Duggan MBChB DipObst MMedSc MD GradCertEd FRANZCOG
Associate Professor of Obstetrics and Gynaecology
University of Adelaide
Adelaide, South Australia, Australia

Eloïse Fraison MD
Specialist Registrar in Obstetrics, Gynaecology and Reproductive Medicine
University of Montpellier
Montpellier, France;
Associate Lecturer
Department of Reproductive Medicine
University of New South Wales
Sydney, New South Wales, Australia

Ian S. Fraser AO DSc MD
Conjoint Professor in Reproductive Medicine
School of Women's and Children's Health,
University of New South Wales
Royal Hospital for Women,
Sydney, New South Wales, Australia

Kevin Hayes MBBS FRCOG
Consultant in Obstetrics and Gynaecology
Reader in Medical Education
St George's University of London
London, UK

Shaylee Iles BA BSc(Med) MBBS(Hons) UNSW GradCertClinEd(Flinders) FRANZCOG
Staff Specialist in Obstetrics and Gynaecology
John Hunter Hospital
Newcastle, New South Wales
Conjoint Lecturer in Obstetrics and Gynaecology
University of Newcastle Australia
Consultant Gynaecologist
Newcastle Gynaecology
Newcastle, New South Wales, Australia

Adonis S. Ioannides MBChB(Hons) PhD FRCSEd
Associate Professor of Clinical Genetics
University of Nicosia Medical School
Nicosia, Cyprus

Jay Iyer MBBS MD DNB MRCOG FRANZCOG
Consultant Obstetrician and Gynaecologist
Townsville and Mater Hospitals
Townsville, Queensland
Adjunct Senior Lecturer, James Cook University
Townsville, Queensland, Australia

David James MA MD FRCOG DCH
Emeritus Professor of Fetomaternal Medicine
University of Nottingham
Nottingham, UK

Mugdha Kulkarni MBBS DRANZCOG RANZCOG Trainee
Urogynaecology Fellow
RANZCOG Trainee
Australia

William Ledger MA DPhil(Oxon) MB ChB FRCOG FRANZCOG CREI
Head and Professor of Obstetrics and Gynaecology
School of Women's and Children's Health
University of New South Wales
Sydney, New South Wales, Australia

Boon H. Lim MBBS FRCOG FRANZCOG
Associate Professor and Senior Staff Specialist
Department of Obstetrics and Gynaecology
Clinical Director
Division of Women, Youth and Children
Canberra Hospital and Health Services
Australian National University
Canberra, Australian Capital Territory, Australia

Tahir Mahmood CBE MD MBA FRCPE FACOG(Hon) FEBCOG FRCOG
Consultant Obstetrician and Gynaecologist
Victoria Hospital
Kirkcaldy, Fife, UK
Senior Lecturer, University of St Andrews
St Andrews, UK

Sambit Mukhopadhyay MD DNB MMedSci FRCOG
Consultant Gynaecologist and Honorary Senior Lecturer
Norwich Medical School
Norfolk and Norwich University Hospitals NHS Foundation Trust
Norwich, UK

Henry G. Murray MB ChB(Hons) DipObstets BMedSci DM DDU MRCOG FRANZCOG DDU CMFM
Clinical Lead and Senior Staff Specialist
Maternity and Gynaecology
John Hunter Hospital
Newcastle, New South Wales, Australia

Hextan Y.S. Ngan MBBS MD FRCOG FHKCOG FHKAM(O&G) CertRCOG(GynOnc)
Tsao Yin-Kai Professor in Obstetrics and Gynaecology
Chair and Head
Department of Obstetrics and Gynaecology
The University of Hong Kong
Hong Kong, China

Roger Pepperell MD MGO FRACP FRCOG FRANZCOG FACOG(Hon)
Professor Emeritus in Obstetrics and Gynaecology
University of Melbourne
Melbourne, Victoria, Australia
Retired Professor of Obstetrics and Gynaecology
Penang Medical College
Malaysia

Ajay Rane OAM MBBS MSc MD PhD FRCS FRCOG FRANZCOG CU GAICD
Professor and Head
Obstetrics and Gynaecology
Consultant Urogynaecologist
James Cook University
Townsville, Queensland, Australia

Ian Symonds MB BS MMedSci DM FRCOG FRANZCOG
Dean of Medicine
University of Adelaide
Head of School
Adelaide Medical School
Visiting Medical Specialist in Obstetrics
Women's and Children's Hospital
Adelaide, South Australia, Australia

Suzanne V.F. Wallace MA BM BCh FRCOG
Consultant Obstetrician
Nottingham University Hospitals NHS Trust
Nottingham, UK

Acknowledgements

The editors would like to acknowledge and offer grateful thanks for the input of all those who have contributed to previous editions of this textbook; without them this new edition would not have been possible. In particular we acknowledge and thank the following who have stepped down after contributing to the fifth edition:

Kirsten Black
Paddy Moore
Margaret R. Oates
E. Malcolm Symonds
The late Aldo Vacca

The editors would also like to thank all those who contributed to the self-assessment questions in previous editions.

This is the sixth edition of the textboook orginally published in 1987 by Emeritus Professor Malcolm Symonds. It was his vision of an accesible concise summary of the clinical and scientific aspects of womens health, equally suited to medical students, midwives and junior trainees, that has ensured the ongoing popularity of the book. The Editors would like to acknowledge his central contribution over more than 30 years to this publication as well as his role as a mentor and teacher to many including ourselves.

To Our Families

Preface

This is the sixth edition of *Essential Obstetrics and Gynaecology,* marking more than 30 years since the first edition was published.

The last 20 years have seen significant changes in both the scientific understanding of human reproduction and clinical practice. Although some aspects have remained constant, the sheer pace of development has made it necessary for us to invite experts within the different fields of the disciplines of obstetrics and gynaecology to contribute to the work. In addition to a complete update of the content, in this edition we have included OSCE stations in the self-assessment section because this is a common modality for undergraduate assessment. We have retained the popular overall structure of division into basic reproductive sciences of obstetrics and gynaecology and continued with the format that was introduced with the fifth edition of defining learning outcomes in alignment with the RCOG national undergraduate curriculum. Our section on further reading provides information on key articles and guidelines for the reader to obtain greater understanding of the subject.

We would like to acknowledge the contributions of all of our authors and particularly to welcome Dr Jo Black who contributed the chapter on psychiatric disorders of childbirth, updating this chapter from our longstanding contributor Dr Margaret Oates.

We would also like to acknowledge Dr Neville Fields for his comments on the gynaecological chapters from the perspective of a trainee medical officer and Associate Professor Paul Duggan who also reviewed this content. In constructing the revision, we sought the views of both students and junior medical officers, and we would like to thank all of our student contributors to this peer review process. We would like the readers to write to us about omissions and controversies so that we can update the book as we go along.

Ian Symonds
Sabaratnam Arulkumaran

Section | 1 |

Essential reproductive science

1

Chapter | 1 |

Anatomy of the female pelvis

Caroline de Costa

LEARNING OUTCOMES

After studying this chapter you should be able to:

Knowledge criteria

- Describe the anatomy of the bony pelvis, external genitalia and internal genital organs
- Describe the blood, lymphatic and nerve supply to the external and internal genital organs
- Describe the pelvic floor and the perineum

Knowledge of the major features of the female pelvis is essential to the understanding of the processes of reproduction and childbearing and to the effect that various pathological processes may have on the pelvic organs and on the health of the woman.

The structure and function of the genital organs vary considerably with the age of the individual and her hormonal status, as will be apparent in Chapter 16, which covers the changes that take place in puberty and menopause. This chapter aims to outline the major structures comprising the female pelvis, predominantly in the sexually mature female.

The bony pelvis

The bony pelvis consists of the paired innominate bones (each consisting of an ilium, ischium and pubis) and the sacrum and coccyx (Fig. 1.1).

The innominate bones are joined anteriorly at the symphysis pubis, and each articulates posteriorly with the sacrum in the sacroiliac joints. All three joints are fixed in the non-pregnant state, but during pregnancy there is

a relaxation of the joints to allow some mobility during labour and birth. The sacrum articulates with the fifth lumbar vertebra superiorly and the coccyx inferiorly.

The bony pelvis is divided into the false pelvis and the true pelvis by the pelvic brim. The true pelvis is divided into three sections: the pelvic inlet (bounded anteriorly by the superior surface of the pubic bones and posteriorly by the promontory and alae of the sacrum); the mid-pelvis (at the level of the ischial spines); and the pelvic outlet (bounded anteriorly by the lower border of the symphysis, laterally by the ischial tuberosities and posteriorly by the tip of the sacrum).

> The ischial spines are easily palpable on vaginal examination during labour and provide the reference point for assessing the descent of the fetal head during labour and birth.

The external genitalia

The term *vulva* is generally used to describe the female external genitalia and includes the mons pubis, the labia majora, the labia minora, the clitoris, the external urinary meatus, the vestibule of the vagina, the vaginal orifice and the hymen (Fig. 1.2).

The **mons pubis,** sometimes known as the *mons veneris,* is composed of a fibrofatty pad of tissue that lies above the pubic symphysis and, in the mature female, is covered with dense pubic hair. The upper border of this hair is usually straight or convex upwards and differs from the normal male distribution. Pubic hair generally begins to appear between the ages of 11 and 12 years.

The **labia majora** consist of two longitudinal cutaneous folds that extend downwards and posteriorly from the

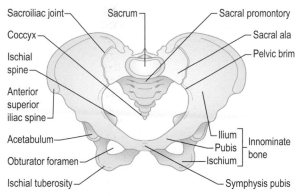

Fig. 1.1 Bony pelvis.

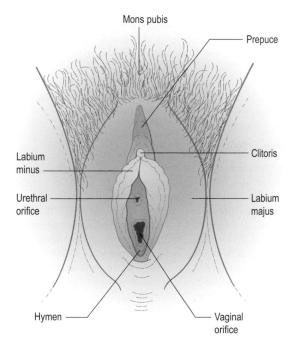

Fig. 1.2 External genital organs of the female.

mons pubis anteriorly to the perineum posteriorly. The labia are composed of an outer surface covered by hair and sweat glands and an inner smooth layer containing sebaceous follicles. The labia majora enclose the pudendal cleft into which the urethra and vagina open.

Posterior to the vaginal orifice, the labia merge to form the posterior commissure, and the area between this structure and the anterior verge of the anus constitutes the obstetric perineum.

The labia majora are homologous with the male scrotum.

The **labia minora** are enclosed by the labia majora and are cutaneous folds that enclose the clitoris anteriorly and fuse posteriorly behind the vaginal orifice to form the posterior fourchette or posterior margin of the vaginal introitus. Anteriorly, the labia minora divide to enclose the clitoris, with the anterior fold forming the prepuce and the posterior fold the frenulum. They are richly vascularized and innervated and are erectile. They do not contain hair but are rich in sebaceous glands.

The **clitoris** is the female homologue of the penis and is situated between the anterior ends of the labia minora. The body of the clitoris consists of two corpora cavernosa of erectile tissue enclosed in a fibrous sheath. Posteriorly, these two corpora divide to lie along the inferior rami of the pubic bones. The free end of the clitoris contains the glans, composed of erectile tissue covered by skin and richly supplied with sensory nerve endings and hence is very sensitive. The clitoris plays an important role in sexual stimulation and function.

The **vestibule** consists of a shallow depression lying between the labia minora. The external urethral orifice opens into the vestibule anteriorly and the vaginal orifice posteriorly. The ducts from the two Bartholin's glands drain into the vestibule at the posterior margin of the vaginal introitus, and the secretions from these glands have an important lubricating role during sexual intercourse.

Skene's ducts lie alongside the lower 1 cm of the urethra and also drain into the vestibule. Although they have some lubricating function, it is minor compared to the function of Bartholin's glands.

The bulb of the vestibule consists of two erectile bodies that lie on either side of the vaginal orifice and are in contact with the surface of the urogenital diaphragm. The bulb of the vestibule is covered by a thin layer of muscle known as the *bulbocavernosus muscle*.

The **external urethral orifice** lies 1.5–2 cm below the base of the clitoris and is often covered by the labia minora, which also function to direct the urinary stream. In addition to Skene's ducts, there are often a number of paraurethral glands without associated ducts, and these sometimes form the basis of paraurethral cysts.

The **vaginal orifice** opens into the lower part of the vestibule and, prior to the onset of sexual activity, is partly covered by the hymenal membrane. The **hymen** is a thin fold of skin attached around the circumference of the vaginal orifice. There are various types of openings within the hymen, and the membrane varies in consistency. Once the hymen has been penetrated, the remnants are represented by the *carunculae myrtiformes*, which are nodules of fibrocutaneous material at the edge of the vaginal introitus.

Bartholin's glands are a pair of racemose glands located at either side of the vaginal introitus and measuring 0.5–1.0 cm in diameter. The ducts are approximately 2 cm in length and open between the labia minora and the vaginal orifice. Their function is to secrete mucus during sexual arousal.

> **!** Cyst formation (Bartholin's cysts) is relatively common but is the result of occlusion of the duct, with fluid accumulation in the duct and not in the gland.

Although it does not strictly lie within the description of the vulva, the **perineum** as described in relation to obstetric function is defined as the area that lies between the posterior fourchette anteriorly and the anus posteriorly; it lies over the perineal body, which occupies the area between the anal canal and the lower one-third of the posterior vaginal wall.

The internal genital organs

The internal genitalia include the vagina, the uterus, the Fallopian tubes and the ovaries. Situated in the pelvic cavity, these structures lie in close proximity to the urethra and urinary bladder anteriorly and the rectum, anal canal and pelvic colon posteriorly (Fig. 1.3).

The vagina

The vagina is a muscular tube some 6–7.5 cm long in the mature female. It is lined by non-cornified squamous epithelium and is more capacious at the vault than at the introitus. In cross-section, the vagina is H shaped and is capable of considerable distension, particularly during parturition when it adapts to accommodate the passage of the fetal head. Anteriorly, it is intimately related to the trigone of the urinary bladder and the urethra. Posteriorly, the lower part of the vagina is separated from the anal canal by the perineal body. In the middle third, it lies in apposition to the ampulla of the rectum, and in the upper segment it is covered by the peritoneum of the rectovaginal pouch (pouch of Douglas).

The uterine cervix protrudes into the vaginal vault. Four zones are described in the vaginal vault: the anterior fornix, the posterior fornix, and the two lateral fornices. The lateral fornices lie under the base of the broad ligament in close proximity to the point where the uterine artery crosses the ureter.

The pH of the vagina in the sexually mature non-pregnant female is between 4.0 and 5.0. This has an important antibacterial function that reduces the risk of pelvic

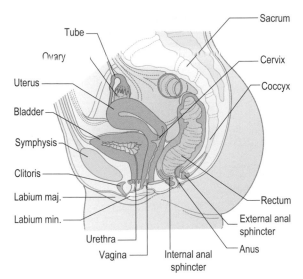

Fig. 1.3 Sagittal section of the female pelvis showing the relationship of the pelvic organs with surrounding structures.

infection. The functions of the vagina are copulation, parturition and the drainage of menstrual loss.

The uterus

The uterus is a hollow, muscular, pear-shaped organ situated in the pelvic cavity between the bladder anteriorly and the rectum and pouch of Douglas posteriorly. The size of the uterus depends on the hormonal status of the female. In the sexually mature female, the uterus is approximately 7.5 cm long and 5 cm across at its widest point. The uterus normally lies in a position of *anteversion* such that the uterine fundus is anterior to the uterine cervix. In about 10% of women, the uterus lies in a position of *retroversion* in the pouch of Douglas. The uterus may also be curved anteriorly in its longitudinal axis, a feature that is described as *anteflexion*, or posteriorly, when it is described as *retroflexion*.

It consists of a body or corpus, an isthmus and a cervix.

The **corpus uteri** consists of a mass of smooth muscle cells, the *myometrium*, arranged in three layers. The external layers contain smooth muscle cells that pass transversely across the uterine fundus into the lateral angles of the uterus, where their fibres merge with the outer layers of the smooth muscle of the Fallopian tubes and the ovarian and round ligaments. The muscle fibres in the middle layer are arranged in a circular manner, and the inner layer contains a mixture of longitudinal, circular and oblique muscle fibres.

The cavity of the uterus is triangular in shape and is flattened anteroposteriorly so that the total volume of the cavity in the non-pregnant state is approximately 2 mL. It is lined by **endometrium** that consists on the surface of mucus-secreting columnar epithelium. The nature of the endometrium depends on the phase of the menstrual cycle. Following menstruation, the endometrium in the proliferative phase is only 1–2 mm thick. By the second half (secretory phase) of the cycle, the endometrium has grown to a thickness of up to 1 cm.

The endometrial cavity is in contact with the vaginal cavity inferiorly via the cervical canal and superiorly with the peritoneal cavity through the Fallopian tubes.

The **cervix** is a barrel-shaped structure extending from the external cervical os, which opens into the vagina at the apex of the vaginal portion of the cervix, to the internal cervical os in its supravaginal portion. The internal os opens into the uterine cavity through the isthmus of the uterus. In non-parous women the external os is round or oval, but it becomes transverse following vaginal birth, and this can be noted in clinical examination when a speculum is passed – for example, when taking cervical specimens.

The cervical canal is fusiform in shape and is lined by ciliated columnar epithelium that is mucus secreting. The transition between this epithelium and the stratified squamous epithelium of the vaginal ectocervix forms the squamocolumnar junction. The exact site of this junction is related to the hormonal status of the woman. Some of the cervical glands in the endocervical lining are extensively branched and mucus secreting. If the opening to these glands becomes obstructed, small cysts may form, known as *nabothian follicles*.

The cervix consists of layers of circular bundles of smooth muscle cells and fibrous tissue. The outer longitudinal layer merges with the muscle layer of the vagina.

The **isthmus** of the uterus joins the cervix to the corpus uteri and in the non-pregnant uterus is a narrow, rather poorly defined area some 2–3 mm in length. In pregnancy, it enlarges and contributes to the formation of the lower segment of the uterus, which is the normal site for the incision of caesarean section. In labour it becomes a part of the birth canal but does not contribute significantly to the expulsion of the fetus.

Supports and ligaments of the uterus

The uterus and the pelvic organs are supported by a number of ligaments and fascial thickenings of varying strength and importance. The pelvic organs also depend for support on the integrity of the pelvic floor: a particular feature in the human female is that, an upright posture having been adopted, the pelvic floor has to contain the downward pressure of the viscera and the pelvic organs.

The **anterior ligament** is a fascial condensation that, with the adjacent peritoneal uterovesical fold, extends from the anterior aspect of the cervix across the superior surface of the bladder to the peritoneal peritoneum of the anterior abdominal wall. It has a weak supporting role.

Posteriorly, the **uterosacral ligaments** play a major role in supporting the uterus and the vaginal vault. These ligaments and their peritoneal covering form the lateral boundaries of the rectouterine pouch (of Douglas). The ligaments contain a considerable amount of fibrous tissue and non-striped muscle and extend from the cervix onto the anterior surface of the sacrum.

Laterally, the **broad ligaments** are reflected folds of peritoneum that extend from the lateral margins of the uterus to the lateral pelvic walls. They cover the Fallopian tubes and the round ligaments, the blood vessels and nerves that supply the uterus, tubes and ovaries, and the mesovarium and ovarian ligaments that suspend the ovaries from the posterior surface of the broad ligament. Like the anterior ligaments, the broad ligaments play only a weak supportive role for the uterus.

The **round ligaments** are two fibromuscular ligaments that extend from the anterior surface of the uterus. In the non-pregnant state, they are a few millimetres thick and are covered by the peritoneum of the broad ligaments. They arise from the anterolateral surface of the uterus just below the entrance of the tubes and extend diagonally and laterally for 10–12 cm to the lateral pelvic walls, where they enter the abdominal inguinal canal and blend into the upper part of the labia majora. These ligaments have a weak supporting role for the uterus but do play a role in maintaining its anteverted position. In pregnancy, they become much thickened and strengthened and during contractions may pull the uterus anteriorly and align the long axis of the fetus in such a way as to improve the direction of entry of the presenting part into the pelvic cavity.

The **cardinal ligaments** (transverse cervical ligaments) form the strongest supports for the uterus and vaginal vault and are dense fascial thickenings that extend from the cervix to the fascia over the obturator fossa on each pelvic side wall. Medially, they merge with the mass of fibrous tissue and smooth muscle that encloses the cervix and the vaginal vault and is known as the *parametrium*. The uterosacral ligaments merge with the parametrium. Close to the cervix, the parametrium contains the uterine arteries, nerve plexuses and the ureter passing through the ureteric canal to reach the urinary bladder. Lower down, the muscular activity of the pelvic floor muscles and the integrity of the perineal body play a vital role in preventing the development of uterine prolapse (see Chapter 21).

The Fallopian tubes

The Fallopian tubes or uterine tubes are the oviducts. They extend from the superior angle of the uterus, where the tubal canal at the tubal ostium opens into the lateral and uppermost part of the uterine cavity. The tubes are approximately 10–12 cm long and lie on the posterior surface of the broad ligament, extending laterally in a convoluted fashion so that, eventually, the tubes open into the peritoneal cavity in close proximity to the ovaries.

The tubes are enclosed in a mesosalpinx, a superior fold of the broad ligament, and this peritoneal fold, apart from the tube, also contains the blood vessels and nerve supply to the tubes and the ovaries. It also houses various embryological remnants such as the epoophoron, the paraoophoron, Gartner's duct and the hydatid of Morgagni. These embryological remnants are significant in that they may form para-ovarian cysts, which are difficult to differentiate from true ovarian cysts. They are generally benign.

The tube is divided into four sections:
- The *interstitial portion* lies in the uterine wall.
- The *isthmus* is a constricted portion of the tube extending from the emergence of the interstitial portion until it widens into the next section. The lumen of the tube is narrow, and the longitudinal and circular muscle layers are well differentiated.
- The *ampulla* is a widened section of the tube, and the muscle coat is much thinner. The widened cavity is lined by thickened mucosa.
- The *infundibulum* of the tube is the outermost part of the ampulla. It terminates at the abdominal ostium, where it is surrounded by a fringe of fimbriae, the longest of which is attached to the ovary.

The tubes are lined by a single layer of ciliated columnar epithelium, which serves to assist the movement of the oocyte down the tube. The tubes are richly innervated and have an inherent rhythmicity that varies according to the stage of the menstrual cycle and whether the woman is pregnant.

The ovaries

The ovaries are paired, almond-shaped organs that have both reproductive and endocrine functions.

They are approximately 2.5–5 cm in length and 1.5–3.0 cm in width. Each ovary lies on the posterior surface of the broad ligaments in a shallow depression known as the *ovarian fossa* in close proximity to the external iliac vessels and the ureter on the lateral pelvic walls. Each has a medial and a lateral surface, an anterior border, a posterior border that lies free in the peritoneal cavity, an upper or tubal pole and a lower or uterine pole.

The anterior border of the ovary is attached to the posterior layer of the broad ligament by a fold in the peritoneum known as the *mesovarium*. This fold contains the blood vessels and nerves supplying the ovary. The tubal pole of the ovary is attached to the pelvic brim by the *suspensory ligament (infundibulopelvic fold)* of the ovary. The lower pole is attached to the lateral border of the uterus by a musculo-fibrous condensation known as the *ovarian ligament*.

The surface of the ovary is covered by a cuboidal or low columnar type of germinal epithelium. This surface opens directly into the peritoneal cavity.

The development of malignant disease in the ovary leads to the shedding of malignant cells directly into the peritoneal cavity as soon as the tumour breaches the surface of the ovary. The disease is silent and often asymptomatic and thus presents late. As a result of these characteristics, the prognosis is generally poor unless the disease is diagnosed when it has not extended beyond the substance of the ovary.

Beneath the germinal epithelium is a layer of dense connective tissue that effectively forms the capsule of the ovary; this is known as the **tunica albuginea**. Beneath this layer lies the **cortex** of the ovary, formed by stromal tissue and collections of epithelial cells that form the **Graafian follicles** at different stages of maturation and degeneration. These follicles can also be found in the highly vascular, central portion of the ovary: the **medulla**. The blood vessels and nerve supply enter the ovary through the medulla.

The blood supply to the pelvic organs

Internal iliac arteries

The major part of the blood supply to the pelvic organs is derived from the internal iliac arteries (sometimes known as the *hypogastric arteries*), which originate from the bifurcation of the common iliac vessels into the external iliac arteries and the internal iliac vessels (Fig. 1.4).

The internal iliac artery arises at the level of the lumbosacral articulation and passes over the pelvic brim, continuing downward on the posterolateral wall of the cavity of the true pelvis beneath the peritoneum until it crosses the psoas major and the piriformis muscles. It then reaches the lumbosacral trunk of the sacral plexus of nerves and, at the upper margin of the greater sciatic notch, it divides into anterior and posterior divisions. It then continues as the umbilical artery, which, shortly after birth, becomes obliterated to form the lateral umbilical ligament. Thus, in fetal life, this is the major vascular network, which delivers blood via the internal iliac anterior division and its continuation as the umbilical artery to the placenta.

The branches of the two divisions of the internal iliac artery are as follows.

Anterior division

The anterior division provides the structure for the umbilical circulation as previously described. It also provides the

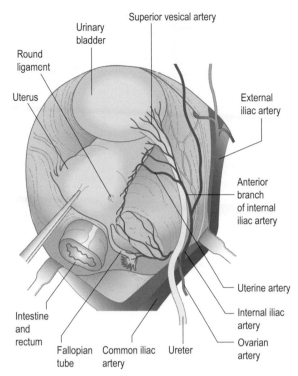

Round ligament

Uterus

Urinary bladder

Superior vesical artery

External iliac artery

Anterior branch of internal iliac artery

Uterine artery

Internal iliac artery

Ovarian artery

Intestine and rectum

Fallopian tube

Common iliac artery

Ureter

Fig. 1.4 Major blood vessels of the female pelvis.

superior, middle and inferior vesical arteries that provide the blood supply for the bladder. The superior and middle branches, having passed medially to the lateral and superior surfaces of the bladder, anastomose with branches from the contralateral vessels and with the branches of the uterine and vaginal arteries.

It also forms the middle haemorrhoidal artery.

The uterine artery becomes the major vascular structure arising from this division during pregnancy, when there is a major increase in uterine blood flow. It initially runs downwards in the subperitoneal fat under the inferior attachment of the broad ligament towards the cervix.

The artery crosses over the ureter shortly before that structure enters the bladder approximately 1.5–2 cm from the lateral fornix of the vagina. At the point of contact with the vaginal fornix, it gives off a vaginal branch that runs downwards along the lateral vaginal wall. The main uterine artery then follows a tortuous course along the lateral wall of the uterus, giving off numerous branches into the substance of the uterus and finally diverging laterally into the broad ligament to anastomose with the ovarian artery, thus forming a continuous loop that provides the blood supply for the ovaries and the tubes as well as the uterine circulation.

There are also parietal branches of the anterior division of the internal iliac artery, and these include the obturator artery, the internal pudendal artery and the inferior gluteal artery.

Posterior division

The posterior division divides into the iliolumbar branch and the lateral sacral and superior gluteal branches and does not play a major function in the blood supply to the pelvic organs.

The ovarian vessels

The other important blood supply to the pelvic organs comes from the ovarian arteries. These arise from the front of the aorta between the origins of the renal and inferior mesenteric vessels. They descend behind the peritoneum on the surface of the corresponding psoas muscle until they reach the brim of the pelvis, where they cross into the corresponding infundibulopelvic fold and from there to the base of the mesovarium and on to anastomose with the uterine vessels. Both the uterine and ovarian arteries are accompanied by a rich plexus of veins.

> The richness of the anastomosis of the uterine and ovarian vessels means that it is possible to ligate both internal iliac arteries and reduce bleeding from the uterus and yet still maintain the viability of the pelvic organs by expanding the blood flow through the ovarian vessels.

The pelvic lymphatic system

The lymphatic vessels follow the course of the blood vessels but have a specific nodal system that is of particular importance in relation to malignant disease of the pelvis (Fig. 1.5).

The lymphatic drainage from the lower part of the vagina, the vulva and perineum and anus passes to the superficial inguinal and adjacent superficial femoral nodes.

The superficial inguinal nodes lie in two groups, with an upper group lying parallel with the inguinal ligament and a lower group situated along the upper part of the great saphenous vein.

Some of these nodes drain into the deep femoral nodes, which lie medial to the upper end of the femoral vein.

One of these nodes, known as the *gland of Cloquet*, occupies the femoral canal.

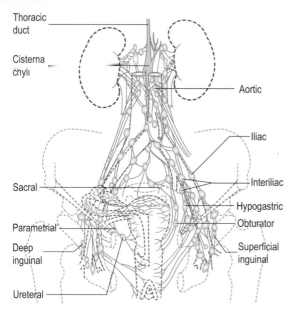

Fig. 1.5 Lymphatic drainage of the female pelvis.

There are also pelvic parietal nodes grouped around the major pelvic vessels. These include the common iliac, external iliac and internal iliac nodes, which subsequently drain to the aortic chain of nodes.

The lymphatics of the cervix, the uterus and the upper portion of the vagina drain into the iliac nodes, whereas the lymphatics of the fundus of the uterus, the Fallopian tubes and the ovaries follow the ovarian vessels to the aortic nodes. Some of the lymphatics from the uterine fundus follow the round ligament into the deep and superficial inguinal nodes.

Nerves of the pelvis

The nerve supply to the pelvis and the pelvic organs has both a somatic and an autonomic component. While the somatic innervation is both sensory and motor in function and relates predominantly to the external genitalia and the pelvic floor, the autonomic innervation provides the sympathetic and parasympathetic nerve supply to the pelvic organs (Fig. 1.6).

Somatic innervation

The somatic innervation to the vulva and pelvic floor is provided by the pudendal nerves that arise from the S2, S3 and S4 segments of the spinal cord. These nerves include both efferent and afferent components.

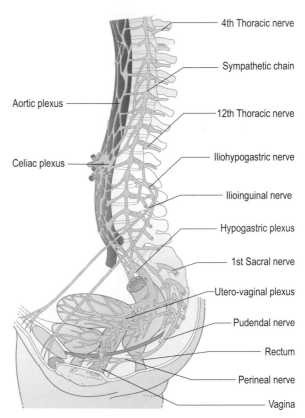

Fig. 1.6 Nerve supply of the pelvis.

The pudendal nerves arise in the lumbosacral plexus and leave the pelvis under the sacrospinous ligament to enter Alcock's canal and pass through the layers of the wall of the ischiorectal fossa to enter the perineum. Motor branches provide innervation of the external anal sphincter muscle, the superficial perineal muscles and the external urethral sphincter.

Sensory innervation is provided to the clitoris through the branch of the dorsal nerve of the clitoris. The sensory innervation of the skin of the labia and of the perineum is also derived from branches of the pudendal nerves. Additional cutaneous innervation of the mons and the labia is derived from the ilioinguinal nerves (L1) and the genito-femoral nerves (L1 and L2) and of the perineum through the posterior femoral cutaneous nerve from the sacral plexus (S1, S2 and S3).

Autonomic innervation

Sympathetic innervation arises from preganglionic fibres at the T10/T11 level and supplies the ovaries and tubes through sympathetic fibres that follow the ovarian vessels.

The body of the uterus and the cervix receive sympathetic innervation through the hypogastric plexus, which accompanies the branches of the iliac vessels, and also contain fibres that signal stretching.

The parasympathetic innervation to the uterus, bladder and anorectum arises from the S1, S2 and S3 segments; these fibres are important in the control of smooth muscle function of the bladder and the anal sphincter system.

Uterine pain is mediated through sympathetic afferent nerves passing up to T11/T12 and L1/L2; the pain is felt in the lower abdomen and the high lumbar spine.

Cervical pain is mediated through the parasympathetic afferent nerves passing backwards to S1, S2 and S3; perineal pain is felt at the site and is mediated through the pudendal nerves.

The pelvic floor

The pelvic floor provides a diaphragm across the outlet of the true pelvis that contains the pelvic organs and some of the organs of the abdominal cavity. The pelvic floor is naturally breached by the vagina, the urethra and the rectum. It plays an essential role in parturition and in urinary and faecal continence (Fig. 1.7). The principal supports of the pelvic floor are the constituent parts of the levator ani muscles. These are described in three sections:

- The iliococcygeus muscle arises from the parietal pelvic fascia, extends from the posterior surface of the pubic rami to the ischial spines and is inserted into the anococcygeal ligament and the coccyx.
- The puborectalis muscle arises from the posterior surface of the pubic rami and passes to the centre of the perineal body anterior to the rectum, with some decussation with muscle fibres from the contralateral muscle.
- The pubococcygeus muscle has a similar origin and passes posteriorly to the sides of the rectum and the anococcygeal ligament.

These muscles play an important role in defecation, coughing, vomiting and parturition.

The perineum

The perineum is the region defined as the inferior aperture of the pelvis and consists of all the pelvic structures that lie below the pelvic floor. The area is bounded anteriorly by the inferior margin of the pubic symphysis, the subpubic arch and the ischial tuberosities. Posteriorly, the boundaries are formed by the sacrotuberous ligaments and the coccyx.

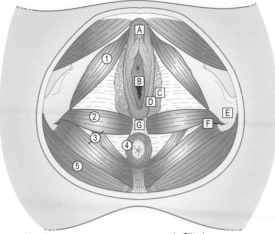

Muscles	A. Clitoris
1. Ischiocavernosus	B. Vagina
2. Superficial transverse perineal	C. Bulb of vestibule
3. Levator ani pubococcygeus iliococcygeus	D. Site of Bartholin's gland
	E. Ischial tuberosity
4. External anal sphincter	F. Pudendal vessels
5. Gluteus maximus	G. Perineal body

Fig. 1.7 Muscles of the pelvic floor.

The perineum is divided into **anterior** and **posterior triangles** by a line drawn between the two ischial tuberosities. The anterior portion is known as the *urogenital triangle* and includes part of the urethra; the urogenital diaphragm is a condensation of fascia below the level of the pelvic floor muscles and is traversed by the vagina. The posterior or anal triangle includes the anus, the anal sphincter and the perineal body. The two triangles have their bases on the deep transverse perineal muscles.

The perineal body is a pyramidal fibromuscular mass in the midline of the perineum at the junction of the urogenital and anal triangles. The muscles comprising the levator ani, the bulbospongiosus, superficial and deep transverse perineal muscles, external anal sphincter and external urethral sphincter are all attached to the perineal body.

> During the second stage of labour, the perineal body plays an important role in supporting the posterior vaginal wall and protecting the external anal sphincter from tearing.

The **ischiorectal fossa** lies between the anal canal and the lateral wall of the fossa formed by the inferior ramus of the ischium covered by the obturator internus muscle and fascia. Posteriorly, the fossa is formed by the gluteus maximus muscle and the sacrotuberous ligament, and anteriorly by the posterior border of the urogenital diaphragm.

The pudendal nerve and internal pudendal vessels pass through the lateral aspect of the fossa enclosed in the fascial layer of Alcock's canal.

Essential information

The external genitalia

- The term *vulva* includes:
  - Mons pubis
  - Labia majora
  - Labia minora
  - Clitoris
  - External urinary meatus
  - Vestibule of the vagina
  - Vaginal orifice and the hymen
- Appearance dependent on age and hormonal status
- Labia majora homologous with the male scrotum
- Clitoris female homologue of the penis
  - Important role in sexual stimulation
- The vestibule contains openings of:
  - Urethral meatus
  - Vaginal orifice
  - Skene's and Bartholin's ducts
- Hymen thin fold of skin attached around the margins of the vaginal orifice

The internal genital organs

- The internal genitalia include:
  - Vagina
  - Uterus
  - Fallopian tubes
  - Ovaries

Vagina

- Muscular tube lined by squamous epithelium
- H shaped in cross-section
- Capable of considerable distension
- Related:
  - Anteriorly with urethra and bladder
  - Posteriorly with anus, perineal body, rectum, pouch of Douglas and pelvic colon

Uterus

- Cervix
  - Musculofibrous cylindrical structure
  - Vaginal portion and supravaginal portion
  - Canal lined by columnar epithelium
  - Ectocervix lined by stratified squamous epithelium
  - External os opens into vagina
  - Internal os opens into uterine cavity
- Isthmus
  - Junctional zone between cervix and corpus uteri
  - Forms lower segment in pregnancy
- Corpus uteri
  - Three layers of smooth muscle fibres:
    - External transverse fibres
    - Middle layer circular fibres
    - Inner layer longitudinal fibres
  - Cavity lined by endometrium
  - Tall columnar epithelium and stromal layers
  - Change with stage of cycle

Supports of the uterus

- Direct supports
  - Weak
    - Round ligaments
    - Broad ligaments
    - Pubocervical ligaments
  - Strong
    - Uterosacral ligaments
    - Cardinal (transverse cervical) ligaments
- Indirect supports – the pelvic floor
  - Levator ani muscles
  - Perineal body
  - Urogenital diaphragm

Fallopian tubes (oviducts)

- Thin muscular tubes
- Lined by ciliated columnar epithelium
- Consist of four sections:
  - Interstitial (intramural)
  - Isthmus
  - Ampulla
  - Infundibulum (fimbriated ends)

The ovaries

- Paired almond-shaped organs
- Surface lies in peritoneal cavity
- Capsule of dense fibrous tissue (tunica albuginea)
- Cortex-stroma and epithelial cells

Continued

Essential information—cont'd

Blood supply

Internal iliac arteries

- Anterior division
  - Visceral
    - Three vesical branches
    - Uterine arteries
  - Parietal
    - Obturator artery
    - Internal gluteal artery
- Posterior division
  - Iliolumbar branch
  - Lateral sacral arteries
  - Inferior gluteal branches

Ovarian arteries

- From aorta below renal arteries
- Rich anastomosis with uterine vessels

Pelvic lymphatic system

- Lymphatic vessels follow blood vessels
- Inguinal nodes (superficial and deep) drain lower vagina, vulva, perineum and anus
- Iliac and then aortic nodes drain cervix, lower part uterus, upper vagina
- Uterine fundus, tubes and ovaries drain to aortic nodes
- Some drainage follows round ligaments to inguinal nodes

Innervation

- Somatic innervation – pudendal nerves from S2, S3, S4
- Autonomic innervation
  - Sympathetic outflow T10, T11, T12, L1, L2
  - Parasympathetic outflow S1, S2, S3
- Pain fibres through T11, T12, L1, L2, S1, S2, S3

Perineum

- Anterior triangle – urogenital triangle includes passage of urethra
- Posterior triangle – includes anus, anal sphincters, perineal body

Chapter | 2 |

Conception and implantation

Roger Pepperell

LEARNING OUTCOMES

After studying this chapter you should be able to:

Knowledge criteria

- Describe the basic principles of the formation of the gametes
- Describe the physiology of the normal menstrual cycle
- Describe the physiology of coitus, fertilization and implantation

Clinical competency

- Counsel a couple about the fertile period

Oogenesis

Primordial germ cells originally appear in the yolk sac and can be identified by the fourth week of fetal development (Fig. 2.1). These cells migrate through the dorsal mesentery of the developing gut and finally reach the genital ridge between 44 and 48 days post-conception. Migration occurs into a genital tubercle consisting of mesenchymal cells that appear over the ventral part of the mesonephros. The germ cells form sex cords and become the cortex of the ovary.

The sex cords subsequently break up into separate clumps of cells and, by 16 weeks, these clumped cells become primary follicles, which incorporate central germ cells.

These cells undergo rapid mitotic activity, and by 20 weeks of intrauterine life, there are about 7 million cells, known as *oogonia*. After this time, no further cell division occurs and no further ova are produced. By birth, the oogonia have already begun the first meiotic division and have become primary oocytes. The number of primary oocytes falls progressively and by birth is down to about 1 million and to about 0.4 million by puberty.

Meiosis

The process of meiosis results in 23 chromosomes being found in each of the gametes, half the number of chromosomes found in normal cells. With the fertilization of the egg by a sperm, the chromosome count is returned to the normal count of 46 chromosomes. Fusion of the sperm and the egg occurs when the first of two meiotic divisions of the oocyte has already been completed; with the second meiotic division occurring subsequently and being completed prior to the 23 chromosomes of the male gamete joining those of the female gamete within the nucleus of the cell, the zygote is formed, which will become the embryo.

In meiosis, two cell divisions occur in succession, each of which consists of prophase, metaphase, anaphase and telophase. The first of the two cell divisions is a reduction division, and the second is a modified mitosis in which the prophase is usually lacking (Fig. 2.2). At the end of the first meiotic prophase, the double chromosomes undergo synapsis, producing a group of four homologous chromatids called a *tetrad*. The two centrioles move to opposite poles. A spindle forms in the middle, and the membrane of the nucleus disappears. During this prophase period of meiosis I, the double chromosomes, which are closely associated in pairs along their entire length, undergo synapsis, crossing over and undergoing chromatid exchange, with these processes accounting for the differences seen between two same-sex siblings despite the fact that the female gametes came from the same mother.

The primary oocytes remain in suspended prophase until sexual maturity is reached, or even much later, with meiosis I not recommencing until the dominant follicle is triggered by luteinizing hormone (LH) to commence

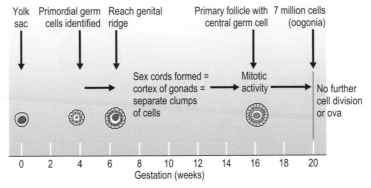

Fig. 2.1 Embryonic and fetal development of oogonia.

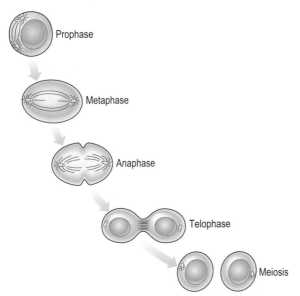

Fig. 2.2 Primary oocytes remain in suspended prophase. Meiotic division resumes under stimulation by luteinizing hormone.

ovulation. In anaphase, the daughter chromatids separate and move towards opposite poles. Meiosis II commences around the time the sperm are attached to the surface of the oocyte and is completed prior to the final phase of fertilization.

Thus, the nuclear events in oogenesis are virtually the same as in spermatogenesis, but the cytoplasmic division in oogenesis is unequal, resulting in only one secondary oocyte. This small cell consists almost entirely of a nucleus and is known as the *first polar body*. As the ovum enters the Fallopian tube, the second meiotic division occurs and a secondary oocyte forms, with

the development of a small second polar body. In the male the original cell containing 46 chromosomes ultimately results in four separate spermatozoa, each being of the same size but containing only 23 chromosomes (see Spermatogenesis, later).

Follicular development in the ovary

The gross structure and the blood supply and nerve supply of the ovary have been described in Chapter 1. However, the microscopic anatomy of the ovary is important in understanding the mechanism of follicular development and ovulation.

The surface of the ovary is covered by a single layer of cuboidal epithelium. The cortex of the ovary contains a large number of oogonia surrounded by follicular cells that become *granulosa* cells. The remainder of the ovary consists of a mesenchymal core. Most of the ova in the cortex never reach an advanced stage of maturation and become atretic early in follicular development. At any given time, follicles can be seen in various stages of maturation and degeneration (Fig. 2.3). About 800 primary follicles are 'lost' during each month of life from soon after puberty until menopause, with only one or two of these follicles resulting in release of a mature ovum each menstrual cycle in the absence of ovarian hyperstimulation therapy. This progressive loss occurs irrespective of whether the patient is pregnant, on the oral contraceptive pill, having regular cycles or amenorrhoeic, with menopause occurring at the same time irrespective of the number of pregnancies or cycle characteristics. The vast majority of the follicles lost have undergone minimal or no actual maturation.

The first stage of follicular development is characterized by enlargement of the ovum with the aggregation of stromal cells to form the thecal cells. When a dominant follicle is selected at about day 6 of the cycle, the

13

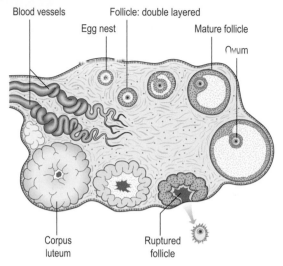

Fig. 2.3 Development and maturation of the Graafian follicle.

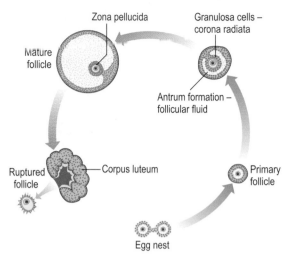

Fig. 2.4 Ovulation and corpus luteum formation.

innermost layers of granulosa cells adhere to the ovum and form the *corona radiata*. A fluid-filled space develops in the granulosa cells, and a clear layer of gelatinous material collects around the ovum, forming the *zona pellucida*. The ovum becomes eccentrically placed, and the Graafian follicle assumes its classic mature form. The mesenchymal cells around the follicle become differentiated into two layers, forming the *theca interna* and the *theca externa*.

As the follicle enlarges, it bulges towards the surface of the ovary and the area under the germinal epithelium thins out. Finally, the ovum, with its surrounding investment of granulosa cells, escapes through this area at the time of ovulation.

The cavity of the follicle often fills with blood but, at the same time, the granulosa cells and the theca interna cells undergo the changes of luteinization to become filled with yellow carotenoid material. The corpus luteum in its mature form shows intense vascularization and pronounced vacuolization of the theca and granulosa cells with evidence of hormonal activity. This development reaches its peak approximately 7 days after ovulation, and thereafter the corpus luteum regresses unless implantation occurs, when human chorionic gonadotropin (hCG) production by the implanting embryo prolongs corpus luteum function until the placenta takes over this role at about 10 weeks of gestation. The corpus luteum degeneration is characterized by increasing vacuolization of the granulosa cells and the appearance of increased quantities of fibrous tissue in the centre of the corpus luteum. This finally develops into a white scar known as the *corpus albicans* (Fig. 2.4).

Hormonal events associated with ovulation

The maturation of oocytes, ovulation and the endometrial and tubal changes of the menstrual cycle are all regulated by a series of interactive hormonal changes (Fig. 2.5).

The process is initiated by the release of the gonadotrophin-releasing hormone (GnRH), a major neurosecretion produced in the median eminence of the hypothalamus. This hormone is a decapeptide and is released from axon terminals into the pituitary portal capillaries. It results in the release of both follicle-stimulating hormone (FSH) and LH from the pituitary.

GnRH is released in episodic fluctuations, with an increase in the number of surges being associated with the higher levels of plasma LH commencing just before mid-cycle and continued ongoing GnRH action required to initiate the huge oestrogen-induced LH surge. Kisspeptin levels in the serum and urine have been studied during the menstrual cycle and found to be useful in the prediction of ovulation. During the first 5 days of the cycle, it is low. There is a surge around the eleventh day when the dominant follicle is about 1.2 cm. The second surge, which is smaller, is around the fourteenth day. Serum kisspeptin levels correlate well with 17-β oestradiol (E_2) levels. It appears that kisspeptin surge may be a good marker of the dominant follicle development prior to ovulation.

The three major hormones involved in reproduction are produced by the anterior lobe of the pituitary gland or adenohypophysis and include FSH, LH and prolactin. Blood levels of FSH are slightly higher during menses and

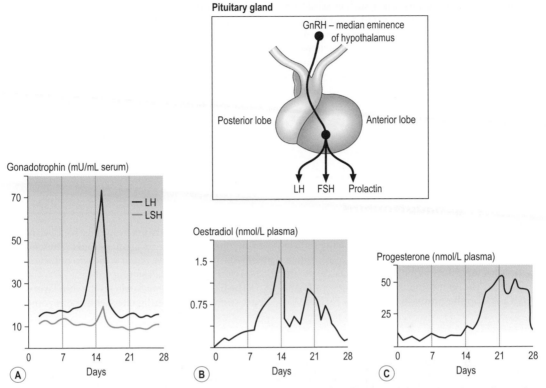

Fig. 2.5 The hormonal regulation of ovulation. Gonadotrophin-releasing hormone (GnRH) stimulates the release of gonadotrophins from the anterior lobe of the pituitary. Blood levels of (A) luteinizing hormone (LH) and follicle-stimulating hormone (FSH); (B) oestradiol; and (C) progesterone during a 28-day menstrual cycle. *LSH*, Lutein-stimulating hormone.

subsequently decline due to the negative feedback effect of the oestrogen production by the dominant follicle. LH levels appear to remain at a relatively constant level in the first half of the cycle; however, there is a marked surge of LH 35–42 hours before ovulation and a smaller coincidental FSH peak (see Fig. 2.5). The LH surge is, in fact, made up of two proximate surges, and a peak in plasma oestradiol precedes the LH surge. Plasma LH and FSH levels are slightly lower in the second half of the cycle than in the preovulatory phase, but continued LH release by the pituitary is necessary for normal corpus luteum function. Pituitary gonadotrophins influence the activity of the hypothalamus by a short-loop feedback system between the gonadotrophins themselves and the effect of the ovarian hormones produced due to FSH and LH action on the ovaries.

Oestrogen production increases in the first half of the cycle, then falls to about 60% of its follicular phase peak following ovulation, and a second peak occurs in the luteal phase. Progesterone levels are low prior to ovulation but then become elevated throughout most of the luteal phase. These features are shown in Fig. 2.5.

Certain feedback mechanisms regulate the release of FSH and LH by the pituitary. This is principally achieved by the oestrogens and progesterone produced by the ovaries. In the presence of ovarian failure, as seen in menopause, the gonadotrophin levels become markedly elevated because of the lack of ovarian oestrogen and progesterone production. Inhibin B levels were thought to predict the ovarian reserve in infertile women but have been shown not to be that useful.

Prolactin is secreted by lactotrophs in the anterior lobe of the pituitary gland. Prolactin levels rise slightly at midcycle but are still within the normal range and remain at similar levels during the luteal phase and tend to follow the changes in plasma oestradiol-17 β levels. Prolactin tends to control its own secretion predominantly through a short-loop feedback system on the hypothalamus, which produces the prolactin-inhibiting factor, dopamine. Oestrogen appears to stimulate prolactin release in addition to the release of various neurotransmitters, such as serotonin, noradrenaline (norepinephrine), morphine and enkephalins, by a central action on the brain. Antagonists to dopamine such as phenothiazine, reserpine and methyltyrosine also stimulate the release of prolactin, whereas dopamine agonists such as bromocriptine and cabergoline have the opposite effect.

 Hyperprolactinaemia prevents ovulation by an inhibitory effect on hypothalamic GnRH production and release and is an important cause of secondary amenorrhoea and infertility.

The action of gonadotrophins

FSH stimulates follicular growth and development and binds exclusively to granulosa cells in the growing follicle. Of the 30 or so follicles that begin to mature in each menstrual cycle, one becomes pre-eminent and is called the *dominant follicle*. The granulosa cells produce oestrogen, which feeds back on the pituitary to suppress FSH release,

with only the dominant follicle then getting enough FSH to continue further development. At the same time, FSH stimulates receptors for LH.

LH stimulates the process of ovulation, the reactivation of meiosis I and sustains the development of the corpus luteum; receptors for LH are found in the theca and granulosa cells and in the corpus luteum. There is a close interaction between FSH and LH in follicular growth and maturation. The corpus luteum produces oestrogen and progesterone until it begins to deteriorate in the late luteal phase (see Fig. 2.4).

The endometrial cycle

The normal endometrium responds in a cyclical manner to the fluctuations in ovarian steroids. The endometrium consists of three zones, and it is the two outer zones that are shed during menstruation (Fig. 2.6).

The basal zone (*zona basalis*) is the thin layer of the compact stroma that interdigitates with the myometrium and

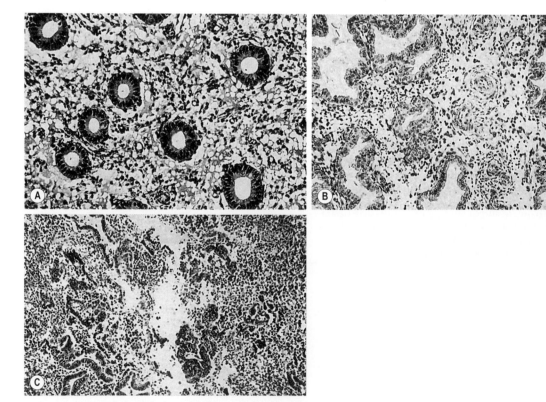

Fig. 2.6 Cyclical changes in the normal menstrual cycle. (A) Proliferative phase. (B) Mid-luteal phase. (C) Menstrual phase.

shows little response to hormonal change. It is not shed at the time of menstruation. The next adjacent zone (*zona spongiosa*) contains the endometrial glands, which are lined by columnar epithelial cells surrounded by loose stroma. The surface of the endometrium is covered by a compact layer of epithelial cells (*zona compacta*) that surrounds the ostia of the endometrial glands. The endometrial cycle is divided into four phases:

1. **Menstrual phase.** This occupies the first 4 days of the cycle and results in shedding of the outer two layers of the endometrium. The onset of menstruation is preceded by segmental vasoconstriction of the spiral arterioles. This leads to necrosis and shedding of the functional layers of the endometrium. The vascular changes are associated with a fall in both oestrogen and progesterone levels, but the mechanism by which these vascular changes are mediated is still not understood. What is clear clinically is that the menstruation due to the shedding of the outer layers of the endometrium occurs whether oestrogen or progesterone, or both, fall, with the loss generally being less if both the oestrogen and progesterone levels fall (as at the end of an ovulatory cycle), and heavier when only the oestrogen level falls (as in an anovulatory cycle).
2. **Phase of repair.** This phase extends from day 4 to day 7 and is associated with the formation of a new capillary bed arising from the arterial coils and with the regeneration of the epithelial surface.
3. **Follicular or proliferative phase.** This is the period of maximal growth of the endometrium and is associated with elongation and expansion of the glands and with stromal development. This phase extends from day 7 until the day of ovulation (generally day 14 of the cycle).
4. **Luteal or secretory phase.** This follows ovulation and continues until 14 days later when menstruation starts

again. During this phase, the endometrial glands become convoluted and 'saw-toothed' in appearance. The epithelial cells exhibit basal vacuolation, and by the mid-luteal phase (about day 20 of a 28-day cycle), there is visible secretion in these cells. The secretion subsequently becomes inspissated and, as menstruation approaches, there is oedema of the stroma and a pseudo-decidual reaction. Within 2 days of menstruation, there is infiltration of the stroma by leukocytes.

It is now clear that luteinization of the follicle can occur in the absence of the release of the oocyte, which may remain entrapped in the follicle. This condition is described as *entrapped ovulation* or luteinized unruptured follicle (LUF) syndrome and is associated with normal progesterone production and an apparently normal ovulatory cycle. Histological examination of the endometrium generally enables precise dating of the menstrual cycle and is particularly important in providing presumptive evidence of ovulation.

Production of sperm

Spermatogenesis

The testis combines the dual function of spermatogenesis and androgen secretion. FSH is predominantly responsible for stimulation of spermatogenesis and LH for the stimulation of Leydig cells and the production of testosterone.

The full maturation of spermatozoa takes about 64–70 days (Fig. 2.7). All phases of maturation can be seen in the testis. Mitotic proliferation produces large numbers of cells (called *spermatogonia*) after puberty until late in life. These spermatogonia are converted to spermatocytes within the testis, and then the first meiotic division commences. As in the female, during this phase, chromatid exchange occurs,

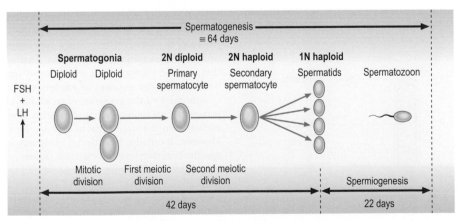

Fig. 2.7 The maturation cycle of spermatozoa.

resulting in all gametes being different despite coming from the same original cell. Spermatocytes and spermatids are produced from the spermatogonia. Spermatozoa are finally produced and released into the lumen of the seminiferous tubules and then into the vas deferens. At the time of this final release, meiosis II has been completed. Full capacitation of the sperm, to enable fertilization to occur, is not achieved until the sperm have passed through the epididymis and seminal vesicles, augmented by a suitable endocrine environment in the uterus or Fallopian tube and finally when the spermatozoon becomes adherent to the oocyte.

Structure of the spermatozoon

The spermatozoon consists of a head, midpiece and tail (Fig. 2.8). The head is flattened and ovoid in shape and is covered by the acrosomal cap, which contains several lysins.

The nucleus is densely packed with the genetic material of the sperm. The midpiece contains two centrioles, proximal and distal, which form the beginning of the tail. The distal centriole is vestigial in mature spermatozoa but is functional in the spermatid. The body contains a coiled helix of mitochondria that provides the 'powerhouse' for sperm motility.

The tail consists of a central core of two longitudinal fibres surrounded by nine pairs of fibres that terminate at various points until a single ovoid filament remains. These contractile fibres propel the spermatozoa.

Seminal plasma

Spermatozoa carry little nutritional reserve and therefore depend on seminal plasma for nutritional support. Seminal plasma originates from the prostate, the seminal vesicles,

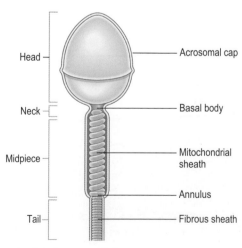

Fig. 2.8 Structure of the mature spermatozoon.

the vas deferens and the bulbourethral glands. There is a high concentration of fructose, which is the major source of energy for the spermatozoa. The plasma also contains high concentrations of amino acids, particularly glutamic acid, and several unique amines such as spermine and spermidine.

Seminal plasma also contains high concentrations of prostaglandins, which have a potent stimulatory effect on uterine musculature. Normal semen clots shortly after ejaculation but liquefies within 30 minutes through the action of fibrinolytic enzymes.

Fertilization

The process of fertilization involves the fusion of the male and female gametes to produce the diploid genetic complement from the genes of both partners.

Sperm transport

Following the deposition of semen near the cervical os, migration occurs rapidly into the cervical mucus. The speed of this migration depends on the presence of receptive mucus in mid-cycle. During the luteal phase, the mucus is not receptive to sperm invasion and, therefore, very few spermatozoa reach the uterine cavity. Under favourable circumstances, sperm migrate at a rate of 6 mm/min. This is much faster than could be explained by the motility of the sperm and must therefore also be dependent on active support within the uterine cavity. Only motile spermatozoa reach the fimbriated end of the tube, where fertilization occurs.

Capacitation

During their passage through the Fallopian tubes, the sperm undergo the final stage in maturation (capacitation), which enables penetration of the zona pellucida. It seems likely that these changes are enzyme induced, and enzymes such as β-amylase or β-glucuronidase may act on the membranes of the spermatozoa to expose receptor sites involved in sperm penetration. In addition, various other factors that may be important in capacitation have been identified, such as the removal of cholesterol from the plasma membrane and the presence of α- and β-adrenergic receptors on the spermatozoa. Until recently, it was thought that capacitation occurred only in vivo in the Fallopian tubes. However, it can also be induced in vitro by apparently nonspecific effects of relatively simple culture solutions.

Inhibitory substances in the plasma of the cauda epididymis and in seminal plasma can prevent capacitation, and these substances also exist in the lower reaches of the female genital tract. It seems likely that these substances protect the sperm until shortly before fusion with the oocyte.

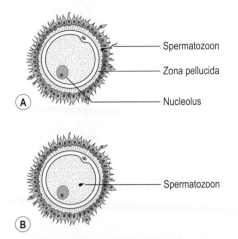

Spermatozoon

Zona pellucida

Nucleolus

(A)

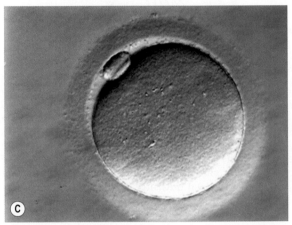

Spermatozoon

(B)

(C)

Fig. 2.9 (A) Adherence of the sperm to the oocyte initiates the acrosome reaction. (B, C) Syngamy involves the passage of the nucleus of the sperm head into the cytoplasm of the oocyte with the formation of the zygote.

Fertilization and implantation

Only a small number of spermatozoa reach the oocyte in the ampulla of the tube and surround the zona pellucida. The adherence of the sperm to the oocyte initiates the *acrosome reaction*, which involves the loss of plasma membrane over the acrosomal cap (Fig. 2.9A).

The process allows the release of lytic enzymes, which facilitate penetration of the oocyte membrane. Generally, only one sperm head fuses with the oocyte plasma membrane, and by phagocytosis the sperm head and midpiece are engulfed into the oocyte.

The sperm head decondenses to form the male pronucleus and eventually becomes apposed to the female pronucleus in the female egg to form the *zygote*. The membranes of the pronuclei break down to facilitate the fusion of male and female chromosomes. This process is known

as *syngamy* (see Fig. 2.9B, C) and is followed almost immediately by the first cleavage division.

During the 36 hours after fertilization, the conceptus is transported through the tube by muscular peristaltic action. The zygote undergoes cleavage and, at the 16-cell stage, becomes a solid ball of cells known as a *morula*. A fluid-filled cavity develops within the morula to form the *blastocyst* (Fig. 2.10). Six days after ovulation, the embryonic pole of the blastocyst attaches itself to the endometrium, usually near to the mid-portion of the uterine cavity. By the seventh post-ovulatory day, the blastocyst has penetrated deeply into the endometrium.

Endometrial cells are destroyed by the cytotrophoblast, and the cells are incorporated by fusion and phagocytosis into the trophoblast. The endometrial stromal cells become large and pale; this is known as the *decidual reaction*.

The processes of fertilization and implantation are now complete.

The physiology of coitus

Normal sexual arousal has been described in four levels in both the male and the female. These levels consist of excitement, plateau, orgasmic and resolution phases. In the male, the *excitement phase* results in compression of the venous channels of the penis, resulting in erection. This is mediated through the parasympathetic plexus through S2 and S3. During the *plateau phase*, the penis remains engorged and the testes increase in size, with elevation of the testes and scrotum. Secretion from the bulbourethral glands results in the appearance of a clear fluid at the urethral meatus. These changes are accompanied by general systemic features, including increased skeletal muscle tension, hyperventilation and tachycardia.

> Erectile dysfunction may result from neurological damage to the spinal cord or the brain and is seen as a result of spina bifida, multiple sclerosis and diabetic neuropathy. However, over 200 prescription drugs are known to cause impotence, and these account for some 25% of all cases. Recreational drugs such as alcohol, nicotine, cocaine, marijuana and LSD may also cause impotence; however, this can usually be improved by the male taking the pharmacological preparation sildenafil citrate (Viagra). Sexual stimulation causes local release of nitric oxide. Inhibition of phosphor diesterase type 5 (PDE5) results in increased levels of cyclic guanosine monophosphate (cGMP) in the corpus cavernosum. This leads to smooth muscle relaxation and inflow of blood to the corpus cavernosum, causing the erection. Hence the drug has no effect in the absence of sexual stimulation.

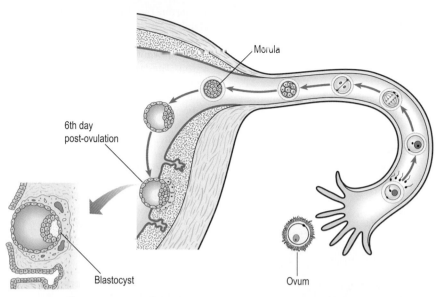

Fig. 2.10 Stages of development from fertilization to implantation.

The *orgasmic phase* is induced by stimulation of the glans penis and by movement of penile skin on the penile shaft. There are reflex contractions of the bulbocavernosus and ischiocavernosus muscles and ejaculation of semen in a series of spurts. Specific musculoskeletal activity occurs that is characterized by penile thrusting. The systemic changes of hyperventilation and rapid respiration persist.

Seminal emission depends on the sympathetic nervous system. Expulsion of semen is brought about by contraction of smooth muscle within the seminal vesicles, ejaculatory ducts and prostate.

During the *resolution phase*, penile erection rapidly subsides, as do the hyperventilation and tachycardia. There is a marked sweating reaction in some 30–40% of individuals. During this phase, the male becomes refractory to further stimulation. The plateau phase may be prolonged if ejaculation does not occur.

In the female, the *excitement phase* involves nipple and clitoral erection, vaginal lubrication (resulting partly from vaginal transudation and partly from secretions from Bartholin's glands), thickening and congestion of the labia majora and the labia minora and engorgement of the uterus. Stimulation of the clitoris and the labia results in progression to the *orgasmic platform*, with narrowing of the outer third of the vagina and ballooning of the vaginal vault. The vaginal walls become congested and purplish in colour, and there is a marked increase in vaginal blood flow. During orgasm, the clitoris retracts below the pubic symphysis and a succession of contractions occurs in the vaginal walls and pelvic floor approximately every second for several seconds. At the same time, there is an increase in pulse rate, hyperventilation and specific skeletal muscular contractions. Blood pressure rises, and there is some diminution in the level of awareness. Both intravaginal and intrauterine pressures rise during orgasm.

The *plateau phase* may be sustained in the female and result in multiple orgasms. Following orgasm, resolution of the congestion of the pelvic organs occurs rapidly, although the tachycardia and hypertension, accompanied by a sweating reaction, may persist.

Factors that determine human sexuality are far more complex than the simple process of arousal by clitoral or penile stimulation. Although the frequency of intercourse and orgasm declines with age, this is in part mediated by loss of interest by the partners. The female remains capable of orgasm until late in life, but her behaviour is substantially determined by the interest of the male partner. Sexual interest and performance also decline with age in the male, and the older male requires more time to achieve excitement and erection. Ejaculation may become less frequent and forceful.

Common sexual problems are discussed in Chapter 19.

Essential information

Oogenesis

- Primordial germ cells appear in the yolk sac
- By 20 weeks, there are 7 million oogonia
- Number of oocytes falls to 1 million by birth
- Number falls to about 0.4 million by puberty
- Chromosome number in gametes is half that of normal cells
- Primary oocyte remains in suspended prophase for 10–50 years
- The second meiotic division commences as the ovum enters the tube

Follicular development in the ovary

- Most ova never reach advanced maturity, and about 800 are lost each month
- Aggregation of stromal cells around follicles become thecal cells
- Innermost layers of granulosa cells form the corona radiata
- After ovulation, the corpus luteum is formed

Hormonal events and ovulation

- FSH stimulates follicular growth
- FSH stimulates LH receptor development
- LH stimulates ovulation and stimulates and sustains development of the corpus luteum
- Follicles produce oestrogen
- Corpus luteum produces oestrogen and progesterone

The endometrial cycle

- Menstrual phase – shedding of functional layer of endometrium
- Phase of repair – day 4–7 of cycle
- Follicular phase – maximum period of growth of endometrial glands due to oestrogen
- Luteal phase – 'saw-toothed' glands, pseudodecidual reaction in stroma

Spermatogenesis

- Full maturation takes 64–70 days
- Mature sperm arise from haploid spermatids

Structure of spermatozoon

- Head is covered by acrosomal cap
- Body contains helix of mitochondria
- Tail consists of two longitudinal fibres and nine pairs of fibres

Seminal plasma

- Originates from the prostate, seminal vesicles and bulbourethral glands
- High concentration of fructose provides energy for sperm motility
- High concentration of prostaglandins

Sperm transport

- Rapid migration into receptive cervical mucus
- Sperm migrate at 6 mm/min
- Only motile sperm reach the fimbriated ends of the tubes

Capacitation

- Final sperm maturation occurs during passage through the oviduct
- Inhibitory substances produced in caudoepididymis and in seminal plasma

Fertilization

- Small number of sperm reaches oocyte
- Adherence of sperm initiates the acrosome reaction
- Sperm head fuses with oocyte plasma membrane
- Sperm head and midpiece engulfed into oocyte
- Fusion of male and female chromosomes is known as *syngamy*
- Thirty-six hours after fertilization, the morula is formed
- Six days after fertilization, implantation occurs

Physiology of coitus

- Penile erection results from compression of venous channels
- Ejaculation mediated by contractions of bulbocavernosus and ischiocavernosus
- Female excitation results in nipple and clitoral erection
- Lubrication comes from vaginal transudation, Bartholin's glands secretions
- Orgasm results in clitoral retraction and contractions of pelvic floor muscles

Chapter | 3 |

Physiological changes in pregnancy

Fiona Broughton Pipkin

LEARNING OUTCOMES

After studying this chapter you should be able to:

Knowledge criteria
- Understand the immunology of pregnancy
- Describe the changes in the uterus, vagina and breasts that take place in pregnancy
- Describe the adaptations of the cardiovascular, endocrine, respiratory, renal and gastrointestinal systems to pregnancy

Clinical competencies
- Interpret the clinical findings and investigatory findings of various tests related to cardiovascular, respiratory, gastrointestinal and renal parameters in pregnancy

Professional skills and attitudes
- Describe the impact of the physiological adaptation to pregnancy on the wellbeing of the mother

Many maternal adaptations to pregnancy, such as an increased heart rate and renal blood flow, are initiated in the luteal phase of every ovulatory cycle and are thus proactive rather than reactive, simply being amplified during the first trimester should conception occur. This suggests very strongly that they are driven by progesterone. All physiological systems are affected to some degree and will also vary within a physiological range because of factors such as age, parity, multiple pregnancy, socioeconomic status and race.

From a teleological point of view, there are two main reasons for these changes:
- To provide a suitable environment for the nutrition, growth and development of the fetus.

- To protect and prepare the mother for the process of parturition and subsequent support and nurture of the newborn infant.

Immunology of pregnancy

Pregnancy defies the laws of transplant immunology. The fetus is an allograft that, according to the laws that protect 'self' from 'non-self', 'should' be rejected by the mother. Furthermore, the mother continues to respond to and destroy other foreign antigens and confers passive immunity to the newborn while not rejecting the fetus. The uterus is not an immunologically privileged site, because other tissues implanted in the uterus are rejected.

Protection must occur from the time of implantation when the endometrium decidualizes. The decidua contains all the common immunological cell types, e.g. lymphocytes and macrophages, but it also contains additional cell types, e.g. large granular lymphocytes. Macrophages appear to initiate and direct almost all immune responses, including those of T and B cells, inducing adaptive immunity. Crudely speaking, they are able to 'kill or repair' tissues by promoting or inhibiting proliferation, depending on whether they metabolize arginine to nitric oxide or to ornithine. Macrophages in the 'kill' state are known as *M1 macrophages* and those in the 'repair' state are known as *M2 macrophages*. The M1 state predominates around the time of implantation, switching to a predominantly M2 state once there is an adequate placento-fetal blood supply.

Only two types of fetoplacental tissue come into direct contact with maternal tissues: the villous and extravillous trophoblast (EVT), and there are effectively no systemic maternal T- or B-cell responses to trophoblast cells in humans. The villous trophoblast, which is bathed by maternal blood, seems to be immunologically inert and never expresses human leucocyte antigen (HLA) class I or class II molecules. EVT, which is directly in contact with endometrial/decidual tissues, does not express the major T-cell ligands, HLA-A or HLA-B, but does express the HLA class I trophoblast-specific HLA-G, which is strongly immunosuppressive; HLA-C; and HLA-E.

The main type of decidual lymphocytes are the uterine natural killer (NK) cells, which differ from those in the systemic circulation. They express surface killer immunoglobulin-like receptors (KIRs), which bind to HLA-C and HLA-G on trophoblasts. The KIRs are highly polymorphic, with two main classes: the KIR-A (non-activating) and KIR-B (multiply activating). HLA-E and HLA-G are effectively monomorphic, but HLA-C is polymorphic, with two main groups: the HLA-C1 and the HLA-C2. Thus, the very polymorphic KIR in maternal tissues and the polymorphic HLA-C in the fetus make up a potentially very variable receptor–ligand system. It has been shown that if the maternal KIR haplotype is AA and the trophoblast expresses any HLA-C2, then the possibility of miscarriage or pre-eclampsia, both associated with shallow invasion, is significantly increased. However, even one KIR-B provides protection. HLA-C2 is highly inhibitory to trophoblast migration and thus appears to need 'activating KIR' to overcome it.

A population of NK-derived, CD56+ granulated lymphocytes is found in first-trimester decidua. They release transforming growth factor-β2, which also has immunosuppressive activity.

The fetus expresses paternal antigens, and these can stimulate the production of maternal antibodies. Conversely, maternal antibodies are present in the fetus, confirming that the placenta is not an impermeable immunological barrier. Pregnancy may also induce blocking antibodies, but these do not appear to be vital to the continuation of pregnancy. Low-grade inflammatory markers such as C-reactive peptide and GlycA are increased, suggesting enhanced maternal innate immunity. Normal pregnancy seems to shift the adaptive immune response towards the Th2 response, with increased circulating interleukin (IL)-18 and lower IL-12p70.

While the fetus needs to avoid attack, this carries a cost, as the partly suppressed immune state in pregnancy makes new infections, parasitic diseases (e.g. malaria) and reactivation of latent viruses potentially more dangerous. Infections are involved in some 40% of pre-term deliveries. The placental and decidual cells express most toll-like receptors (TLRs), and when there is TLR–ligand activation, various cytokines and chemokines, such as the interleukins, are expressed.

The thymus shows some reversible involution during pregnancy, apparently caused by the progesterone-driven exodus of lymphocytes from the thymic cortex, and the Th1:Th2 cytokine ratio shifts towards Th2. Conversely, the spleen enlarges

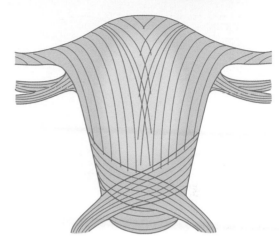

Fig. 3.1 Decussation of muscle fibres in the various layers of the human uterus.

during pregnancy possibly due to the accelerated production of erythrocytes and immunoglobulin-producing cells. The lymph nodes in the para-aortic chain draining the uterus may increase in size, although the germinal centres of these nodes may shrink, with the shrinkage reversing after delivery.

The uterus

The non-pregnant uterus weighs ≈40–100 g, increasing during pregnancy to 300–400 g at 20 weeks and 800–1000 g at term. Involution is rapid over the first 2 weeks after delivery but slows thereafter and is not complete by 2 months. The uterus consists of bundles of smooth muscle cells separated by thin sheets of connective tissue composed of collagen, elastic fibres and fibroblasts. All hypertrophy during pregnancy. The muscle cells are arranged as an innermost longitudinal layer, a middle layer with bundles running in all directions and an outermost layer of both circular and longitudinal fibres partly continuous with the ligamentous supports of the uterus (Fig. 3.1). Myometrial growth is almost entirely due to muscle hypertrophy and elongation of the cells from 50 μm in the non-pregnant state to 200–600 μm at term, although some hyperplasia may occur during early pregnancy. The stimulus for myometrial growth and development is the effect of the growing conceptus and oestrogens and progesterone.

The uterus is functionally and morphologically divided into three sections: the cervix, the isthmus and the body of the uterus (corpus uteri).

The cervix

The cervix is predominantly a fibrous organ with only 10% of uterine muscle cells in the substance of the cervix.

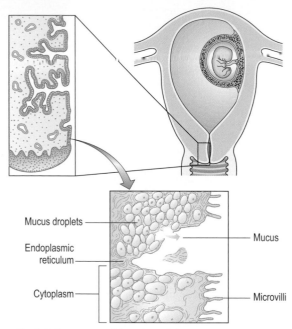

Mucus droplets

Endoplasmic
reticulum

Cytoplasm

Mucus

Microvilli

Fig. 3.2 Structure and function of the cervix in pregnancy.

Eighty percent of the total protein in the non-pregnant state consists of collagen but, by the end of pregnancy, the concentration of collagen is reduced to one-third of the amount present in the non-pregnant state. The principal function of the cervix is to retain the conceptus (Fig. 3.2).

The characteristic changes in the cervix during pregnancy are:

- Increased vascularity.
- Hypertrophy of the cervical glands producing the appearance of a cervical erosion; an increase in mucous secretory tissue in the cervix during pregnancy leads to a thick mucus discharge and the development of an antibacterial plug of mucus in the cervix.
- Reduced collagen in the cervix in the third trimester and the accumulation of glycosaminoglycans and water, leading to the characteristic changes of cervical ripening. The lower section shortens as the upper section expands, while during labour there is further stretching and dilatation of the cervix.

The isthmus

The isthmus of the uterus is the junctional zone between the cervix and the body of the uterus. It joins the muscle fibres of the corpus to the dense connective tissue of the cervix both functionally and structurally. By the twenty-eighth week of gestation, regular contractions produce some stretching and thinning of the isthmus, resulting in the early formation of the lower uterine segment.

The lower segment is fully formed during labour and is a thin, relatively inert part of the uterus. It contributes little to the expulsive efforts of the uterus and becomes, in effect, an extension of the birth canal. Because of its relative avascularity and quiescence in the puerperium, it is the site of choice for the incision for a caesarean delivery.

The corpus uteri

The uterus changes throughout pregnancy to meet the needs of the growing fetus both in terms of physical size and in vascular adaptation to supply the nutrients required:

- As progesterone concentrations rise in the mid-secretory phase of an ovulatory menstrual cycle, endometrial epithelial and stromal cells stop proliferating and begin to differentiate, with an accumulation of maternal leukocytes, mainly NK cells (see Immunology earlier). This decidualization is essential for successful pregnancy.
- The uterus changes in size, shape, position and consistency. In later pregnancy, the enlargement occurs predominantly in the uterine fundus so that the round ligaments tend to emerge from a relatively caudal point in the uterus. The uterus changes from a pear shape in early pregnancy to a more globular and ovoid shape in the second and third trimesters. The cavity expands from some 4 mL to 4000 mL at full term. The myometrium must remain relatively quiescent until the onset of labour.
- All the vessels supplying the uterus undergo massive hypertrophy. The uterine arteries dilate so that the diameters are 1.5 times those seen outside pregnancy. The arcuate arteries, supplying the placental bed, become 10 times larger, and the spiral arterioles reach 30 times the pre-pregnancy diameter (see later). Uterine blood flow increases from 50 mL/min at 10 weeks' gestation to 500–600 mL/min at term.

In the non-pregnant uterus, blood supply is almost entirely through the uterine arteries, but in pregnancy 20–30% is contributed through the ovarian vessels. A small contribution is made by the superior vesical arteries. The uterine and radial arteries are subject to regulation by the autonomic nervous system and by direct effects from vasodilator and vasoconstrictor humoral agents.

The final vessels delivering blood to the intervillous space (Fig. 3.3) are the 100–150 spiral arterioles. Two or three spiral arterioles arise from each radial artery, and each placental cotyledon is provided with one or two. The remodelling of these spiral arteries is very important for a successful pregnancy. Cytotrophoblast differentiates into villous or EVT. The latter can differentiate further into invasive EVT, which in turn is either interstitial, migrating into the decidua and later differentiating into myometrial giant cells, or endovascular and invades the lumen of the spiral arteries. The intrauterine oxygen tension is very low in the first trimester, stimulating EVT invasion.

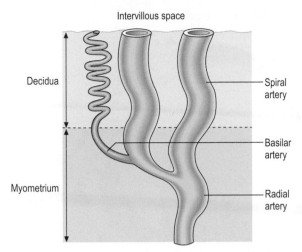

Intervillous space

Decidua

Myometrium

Spiral artery

Basilar artery

Radial artery

Fig. 3.3 Vascular structure in the uteroplacental bed.

In the first 10 weeks of normal pregnancy, EVT invades the decidua and the walls of the spiral arterioles, destroying the smooth muscle in the wall of the vessels, which then become inert channels unresponsive to humoral and neurological control (Fig. 3.4). From 10 to 16 weeks, a further wave of invasion occurs, extending down the lumen of the decidual portion of the vessel; from 16 to 24 weeks this invasion extends to involve the myometrial portion of the spiral arterioles. The net effect of these changes is to turn the spiral arterioles into flaccid sinusoidal channels.

Failure of this process, particularly in the myometrial portion of the vessels, means that this portion of the vessels remains sensitive to vasoactive stimuli with the potential for a reduction in blood flow. This is a feature of pre-eclampsia and intrauterine growth restriction, with or without pre-eclampsia.

The uterus has both afferent and efferent nerve supplies, although it can function normally in a denervated state. The main sensory fibres from the cervix arise from S1 and S2, whereas those from the body of the uterus arise from the dorsal nerve routes on T11 and T12. There is an afferent pathway from the cervix to the hypothalamus so that stretching of the cervix and upper vagina stimulates the release of oxytocin (*Ferguson's reflex*). The cervical and uterine vessels are well supplied by adrenergic nerves, whereas cholinergic nerves are confined to the blood vessels of the cervix.

Uterine contractility

The continuation of a successful pregnancy depends on the fact that the myometrium remains quiescent until the fetus is mature and capable of sustaining extrauterine life. Pregnant myometrium has a much greater compliance than non-pregnant myometrium in response to

distension. Thus, although the uterus becomes distended by the growing conceptus, intrauterine pressure does not increase, even though the uterus does maintain the capacity to develop maximal active tension. Progesterone maintains quiescence by increasing the resting membrane potential of the myometrial cells while at the same time impairing the conduction of electrical activity and limiting muscle activity to small clumps of cells. Progesterone receptor function appears to decrease towards term. Progesterone antagonists such as mifepristone can induce labour from the first trimester, as can prostaglandin F2$_\alpha$, which is luteolytic. Other mechanisms include locally generated nitric oxide, probably acting through cyclic guanosine monophosphate (cGMP) or voltage-gated potassium channels, while several relaxatory hormones such as prostacyclin (PGI$_2$), prostaglandin (PGE$_2$) and calcitonin gene-related peptide, which act through the G$_s$ receptors, increase in pregnancy.

The development of myometrial activity

The myometrium functions as a syncytium so that contractions can pass through the gap junctions linking the cells and produce coordinated waves of contractions. Uterine activity occurs throughout pregnancy and is measurable as early as 7 weeks' gestation, with frequent, low-intensity contractions. As the second trimester proceeds, contractions increase in intensity but remain of relatively low frequency. In the third trimester, they increase in both frequency and intensity, leading up to the first stage of labour. Contractions during pregnancy are usually painless and are felt as 'tightenings' (*Braxton Hicks contractions*) but may sometimes be sufficiently powerful to produce discomfort. They do not produce cervical dilatation, which occurs with the onset of labour.

In late gestation, the fetus continues to grow, but the uterus stops growing, so tension across the uterine wall increases. This stimulates expression of a variety of gene products such as oxytocin and prostaglandin F2$_\alpha$ receptors, sodium channels and the gap junction protein. Pro-inflammatory cytokine expression also increases. Once labour has begun, the contractions in the late first stage may reach pressures up to 100 mmHg and occur every 2–3 minutes (Fig. 3.5). See Chapter 11 for a discussion of labour and delivery.

The vagina

The vagina is lined by stratified squamous epithelium, which hypertrophies during pregnancy. The three layers of superficial, intermediate and basal cells change their relative proportions so that the intermediate cells predominate

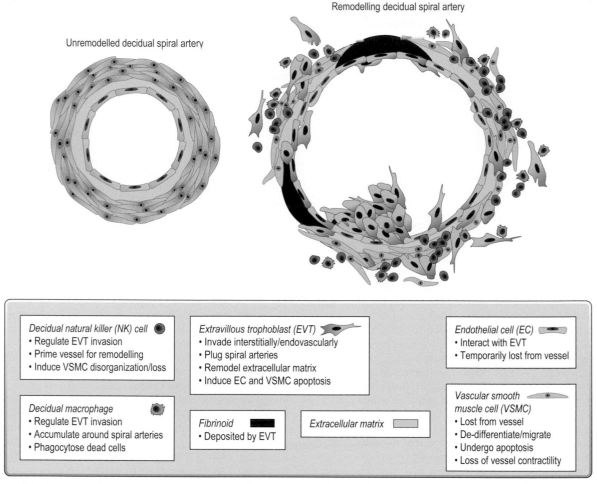

Fig. 3.4 During spiral artery remodelling, vascular cells are lost, increasing the size of the arteries and creating a high-flow, low-resistance vessel. These changes are brought about by both maternal immune cells (decidual NK cells and macrophages) and by invading interstitial and endovascular EVT. (Adapted from Cartwright JE et al. (2010) Reproduction 140:803–813. © Society for Reproduction and Fertility. Reproduced by permission.)

and can be seen in the cell population of normal vaginal secretions. The musculature in the vaginal wall also becomes hypertrophic. As in the cervix, the connective tissue collagen decreases, while water and glycosaminoglycans increase. The rich venous vascular network in the vaginal walls becomes engorged and gives rise to a slightly bluish appearance.

Epithelial cells generally multiply and enlarge and become filled with vacuoles rich in glycogen. High oestrogen levels stimulate glycogen synthesis and deposition, and as these epithelial cells are shed into the vagina, lactobacilli known as *Döderlein's bacilli* break down the glycogen to produce lactic acid. The vaginal pH falls in pregnancy to 3.5–4.0, and this acid environment serves to keep the vagina clear of bacterial infection. Unfortunately, yeast infections may thrive in this environment, and *Candida* infections are common in pregnancy.

The cardiovascular system

The cardiovascular system is one of those that shows proactive adaptations for a potential pregnancy during the luteal phase of every ovulatory menstrual cycle, long before there is any physiological 'need' for them. Many of these changes are almost complete by 12–16 weeks' gestation (Fig. 3.6 and Table 3.1).

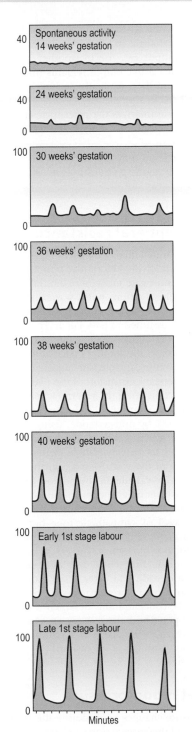

Fig. 3.5 The evolution of uterine activity during pregnancy.

Spontaneous activity 14 weeks' gestation

24 weeks' gestation

30 weeks' gestation

36 weeks' gestation

38 weeks' gestation

40 weeks' gestation

Early 1st stage labour

Late 1st stage labour

Minutes

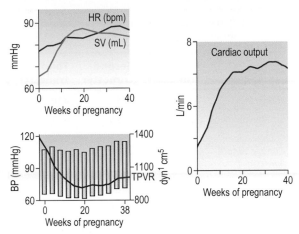

Fig. 3.6 Major haemodynamic changes associated with normal human pregnancy. The marked increase in cardiac output results from asynchronous rises in heart rate (HR) and stroke volume (SV). Despite the rise in cardiac output, blood pressure (BP) falls in the first half of pregnancy, implying a very substantial reduction in total peripheral resistance (TPR). (Adapted from Broughton Pipkin F (2007) Maternal physiology. In: Edmonds DK (ed) Dewhurst's Textbook of Obstetrics and Gynaecology, 8th edn. Blackwell, Oxford.)

Cardiac position and size

As the uterus grows, the diaphragm is pushed upwards and the heart is correspondingly displaced: the apex of the heart is displaced upwards and left laterally, with a deviation of ≈15%. Radiologically, the upper left cardiac border is straightened with increased prominence of the pulmonary conus. These changes result in an inverted T wave in lead III and a Q wave in leads III and aVF.

The heart enlarges by 70–80 mL, some 12%, between early and late pregnancy, due in part to a small increase in wall thickness but predominantly to increased venous filling. The increase in ventricular volume results in dilatation of the valve rings and hence an increase in regurgitant flow velocities. Myocardial contractility is increased during pregnancy, as indicated by a shortening of the pre-ejection period, and this is associated with lengthening of the myocardial muscle fibres.

Cardiac output

Non-invasive methods, such as Doppler velocimetry, echocardiography and impedance cardiography, are now available, allowing standardized sequential studies of cardiac output throughout pregnancy.

There is a small rise in heart rate during the luteal phase, increasing to 10–15 beats/min by mid-pregnancy; this may be related to the progesterone-driven hyperventilation (see later). There is probably a fall in baro-reflex sensitivity as

Table 3.1 Percentage change in some cardiovascular variables during pregnancy

	First trimester	Second trimester	Third trimester
Heart rate	+11	+13	+16
Stroke volume (mL)	+31	+29	+27
Cardiac output (L/min)	+45	+47	+48
Systolic BP (mmHg)	−1	+1	+6
Diastolic BP (mmHg)	−6	−3	+7
MPAP (mmHg)	+5	+5	+5
Total peripheral resistance (resistance units)	−27	−27	−29

BP, Blood pressure; MPAP, mean pulmonary artery pressure.

Data are derived from studies in which pre-conception values were determined. The mean values shown are those at the end of each trimester and are thus not necessarily the maximal. Note that the changes are near maximal by the end of the first trimester.

Data from Robson S, Robson SC, Hunter S, et al. (1989) Serial study of factors influencing changes in cardiac output during human pregnancy. Am J Physiol 1989; 256:H1060. Table reproduced from Broughton Pipkin F (2001) Maternal physiology. In: Chamberlain GV, Steer P (eds) Turnbull's Obstetrics, 3rd edn. Churchill Livingstone, London; with permission from Elsevier.

weights below the tenth centile show much smaller pregnancy-related changes in haemodynamics.

Cardiac output can rise by another third (≈2 L/min) in labour. The cardiac output remains high for ≈24 hours postpartum and then gradually declines to non-pregnant levels by ≈2 weeks after delivery.

Table 3.1 summarizes the percentage changes in some cardiovascular variables during pregnancy.

> Pregnancy imposes a significant increase in cardiac output and is likely to precipitate heart failure in women with heart disease.

Total peripheral resistance

TPR is not measured directly but is calculated from the mean arterial pressure divided by cardiac output. The augmentation index, a surrogate measure of arterial stiffness, is also measured indirectly from pulse wave analysis. Measured TPR and augmentation index both fall by 6 weeks' gestation, so afterload is assumed to have fallen. This is 'perceived' as circulatory under-filling, which is thought to be one of the primary stimuli to the mother's circulatory adaptations. It activates the renin–angiotensin–aldosterone system and allows the necessary expansion of the plasma volume (PV; see Renal function later). In a normotensive non-pregnant woman, the TPR is around 1700 dyn/s/cm; this falls to a nadir of 40–50% by mid-gestation, rising slowly thereafter towards term, reaching 1200–1300 dyn/s/cm in late pregnancy. The fall in systemic TPR is partly associated with the expansion of the vascular space in the utero-placental bed and the renal vasculature; blood flow to the skin is also greatly increased in pregnancy as a result of vasodilatation.

The vasodilatation that causes the fall in TPR is not due to a withdrawal of sympathetic tone but is hormonally driven by a major shift in the balance from vasoconstrictor to vasodilator hormones. The vasodilators involved in early gestation include circulating PGI_2 and locally synthesized nitric oxide and, later, atrial natriuretic peptide. There is also a loss of pressor responsiveness to angiotensin II (AngII), concentrations of which rise markedly (see Endocrinology). The balance between vasodilatation and vasoconstriction in pregnancy is a critical determinant of blood pressure and lies at the heart of the pathogenesis of pre-eclampsia.

Arterial blood pressure

Blood pressure changes occur during the menstrual cycle. Systolic blood pressure increases during the luteal phase of the cycle and reaches its peak at the onset of menstruation, whereas diastolic pressure is 5% lower during the luteal phase than in the follicular phase of the cycle.

pregnancy progresses and heart rate variability falls. Stroke volume rises a little later in the first trimester than heart rate, increasing from about 64 to 71 mL during pregnancy. Women who have an artificial pacemaker and thus a fixed heart rate compensate well in pregnancy based on increased stroke volume alone.

These two factors push up the cardiac output and cardiac index (cardiac output related to body surface area). Most of the rise in cardiac output occurs in the first 14 weeks of pregnancy, with an increase of 1.5 L from 4.5 to 6.0 L/min. The non-labouring change in cardiac output is 35–40% in a first pregnancy and ≈50% in later pregnancies. Twin pregnancies are associated with a 15% greater increase throughout pregnancy. In a healthy pregnancy, the birth weight is associated with the increase in cardiac output and fall in total peripheral resistance (TPR) and augmentation index. Conversely, women with any type of hypertension in pregnancy who deliver babies with birth

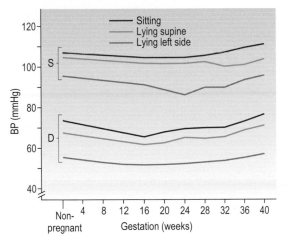

Fig. 3.7 The effect of posture on blood pressure (BP) during pregnancy.

The fall in TPR during the first half of pregnancy causes a fall of some 10 mmHg in mean arterial pressure; 80% of this fall occurs in the first 8 weeks of pregnancy. Thereafter, a small additional fall occurs until arterial pressure reaches its nadir by 16–24 weeks' gestation. It rises again after this and may return to early pregnancy levels. The rate of rise is amplified in women who go on to develop pre-eclampsia.

Posture has a significant effect on blood pressure in pregnancy; pressure is lowest with the woman lying supine on her left side. The pressure falls during gestation in a similar way whether the pressure is recorded sitting, lying supine or in the left lateral supine position, but the levels are significantly different (Fig. 3.7). This means that mothers attending for antenatal visits must have their blood pressure recorded in the same position at each visit if the pressures are to be comparable. Special care must be taken to use an appropriate cuff size for the measurement of brachial pressures. This is especially important with the increasing incidence of obesity among young women. The gap between the fourth and fifth Korotkoff sounds widens in pregnancy, and the fifth Korotkoff sound may be difficult to define. Both these factors may cause discrepancies in the measurement of diastolic pressure in pregnancy. Although most published studies of blood pressure are based on the use of the Korotkoff fourth sound, it is now recommended to use the fifth sound where it is clear and the fourth sound only where the point of disappearance is unclear. Automated sphygmomanometers are unsuitable for use in pregnancy when the blood pressure is raised, as in pre-eclampsia.

Profound falls in blood pressure may occur in late pregnancy when the mother lies on her back. This phenomenon is described as the *supine hypotension syndrome*. It results from the restriction of venous return from the lower limbs due to compression of the inferior vena cava and hence a fall in stroke volume. It must be remembered that aortic compression also occurs and that this will result in conspicuous differences between brachial and femoral blood pressures in pregnancy. When a woman turns from a supine to a lateral position in late pregnancy, the blood pressure may fall by 15%, although some of this fall is a measurement artefact caused by the raising of the right arm above the level of the heart.

There is progressive venodilatation and rises in venous distensibility and capacitance throughout a normal pregnancy. Central venous pressure and pressure in the upper arms remain constant in pregnancy, but the venous pressure in the lower circulation rises progressively on standing, sitting or lying supine because of pressure from the uterus and the fetal presenting part in late pregnancy. The pulmonary circulation can absorb high rates of flow without an increase in pressure, so pressure in the right ventricle and the pulmonary arteries and capillaries does not change. Pulmonary resistance falls in early pregnancy and does not change thereafter.

The blood

Blood volume is a measurement of PV and red cell mass. The indices are under separate control mechanisms. PV changes are considered later (see Renal function).

Erythrocytes

There is a steady increase in red cell mass in pregnancy, and the increase appears to be linear throughout pregnancy. Both cell number and cell size increase. The circulating red cell mass rises from around 1400 mL in non-pregnant women to ≈1700 mL during pregnancy in women who do not take iron supplements. It rises more in women with multiple pregnancies, and substantially more with iron supplementation (≈29% compared with 18%). Erythropoietin rises in pregnancy, more if iron supplementation is not taken (55% compared with 25%), but the changes in red cell mass antedate this; human placental lactogen may stimulate haematopoiesis.

Haemoglobin concentration, haematocrit and red cell count fall during pregnancy because the PV rises proportionately more than the red cell mass ('physiological anaemia'; see Table 9.1). However, in normal pregnancy, the mean corpuscular haemoglobin concentration remains constant. Serum iron concentration falls, but the absorption of iron from the gut rises and iron-binding capacity rises in a normal pregnancy, since there is increased synthesis of the β1-globulin, transferrin. Maternal dietary iron requirements more than double. Plasma folate concentration halves by term because

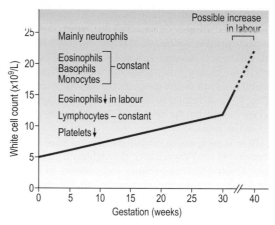

Fig. 3.8 Pregnancy is associated with an increased white cell count; the increase occurs predominantly in polymorphonuclear leukocytes.

of greater renal clearance, although red cell folate concentrations fall less. In the late 1990s, 20% of the female population aged 16–64 years in the UK was estimated to have serum ferritin levels below 15 μg/L, indicating low iron stores; no similar survey appears to have been undertaken since then. Pregnant adolescents seem to be at risk of iron deficiency. Even relatively mild maternal anaemia is associated with increased placental:birth weight ratios and decreased birth weight.

The white cells

The total white cell count rises during pregnancy. This increase is mainly due to an increase in neutrophil polymorphonuclear leukocytes that peaks at 30 weeks' gestation (Fig. 3.8). A further massive neutrophilia normally occurs during labour and immediately after delivery, with a fourfold increase in the number of polymorphs.

A massive neutrophilia is normal during labour and the immediate puerperium and cannot be assumed to be due to infection.

There is also an increase in the metabolic activity of granulocytes during pregnancy, which may result from the action of oestrogens. This can be seen in the normal menstrual cycle, where the neutrophil count rises with the oestrogen peak in mid-cycle. Eosinophils, basophils and monocytes remain relatively constant during pregnancy, but there is a profound fall in eosinophils during labour, and they are virtually absent at delivery. The lymphocyte count remains constant, and the numbers of T and B cells do not alter, but lymphocyte function and cell-mediated immunity in particular are depressed, possibly by the increase in concentrations of glycoproteins coating the surface of the lymphocytes, reducing the response to stimuli.

There is, however, no evidence of suppression of humoral immunity or the production of immunoglobulins.

Platelets

Longitudinal studies show a significant fall in platelet count during pregnancy. The fall in platelet numbers may be a dilutional effect, but the substantial increase in platelet volume from ≈28 weeks suggests that there is increased destruction of platelets in pregnancy with an increase in the number of larger and younger platelets in the circulation. The platelet count falls below 150,000 ×10⁹/L in ≈10% of otherwise normal women in late gestation. Platelet reactivity is increased in the second and third trimesters and does not return to normal until ≈12 weeks after delivery.

Clotting factors

There are major changes in the coagulation system in pregnancy, with an increased tendency towards clotting (Box 3.1). In a situation where haemorrhage from the uterine vascular bed may be sudden, profuse and life threatening, the increase in coagulability may play a lifesaving role. On the other hand, it increases the risk of thrombotic disease.

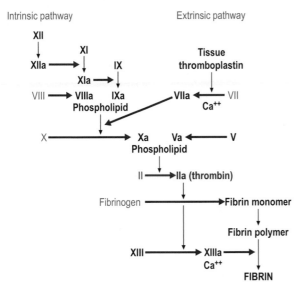

Intrinsic pathway   Extrinsic pathway

Fig. 3.9 Alterations in the coagulation pathways associated with human pregnancy. Factors that increase during normal pregnancy are shown in bold type. (Adapted from Broughton Pipkin F (2007) Maternal physiology. In: Edmonds DK (ed) Dewhurst's Textbook of Obstetrics and Gynaecology, 8th edn. Blackwell, Oxford.)

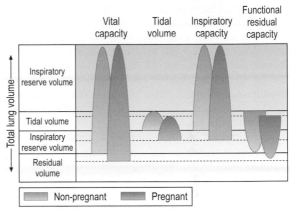

Fig. 3.10 Alterations in lung volumes associated with human pregnancy. Overall, inspiratory reserve and tidal volumes increase at the expense of expiratory reserve and residual volumes. (Adapted from Broughton Pipkin F (2007) Maternal physiology. In: Edmonds DK (ed) Dewhurst's Textbook of Obstetrics and Gynaecology, 8th edn. Blackwell, Oxford.)

Many clotting factors remain constant in pregnancy, but there are notable and important exceptions (Fig. 3.9). Factors VII, VIII, VIII:C, X and IX (Christmas factor) all increase during pregnancy, whereas factors II and V tend to remain constant. Factor XI falls to 60–70% of the non-pregnant values, and concentrations of factor XIII fall by 50%. Protein C, which inactivates factors V and VIII, is probably unchanged in pregnancy, but concentrations of protein S, one of its co-factors, fall during the first two trimesters.

Plasma fibrinogen levels increase from non-pregnant values of 2.5–4.0 g/L to levels as high as 6.0 g/L in late pregnancy, and there is an increase in the concentration of high-molecular-weight fibrin/fibrinogen complexes during normal pregnancy. The erythrocyte sedimentation rate rises early in pregnancy, mainly due to the increase in fibrinogen. An estimated 5–10% of the total circulating fibrinogen is consumed during placental separation, and thromboembolism is one of the main causes of maternal death in the UK. On the other hand, there is a reduction in plasma fibrinolytic activity during pregnancy; the rapid return to non-pregnant levels of activity within 1 hour of delivery suggests that this inhibition is mediated through the placenta.

> There is an increased tendency to clotting in pregnancy and the puerperium.

Respiratory function

The level of the diaphragm rises and the intercostal angle increases from 68 degrees in early pregnancy to 103 degrees in late pregnancy. Although there is upward pressure on the diaphragm in late pregnancy, the costal changes occur well before they could be attributed to pressure from the enlarging uterus. Nevertheless, breathing in pregnancy is more diaphragmatic than costal.

Vital capacity describes the maximum amount of gas that can be expired after maximum inspiration. Since residual volume decreases slightly in pregnancy (Fig. 3.10), vital capacity increases slightly. Vital capacity is related to body weight and is reduced by obesity. Inspiratory capacity measures tidal volume plus inspiratory reserve volume. It increases progressively during pregnancy by ≈300 mL, while residual volume decreases by about 300 mL. This improves gas mixing. Forced expiratory volume in 1 second (FEV_1) and peak expiratory flow remain constant in pregnancy, and women with asthma do not appear to be affected by pregnancy.

Progesterone sensitizes the medulla oblongata to P_aCO_2, and so stimulates some over-breathing in the luteal phase and in pregnancy. Respiratory rate remains constant during pregnancy at 14–15 breaths/min, whereas tidal volume increases from about 500 mL in the non-pregnant state to about 700 mL in late pregnancy. Thus, there is ≈40% increase during pregnancy, so the minute ventilation (the product of tidal volume and respiratory rate) also increases by 40%, from about 7.5 to 10.5 L/min.

Because of the increase in minute ventilation and the effect of progesterone increasing the level of carbonic anhydrase B in red cells, arterial PCO_2 falls in pregnancy. At the same time, there is a fall in plasma bicarbonate concentration, and the arterial pH therefore remains constant. Carbon dioxide production rises sharply during the third trimester as fetal metabolism increases. The low maternal P_aCO_2 allows more efficient placental transfer of carbon dioxide from the fetus.

The increased alveolar ventilation results in a small ($\approx$5%) rise in maternal PO_2. This increase is offset by the rightward shift of the maternal oxyhaemoglobin dissociation curve caused by an increase in 2,3-diphosphoglycerate (2,3-DPG) in the erythrocytes. This facilitates oxygen unloading to the fetus, which has both a much lower PO_2 and a marked leftwards shift of the oxyhaemoglobin dissociation curve due to the lower sensitivity of fetal haemoglobin to 2,3-DPG.

There is an increase of $\approx$16% in oxygen consumption by term due to increasing maternal and fetal demands. Since the increase in oxygen-carrying capacity of the blood (see earlier) is $\approx$18%, there is actually a fall in arteriovenous oxygen difference.

Overall, respiratory diseases and especially obstructive airway diseases have far fewer implications for the mother's health than cardiac disorders, with the exception of conditions such as severe kyphoscoliosis, where the lung space is severely restricted.

Pregnancy does not generally impose any increased risk on women with respiratory disease.

Renal function

Anatomy

Renal parenchymal volume increases by 70% by the third trimester, and there is marked dilatation of the calyces, renal pelvis and ureters in most women. This, together with the expansion of vascular volume, results in increased renal size. The changes occur in the first trimester under the influence of progesterone rather than the effect of back pressure. This is physiological. However, the ureteric dilatation ends at the pelvic brim, suggesting that there may be some effect from back pressure in later pregnancy. These changes are invariably more pronounced on the right side, suggesting an anatomical contribution. The ureters are not hypotonic or hypomotile, and there is hypertrophy of the ureteral smooth muscle and hyperplasia of the connective tissue. Vesicoureteric reflux occurs sporadically, and the combination of reflux and ureteric dilatation is associated with a high incidence of urinary stasis and urinary tract infection.

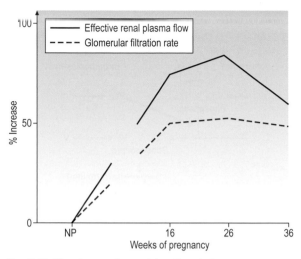

Fig. 3.11 The changes in renal function during pregnancy are largely complete by the end of the first trimester. (Adapted from Broughton Pipkin F (2007) Maternal physiology. In: Edmonds DK (ed) Dewhurst's Textbook of Obstetrics and Gynaecology, 8th edn. Blackwell, Oxford.)

Physiology

Both renal blood flow (RBF) and glomerular filtration rate (GFR) increase during an ovulatory menstrual cycle, and this increase is maintained should conception occur. RBF increases by 50–80% in the first trimester, is maintained at these levels during the second trimester and falls by $\approx$15% thereafter (Fig. 3.11). Creatinine clearance is a useful indicator of GFR but gives values that are significantly less than those obtained by inulin clearance (gold standard). The 24-hour creatinine clearance has increased by 25% 4 weeks after the last menstrual period and by 45% at 9 weeks. In the third trimester, there is some decrease towards non-pregnant values, but less than the fall in RBF. The filtration fraction thus falls in the first trimester, is stable in the second and rises towards non-pregnant values towards term.

Water retention must occur to allow the increase in plasma volume. The osmotic threshold for drinking falls between weeks 4 and 6, which stimulates water intake and thus dilution of body fluids. There is a marked fall in plasma osmolality ($\approx$10 mOsm/kg). However, arginine vasopressin (AVP) continues to circulate at concentrations that allow water to be reabsorbed in the renal medullary collecting ducts until the P_{osm} falls below the new osmotic thirst threshold, when a new steady state is established. Water retention is facilitated by the sodium retention of pregnancy (see later). Standing upright is significantly more antidiuretic than in non-pregnant subjects.

PV increases in pregnancy to a peak between 32 and 34 weeks, from a non-pregnant level of 2600 mL, and returns to non-pregnant levels by 4 weeks after delivery. The total increase is ≈50% in a first pregnancy and 60% in a second or subsequent pregnancy. The bigger the expansion is, the bigger, on average, the birth weight of the baby. The total extracellular fluid volume rises by about 16% by term, so the percentage rise in PV is disproportionately large. Multiple pregnancies are associated with a significantly higher increase in plasma volume. Women with established gestational hypertension or pre-eclampsia have lower plasma volumes, as do pregnancies exhibiting impaired fetal growth, but it is not yet established when the decrease occurs.

> The marked increase in GFR and the expansion of the PV mean that plasma concentrations of a variety of solutes, such as creatinine and urea, fall in normal pregnancy. This should be remembered when interpreting laboratory reports.

The filtered load of sodium increases by 5000–10,000 mmol/day because of the increase in the GFR. Tubular reabsorption increases in parallel with the GFR (see Renin–angiotensin system later), with the retention of 3–5 mmol of sodium per day into the fetal and maternal stores. The total net sodium gain amounts to 950 mmol, mainly stored in the maternal compartment. However, the plasma concentration of sodium falls slightly in pregnancy because of the marked rise in plasma volume. A similar change occurs with potassium ions, with a net gain of approximately 350 mmol.

Renal tubular function also changes significantly during pregnancy. Uric acid is freely filtered through the glomerulus, but most is later reabsorbed. However, in pregnancy, uric acid filtration doubles, following the GFR, and there is a decrease in net tubular reabsorption, so serum uric acid concentrations fall by 25% to mid-pregnancy. The normal values in pregnancy range from 148–298 µmol/L, with an upper limit of ≈330 µmol/L. In later gestation, the kidney excretes a progressively smaller proportion of the filtered uric acid, so some rise in serum uric acid concentration during the second half of pregnancy is normal. A similar pattern is seen in relation to urea, which is also partly reabsorbed in the nephron.

Glucose excretion increases during pregnancy, and intermittent glycosuria is common in normal pregnancy, unrelated to blood glucose levels. Tubular reabsorption is probably less complete during pregnancy. The excretion of other sugars, such as lactose and fructose, is also increased.

> Glycosuria may be a feature of normal pregnancy.

The tubular reabsorption of calcium is enhanced, presumably under the influence of the increased concentrations of 1,25-dihydroxyvitamin D. Even so, urinary calcium excretion is twofold to threefold higher in normal pregnancy than in the non-pregnant woman. Renal bicarbonate reabsorption and hydrogen ion excretion appear to be unaltered during pregnancy. Although pregnant women can acidify their urine, it is usually mildly alkaline.

Both total protein and albumin excretion rise from the first trimester to at least 36 weeks. Thus in late pregnancy, an upper limit of normal of 200 mg total protein excretion/24 hour collection is accepted. Overall, at least one woman in eight will show significant proteinuria without clinically defined hypertension by term ('gestational proteinuria'), although their blood pressure increases more than that of women who do not show clinically significant rises in proteinuria. This may reflect increased glomerular permeability or altered tubular handling. Using dipsticks to assess proteinuria in pregnancy gives highly variable data.

The alimentary system

Gastric secretion is reduced in pregnancy and gastric motility is low, so gastric emptying is delayed. Decreased motility also occurs in both the small and large bowel, and the colonic absorption of water and sodium is increased, leading to a greater likelihood of constipation. Heartburn is common and may be related to the displacement of the lower oesophageal sphincter through the diaphragm and its decreased response as the intra-abdominal pressure rises. Pregnant women are more prone to aspiration of the gastric contents during the induction of general anaesthesia.

Hepatic synthesis of albumin, plasma globulin and fibrinogen increases under oestrogen stimulation – the latter two increase sufficiently to give increased plasma concentrations despite the increase in plasma volume. There are marked individual differences in the globulin fractions.

Hepatic extraction of circulating amino acids is decreased. The gallbladder increases in size and empties more slowly during pregnancy, but bile secretion is unchanged.

Nutrients in blood

Maternal carbohydrate metabolism

Glucose is the major substrate for fetal growth and nutrition, so carbohydrate metabolism in pregnancy is very important for fetal development. Neither the absorption of glucose from the gut nor the half-life of insulin seem to change. However, by 6–12 weeks' gestation, fasting plasma glucose

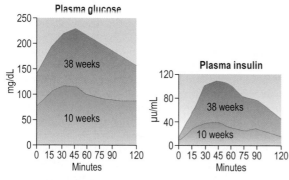

Fig. 3.12 Responses in normal pregnant women to a 50-g oral glucose load during early and late gestation. During early pregnancy there is a normal plasma insulin response, with a relative reduction in plasma glucose concentrations compared with the non-pregnant state. However, during late pregnancy, plasma glucose concentrations reach higher levels after a delay, despite a considerably enhanced plasma insulin response, a pattern that could be explained by relative resistance to insulin. (Adapted from Broughton Pipkin F (2007) Maternal physiology. In: Edmonds DK (ed) Dewhurst's Textbook of Obstetrics and Gynaecology, 8th edn. Blackwell, Oxford.)

concentrations have fallen to about 0.5–1 mmol/L lower than non-pregnant values; fetal concentrations run ≈20% lower than this. The mother's plasma insulin concentrations rise, favouring fat accumulation. By the end of the first trimester, the increase in blood glucose following a carbohydrate load is less than outside pregnancy (Fig. 3.12). Pregnant women develop insulin resistance later in pregnancy, so any given glucose challenge will produce extra insulin, which does not reduce the blood glucose levels as quickly as the response in non-pregnant women. This results in a catabolic state, with raised maternal blood glucose and free fatty acid (FFA) concentrations, both of which are needed for fetal growth. The insulin resistance is hormonally driven, possibly via human placental lactogen or cortisol. The management of the pregnant woman with diabetes is discussed in Chapter 9.

As well as moving glucose into the cells, insulin reduces the circulating level of amino acids and FFAs (see Endocrinology later).

Changes in plasma proteins

The total protein concentration falls by about 1 g/dL during the first trimester from 7 to 6 g/dL, even though there is increased nitrogen retention. This is partly due to the increased insulin concentrations, but also because of placental uptake and transfer of amino acids to the fetus for gluconeogenesis and protein synthesis. This fall is largely proportional to the fall in albumin concentration and is associated with a corresponding fall in colloid osmotic pressure. The fall is insufficient to affect drug-carrying capacity.

Amino acids

With the exception of alanine and glutamic acid, amino acid levels in maternal plasma decrease below non-pregnant values. There is active transport of amino acids to the fetus as building blocks for protein synthesis and gluconeogenesis.

Lipids

The total serum lipid concentration rises from about 600 to 1000 mg per 100 mL. The greatest changes are the approximate threefold increases in very-low-density lipoprotein (VLDL) triglycerides and a 50% increase in VLDL cholesterol by 36 weeks. Birth weight and placental weight are directly related to maternal VLDL triglyceride levels at term. Total fatty acid (FA) concentration rises throughout pregnancy, as does the proportion of saturated and monounsaturated FAs, but the proportion of omega-6 FAs falls. Levels of FFAs are particularly unstable in pregnancy and may be affected by fasting, exertion, emotional stress and smoking. Lipid oxidation is higher throughout pregnancy in women who are overweight than in those with normal body mass index (BMI).

The hyperlipidaemia of normal pregnancy is not atherogenic, although pregnancy can unmask pathological hyperlipidaemia. Mothers are usually protected from the potentially harmful effects of increasing lipid peroxidation in pregnancy by an increase in endogenous antioxidants, although this may be inadequate in pre-eclampsia. An adequate dietary intake of antioxidants such as vitamin A, the carotenoids and provitamin A carotenoids is also needed. Levels of fat-soluble vitamins rise in pregnancy, whereas levels of water-soluble vitamins tend to fall.

Bile salts facilitate the absorption of dietary fats and fat-soluble vitamins. Serum bile acids rise as pregnancy progresses, with the primary bile acids showing the greatest increase. The nuclear Farnesoid X receptor (FXR) is mainly responsible for bile acid homeostasis; its activity is reduced during pregnancy.

Fat is deposited early in pregnancy. It is also used as a source of energy, mainly by the mother from mid to late pregnancy for the high metabolic demands and during lactation so that glucose is available for the growing fetus. Total fat accretion is ≈2–6 kg, mainly laid down in the second trimester, and is regulated by the hormone leptin. It is deposited mainly over the back, the upper thighs, the buttocks and the abdominal wall.

Calcium

Maternal total plasma calcium falls because albumin concentration falls, but unbound ionized calcium is unchanged. Synthesis of 1,25-dihydroxycholecalciferol increases, promoting enhanced gastrointestinal calcium absorption, which doubles by 24 weeks, after which it stabilizes.

Maternal weight gain

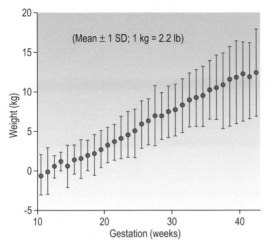

Fig. 3.13 Maternal weight gain (mean ± 1 SD [standard deviation]) in normal pregnancy. (From James D, Steer P, Weiner C, et al (2010) High Risk Pregnancy: Management Options. Elsevier Saunders, St Louis © Elsevier. Reproduced by permission.)

Pregnancy is an anabolic state. The average weight gain over pregnancy in a woman of normal BMI is ≈12.5 kg. Many women during the first trimester do not gain any weight because of reduced food intake associated with loss of appetite and morning sickness. However, in normal pregnancy, the average weight gain is 0.3 kg/week up to 18 weeks, 0.5 kg/week from 18 to 28 weeks and thereafter a slight reduction with a rate of ≈0.4 kg/week until term (Fig. 3.13). The range of maternal weight gain in normal pregnancy may vary from near zero to twice the mean weight gain because of variation in the multiple contributory factors. The respiratory quotient (RQ: carbon dioxide production/oxygen consumption; used to calculate basal metabolic rate (BMR)) gives an idea of changes in the proportion of carbohydrate vs. fat oxidized during pregnancy. The BMR rises by ≈5% by the end of pregnancy in a woman of normal weight. Figure 3.14 summarizes the relative maternal and fetal contributions to weight gain at term.

Much of this weight increase in all systems arises from the retention of water; the mean total increase is ≈8.5 L and is the same in primigravid and multiparous women. The increased hydration of connective tissue results in laxity of the joints, particularly in the pelvic ligaments and the pubic symphysis. Tissues such as the uterus and breasts increase in size.

High weight gain is commonly associated with oedema and fluid retention. However, overall weight gain has a positive association with birth weight, although this may relate

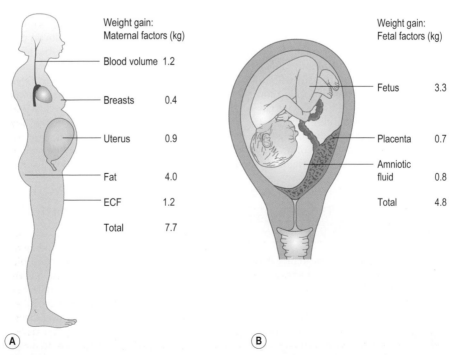

Fig. 3.14 (A) Maternal and (B) fetal contributions to weight gain at term. *ECF*, Extracellular fluid.

to the underlying rise in plasma volume. Although acute excessive weight gain may be associated with the development of pre-eclampsia, mild oedema is associated with a good fetal outcome.

Far more sinister is failure to gain weight, which may be associated with reduced amniotic fluid volume, small placental size, impaired fetal growth and an adverse outcome.

> Acute excess weight gain indicates fluid retention. Poor weight gain is associated with fetal growth restriction. **!**

No more protein is laid down than can be accounted for by fetal and placental growth and by the increase in size in specific target organs such as the uterus and the breasts.

Between 20% and 40% of pregnant women in Europe are gaining more weight than recommended. Surprisingly, the correlation between energy intake and maternal weight gain is poor, and it is generally not advisable to attempt to promote weight loss in pregnancy, as it may result in a parallel restriction of essential nutrients, which in turn may have undesirable effects on fetal growth and development.

Postpartum weight

Immediately following delivery, there is a weight loss of ≈6 kg, which is accounted for by water and fluid loss and by the loss of the products of conception. Diuresis occurs during the early puerperium, removing the water retained during pregnancy. From approximately day 3, body weight falls by ≈0.3 kg/day until day 10, stabilizing by week 10 at ≈2.3 kg above pre-pregnancy weight, or 0.7 kg in women who are continuing to lactate. By 6–18 months after delivery, 1–2 kg of pregnancy-related weight gain will still be retained, but in about one-fifth of women, 5 kg or more can be retained. Obese women usually put on less weight during pregnancy but retain more postpartum.

Weight gain is about 0.9 kg less in multigravidae than in primigravidae. However, a 5-year follow-up of nearly 3000 women found that parous women gained 23 kg more than nulliparae during this time.

The breasts

Some of the first signs and symptoms of pregnancy occur in the breasts, including breast tenderness, an increase in size, enlargement of the nipples and increased vascularity and pigmentation of the areola.

The areola contains sebaceous glands that hypertrophy during pregnancy (Montgomery's tubercles). The areola is richly supplied with sensory nerves, which ensures that suckling sends impulses to the

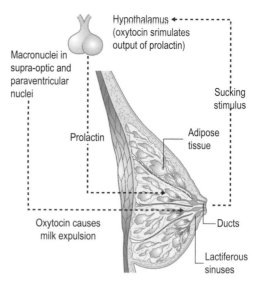

Fig. 3.15 Factors regulating milk production and expulsion.

hypothalamus and thus stimulates the release of oxytocin from the posterior lobe of the pituitary gland and the expulsion of milk.

Breast development during pregnancy

High oestrogen concentrations, with growth hormone and glucocorticoids, stimulate ductal proliferation during pregnancy (Fig. 3.15). Alveolar growth is stimulated in the oestrogen-primed breast by progesterone and prolactin. Secretory activity is initiated during pregnancy and is promoted by prolactin and placental lactogen so that from 3 to 4 months onwards and for the first 30 hours after delivery, a thick, glossy, protein-rich fluid known as *colostrum* can be expressed from the breast. However, full lactation is inhibited during pregnancy by the high levels of oestrogen and progesterone that block the alveolar transcription of α-lactalbumin.

The initiation of lactation

Prolactin acts directly on alveolar cells to stimulate the synthesis of all milk components, including casein, lactalbumin and fatty acids. The sudden reduction of progesterone and oestrogen levels following parturition allows prolactin to act in an uninhibited manner, and its release is promoted by suckling, with the development of the full flow of milk by day 5 and a further gradual increase over the next 3 weeks. Some 500–1000 mL of milk is produced daily, and the mother needs about 500 kcal extra per day to maintain this; a further 250 kcal/day are derived from the maternal fat stores. The visceral fat accumulation and increased insulin resistance, lipid and triglyceride levels of later pregnancy reverse more quickly, and more completely, in breast-feeding mothers.

Suckling also promotes the release of oxytocin from specialized neurons in the supraoptic and paraventricular nuclei of the hypothalamus, and this in turn results in the milk-ejection reflex as the oxytocin stimulates the myoepithelial cells to contract. The milk-ejection reflex can also be stimulated by the mother seeing the infant or hearing its cry or just thinking about feeding! It may also be inhibited by catecholamine release or by adverse emotional and environmental factors. The administration of a dopamine agonist such as bromocriptine inhibits the release of prolactin and abolishes milk production.

The skin

The characteristic feature of skin changes in pregnancy are the appearance of melanocyte-stimulating hormone (MSH)–stimulated pigmentation on the face, known as *chloasma*, the areola of the nipples and the linea alba of the anterior abdominal wall, giving rise to the *linea nigra*. Stretch marks (*striae gravidarum*) predominantly occur in the lines of stress of the abdominal wall but also occur on the lateral aspects of the thighs and breasts. Striae gravidarum result from the disruption of collagen fibres in the subcuticular zone and are related more to the increased production of adrenocortical hormones in pregnancy than to the stress and tension in the skin folds associated with the expansion of the abdominal cavity.

Skin blood flow increases markedly, and flow-mediated dilatation is increased. These changes allow more efficient heat loss, especially in late pregnancy, when the developing fetus, whose core temperature is $\approx 1\,^{\circ}\text{C}$ higher than the mother's, contributes to increasing heat production.

Endocrine changes

Massive production of sex steroids by the placenta tends to dominate the endocrine picture, but there are also significant changes in all the maternal endocrine organs during pregnancy. It is important to be aware of these changes so that they are not interpreted as indicating abnormal function.

Placental hormones

Human chorionic gonadotrophin is the signal for pregnancy. The fetoplacental unit synthesizes very large amounts of oestrogen and progesterone, both being needed for uterine growth and quiescence and for breast development. However, oestrogen also stimulates the synthesis of binding globulins for thyroxine and corticosteroids; cortisol-binding globulin (CBG) increases throughout pregnancy to reach twice non-pregnant levels, while thyroid-binding globulin (TBG) is doubled by the end of the first trimester and remains elevated throughout pregnancy. Oestrogens also stimulate vascular endothelial growth factor (VEGF) and its receptors and angiogenesis. In turn, VEGF appears to interact with other placentally produced hormones and angiopoietin-2 in the development of the placental villous capillary bed. The placentally specific form of the anti-angiogenic soluble fms-like tyrosine kinase-1 (sFLT-1) e15a antagonizes the activity of VEGF and placental growth factor. In excess, this can lead to endothelial dysfunction. The peroxisome proliferator-activated receptor-γ (PPARγ) is expressed in human villous and extravillous cytotrophoblast and binds to, and is activated by, natural ligands such as eicosanoids, FAs and oxidized low-density lipoproteins.

The pituitary gland

Anatomy

The anterior and posterior pituitary glands have different embryological origins, with the anterior pituitary arising from Rathke's pouch in the developing oral cavity, while the posterior pituitary is derived from a down-growth of neural tissue that forms the floor of the third ventricle. A specialized vascular portal system connects the two parts. The pituitary gland enlarges during pregnancy by $\approx 30\%$ in primigravid women and 50% in multiparous women. The weight increase is largely due to changes in the anterior lobe.

Anterior pituitary

The anterior pituitary produces three glycoproteins (luteinizing hormone, follicular-stimulating hormone and thyroid-stimulating hormone) and three polypeptide and peptide hormones (growth hormone, prolactin and adrenocorticotrophic hormone (ACTH)). The increased oestrogen levels stimulate the number and secretory activity of the lactotrophs. Prolactin release is controlled by prolactin inhibitory factors such as dopamine. There is a steady rise in prolactin synthesis and plasma concentration, with a surge at the time of delivery, and a subsequent fall with the disappearance of placental oestrogens. Levels of prolactin remain raised above basal in women who continue to breast-feed.

Plasma levels of ACTH rise in pregnancy but remain within the normal non-pregnant range. Some of the increase may be the result of placental production. Melanocyte-stimulating hormone (MSH), synthesized in the pituitary intermediate lobe, shares a precursor (pro-opiomelanocortin) with ACTH and rises in pregnancy.

Gonadotrophin secretion is inhibited by the rising chorionic gonadotrophin, as is the secretion of growth hormone. Thyrotrophin levels remain constant in pregnancy.

Posterior pituitary

The posterior pituitary releases AVP and oxytocin. Plasma osmolality falls in early pregnancy and clearance of AVP increases fourfold because of a placentally produced leucine aminopeptidase (PLAP). However, AVP responds appropriately to over- and under-hydration once the new baseline osmolality is reached (see Plasma volume earlier).

Oxytocin stimulates uterine contractions. Concentrations are low during gestation, again because of the high concentrations of PLAP. Oxytocin levels are not raised in labour, but there is an upregulation of uterine oxytocin receptors, so there is enhanced sensitivity to oxytocin. This appears to be related to the oestrogen:progesterone ratio, as oestrogen upregulates binding sites and progesterone downregulates them. In addition, dilatation of the cervix stimulates the release of oxytocin, thus reinforcing uterine activity. Oxytocin also plays an important role in lactation, as it is released following stimulation of the nipples. It then acts on the myoepithelial cells surrounding the breast alveoli, causing these cells to contract and eject milk.

Hypothalamus

The hypothalamus synthesizes a variety of 'releasing hormones' such as thyrotropin-releasing hormone (TRH) and gonadotropin-releasing hormone. The mean serum prolactin and thyroid-stimulating hormone (TSH) responses to TRH in pregnancy are somewhat smaller than the non-pregnant response and are similar across pregnancy. Corticotrophin-releasing hormone (CRH) stimulates the release of ACTH. Both hypothalamus and placenta synthesize CRH. Plasma levels of CRH increase greatly in the third trimester and may be one of the triggers for the onset of labour.

The thyroid

The thyroid gland enlarges in up to 70% of pregnant women, the percentage varying depending on iodine intake. In normal pregnancy, there is increased urinary excretion of iodine and transfer of iodothyronines to the fetus. This in turn results in a fall of plasma inorganic iodide levels in the mother. At the same time, the thyroid gland triples its uptake of iodide from the blood, creating a relative iodine deficiency, which is probably responsible for the compensatory follicular enlargement of the gland (Fig. 3.16).

As a result of the increase in TBG, total tri-iodothyronine (T_3) and thyroxine (T_4) levels increase in pregnancy, although free T_3 and T_4 rise in early pregnancy and then fall to remain

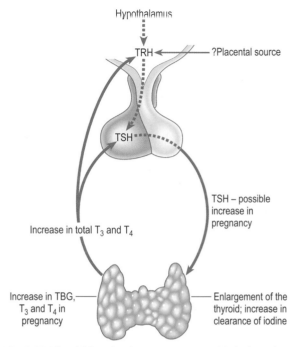

Fig. 3.16 Thyroid function in pregnancy. *T_3*, Tri-iodothyronine; *T_4*, thyroxine; *TBG*, thyroid-binding globulin; *TRH*, thyrotropin-releasing hormone; *TSH*, thyroid-stimulating hormone.

in the non-pregnant range. TSH may increase slightly but tends to remain within the normal range. T_3, T_4 and TSH do not cross the placental barrier, and there is therefore no direct relationship between maternal and fetal thyroid function. However, iodine and anti-thyroid drugs do cross the placenta, as does the long-acting thyroid stimulator (LATS). Hence, the fetus may be affected by the level of iodine intake and by the presence of autoimmune disease in the mother.

Calcitonin is another thyroid hormone. It rises during the first trimester, peaks in the second and falls thereafter, although the changes are not large. It may contribute to the regulation of 1,25-di-hydroxy vitamin D.

The parathyroids

Parathyroid hormone (PTH) regulates the synthesis of 1,25-dihydroxy vitamin D in the proximal convoluted tubule. There is a fall in intact PTH during pregnancy but a doubling of 1,25-dihydroxy vitamin D. Placentally derived PTH-related protein (PTHrP) is also present in the maternal circulation and affects calcium homeostasis by acting through the PTH receptor.

The renin–angiotensin system (RAS)

The RAS is activated in the luteal phase and is one of the first hormones to 'recognize' pregnancy. The increased GFR and high progesterone cause an increased sodium load at the macula densa, which stimulates renin release. At the same time, oestrogens stimulate angiotensinogen synthesis. The resultant increase in AngII stimulates aldosterone synthesis and release from the adrenal cortex, which counters the natriuretic effect of progesterone at the distal tubule and results in sodium retention and PV expansion. The potential effect of the raised AngII on blood pressure is offset by a parallel, specific reduction in vascular sensitivity to AngII. The decreased sensitivity to AngII in normal pregnancy is lost in pre-eclampsia, where sensitivity increases even before the onset of hypertension.

AngII acts through two directly opposing receptors, the AT1 and AT2 subtypes. AT1 receptors promote angiogenesis, hypertrophy and vasoconstriction, and AT2 receptors promote apoptosis. AT2 expression dominates in the early placenta, where the system may be involved in implantation and vascular re-modelling.

The adrenal gland

The adrenal glands remain constant in size but exhibit changes in function. Like the pituitary gland, the adrenal gland has two distinct embryological origins: the mesenchymal cortex and the adrenal medulla, which originates from migratory neural crest cells. Cortical hormones can influence medullary ones (e.g. glucocorticoids stimulate adrenaline synthesis); conversely, adrenaline may increase ACTH release under 'stress'.

The rising ACTH stimulates cortisol synthesis, and plasma total cortisol concentrations rise from 3 months to term. Much of this cortisol is bound to CBG or to albumin; even so, mean free (active) cortisol concentrations do also increase during pregnancy, with the loss of diurnal variation. The normal placenta synthesizes a pregnancy-specific 11 β-hydroxysteroid dehydrogenase, which inhibits transfer of maternal cortisol to the fetus; excess transfer is thought to inhibit fetal growth.

Plasma aldosterone from the zona glomerulosa rises progressively throughout pregnancy (see The renin–angiotensin system earlier); there is also a substantial increase in the weak mineralocorticoid deoxycorticosterone that is apparent by 8 weeks' gestation and may reflect production by the fetoplacental unit.

The oestrogen-induced increase in the production of sex hormone–binding globulin (SHBG) results in an increase in total testosterone levels.

Improved measurement techniques have shown that plasma catecholamine concentrations fall from the first to the third trimester. There is some blunting of the rise in noradrenaline (reflecting mainly sympathetic nerve activity) seen on standing and isometric exercise in pregnancy, but the adrenaline response (predominantly adrenal) is unaltered. However, there are often massive increases in both adrenaline and noradrenaline concentrations during labour as the result of stress and muscle activity.

Conclusion

Many of the sometimes very large, inter-dependent and integrated changes in maternal physiology begin even before conception. One needs a good understanding of the normal changes to understand the abnormal.

Essential information

General

- Many pregnancy adaptations are initiated in the luteal phase, i.e. are proactive

Immunological responses

- The uterus is not an immunologically privileged site
- Trophoblast does not elicit allogeneic responses
- Fetus has a non-immunogenic interface with maternal circulation
- Maternal immune response is locally manipulated
- Thymus involutes in pregnancy
- Lymph nodes draining the uterus enlarge

Changes in the cervix

- Increased vascularity
- Reduction in collagen

- Accumulation of glycosaminoglycans and water
- Hypertrophy of cervical glands
- Increased mucus secretions

Vascular changes in the pregnant uterus

- Hypertrophy of the uterine vessels
- Uterine blood flow from 50 to 500 mL/min 10 weeks to term
- Trophoblast invasion of spiral arterioles up to 24 weeks
- 100–150 spiral arterioles supply intervillous space
- One spiral arteriole per placental cotyledon

Uterine contractility

- Suppressed by progesterone
- Increased resting membrane potential
- Impaired conduction
- Contractions by 7 weeks – frequent low intensity

Continued

Essential information—cont'd

- Late pregnancy – stronger and more frequent
- In labour, contractions produce cervical dilatation

Cardiac output

- 40% increase in the first trimester
- Further increase of up to 2 L/min in labour
- 15% increment with twin pregnancy
- Heart rate increased by 15 beats/min
- Stroke volume increases from 64 to 71 mL

Total peripheral resistance

- Falls in first 4–6 weeks, halving by mid-pregnancy
- Allows expansion of blood volume
- Hormonally driven

Arterial blood pressure

- Korotkoff sound 5 is now preferred for diastolic pressure measurement
- Mean blood pressure falls to mid-pregnancy
- Supine hypotension is common in the second half of pregnancy

The blood

- Red cell mass rises by ≈20–30% depending on iron intake
- Concentration measures fall, e.g. haematocrit
- White cell count rises slowly, but massive neutrophilia is usual around labour and delivery
- There is an increased tendency to clotting in pregnancy and the puerperium

Respiratory function

- Minute ventilation rises by 40%
- Maternal P_aCO_2 falls, allowing better gas exchange from the fetus

- Pregnancy is not usually a problem for women with respiratory disease

Renal function

- GFR rises by ≈50% and RPF by 50% in the first trimester
- Plasma concentration of many solutes falls – effect on interpretation of lab results
- Some glycosuria and mild proteinuria (≤200 mg/mL) are common in pregnancy

Nutrients in blood

- Glucose is the major fetal energy substrate
- Albumin falls throughout pregnancy; globulin rises by ≈10%
- Amino acids decrease, except alanine and glutamic acid
- Pregnancy is a hyperlipidaemic state
- Free fatty acids are raised
- Concentration of fat-soluble vitamins rises; that of water-soluble vitamins falls

Endocrine changes

- Placenta is an endocrine powerhouse, synthesizing steroids, polypeptides and prostanoids
- Placenta produces CRH and ACTH
- Placental leucine aminopeptidase lowers oxytocin during pregnancy
- Growth hormone, LH and FSH levels are suppressed by placental gonadotrophins
- Pituitary gland enlarges
- Increased secretion of prolactin
- Thyroid function increases
- Aldosterone and deoxycorticosterone levels rise

Chapter 4

Placental and fetal growth and development

Adonis S. Ioannides

LEARNING OUTCOMES

After studying this chapter you should be able to:

Knowledge criteria

- Describe normal placental development
- Describe the structure of the umbilical cord and uteroplacental blood flow
- List the placental transfer mechanisms and functions
- Describe the sequence of normal fetal development
- Understand the formation and clinical significance of amniotic fluid

Early placental development

After fertilization and egg cleavage, the *morula* is transformed into a *blastocyst* by the formation of a fluid-filled cavity within the ball of cells.

The outer layer of the blastocyst consists of primitive cytotrophoblast, and by day 7, the blastocyst penetrates the endometrium as a result of trophoblastic invasion (Fig. 4.1). The outer layer of the trophoblast becomes a syncytium. In response to contact with the syncytiotrophoblast, the endometrial stromal cells become large and pale, a process known as the *decidual reaction*. Some endometrial cells are phagocytosed by the trophoblastic cells.

The nature and function of the decidual reaction remain uncertain, but it seems likely that the decidual cells both limit the invasion of trophoblastic cells and serve an initial nutritional function for the developing placenta.

During development of the placenta, cords of cytotrophoblast, or *Langhans cells*, grow down to the basal layers of decidua and penetrate some of the endometrial venules and capillaries. The formation of lacunae filled with maternal blood presages the development of the intervillous space.

The invading cords of trophoblast form the primary villi, which later branch to form secondary villi and, subsequently, free-floating tertiary villi.

The central core of these villi is penetrated by a column of mesoblastic cells that become the capillary network of the villi. The body stalk attaching the developing fetus to the placenta forms the umbilical vessels, which advance into the villi to join the villous capillaries and establish the placental circulation.

Although trophoblastic cells surround the original blastocyst, the area that develops into the placenta becomes thickened and extensively branched and is known as the *chorion frondosum*. However, in the area that subsequently expands to form the outer layer of the fetal membranes, or *chorion laeve,* the villi become atrophic and the surface becomes smooth (Fig. 4.2). The decidua underlying the placenta is known as the *decidua basalis* and the decidua between the membranes and the myometrium is known as as the *decidua capsularis*.

Further placental development

By 6 weeks after ovulation, the trophoblast has invaded some 40–60 spiral arterioles. Blood from the maternal vasculature pushes the free-floating secondary and tertiary capillaries into a tent-shaped *maternal cotyledon*. The tents are held down to the basal plate of the decidua by anchoring villi, and the blood from arterioles spurts towards the chorionic plate and then returns to drain through maternal veins in the basal plate. There are eventually about 12 large maternal cotyledons and 40–50 smaller ones (Fig. 4.3).

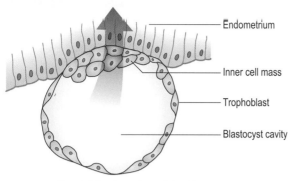

Fig. 4.1 Implantation of the blastocyst.

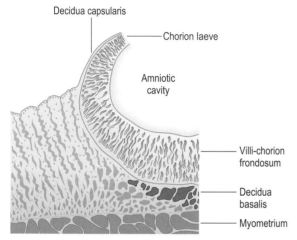

Fig. 4.2 Development of early placentation. The chorion frondosum forms the placental villi. The chorion laeve forms the chorionic portion of the fetal membranes.

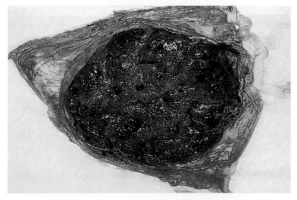

Fig. 4.3 Maternal surface of the full-term placenta showing cotyledons.

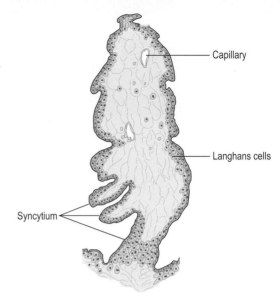

Fig. 4.4 The chorionic villus is the functional unit of the placenta.

The villus

Despite the arrangement of villi into maternal cotyledons, the functional unit of the placenta remains the *stem villus* or *fetal cotyledon*. The end unit of the stem villus, sometimes known as the terminal or chorionic villus, is shown in Fig. 4.4. There are initially about 200 stem villi arising from the chorion frondosum. About 150 of these structures are compressed at the periphery of the maternal cotyledons and become relatively functionless, leaving a dozen or so large cotyledons and 40–50 smaller ones as the active units of placental function.

The estimated total surface area of the chorionic villi in the mature placenta is approximately $11\,m^2$. The surface area of the fetal side of the placenta and of the villi is enlarged by the presence of numerous microvilli. The core of the villus consists of a stroma of closely packed spindle-shaped fibroblasts and branching capillaries. The stroma also contains phagocytic cells known as *Hofbauer cells*. In early pregnancy, the villi are covered by an outer layer of syncytiotrophoblast and an inner layer of cytotrophoblast. As pregnancy advances, the cytotrophoblast disappears until only a thin layer of syncytiotrophoblast remains. The formation of clusters of syncytial cells, known as *syncytial knots*, and the reappearance of cytotrophoblast in late pregnancy are probably the result of hypoxia. There is evidence that the rate of apoptosis of syncytial cells accelerates towards term and is particularly increased where there is evidence of fetal growth impairment.

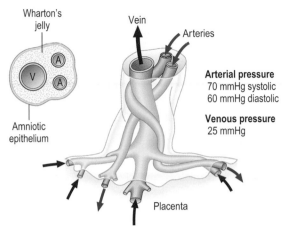

Fig. 4.5 Vascular structure of the umbilical cord. The vein carries oxygenated blood, and the two arteries carry deoxygenated blood.

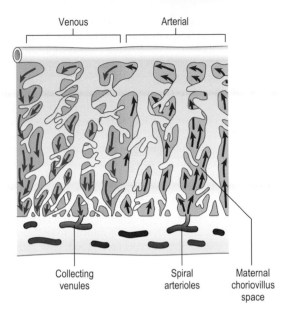

Fig. 4.6 Blood from the spiral arterioles spurts towards the chorionic plate and returns to the collecting venules.

Structure of the umbilical cord

The umbilical cord contains two arteries and one vein (Fig. 4.5). The two arteries carry deoxygenated blood from the fetus to the placenta and the oxygenated blood returns to the fetus via the umbilical vein. Absence of one artery occurs in about 1 in 200 deliveries and is associated with a 10–15% incidence of cardiovascular anomalies. The vessels are surrounded by a hydrophilic mucopolysaccharide known as *Wharton's jelly*, and the outer layer covering the cord consists of amniotic epithelium. The cord length varies between 30 and 90 cm.

The vessels grow in a helical shape. This configuration has the functional advantage of protecting the patency of the vessels by absorbing torsion without the risk of kinking or snarling of the vessels.

The few measurements that have been made in situ of blood pressures in the cord vessels indicate that the arterial pressure in late pregnancy is around 70 mmHg systolic and 60 mmHg diastolic, with a relatively low pulse pressure and a venous pressure that is exceptionally high, at approximately 25 mmHg. This high venous pressure tends to preserve the integrity of the venous flow and indicates that the pressure within the villus capillaries must be in excess of the cord venous pressures.

> The high capillary pressures imply that, at the point of proximity, the fetal pressures exceed the pressures in the choriodecidual space so that any disruption of the villus surface means that fetal blood cells enter the maternal circulation and only rarely do maternal cells enter the fetal vascular space.

The cord vessels often contain a false knot consisting of a refolding of the arteries; occasionally, blood flow is threatened by a true knot, although such formations are often seen without any apparent detrimental effects on the fetus.

In the full-term fetus, the blood flow in the cord is approximately 350 mL/min.

Uteroplacental blood flow

Trophoblastic cells invade the spiral arterioles within the first 10 weeks of pregnancy and destroy some of the smooth muscle in the wall of the vessels, which then become flaccid dilated vessels. Maternal blood enters the intervillous space, and during maternal systole, blood spurts from the arteries towards the chorionic plate of the placenta and returns to the venous openings in the placental bed. The intervillous space is characterized by low pressures, with a mean pressure estimated at 10 mmHg and high flow. Assessments of uterine blood flow at term indicate values of 500–750 mL/min (Fig. 4.6).

Factors that regulate fetoplacental and uterine blood flow

The fetoplacental circulation is affected by the fetal heart and aorta, the umbilical vessels and the vessels of the chorionic villi, so factors that affect these structures may affect the fetal circulation. Such factors as oedema of the cord, intra-mural thrombosis and calcification within the large fetal vessels or acute events such as acute cord compression or obstruction of the umbilical cord may have immediate and lethal consequences for the fetus. However, the more common factors that influence the welfare of the fetus arise in the uteroplacental circulation. Access to these factors by the use of Doppler ultrasound has greatly improved our understanding of the control mechanisms of uterine blood flow.

The regulation of uterine blood flow is of critical importance to the welfare of the fetus. The uteroplacental blood flow includes the uterine arteries and their branches down to the spiral arterioles, the intervillous blood flow and the related venous return.

Impairment of uterine blood flow leads to fetal growth impairment and, under severe circumstances, to fetal death. Factors that influence uteroplacental blood flow acutely include maternal haemorrhage, tonic or abnormally powerful and prolonged uterine contractions and substances such as noradrenaline (norepinephrine) and adrenaline (epinephrine). Angiotensin II increases uterine blood flow at physiological levels, as it has a direct effect on the placental release of vasodilator prostaglandins, but in high concentrations it produces vasoconstriction.

At the simplest level, acute fetal asphyxia can be produced by the effect of the mother lying in the supine position in late pregnancy, causing compression of the maternal inferior vena cava and hence a sudden reduction in blood flow through the uteroplacental bed.

In terms of chronic pathology, the main causes of impaired uteroplacental circulation are inadequate trophoblast invasion and acute atherosis affecting the spiral arterioles, resulting in placental ischaemia, advanced maturation and placental infarction.

Placental transfer

The placenta plays an essential role in the growth and development of the fetus and in regulating maternal adaptation to pregnancy. The placenta is an organ of fetal nutrition, excretion, respiration and hormone synthesis.

Transfer of materials across the placental membrane is governed by molecular mass, solubility and the ionic charge of the substrate involved. Actual transfer is achieved by simple diffusion, facilitated diffusion, active transport and pinocytosis (Fig. 4.7).

Simple diffusion

Transfer between maternal and fetal blood is regulated by the trophoblast, and it must be remembered that the layer

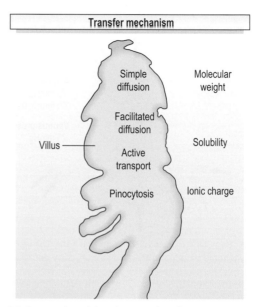

Fig. 4.7 Factors that determine transfer of materials and gases across the placenta.

separating fetal from maternal blood in the chorionic villus is not a simple semipermeable membrane but a metabolically active cellular layer. However, with regard to some substances, it does behave like a semipermeable membrane, and substances pass by simple diffusion.

Although there are some exceptions, small molecules generally cross the placenta in this way, and movement is determined by chemical or electrochemical gradients. The quantity of solute transferred is described by the Fick diffusion equation:

$$\frac{Q}{t} = \frac{KA\left(C^1 - C^2\right)}{L}$$

where Q/t is the quantity transferred per unit of time, K is a diffusion constant for the particular substance, A is the total surface area available, C^1 and C^2 indicate the difference in concentrations of solute and L represents the thickness of the membrane.

This method is applicable particularly to transfer of gases, although the gradient of oxygen, for example, is exaggerated by the fact that oxygen is extracted by the villous trophoblast.

Facilitated diffusion

Some compounds are transported across the placenta at rates that are considerably enhanced above the rate that would be anticipated by simple diffusion. Transport always occurs in favour of the gradient, but at an accelerated rate.

This mechanism pertains to glucose transport and can only be explained by the active involvement of enzyme processes and specific transport systems.

Active transport

Transfer against a chemical gradient occurs with some compounds and must involve an active transport system that is energy dependent. This process occurs with amino acids and water-soluble vitamins and can be demonstrated by the presence of higher concentrations of the compound in the fetal blood as compared with maternal blood. Such transfer mechanisms can be inhibited by cell poisons and are stereo-specific.

Pinocytosis

Transfer of high-molecular-mass compounds is known to occur even where such transfer would be impossible through the villus membrane because of the molecular size. Under these circumstances, microdroplets are engulfed into the cytoplasm of the trophoblast and then extruded into the fetal circulation. This process applies to the transfer of globulins, phospholipids and lipoproteins and is of particular importance in the transfer of immunologically active material. The major source of materials for protein synthesis, which also accounts for some 10% of energy supplies, is amino acids transferred by active transport.

Transport of intact cells

Fetal red cells are commonly seen in the maternal circulation, particularly following delivery. This transfer occurs through fractures in the integrity of the trophoblastic membrane and may also therefore occur at the time of abortion or following placental abruption. Although some maternal cells can be found in the fetal circulation, this is much less common. As previously mentioned, the pressure gradient favours movement from the relatively high pressure of the fetal capillaries to the low-pressure environment of the intervillous space.

Water and electrolyte transfer

Water passes easily across the placenta, and a single pass allows equilibrium. The driving forces for movement of water across the placenta include hydrostatic pressure, colloid osmotic pressure and solute osmotic pressure.

Sodium

The concentration of sodium is higher in the venous plasma of the fetus than in the maternal venous plasma. It therefore seems that the placenta actively regulates sodium transfer, probably through the action of Na/K ATPase on the fetal surface of the villus trophoblast.

Potassium

The transfer of potassium is also controlled at the cell membrane level, but the mechanism remains obscure. Fetal plasma potassium levels are significantly higher than maternal plasma levels. In particular, fetal plasma levels become significantly raised in the presence of fetal hypoxia and fetal acidosis with an exaggerated gradient if the acid–base balance remains normal. There is evidence for a carrier-mediated transfer at the maternal surface of the placenta, and the transfer of placental potassium may also be modulated by intracellular Ca^{2+}.

Calcium

Calcium is actively transported across the placenta, and there are higher concentrations in fetal plasma than in maternal plasma.

Placental function

The placenta has three major functions:
- gaseous exchange
- fetal nutrition and removal of waste products
- endocrine function

Gaseous exchange

As the transfer of gases occurs by simple diffusion, the major determinants of gaseous exchange are the efficiency and flow of the fetal and maternal circulation, the surface area of the placenta that is available for transfer and the thickness of the placental membrane.

Oxygen transfer

The average oxygen saturation of maternal blood entering the intervillous space is 90–100% at a Po_2 of 90–100 mmHg, and these high levels of oxygen favour transfer to the fetal circulation. After the placenta itself has utilized some of this oxygen, the remainder is available to the fetal circulation. Fetal haemoglobin has a higher affinity for oxygen than does adult haemoglobin, and haemoglobin concentration is higher in the fetus. All of these factors favour the rapid uptake of oxygen by the fetus at Po_2 levels as low as 30–40 mmHg. The extent to which haemoglobin can be saturated by oxygen is affected

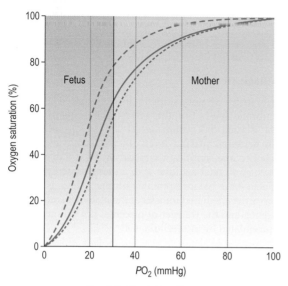

Fig. 4.8 The Bohr effect.

by hydrogen ion concentration. The increase that occurs in deoxygenated blood arriving in the placental circulation from the fetus favours the release of maternal oxygen in the fetoplacental bed. The oxygen dissociation curve is shifted to the right by the increase in H^+ concentration, P_{CO_2} and temperature, and this is known as the *Bohr effect* (Fig. 4.8). Oxygen is predominantly transported in the form of oxyhaemoglobin, as there is little free oxygen in solution.

Carbon dioxide transfer

Carbon dioxide is readily soluble in blood and transfers rapidly across the placenta. The partial pressure difference is about 5 mmHg. Transport of carbon dioxide may occur in solution as either bicarbonate or carbonic acid. It is also transported as carbamino-haemoglobin. The binding of CO_2 to haemoglobin is affected by factors that influence oxygen release. Thus, an increase in carbamino-haemoglobin results in the release of oxygen. This is known as the *Haldane effect*.

Acid–base balance

Factors involved in the regulation of acid–base balance such as H^+, lactic acid and bicarbonate ions also move across the placenta. As a consequence, acidosis associated with starvation and dehydration in the mother may also result in acidosis in the fetus. However, the fetus may become acidotic as the result of oxygen deprivation in the presence of normal maternal acid–base balance.

Fetal nutrition and removal of waste products

Carbohydrate metabolism

Glucose transferred from the maternal circulation provides the major substrate for oxidative metabolism in the fetus and placenta and provides 90% of the energy requirements of the fetus. Facilitated diffusion ensures that there is rapid transfer of glucose across the placenta. In late pregnancy, the fetus retains some 10 g/kg body weight, and any excess glucose is stored as glycogen or fat. Glycogen is stored in the liver, muscle, placenta and heart, whereas fat is deposited around the heart and behind the scapulae.

Animal studies have shown that the transfer of sugars is selective. Generally, glucose and the monosaccharides cross the placenta readily, whereas it is virtually impermeable to disaccharides such as sucrose, maltose and lactose. The placenta is also impermeable to sugar alcohols such as sorbitol, mannitol, deleitol and meso-inositol.

In the fasting normal pregnant woman, blood glucose achieves a concentration of approximately 4.0 mmol/L in the maternal venous circulation and 3.3 mmol/L in the fetal cord venous blood. Infusion of glucose into the maternal circulation results in a parallel increase in both maternal and fetal blood until the fetal levels reach 10.6 mmol/L, when no further increase occurs, regardless of the values in the maternal circulation.

The hormones that are important in glucose homeostasis – insulin, glucagon, human placental lactogen and growth hormone – do not cross the placenta, and maternal glucose levels appear to be the major regulatory factor in fetal glucose metabolism. The placenta itself utilizes glucose and may retain as much as half of the glucose transferred to the fetoplacental unit.

In mid-pregnancy, approximately 70% of this glucose is metabolized by glycolysis and 10% via the pentose phosphate pathway; the remainder is stored by glycogen and lipid synthesis. By full term, the rate of placental glucose utilization has fallen by 30%.

Glycogen storage in the fetal liver increases steadily throughout pregnancy and by full term is twice as high as the storage in the maternal liver. A rapid fall to adult levels occurs within the first few hours of life.

Fetal glycogen reserves are particularly important in providing an energy source in the asphyxiated fetus when anaerobic glycolysis is activated.

Fat metabolism

Fats are insoluble in water and are therefore transported in blood either as free fatty acids bound to albumin or as lipoproteins consisting of triglycerides attached to other lipids or proteins and packaged in chylomicrons.

The fetus needs fatty acids for cell membrane construction and for deposition in adipose tissue. This is particularly important as a source of energy in the immediate neonatal period.

There is evidence that free fatty acids cross the placenta and that this transfer is not selective. Essential fatty acids are also transferred from the maternal circulation, and there is evidence to suggest that the placenta has the ability to convert linoleic acid to arachidonic acid. Starvation of the mother increases mobilization of triglycerides in the fetus.

Protein metabolism

Fetal proteins are synthesized by the fetus from free amino acids transported across the placenta against a concentration gradient. The concentration of free amino acids in fetal blood is higher than in the maternal circulation.

The placenta takes no part in the synthesis of fetal proteins, although it does synthesize some protein hormones that are transferred into the maternal circulation: chorionic gonadotrophin and human placental lactogen. By full term, the human fetus has accumulated some 500 g of protein.

Immunoglobulins (Ig) are synthesized by fetal lymphoid tissue, and IgM first appears in the fetal circulation by 20 weeks' gestation, followed by IgA and finally IgG.

IgG is the only gamma-globulin to be transferred across the placenta, and this appears to be selective for IgG. There is no evidence of placental transfer of growth-promoting hormones.

Urea and ammonia

Urea concentration is higher in the fetus than in the mother by a margin of about 0.5 mmol/L, and the rate of clearance across the placenta is approximately 0.54 mg^{-1} min^{-1} kg fetal weight at term.

Ammonia transfers readily across the placenta, and there is evidence that maternal ammonia provides a source of fetal nitrogen.

Placental hormone production

The placenta plays a major role as an endocrine organ and is responsible for the production of both protein and steroid hormones. The fetus is also involved in many of the processes of hormone production, and in this capacity the conceptus functions as a unit involving both fetus and placenta.

Protein hormones

Chorionic gonadotrophin

Human chorionic gonadotrophin (hCG) is produced by trophoblast and has a structure that is chemically very similar to that of luteinizing hormone. It is a glycoprotein with two non-identical α and β subunits and reaches a peak in maternal urine and blood between 10 and 12 weeks' gestation. A small sub-peak occurs between 32 and 36 weeks. The β subunit of hCG can be detected in maternal plasma within 7 days of conception.

The only known function of the hormone appears to be the maintenance of the corpus luteum of pregnancy, which is responsible for the production of progesterone until such time as this production is taken over by the placenta.

The hormone is measured by agglutination inhibition techniques using coated red cells or latex particles, and this forms the basis for the standard modern pregnancy test (see Chapter 18). This will be positive in urine by 2 weeks after the period is missed in 97% of pregnant women. Home pregnancy test kits are able to detect 25–50 IU/L of β hCG.

Human placental lactogen

Human placental lactogen (hPL), or chorionic somato-mammotrophin, is a peptide hormone with a molecular weight of 22,000 that is chemically similar to growth hormone. It is produced by syncytiotrophoblast, and plasma hPL levels rise steadily throughout pregnancy. The function of the hormone remains uncertain. It increases levels of free fatty acids and insulin. The level tends to rise steeply in the third trimester and is linked to higher blood sugars and abnormal glucose tolerance tests, i.e. helping to unmask late-onset diabetes.

Plasma hPL levels have been extensively used in the assessment of placental function, as the levels are low in the presence of placental failure. In the last 2 weeks of gestation, the levels in the serum fall in normal pregnancy. However, the use of these measurements as placental function tests has largely fallen into disfavour because of their low discriminant function. The hormone is measured by immunoassay.

Steroid hormones

Progesterone

The placenta becomes the major source of progesterone by the seventeenth week of gestation, and the biosynthesis of progesterone is mainly dependent on the supply of maternal cholesterol. In maternal plasma, 90% of progesterone is bound to protein and is metabolized in the liver and the kidneys. Some 10–15% of progesterone is excreted in the urine as pregnanediol. The placenta produces about 350 mg of progesterone per day by full term, and plasma progesterone levels increase throughout pregnancy to achieve values around 150 mg/mL by full term. The measurement of urinary pregnanediol or plasma progesterone has been used in the past as a method of assessing placental function but has not proved to be particularly useful because of the wide scatter of values in normal pregnancies.

Oestrogens

Over 20 different oestrogens have been identified in the urine of pregnant women, but the major oestrogens are oestrone, oestradiol-17β and oestriol. The largest increase in urinary oestrogen excretion occurs in the oestriol fraction. Whereas oestrone excretion increases 100-fold, urinary oestriol increases 1000-fold.

The ovary makes only a minimal contribution to this increase, as the placenta is the major source of oestrogens in pregnancy. The substrate for oestriol production comes from the fetal adrenal gland. Dehydroepiandrosterone (DHEA) synthesized in the fetal adrenal cortex passes to the fetal liver, where it is 16-hydroxylated. Conjugation of these precursors with phosphoadenosyl phosphosulphate aids solubility, and active sulphatase activity in the placenta results in the release of free oestriol.

Oestradiol and oestrone are directly synthesized by the syncytiotrophoblast. Urinary and plasma oestriol levels increase progressively throughout pregnancy until 38 weeks' gestation, when some decrease occurs.

The use of oestriol measurements has now largely been replaced by the use of various forms of ultrasound assessment.

Corticosteroids

There is little evidence that the placenta produces corticosteroids. In the presence of Addison's disease or following adrenalectomy, 17-hydroxycorticosteroids and aldosterone disappear from the maternal urine. In normal pregnancy, there is a substantial increase in cortisol production, and this is at least in part due to the raised levels of transcortin in the blood so that the capacity for binding cortisol increases substantially.

Corticotrophin-releasing hormone

A progressive increase in the levels of corticotrophin-releasing hormone (CRH) in maternal plasma has been noted in the final two trimesters of pregnancy. Any biological effects of CRH are diminished by the presence of a high-affinity CRH-binding protein (CRH-BP) in maternal plasma, although the concentrations of CRH-BP fall in the last 4–5 weeks of pregnancy, and as a consequence, free levels of CRH appear to rise.

Fetal development

Growth

Up to 10 weeks' gestation, a massive increase in cell numbers occurs in the developing embryo, but the actual gain in weight is small. Thereafter a rapid increase in weight occurs until the full-term fetus reaches a final weight of around 3.5 kg.

Protein accumulation occurs in the fetus throughout pregnancy. However, the situation is very different as far as fetal adipose tissue is concerned. Free fatty acids are stored in brown fat around the neck, behind the scapulae and the sternum and around the kidneys. White fat forms the subcutaneous fat covering the body of the full-term fetus. Fat stores in the fetus between 24 and 28 weeks' gestation make up only 1% of the body weight, whereas by 35 weeks, it makes up 15% of body weight.

The rate of fetal growth diminishes towards term. Actual fetal size is determined by a variety of factors, including the efficiency of the placenta, the adequacy of the uteroplacental blood flow and inherent genetic and racial factors in the fetus.

Normal fetal growth and birth weight are determined by gestational age as well as constitutional variables such as maternal height, weight, parity and ethnic origin. The projected birth weight depends on a combination of these factors and is different for each pregnancy. The computer-generated 'customized' growth curve outlines how this weight is to be reached, together with upper and lower limits. Fig. 4.9 shows two growth charts, for 'Mrs Small' and 'Mrs Average', respectively, based on the sets of characteristics displayed in the top-left corner. The median as well as the 90th and 70th centile lines are shown, outlining different normal ranges for fundal height and fetal weight measurements for each pregnancy. The same series of fetal weight measurements is plotted on each chart and shows an acceptable growth trajectory for 'Mrs Small' but slow growth for 'Mrs Average', which should raise concern for the fetus and prompt further investigation and/or intervention.

The characteristic appearance of the fetus at 12 weeks' gestation is shown in Fig. 4.10. The skin is translucent, and there is virtually no subcutaneous fat so that the blood vessels in the skin are easily seen, but even at this stage, the fetus reacts to stimuli. The upper limbs have already reached their final relative length, and the external genitals are distinguishable externally but remain undifferentiated.

By 16 weeks' gestation (Fig. 4.11), the crown–rump length is 122 mm and the lower limbs have achieved their final relative length. The external genitalia can now be differentiated.

By 24 weeks' gestation (Fig. 4.12), the crown–rump length is 210 mm. The eyelids are separated, the skin is opaque but wrinkled because of the lack of subcutaneous fat and there is fine hair covering the body. By 28 weeks, the eyes are open and the scalp is growing hair.

The cardiovascular system

The paired endocardial tubes that develop in the mesoderm towards the end of the third week of gestation are brought closer together as a result of embryonic folding and fuse

Antenatal growth chart for Mrs Small

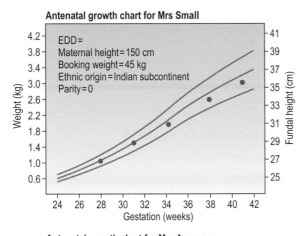

EDD=
Maternal height=150 cm
Booking weight=45 kg
Ethnic origin=Indian subcontinent
Parity=0

Antenatal growth chart for Mrs Average

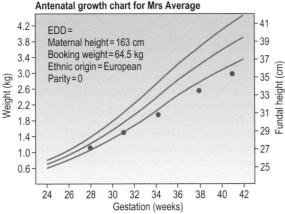

EDD=
Maternal height=163 cm
Booking weight=64.5 kg
Ethnic origin=European
Parity=0

Fig. 4.9 Fetal weight and gestational age plotted on the basis of parity, maternal height and weight and ethnic group. *EDD*; Estimated date of delivery. (Courtesy Jason Gardosi. Adapted from Gardosi, J., Chang A., Kalyan B., et al (1992) Customised antenatal growth charts. The Lancet, 339 (8788):283–287.)

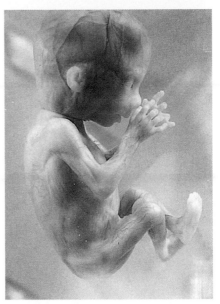

Fig. 4.10 At 12 weeks' gestation, the fetus reacts to stimuli. The upper limbs reach their final relative length, and the sex of the fetus is distinguishable externally.

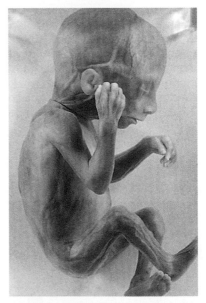

Fig. 4.11 At 16 weeks' gestation, the crown–rump length is 122 mm. The lower limbs achieve their final relative length, and the eyes face anteriorly.

to form a single cardiac tube during week 4. By 4–5 weeks' gestation, a heartbeat is present at a rate of 65 beats/min. A number of grooves (sulci) and expansions form in this single tube, marking the precursors of the cardiac chambers and outflow tract, which are rearranged by a process of folding and looping resulting in the spatial relationships of the adult heart. Septation and valvular development complete the definition of the chambers.

The definitive circulation has developed by 11 weeks' gestation, and the heart rate increases to around 140 beats/min. In the mature fetal circulation, about 40% of the venous return entering the right atrium flows directly into the left atrium through the foramen ovale (Fig. 4.13). Blood pumped from the right atrium into the right ventricle is expelled into the pulmonary artery, where it passes either into the aorta via the ductus arteriosus or into the pulmonary vessels. These two connections allow oxygenated blood entering the heart via the umbilical vein to largely bypass the constricted pulmonary circulation and be pumped into the systemic circulation instead.

49

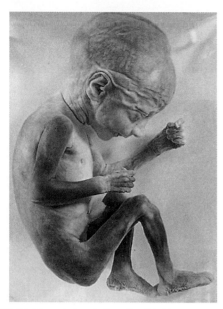

Fig. 4.12 At 24 weeks' gestation, the fetal lungs start to secrete surfactant. The eyelids are separated, and fine hair covers the body.

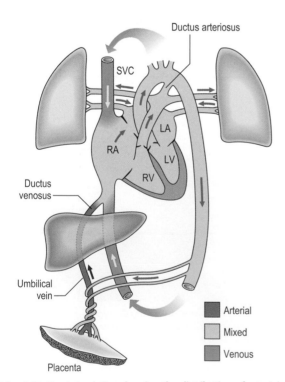

Fig. 4.13 Fetal circulation showing the distribution of arterial, venous and mixed blood. *LA*, Left atrium; *LV*, left ventricle; *RA*, right atrium; *RV*, right ventricle; *SVC*, superior vena cava.

In the mature fetus, the fetal cardiac output is estimated to be 200 mg^{-1} min^{-1} kg body weight. Unlike the adult circulation, fetal cardiac output is entirely dependent on heart rate and not on stroke volume. Autonomic control of the fetal heart rate matures during the third trimester, and parasympathetic vagal tonus tends to reduce the basal fetal heart rate.

The respiratory system

The respiratory system develops from the primitive foregut tube as a ventral evagination, the laryngotracheal groove, at the start of the fourth week of gestation. By the end of the fourth week, the primordia of the future bronchi and lungs appear as a bifurcation at the caudal end of the laryngotracheal groove. Respiratory morphogenesis involves the separation of the ventral trachea from the dorsal oesophagus cranial to the bifurcation and successive branching of the bronchopulmonary buds to form the respiratory tree and alveoli. Branching morphogenesis comprises the embryonic, pseudoglandular, canalicular and saccular phases, followed by a period of alveolar maturation that starts at about the thirty-sixth week of gestation and continues into the postnatal period.

Fetal respiratory movements can be detected from as early as 12 weeks' gestation, and by mid-trimester, a regular respiratory pattern is established. By 34 weeks' gestation, respiration occurs at a rate of 40–60 movements/min with intervening periods of apnoea. These respiratory movements are shallow, with movement of amniotic fluid only into the bronchioles. There are occasional larger flows of fluid into the bronchial tree, but this does not extend into the alveoli because of the high pressure maintained in the developing alveoli from the secretion of alveolar fluid. An exception to this situation may result from episodes of hypoxia, when gasping may lead to the inhalation of amniotic fluid deeper into the alveoli. This fluid may often, under these circumstances, be meconium stained.

Fetal breathing is stimulated by hypercapnia and by raised maternal glucose levels, as in the post-prandial state, whereas hypoxia reduces the number of respiratory movements, as does maternal smoking.

The occurrence of fetal apnoea increases towards term, when breathing movements may be absent for as long as 120 minutes in a normal fetus.

The fetal pulmonary alveoli are lined by two main types of alveolar epithelial cell. Gaseous exchange occurs across the type I cells, and the type II cells secrete a surface-active phospholipid surfactant that is essential in maintaining the functional patency of the alveoli. The principal surfactants are sphingomyelin and lecithin; production of lecithin reaches functional levels by 32 weeks' gestation, although it may begin as early as 24 weeks. In some circumstances, such as in the diabetic pregnancy, the production of surfactant may be delayed, and the process can be accelerated by the administration of corticosteroids to the mother.

The measurement of lecithin concentration in the amniotic fluid provides a useful method of assessing functional fetal lung maturity.

The gastrointestinal tract

Embryonic folding converts the flat endodermal layer into the primitive gastrointestinal tube during the fourth week of gestation. The tube is initially connected to the yolk sac by the vitellointestinal duct and is closed at both its cranial and caudal ends by the oropharyngeal and cloacal membranes, respectively. The mouth is formed by the breakdown of the oropharyngeal membrane, and in the hindgut, the developing urorectal septum divides the cloaca into a ventral urogenital sinus and a dorsal rectum. The foregut, midgut and hindgut regions are defined by the boundaries of their corresponding blood supply. Rapid growth of the midgut leads to a physiological herniation of part of the intestine into the base of the umbilical cord during the period between the sixth and the tenth to eleventh weeks of gestation. The final anatomical position of the bowel in the abdominal cavity is the result of intestinal rotation during this period. Thickening of the duodenal endoderm and subsequent budding lead to the development of the pancreas, liver and gallbladder.

The development of the fetal gut and gut function proceeds throughout pregnancy, and by 16–20 weeks' gestation, mucosal glands appear, heralding the earliest onset of gut function. By 26 weeks' gestation most of the digestive enzymes are present, although amylase activity does not appear until the neonatal period. The fetus swallows amniotic fluid, and peristaltic gut movement is established by mid-pregnancy. The digestion of cells and protein in amniotic fluid results in the formation of fetal faeces known as *meconium*.

Meconium normally remains in the gut and appears in the amniotic fluid with increasing maturity and also under conditions of fetal stress and asphyxia when the quantity of amniotic fluid may be less.

The kidney

The kidneys start developing in the intermediate mesoderm at the beginning of the fourth week of gestation. Three distinct phases of nephrogenesis have been described with the sequential development of the pronephros, mesonephros and metanephros (the definitive kidney) in a craniocaudal direction. The pronephros is not functional and regresses. The mesonephros consists of multiple mesonephric tubules that develop into functional units and drain into paired mesonephric (Wolffian) ducts, which themselves caudally connect to the primitive urogenital sinus. In the female, the mesonephric duct all but degenerates in contrast to the male, where its caudal-most part develops into the efferent ducts, epididymis, vas deferens and seminal vesicle. Development of the metanephros begins at the start of the fifth week of gestation with the budding of ureteric buds from the mesonephric duct. The ureteric buds will form the collecting system of the kidneys and connect to the part of the urogenital sinus that will form the future urinary bladder. The ureteric buds grow laterally and induce development of the renal parenchyma through a series of reciprocal epithelial–mesenchymal interactions with a mass of cells in the intermediate mesoderm known as the *metanephric blastema*.

Functional renal corpuscles first appear in the juxtaglomerular zone of the renal cortex at 22 weeks' gestation, and filtration begins at this time. The formation of the kidney is completed by 36 weeks' gestation. Glomerular filtration increases towards term as the number of glomeruli increases and fetal blood pressure rises.

In the fetus, only 2% of the cardiac output perfuses the kidney, as most of the excretory functions normally served by the kidney are met by the placenta.

The fetal renal tubules are capable of active transport before any glomerular filtrate is received, and thus some urine may be produced within the tubules before glomerular filtration starts. The efficiency of tubular reabsorption is low, and glucose in the fetal circulation spills into fetal urine at levels as low as 4.2 mmol/L.

Fetal urine makes a significant contribution to amniotic fluid.

The special senses

The embryology of the ear is complex with the external and middle ear deriving from the first and second pharyngeal arches and the associated cleft and pouch and the internal ear from an ectodermal structure known as the *otic placode*. The external ear can be visualized using ultrasound from 10 weeks onwards. The middle ear and the three ossicles are fully formed by 18 weeks, when they also become ossified; the contents of the inner ear, including the cochlear and the membranous and bony labyrinth, are all fully developed by 24 weeks' gestation. The perception of sound by the fetus has to be gauged by behavioural responses, and it is generally agreed that the first responses to acoustic stimuli occur at 24 weeks' gestation, although some observations have suggested that there may be perception as early as 16 weeks. In view of the developmental timetable of the inner ear, this seems unlikely.

There is good evidence that the fetus can hear the mother's voice, and indeed sounds delivered internally are much louder than sounds delivered from outside the maternal abdominal wall. Studies with echoplanar functional magnetic resonance imaging have demonstrated temporal lobe vascular changes in the fetus in response to the mother reciting nursery rhymes in late pregnancy. Perhaps mothers should beware what they say to the fetus in late pregnancy!

The eye develops both from ectoderm (neuroectoderm, neural crest and surface ectoderm) and mesoderm. Visual perception is much more difficult to assess, but it seems likely that some perception to light through the maternal abdominal wall does develop in late pregnancy. Certainly, fetal eye movements can be observed during pregnancy and form an important part of the observations made concerning various fetal behavioural states, a subject that is discussed in Chapter 10.

Amniotic fluid

Formation

The amniotic sac develops in early pregnancy and has been identified in the human embryo as early as 7 days. The first signs of the development of the amniotic cavity can be seen in the inner cell mass of the blastocyst.

Early in pregnancy, amniotic fluid is probably a dialysate of the fetal and maternal extracellular compartments and therefore is 99% water. It does have a cellular and protein content as well. There is evidence that up to 24 weeks' gestation, when keratinization of fetal skin begins, significant transfer of water may occur by transudation across the fetal skin. In the second half of pregnancy after the onset of kidney function, fetal urine provides a significant contribution to amniotic fluid volume. Certainly, when the kidneys are missing, as in renal agenesis, the condition is invariably associated with minimal amniotic fluid volume, a condition known as *oligohydramnios*.

The role of the fetus in the regulation of amniotic fluid volume in normal pregnancy is poorly understood, but the fetus swallows amniotic fluid, absorbs it in the gut and, in later pregnancy, excretes urine into the amniotic sac (Fig. 4.14).

It must be noted that this is a highly dynamic state, as the total volume of water in the amniotic sac is turned over every 2–3 hours. Any factor that interferes with either formation or removal of amniotic fluid may therefore result in a rapid change in amniotic fluid volume.

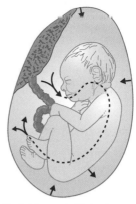

Fig. 4.14 Amniotic fluid secreted into the amniotic sac is swallowed by the fetus, absorbed through the gut and excreted through fetal urine.

Congenital abnormalities that are associated with impaired ability to ingest amniotic fluid are commonly associated with excessive amniotic fluid volume, a condition known as *polyhydramnios*.

In summary, amniotic fluid is formed by the secretion and transudation of fluid through the amnion and fetal skin and from the passage of fetal urine into the amniotic sac. Circulation of amniotic fluid occurs by reabsorption of fluid through the fetal gut, skin and amnion.

Volume

By 8 weeks' gestation, 5–10 mL of amniotic fluid has accumulated. Thereafter, the volume increases rapidly in parallel with fetal growth and gestational age up to a maximum volume of 1000 mL at 38 weeks. Subsequently, the volume diminishes so that by 42 weeks, it may fall below 300 mL. The estimation of amniotic fluid volume forms a standard part of the ultrasound assessment of fetal wellbeing.

Clinical significance of amniotic fluid volume

Oligohydramnios

The diminution of amniotic fluid volume is most commonly associated with impaired secretion of fluid and therefore is a sign of the impairment of placental function, with the exception of the effect of post-maturity. It may be associated with the pre-term rupture of the membranes with chronic loss of amniotic fluid.

Oligohydramnios is commonly associated with intrauterine fetal growth restriction and is therefore an important sign of fetal jeopardy.

It is also associated with congenital abnormalities such as renal agenesis, where there is no production of fetal urine.

Oligohydramnios is associated with various structural and functional problems in the fetus. It may be associated with pulmonary hypoplasia and respiratory difficulties at birth. It may also cause physical deformities such as club foot, skull deformities and wry neck. In labour it has been associated with abnormal cord compression during contractions and hence with fetal hypoxia. Amniotic fluid infusions are used in some units to try and avoid these problems, but the efficacy of these techniques remains in doubt.

Polyhydramnios

The presence of excessive fluid commonly arises as a chronic condition but may on occasions be acute.

Acute polyhydramnios is a rare condition that tends to arise in the second trimester or the early part of the third trimester and commonly results in the onset of pre-term labour. The condition is painful for the mother and may cause dyspnoea and vomiting. The uterus becomes acutely distended, and it may be necessary to relieve the pressure by amniocentesis. However, this only gives short-term relief and nearly always requires repeated procedures. There is often an underlying congenital abnormality. A rare cause is congenital diabetes insipidus. It could also be managed medically with indomethacin to the mother at a dose of 1–3 mg/kg body weight per day. Indomethacin over a prolonged period may cause renal and pulmonary arterial vasoconstriction and hence should be used only for a few days.

Chronic hydramnios may arise in those pregnancies where there is a large placenta, such as occurs in multiple pregnancy, chorioangioma of the placenta or a mother with diabetes. It may also be idiopathic, with no obvious underlying cause, and the fetus may be entirely normal. However, in approximately 30% of all cases, there is a significant congenital anomaly. Chronic hydramnios is seen with the following fetal or placental anomalies, in decreasing order of frequency:
- anencephaly
- oesophageal atresia
- duodenal atresia
- iniencephaly
- hydrocephaly
- diaphragmatic hernia
- chorioangioma of the placenta

Hydramnios itself is associated with certain complications, and these include the following:
- unstable lie
- cord prolapse or limb prolapse
- placental abruption if there is sudden release of amniotic fluid
- postpartum haemorrhage associated with over-distension of the uterus
- maternal discomfort and dyspnoea

Clinical value of tests on amniotic fluid

Both the biochemical and cytological components of amniotic fluid can be used for a variety of clinical tests. However, many of the tests previously used have been replaced by ultrasonography and procedures such as cordocentesis and chorionic villus biopsy.

Amniotic fluid contains two distinct types of cells. The first group is derived from the fetus and the second from the amnion. Cells of fetal origin are larger and more likely to be anucleate, whereas those derived from the amnion are smaller, with a prominent nucleolus contained within the vesicular nucleus, and are found in proportionately greater numbers prior to the thirty-second week of gestation.

Cells that stain with eosin are most prominent in early gestation and are derived from the amnion. After 38 weeks' gestation, numbers of these cells fall to less than 30% of the total cell population.

Basophilic cells increase in number as pregnancy progresses but also tend to decrease after 38 weeks. The presence of large numbers of these cells has been related to the presence of a female fetus; the fetal vagina is thought to be the possible source.

After 38 weeks, a large number of eosinophilic anucleate cells appear. These cells stain orange with Nile blue sulphate and are thought to be derived from maturing sebaceous cells.

These cells have been used in the past as a method of assessing gestational age, but this has now been replaced as a method by ultrasound imaging and the assessment of fetal growth.

Amniocentesis

Amniotic fluid is obtained by the procedure of amniocentesis. This procedure involves inserting a fine-gauge needle under aseptic conditions through the anterior abdominal wall of the mother under local anaesthesia. The procedure, when used for diagnostic testing for chromosomal abnormalities, is commonly performed at 14–16 weeks' gestation. The procedure must be performed under ultrasound guidance in order to identify the best and most accessible pool of amniotic fluid and, where possible, to avoid the placenta and the fetus. Up to 10 mL of fluid is withdrawn, and the presence of a fetal heartbeat is checked both before and after the procedure (Fig. 4.15).

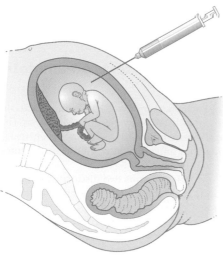

Fig. 4.15 Amniotic fluid is obtained by the procedure of amniocentesis by inserting a needle into the amniotic sac under ultrasound guidance, avoiding the placenta where possible.

Indications for amniocentesis

Chromosomal abnormalities and sex-linked diseases

The fetal karyotype can be determined by the culture of fetal cells obtained from amniotic fluid. This can reveal chromosome abnormalities such as those found in Down syndrome, Turner syndrome and various mosaics. In the past, it was used for the determination of fetal sex to assist in the management of sex-linked disorders such as, haemophilia and Duchenne muscular dystrophy, but this is not common in current practice. Fetal sex can be determined non-invasively using free fetal DNA, even before 10 weeks, and this is supported towards the end of the first trimester by assessing the angle of the genital tubercle.

Metabolic disorders

There are a number of rare metabolic disorders, such as Tay–Sachs disease and galactosaemia, that can be diagnosed using fetal cells obtained from amniotic fluid.

Estimation of fetal lung maturity

The estimation of lecithin or the lecithin/sphingomyelin ratio in amniotic fluid has been used to measure functional lung maturity in the fetus after 28 weeks' gestation and prior to premature delivery and where there is a significant risk of the child developing respiratory distress syndrome. However, it is now routine practice to give the mother corticosteroids under these circumstances. Such is the efficacy of this procedure that it has reduced the need to use the test. Other tests for fetal maturity based on amniotic fluid have now been abandoned in favour of ultrasound techniques.

Essential information

Early placental development

- Implantation of the blastocyst occurs by day 7
- Formation of placental villi takes place from Langhans cells

Further placental development

- Maternal cotyledons form by 6 weeks after ovulation
- Stem villi remain the functional unit of the placenta

Umbilical cord structure

- Contains two arteries and a vein surrounded by Wharton's jelly and covered in epithelium

Uteroplacental blood flow

- Mean pressure 10 mmHg and flow at term 500–750 mL/min
- Can be impaired by haemorrhage, uterine contractions and adrenaline/noradrenaline
- Impairment leads to fetal growth restriction and possible asphyxia

Placental transfer and function

- Gaseous exchange comes about by simple diffusion
- Oxygen rapidly taken up by the fetal circulation even at low pressure
- Fetal nutrition/excretion

Endocrine function

- hCG – reaches peak between 10 and 12 weeks' gestation
- hPL
- Progesterone – placenta produces about 350 mg/day at term
- Oestrogens – placenta major source, 20 different hormones

Fetal development

- Rate of fetal growth increases after 10 weeks and diminishes again towards term
- Heartbeat present at 4–5 weeks

Essential information—cont'd

- Cardiac output at term 200 mL^{-1} min^{-1} kg, entirely dependent on heart rate
- Regular respiratory pattern by mid-trimester
- 40–60 movements/min at 34 weeks
- Principal surfactants sphingomyelin and lecithin
- Production of lecithin reaches functional levels by 32 weeks
- Surfactant production may be delayed by maternal diabetes
- Most digestive enzymes present by 26 weeks
- Fetal kidney completely formed by 36 weeks, but most excretory functions performed by the placenta
- Perception of sound begins between 16 and 24 weeks

Amniotic fluid

- Fetal urine major contributor
- Total volume turned over every 2–3 hours

- Oligohydramnios
  - Associated with intrauterine growth restriction and congenital abnormalities, e.g. renal agenesis
  - May cause pulmonary hypoplasia, club foot, skull deformity, wry neck and fetal hypoxia in labour
- Polyhydramnios
  - May be associated with multiple pregnancy, diabetes or congenital abnormality
  - May cause unstable lie, cord prolapse, placental abruption or postpartum haemorrhage

Clinical tests

- Amniocentesis may help to detect chromosome abnormalities
- Amniocentesis also detects fetal sex
- Can be used to estimate fetal lung maturity where premature delivery is likely

Chapter | 5 |

Perinatal and maternal mortality

Boon H. Lim

LEARNING OUTCOMES

After studying this chapter you should be able to:

Knowledge criteria

- Understand the definitions of maternal and perinatal mortality
- List the main causes of maternal and perinatal mortality
- Describe the socioeconomic factors that affect perinatal and maternal mortality

Clinical competencies

- Interpret maternal and perinatal data and the implications on the various health services

Professional skills and attitudes

- Reflect on the differences in the direct and indirect causes and the sociodemographic factors that influence these in different countries and cultures

Perinatal mortality

Introduction

Perinatal mortality is an important indicator of maternal care, health and nutrition; it also reflects the quality of obstetric, neonatal and paediatric care. The understanding of perinatal mortality statistics is vital in enabling the development of a high-quality approach to the surveillance of the causes of deaths, allowing health care systems to develop prevention strategies and to help clinicians and parents to understand the cause of death of their newborn in order to plan effective monitoring strategies for future pregnancies.

Definitions

The World Health Organization (WHO), in recognizing the importance of international comparison of perinatal and neonatal mortality, coordinates the compilation of health statistics and encourages member countries to rely on the same definitions when comparing the statistics. However, there remain differences in the definitions of perinatal mortality between some countries, reflecting the definition of viability and resources in the individual countries.

The definitions are drawn from the tenth revision of the *International Classification of Diseases* (ICD-10). The key definitions are:

Live birth: Complete expulsion or extraction from its mother of a product of conception, irrespective of the duration of the pregnancy, which, after such separation, breathes or shows any other evidence of life, such as beating of the heart, pulsation of the umbilical cord or definite movement of voluntary muscles, whether or not the umbilical cord has been cut or the placenta is attached; each product of such a birth is considered liveborn.

Stillbirth or **fetal death:** Death prior to the complete expulsion or extraction from its mother of a product of conception, irrespective of the duration of pregnancy; the death is indicated by the fact that after such separation the fetus does not breathe or show any other evidence of life, such as beating of the heart, pulsation of the umbilical cord or definite movement of voluntary muscles.

The definition recommended by the WHO for international comparison is a baby born with no signs of life at or after 28 weeks' gestation (or birth weight of 1000 g). Further definition provided by ICD-10 gave priority of birth weight over gestation as follows:

- Late fetal death – 1000 g or more, 28 weeks or more or 35 cm or more

- Early fetal death – 500 g or more or 22 weeks or more or 25 cm or more
- Miscarriage as a pregnancy loss before 22 completed weeks of gestational age

Perinatal period: Commences at 22 completed weeks (154 days) of gestation and ends 7 completed days after birth.

Neonatal period: Begins with birth and ends 28 complete days after birth. Neonatal deaths may be subdivided into **early neonatal deaths**, occurring during the first 7 days of life (0–6 days), and **late neonatal deaths**, occurring after the seventh day but before the twenty-eighth day of life (7–27 days).

In the UK, the definitions are different, reflecting the survival rates and concept of viability. The present legal definitions that apply to England and Wales are as follows:

Stillbirth: A baby delivered at or after 24+0 weeks gestational age showing no signs of life, irrespective of when the death occurred.

- *Antepartum stillbirth:* A baby delivered at or after 24+0 weeks gestational age showing no signs of life and known to have died before the onset of care in labour.
- *Intrapartum stillbirth:* A baby delivered at or after 24+0 weeks gestational age showing no signs of life and known to have been alive at the onset of care in labour.

Neonatal death: A liveborn baby (born at 20+0 weeks gestational age or later, or with a birth weight of 400 g or more where an accurate estimate of gestation is not available) who died before 28 completed days after birth.

- *Early neonatal death:* A liveborn baby (born at 20+0 weeks gestational age or later, or with a birth weight of 400 g or more where an accurate estimate of gestation is not available) who died before 7 completed days after birth.
- *Late neonatal death:* A liveborn baby (born at 20+0 weeks gestational age or later, or with a birth weight of 40 g or more where an accurate estimate of gestation is not available) who died after 7 completed days but before 28 completed days after birth.

Perinatal death: Death of a fetus or a newborn in the perinatal period that commences at 24 completed weeks' gestation and ends before 7 completed days after birth.

In Australia and New Zealand, stillbirth is defined as 'Death prior to the complete expulsion or extraction from its mother of a product of conception of 20 or more completed weeks of gestation or of 400 g or more birth weight where gestation is not known. The death is indicated by the fact that after such separation the fetus does not breathe or show any other evidence of life, such as beating of the heart, pulsation of the umbilical cord, or definite movement of voluntary muscles'.

In Australia, the perinatal period commences at 20 completed weeks (140 days) of gestation and ends 28 completed days after birth.

Mortality rates

The current definitions are as follows:

Stillbirth rate (SBR): The number of stillbirths per 1000 total births

Neonatal mortality rate (NMR): The number of neonatal deaths occurring within the first 28 days of life per 1000 live births

Perinatal mortality rate (PNMR): The number of stillbirths and early neonatal deaths (those occurring in the first week of life) per 1000 total births (live births and stillbirths)

The global picture

In 2000, the United Nations (UN) member states pledged to work towards a series of Millennium Development Goals (MDGs), including the target of a three-quarters reduction in the 1990 maternal mortality ratio (MMR; maternal deaths per 100,000 live births), to be achieved by 2015. This target (MDG 5A) and that of achieving universal access to reproductive health (MDG 5B) together formed the two targets for MDG 5: Improve maternal health. Disappointingly, at the end of the MDG era, stillbirth rates declined more slowly since 2000 than either maternal mortality or mortality in children younger than 5 years. Worldwide, the number of stillbirths declined by 19.4% between 2000 and 2015, representing an annual reduction rate (ARR) of 2%. This rate of reduction was lower when compared with that for MMR (ARR = 3.0%) and under-5 mortality rate (ARR = 3.9%) for the same period.

In an attempt to improve the classification of maternal deaths, the WHO applied some modifications to the definitions of ICD-10. This is known as *ICD-Maternal Mortality (MM)*.

This defined death occurring during pregnancy, childbirth and the puerperium as the death of a woman while pregnant or within 42 days of termination of pregnancy, irrespective of the cause of death (obstetric and non-obstetric).

In 2015, there were 2.6 million stillbirths globally, with more than 7178 deaths a day, representing a stillbirth rate (SBR) of 18.4 per 1000 births. Ninety-eight percent occurred in low- and middle-income countries. The highest stillbirth rates are in conflict and emergency areas. About 60% of stillbirths are in rural areas. The SBR in sub-Saharan Africa is approximately 10 times that of developed countries (29 versus 3 per 1000 births). Among the 133 million babies born alive each year, 2.8 million die in the first week of life. The patterns of these deaths are similar to the patterns for maternal deaths; this correlates with areas of low-skilled health professional attendants at birth. Ten countries, many of these in Africa and South Asia, account for two-thirds of stillbirths and most neonatal (62%) and maternal (58%) deaths estimated in 2015.

In an effort to continue to improve the perinatal mortality rates worldwide, the Every Newborn Action Plan (ENAP) was launched in mid-2014 with a World Health Assembly

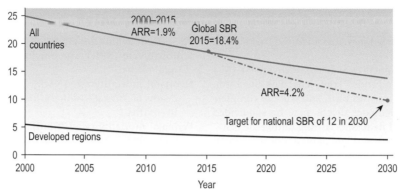

Fig. 5.1 Global progress towards Every Newborn Action Plan target to end preventable stillbirths by 2030. *ARR*, Annual reduction rate; *SBR*, stillbirth rate. (Reproduced with permission. From www.thelancet.com/pb/assets/raw/Lancet/stories/series/stillbirths2016-exec-summ.pdf (Accessed 10 October 2018)).

resolution, endorsed by all countries. ENAP targets the reduction of the NMR to 12 or fewer per 1000 live births and stillbirths to 12 or fewer per 1000 births in all countries by 2030. Both the neonatal and stillbirth reduction targets are included as core indictors in the Every Woman, Every Child Global Strategy for Women's, Children's and Adolescents' Health (2015–2030) (Fig. 5.1).

Developed countries have seen a steady fall in the PNMR over the last 30 years. In the United Kingdom, MBRRACE-UK (Mothers and Babies: Reducing Risks through Audits and Confidential Enquiries across the UK) published the third annual report of the national perinatal mortality statistics for 2015. This showed a PNMR of 5.61 per 1000 births, comprising an SBR of 3.87 and an NMR of 1.74 per 1000 births. Whilst the SBR has shown a downward trend since 2013, the NMR has only marginally reduced.

The perinatal-related mortality rate in 2015 in New Zealand was reported as 9.7/1000 births. Whilst this rate was the lowest since data were collected by the Perinatal and Maternal Mortality Review Committee in 2007, it did not show a statistically significant trend in improvement.

The Australian Institute of Health and Welfare (AIHW, 2017) reported that in the 20-year period from 1993 to 2012, the overall PNMR remained stable at around 10 deaths per 1000 live births. In 2015, there were 9 perinatal deaths for every 1000 births, a total of 2849 perinatal deaths. This included 2160 fetal deaths (stillbirths), or 7 fetal deaths per 1000 births, and 689 neonatal deaths, a rate of 2 neonatal deaths per 1000 live births.

Factors that influence perinatal mortality rates

PNMRs are influenced by maternal care, health and nutrition. Factors include socio-demographic characteristics, maternal age, deprivation and remoteness, ethnicity and

obesity. Smoking also has a significant adverse effect on birth weight and perinatal mortality.

Sociodemographic characteristics

Like many developed nations, such as those in North America and New Zealand, the PNMRs of the indigenous populations in Australia remain high. The Aboriginal and Torres Strait Islander populations have, on average, 2.3 times the disease burden of non-indigenous people. Whilst there was a 20% decrease in the perinatal death rate of babies born to indigenous mothers between 1993 and 2012, the PNMR of babies born to mothers who identified as Aboriginal or Torres Strait Islander was almost double that of babies of non-indigenous mothers (17.1 versus 9.6 deaths per 1000 births).

Maternal age

Maternal age at both extremes is associated with an increase in perinatal mortality. In Australia, the stillbirth rates for babies of teenage mothers and mothers older than 45 was more than double that for mothers aged 30–34 (13.9 and 17.1 versus 6.4 deaths per 1000 births, respectively). In the UK, a slightly different trend was noted. Whilst there has been a reduction in the rate of stillbirth for the youngest mothers (<20 years of age) over the period 2013–2015 (from 5.28 to 4.65 stillbirths per 1000 total births), a similar-sized increase in the NMR occurred over the same period (2.35–2.95 per 1000 live births). For older mothers (>40 years age), the SBR has remained static over this period, whereas the NMR has shown a small reduction (from 2.66 to 2.52 per 1000 live births). It is important to note this effect as more women are delaying childbearing in developed countries.

Deprivation

The socioeconomic status of the mothers also has a statistically significant effect on the perinatal mortality rates in the UK. Mothers in the most deprived areas were 1.7 times (5.05 versus 3.0 per 1000 births) more likely to have a stillbirth and 1.6 times (2.28 versus 1.41 per 1000 births) more likely to have a neonatal death compared with mothers in the least deprived areas (Table 5.1).

Ethnicity

A statistically significant ethnic distribution compared with the general maternity population in the rates of stillbirths and neonatal mortality, with mothers of black and Asian ethnic origins being at highest risks, was noted in the UK report. Ethnic differences may be linked to employment and deprivation status. Whilst a small reduction in mortality rates over time can be seen for most of the characteristics for both stillbirth and NMR, an increase was noted in the rate of stillbirth for the black British ethnic group from 7.02 to 8.17 per 1000 total births in the period of 2013–2015.

Other maternal characteristics

Smoking is an important independent risk factor. In Australia, the PNMR was almost 50% higher among babies whose mothers smoked compared with those who did not (13.3 versus 8.9 deaths per 1000 births). In the UK, around one-fifth of the mothers of both stillbirths and neonatal deaths were identified as smoking throughout pregnancy in 2015. The National Institute for Health and Care Excellence (NICE, 2010) recommends the use of routine carbon monoxide (CO) monitoring in all pregnant women. This forms part of the Stillbirth Care Bundle in the National Health Service to determine the smoking status of women at booking and to help encourage them to quit. The effect of this on the stillbirth rates is still being monitored.

Body mass index (BMI) may be a factor in contributing to the PNMR, but the data are not universally collected for all births. In the UK, in 2015, 25% of mothers who had stillbirths and 19% of mothers who had neonatal deaths fell into the obese group. There was no statistical difference in outcomes when parity, early booking, presentation at birth or mode of delivery was compared. Past obstetric history such as pre-term birth, mid-trimester loss, recurrent miscarriage and pre-eclampsia were important factors.

Table 5.1 Ratios of mortality rates for stillbirth and neonatal death by mother's age and socioeconomic deprivation quintile of residence: United Kingdom & Crown Dependencies, for births in 2015

Mother's characteristics	Ratio of mortality rates (RR)[§] 2015	
Mother's age (in years)	**Stillbirths**	**Neonatal deaths**
<20	1.28 (1.06–1.55)	1.85 (1.44–2.36)
20–24	1.17 (1.04–1.30)	1.27 (1.08–1.49)
25–29	1.03 (0.94–1.13)	1.05 (0.91–1.21)
30–34	–	–
35–39	1.20 (1.08–1.34)	1.16 (0.99–1.36)
≥40	1.55 (1.32–1.82)	1.58 (1.24–2.01)
Socioeconomic deprivation quintile*		
1 – Least deprived	Reference	Reference
2	1.08 (0.96–1.23)	1.07 (0.89–1.28)
3	1.23 (1.09–1.39)	1.13 (0.94–1.36)
4	1.48 (1.31–1.66)	1.42 (1.19–1.68)
5 – Most deprived	1.68 (1.50–1.89)	1.61 (1.36–1.91)

[§]Excluding terminations of pregnancy and births <24+0 weeks gestational age.
*Based on mothers' postcodes at time of delivery, using the Children in Low-Income Families Local Measure.
From MBRRACE-UK Perinatal Mortality Surveillance Report, UK Perinatal Deaths for Births from January to December 2015. Leicester: The Infant Mortality and Morbidity Studies, Department of Health Sciences, University of Leicester. 2017.

Causes of stillbirths

Stillbirths are the largest contributor to perinatal mortality. It is important to classify the causes of stillbirths in order to help with the understanding of the antecedents. The traditionally used systems such as the Wigglesworth and the Aberdeen (Obstetric) classifications consistently reported up to two-thirds of stillbirths as being from unexplained causes. Many newer classifications have been developed that have resulted in a significant reduction of the numbers of stillbirths being classified as unexplained.

In Australia and New Zealand, the Perinatal Society of Australia and New Zealand Perinatal Death Classification (PSANZ-PDC) and the Perinatal Society of Australia and New Zealand Neonatal Death Classification (PSANZ-NDC) are used to classify all stillbirths and neonatal deaths. Using this classification, the leading cause of stillbirths in Australia was noted to be congenital abnormalities (26.3% of stillbirths) during the period 2011–2012. The leading cause of perinatal deaths among babies of Aboriginal and Torres Strait Islander mothers was spontaneous pre-term birth (26.8% of stillbirths and 48.0% of neonatal deaths). MBR-RACE-UK uses the Cause of Death & Associated Conditions (CODAC) classification system to classify both stillbirths and neonatal deaths. The CODAC system has a three-level hierarchical tree of coded causes of death. Using this system, a revision of the cause of death classification for congenital anomalies in 2015 has resulted in an increase in the percentage for stillbirths and neonatal deaths from congenital abnormalities when compared with the MBR-RACE-UK perinatal mortality surveillance report for births in 2014: 8.8% of stillbirths and 33.1% of neonatal deaths compared with 6.4% and 27.9%, respectively, in 2014. Placental causes account for 27.1% of all stillbirths in 2015, but 39.5% still fall into the 'Unknown' group (Fig. 5.2). Further analysis of the data showed that almost one-third of stillbirths with an unknown primary cause of death were potentially growth restricted (360 out of 1190, 30.2%), highlighting the importance of close monitoring of growth during pregnancy.

On a global scale, the WHO report (2015) states that the major causes of stillbirth include:
- childbirth complications
- post-term pregnancy
- maternal infections in pregnancy (malaria, syphilis and HIV)
- maternal disorders (especially hypertension, obesity and diabetes)
- fetal growth restriction
- congenital abnormalities

Stillbirths are often preceded by maternal perception of decreased fetal movement (DFM). DFM is also strongly linked to adverse perinatal outcomes. While evidence is still emerging in this area, some studies indicate that a reduction in stillbirth rates may be achieved by increasing maternal, clinician and community awareness about the importance of DFM.

Intrapartum stillbirth

The WHO estimations have shown that intrapartum stillbirths account for half of all stillbirths worldwide. Estimated proportions of intrapartum stillbirths vary from 10% (5.3% in the UK) in developed regions to 59% in South Asia. Improved care at birth is essential to prevent 1.3 million intrapartum stillbirths, most of which are preventable.

Complications of childbirth are the cause of almost all the intrapartum deaths; these are largely avoidable through the provision of appropriately trained birth attendants and facilities. Most deliveries in developed countries take place in institutions and in the presence of qualified health personnel. Globally, coverage of skilled attendants during childbirth increased from 61% in 2000 to 78% in 2016. However, despite steady improvement globally and within regions, millions of births were not assisted by a midwife, a doctor or a trained nurse. In sub-Saharan Africa, approximately only half of all live births were delivered with the assistance of a skilled birth attendant in 2016.

Causes of neonatal deaths

Newborn deaths dropped from 4.6 million in 1990 to 3.3 million in 2009, but fell only slightly during the last decade. More investment into health care for women and children since 2000, when the UN MDGs were set, resulted in more rapid progress for the survival of mothers (2.3% per year) and children under 5 years (2.1% per year) than for newborns (1.7% per year). Every year nearly 41% of all under-5 child deaths are among newborn infants, babies in their first 28 days of life or infants in the neonatal period. Three-quarters of all newborn deaths occur in the first week of life. In developing countries, nearly half of all mothers and newborns do not receive skilled care during and immediately after birth. Virtually all (99%) newborn deaths occur in low- and middle-income countries, especially in Africa and South Asia, where the least progress in reducing neonatal deaths has been made. Globally, the three major causes of neonatal deaths are infections (36%, which includes sepsis/pneumonia, tetanus and diarrhoea), pre-term (28%) and birth asphyxia (23%). There is some variation between countries depending on their care configurations.

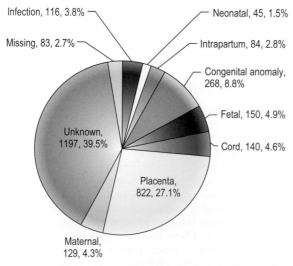

Fig. 5.2 Stillbirths by CODAC Level 1 cause of death: United Kingdom & Crown Dependencies, for births in 2015. (From MBRRACE-UK Perinatal Mortality Surveillance Report, UK Perinatal Deaths for Births from January to December 2015. Leicester: The Infant Mortality and Morbidity Studies, Department of Health Sciences, University of Leicester. 2017.)

In the UK, approximately 44% of the neonatal deaths in 2015 were attributed to a neonatal cause. The classifications for causes of death with the largest numbers of neonatal deaths were extreme prematurity, neurological and cardio-respiratory conditions (Fig. 5.3). In Australia, the leading cause of neonatal deaths (2011–2012) was congenital abnormality (33.1%). An additional PSANZ-NDC of extreme prematurity was the leading condition contributing to deaths in the neonatal period (33.5%). Low birth weight, although not a direct cause of neonatal death, is an important association. Around 15–20% of newborn infants weigh less than 2500 g, ranging from 6% in developed countries to more than 30% in the poorly developed countries.

Many strategies have been implemented in an attempt to improve the PNMRs across the world. Yet disparities in outcomes still persist. The objectives of the various MDGs have been realized with varying degrees of success. The key to improving outcomes remains in the provision of high coverage of high-quality care during labour and birth. This gives a quadruple return on investment by preventing maternal and neonatal deaths, and also stillbirths and disability, with improvements in child development. Improved quality of antenatal care and family planning are also important to maximize maternal and fetal wellbeing and the long-term wellbeing of the child.

Maternal mortality

The Tenth Revision of the ICD defines a maternal death as the death of a woman while pregnant or within 42 days of termination of pregnancy, irrespective of the duration and the site of the pregnancy, from any cause related to or aggravated by the pregnancy or its management but not from accidental or incidental causes.

Maternal deaths are subdivided into two groups:
- *Direct obstetric deaths:* Those resulting from obstetric complications of the pregnancy state (pregnancy, labour and the puerperium); from interventions, omissions or incorrect treatment; or from a chain of events resulting from any of the above.
- *Indirect obstetric deaths:* Those resulting from pre-existing disease or a disease that developed during pregnancy and which was not due to direct obstetric causes but which was aggravated by the physiological effects of pregnancy.

Late maternal death is the death of a woman from direct or indirect causes more than 42 days but less than 1 year after termination of pregnancy.

Coincidental (fortuitous): Deaths from unrelated causes that occur in pregnancy or the puerperium (from ICD-10).

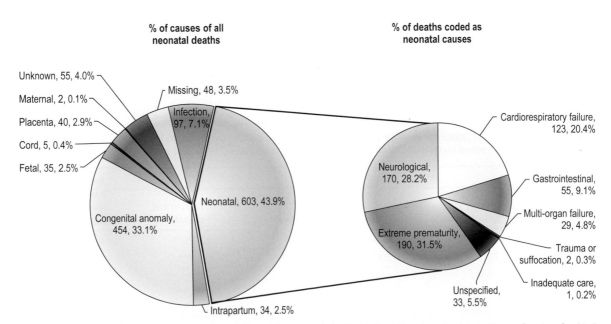

% of causes of all neonatal deaths

% of deaths coded as neonatal causes

Unknown, 55, 4.0%
Maternal, 2, 0.1%
Placenta, 40, 2.9%
Cord, 5, 0.4%
Fetal, 35, 2.5%
Missing, 48, 3.5%
Infection, 97, 7.1%
Neonatal, 603, 43.9%
Congenital anomaly, 454, 33.1%
Intrapartum, 34, 2.5%

Cardiorespiratory failure, 123, 20.4%
Neurological, 170, 28.2%
Gastrointestinal, 55, 9.1%
Multi-organ failure, 29, 4.8%
Extreme prematurity, 190, 31.5%
Trauma or suffocation, 2, 0.3%
Inadequate care, 1, 0.2%
Unspecified, 33, 5.5%

Fig. 5.3 Neonatal deaths by CODAC Level 1 and Level 2 cause of death: United Kingdom & Crown Dependencies, for births in 2015. (From MBRRACE-UK Perinatal Mortality Surveillance Report, UK Perinatal Deaths for Births from January to December 2015. Leicester: The Infant Mortality and Morbidity Studies, Department of Health Sciences, University of Leicester. 2017.)

In an attempt to improve the classification of maternal deaths, the WHO applied some modifications to the definitions of ICD-10. This is known as *ICD-Maternal Mortality (ICD-MM)*.

This defined death occurring during pregnancy, childbirth and the puerperium as the death of a woman while pregnant or within 42 days of termination of pregnancy, irrespective of the cause of death (obstetric and non-obstetric).

The proposals for the new codes are likely to be incorporated into the 11th Revision of the ICD (ICD-11).

Maternal mortality rates

The international definition of the MMR is the number of direct and indirect deaths per 100,000 live births.

Obtaining accurate MMR data remains a global challenge due to a lack of accurate reporting of maternal deaths. Planning and accountability for improving maternal health require accurate and internationally comparable measures of maternal mortality. Many countries have made notable progress in collecting data through civil registration systems, surveys, censuses and specialized studies over the past decade. This laudable increase in efforts to document maternal deaths provides valuable new data, but the diversity of methods used to assess maternal mortality in the absence of civil registration systems prevents direct comparisons among indicators generated. To date, insufficient progress has been made, as many countries still lack civil registration systems, and where such systems do exist, underreporting continues to pose a major challenge to data accuracy.

Given the challenges of obtaining accurate and standardized direct measures of maternal mortality, the Maternal Mortality Estimation Inter-Agency Group (MMEIG),

comprising WHO and many non-governmental organizations and universities across the world, was established to provide better estimates for 1990–2015 to examine the global, regional and country progress of MM. To provide increasingly accurate estimates of MMR, previous estimation methods have been refined to optimize use of country-level data.

Developed countries such as the UK have the advantage of accurate denominator data, including both live births and stillbirths, and have defined their MMRs as the number of direct and indirect deaths per 100,000 maternities as a more accurate denominator to indicate the number of women at risk.

Maternities are defined as the number of pregnancies that result in a live birth at any gestation or stillbirths occurring at or after 24 completed weeks of gestation and are required to be notified by law. This enables a more detailed picture of MMRs to be established and is used for the comparison of trends over time.

Improving maternal health is one of the eight MDGs adopted at the WHO 2000 Millennium Summit. The two targets for assessing progress in improving maternal health (MDG 5) are reducing MMR by 75% between 1990 and 2015 and achieving universal access to reproductive health by 2015.

In the 2015 report issued by the WHO, the United Nations Children's Fund (UNICEF), the United Nations Population Fund (UNFPA), the World Bank Group and the United Nations Population Division (UNPD) entitled *Trends in Maternal Mortality: 1990–2015*, it is encouraging to note that from 1990, the global MMR declined by 44% – from 385 deaths to 216 deaths per 100,000 live births (from an estimated 532,000 to an estimated 303,000), representing an average annual rate of reduction of 2.3% (Table 5.2). While impressive, this is less than half of the 5.5% annual rate needed to achieve the three-quarters

Table 5.2 Comparison of maternal mortality ratio (MMR, maternal deaths per 100,000 live births) and number of maternal deaths, by United Nations Millennium Development Goal region, 1990 and 2015

United Nations Millennium Development Goal region	1990		2015		Percentage change between 1990 and 2015
	MMR	Maternal deaths	MMR	Maternal deaths	
World	385	532,000	216	303,000	44
Developed regions	23	3,500	12	1,700	48
Developing regions	430	529,000	239	302,000	44

From Trends in Maternal Mortality 1990 to 2015: Estimates by WHO, UNICEF, UNFPA, World Bank Group and the United Nations Population Division (WHO 2015).

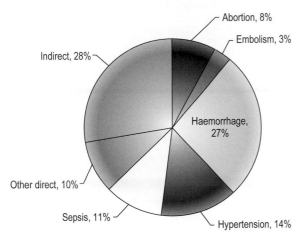

Fig 5.4 Causes of maternal mortality – the global picture. (Reproduced with permission. From Trends in maternal mortality: 1990 to 2015: estimates by WHO, UNICEF, UNFPA, World Bank Group and the United Nations Population Division, 2015.)

reduction in MM targeted for 2015 in MDG 5. Improvements in MMR have been achieved in every region. Almost all maternal deaths are preventable. However, disparities still occur between the richest and poorest countries, with levels of MM remaining unacceptably high in sub-Saharan Africa, which accounts for approximately 66% (201,000), and southern Asia (22% (66,000)), of the global maternal deaths in 2015. The lifetime risk of maternal death in high-income countries is 1 in 3300, compared with 1 in 41 in low-income countries.

Globally, the major causes of maternal death are (Fig. 5.4):
- haemorrhage, the leading cause, accounting for 27% of all deaths
- hypertensive disorders
- sepsis
- unsafe abortion
- embolism

In the UK, the Confidential Enquiry into Maternal Deaths has been publishing triennial reports since it was introduced in England and Wales in 1952 and has represented a gold standard internationally for detailed investigation and improvement in maternity care for over 60 years. Since 2012, MBRRACE-UK has been publishing the Confidential Enquiries into Maternal Mortality and Morbidity from the UK and Ireland entitled *Saving Lives, Improving Mothers' Care*. In the fourth annual report released in December 2017, surveillance data on maternal deaths from 2013 to 2015 were published. In Australia, similar data on MM are reported every 3 years by the AIHW. The latest report was published in 2017, covering the period 2012–2014.

In the UK, 240 women died in 2013–2015 during or within 42 days of the end of pregnancy. The deaths of 38 women were classified as coincidental. Thus, in this triennium, 202 women died from direct and indirect causes among 2,305,920 maternities, a maternal death rate of 8.76 per 100,000 maternities. This is comparable to the rate of 8.54 per 100,000 maternities in 2012–2014.

There was an overall 37% decrease in maternal death rates between 2003–2005 and 2013–2015. The direct maternal death rate has decreased by 44% since 2003–2005, and there was a 31% decrease in the rate of indirect maternal deaths. The rates of overall mortality and direct maternal death in the 2013–2015 triennium were not significantly different from the rates in 2010–2012. However, the indirect maternal death rate was significantly lower in 2013–2015 than 2010–2012 (Fig. 5.5).

Major causes of maternal death in the UK

The five major direct causes of maternal death in the UK (2013–2015), in order of importance, are as follows:
1. thrombosis and thromboembolism
2. haemorrhage
3. psychiatric causes – suicides
4. pregnancy-related infections – sepsis
5. amniotic fluid embolism

The number of indirect maternal deaths has remained largely unchanged since the last triennium. The three commonest indirect causes of maternal death in the year following delivery are cardiac disease, other indirect causes and neurological conditions. Many of the women with cardiac disease had lifestyle-related risk factors such as obesity, smoking and maternal age.

The situation in Australia

Similar trends have occurred in Australia, with a fall in the MMR from 8.4 per 100,000 women giving birth in 2003–2005 to 6.8 in 2012–2014. The MMR in indigenous women (18.7 per 100,000 women giving birth) remains three times higher than in the non-indigenous population (6.3 per 100,000).

In Australia (2012–2014), direct maternal deaths were most frequently due to pulmonary thromboembolism, obstetric haemorrhage and hypertensive disorders. Non-obstetric haemorrhage and cardiovascular disease were the most common groups of indirect maternal death causes. Since 2000, Aboriginal and Torres Strait Islander women have been significantly more likely than other Australian women to die in relation to pregnancy from cardiovascular causes, suicide, hypertensive disorders, obstetric haemorrhage, sepsis and in early pregnancy.

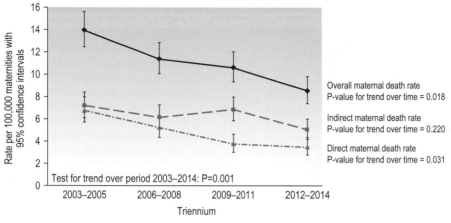

Fig. 5.5 Direct and indirect maternal mortality rates per 100,000 maternities, UK 2003–2014 (using ICD-MM). (Reproduced with permission. From MBRRACE-UK. Saving Lives, Improving Mothers' Care - Lessons learned to inform maternity care from the UK and Ireland Confidential Enquiries into Maternal Deaths and Morbidity 2013–15. Oxford: National Perinatal Epidemiology Unit, University of Oxford 2017.)

Essential information

Perinatal mortality

- Global stillbirth rate: 18.4/1000 births
- UK stillbirth rate, 2015: 3.87/1000 births
- Neonatal death rate: 1.74/1000 births
- Perinatal mortality rate: 5.61/1000 births
- Australian perinatal mortality rate, 2015: 7.0/1000 births

Aetiology (MBRRACE-UK 2015)

- Stillbirths
  - Unexplained: 39.5%
  - Placental: 27.1%
  - Congenital anomaly: 8.8%
- Neonatal deaths
  - Neonatal causes, including extreme prematurity, neurological and cardio-respiratory causes: 43.9%
  - Congenital anomaly: 33.1%
  - Infection: 7.1%

Maternal mortality

- UK Confidential Enquiry 2013–2015
  - Direct deaths: 3.82 per 100,000 maternities
  - Indirect deaths: 4.94 per 100,000 maternities
- AIHW 2012–2014
  - Direct deaths: 3.45 per 100,000 women giving birth
  - Indirect deaths: 3.35 per 100,000 women giving birth

Commonest causes of direct deaths in the UK

1. Thrombosis and thromboembolism
2. Haemorrhage
3. Psychiatric causes – suicides
4. Pregnancy-related infections – sepsis
5. Amniotic fluid embolism

Commonest indirect causes in the UK

- Cardiac disease
- Other indirect causes
- Neurological conditions

Section | 2 |

Essential obstetrics

Chapter | 6 |

History taking and examination in obstetrics

Petra Agoston and Edwin Chandraharan

LEARNING OUTCOMES

After studying this chapter you should be able to:

Knowledge criteria

- Explain the relevance of a detailed history of the index pregnancy
- Discuss the importance of previous obstetric, medical, gynaecological and family history
- Explain how to conduct a detailed, general, obstetric and pelvic examination
- Discuss the pathophysiological basis of symptoms and physical signs in pregnancy

Clinical competency

- Take a detailed obstetric history in a normal pregnancy and a pregnancy with complications in the index or previous pregnancy
- Carry out general and obstetric examination in a normal pregnancy and that with maternal or fetal complications, including:
  - Measure blood pressure in pregnancy
  - Perform and interpret urinalysis in pregnancy
  - Perform an abdominal examination in women during pregnancy (over 20 weeks)
  - Auscultate the fetal heart
- Summarize and integrate the history, examination and investigation results and formulate a management plan
- Provide explanations to patients in a language they can understand

Professional skills and attitudes

- Reflect on the components of effective verbal and non-verbal communication
- Understand the need to be flexible and be willing to take advice in the light of new information
- Recognize the acutely unwell patient in obstetrics

It is vital to differentiate the normal anatomical and physiological changes associated with pregnancy from pathological conditions whilst managing a woman during pregnancy, childbirth and puerperium. Basic clinical skills in obstetrics include effective verbal and non-verbal communication in a logical sequence: history, eliciting physical signs (general, systemic and obstetric examinations), differentiating normal pregnancy-associated changes from abnormal deviation and arriving at a provisional diagnosis. Contemporaneous, accurate, detailed and legible clinical note-keeping is a cornerstone of 'basic clinical skills'. Such a systematic approach will aid effective management by ensuring a multidisciplinary input when required.

Taking a relevant and comprehensive history

Taking a relevant and accurate history forms a cornerstone of good clinical practice, as it helps arrive at a diagnosis. It is essential to appreciate that taking a comprehensive history in obstetrics and gynaecology involves eliciting confidential and often very 'personal' information. Therefore, it is essential to build a good rapport with the woman during the consultation and ask confidential and sensitive information towards the end of this history-taking process, after establishing mutual trust and confidence.

Obstetric history

It is advisable to commence obstetric history taking by eliciting details of the current (or *index*) pregnancy followed by previous obstetric (including modes of birth and complications) and previous gynaecological history.

History of present pregnancy

The date of the first day of the last menstrual period (LMP) provides the clinician with an idea of how advanced the current pregnancy is, i.e. period of gestation. However, this information is often inaccurate, as many women do not record the days on which they menstruate unless the date of the period is associated with a significant life event or the woman has been actively trying to conceive. Hence, in addition to LMP, an ultrasound scan in the first or early second trimester should be used to date the pregnancy and to confirm the gestational age.

Menstrual history should also include the duration of the menstrual cycle, as ovulation occurs on the fourteenth day before menstruation. The time interval between menstruation and ovulation (the proliferative phase of the menstrual cycle) may vary substantially, whereas the post-ovulatory phase (secretory phase) is fairly constant (12–14 days).

The length of the menstrual cycle refers to the time interval between the first day of the period and the first day of the subsequent period. This may vary from 21 to 35 days in normal women, but menstruation usually occurs every 28 days.

It is important to note the method of contraception prior to conception, as hormonal contraception may be associated with a delay in ovulation in the first cycle after discontinuation. The age of onset of menstruation (the *menarche*) may be relevant in teenage pregnancies to determine the onset of fertility.

The estimated date of delivery (EDD) can be calculated from the first day of the LMP by adding 9 months and 7 days to this date. However, to apply this Naegele's rule, the first day of the menstrual period should be accurate and the woman should have had regular 28-day menstrual cycles (Fig. 6.1). The average duration of human gestation is 269 days from the date of conception. Therefore, in a woman with a 28-day cycle, this is 283 days from the first day of the LMP (14 days are added for the period between menstruation and conception). In a 28-day cycle, the EDD can be calculated by subtracting 3 months from the first day of the LMP and adding on 7 days (or alternatively, adding 9 months and 7 days). It is important to appreciate that only 40% of women will deliver within 5 days of the EDD and about two-thirds of women deliver within 10 days of the EDD. The calculation of the EDD based on a woman's LMP is therefore, at best, a guide to a woman as to the date around which her delivery is likely to occur.

If a woman's normal menstrual cycle is less than 28 days or is greater than 28 days, an appropriate number of days should be subtracted from or added to the EDD. For example, if the normal cycle is 35 days, 7 days should be added to the EDD.

Symptoms of pregnancy

A history of secondary amenorrhoea in a woman who has been having a regular menstrual cycle serves as a

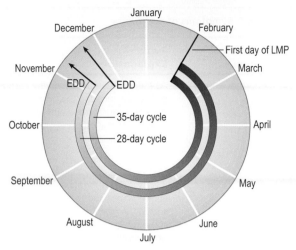

Fig. 6.1 Calculation of the estimated date of delivery (EDD). *LMP*, Last menstrual period.

self-diagnostic tool for pregnancy. In addition to this, anatomical, physiological, biochemical, endocrine and metabolic changes associated with pregnancy may result in the following symptoms (Table 6.1).

Pseudocyesis

Pseudocyesis refers to development of symptoms and many of the signs of pregnancy in a woman who is not pregnant. This is often due to an intense desire for or fears of pregnancy that may result in hypothalamic amenorrhoea. In modern obstetric practice, with the widespread use of ultrasound scanning in early pregnancy, it is unlikely to proceed into late pregnancy unless the woman presents late to a booking clinic.

The presence of a negative pregnancy test and ultrasound scan information will provide confirmation that the woman is not pregnant. However, a sympathetic approach and support are essential to resolve the underlying anxieties that led to pseudocyesis. Menstruation usually returns after the woman is informed of her condition.

Previous obstetric history

The term *gravidity* refers to the number of times a woman has been pregnant, irrespective of the outcome of the pregnancy, i.e. termination, miscarriage or ectopic pregnancy. A *primigravida* is a woman who is pregnant for the first time; and a *multigravida* is a woman who has been pregnant on two or more occasions.

This term *gravidity* must be distinguished from the term *parity*, which describes the number of live-born children and stillbirths a woman has delivered after 24 weeks or with a birth weight of 500 g. Thus, a *primipara* is a woman who has given birth to one infant after 24 weeks.

A multiparous woman is one who has given birth to two or more infants, whereas a nulliparous woman has not

Table 6.1 Symptoms of pregnancy

Symptoms of pregnancy	Explanation	Deviation from normal
Amenorrhoea	As the fertilization occurs, the corpus luteum enlarges and will increase the production of progesterone. As both progesterone and oestrogen levels rise in pregnancy, they suppress further ovulation, leading to amenorrhoea.	Hypothalamo-hypophyseal hormonal changes Ovarian changes (polycystic ovarian syndrome (PCOS), premature menopause, etc.) Uterine scarring, intrauterine adhesions Contraception Low/high body mass index (BMI) Stress
Nausea and vomiting	It is believed to be secondary to a rise in human chorionic gonadotropin (hCG) and commonly occurs within the first 2 weeks of missing the first period. Although it is commonly described as morning sickness, vomiting may occur at any time of the day and is often precipitated by the smell or sight of food.	*Hyperemesis gravidarum* is severe or persistent vomiting leading to maternal dehydration, ketonuria and electrolyte imbalance. This condition needs prompt diagnosis, rehydration and correction of metabolic and electrolyte derangements. Gastrointestinal infections and food poisoning can also present with these symptoms.
Frequent micturition	It is considered to be due to the pressure on the bladder exerted by the gravid uterus. It tends to diminish after the first 12 weeks of pregnancy as the uterus rises above the symphysis pubis. Plasma osmolality falls soon after conception, and the ability to excrete a water load is altered in early pregnancy. There is an increased diuretic response after water loading when the woman is sitting in the upright position, and this response declines by the third trimester. However, it may be sufficient to cause urinary frequency in early pregnancy.	Urinary tract infections (UTIs) can present with persistence of increased frequency, as well as associated symptoms (dysuria, haematuria).
Excessive lassitude or lethargy	It is thought that progesterone can cause lethargy and fatigue. It is a common symptom in early pregnancy and may become apparent even before the first period is missed. Often, it disappears after 12 weeks of gestation.	Hypothyroidism can have similar effects, and expectant mothers with excessive fatigue should be tested for it.
Breast tenderness and heaviness	It is due to the effect of increasing serum progesterone and prolactin increasing the breast tissues to be ready for lactation, as well as an increased retention of water.	This can be experienced in the premenstrual phase of the cycle. It can also be caused by infections, abscesses or injuries and sprains. It can also be a side effect of some medicines (contraceptives, antidepressants).
Fetal movements	First perception of fetal movements is called *quickening*. It is not usually noticed until 20 weeks' gestation during the first pregnancy and 18 weeks in the second or subsequent pregnancies. However, many women may experience fetal movements earlier than 18 weeks, and others may progress beyond 20 weeks of gestation without being aware of fetal movements at all.	Both the lack of fetal movements and a sudden increase in their activity can be abnormal in pregnancy. A decrease can be caused by chronic fetal distress, as in pre-eclampsia, while a sudden increase may be a sign of placental abruption, although this is not well documented.
Pica	Pica is an abnormal desire for a particular food. In pregnancy, particular cravings are considered to be normal; they are thought to be due to hormonal changes.	Its subject can also be a non-nutrient, like soil, metals, paper or wall paint. It can be a sign of iron deficiency.

given birth after 24 weeks. The term *grand multipara* has been used to describe a woman who has given birth to five or more infants.

Thus, a pregnant woman who has given birth to three viable singleton pregnancies and has also had two miscarriages would be described as gravida 5 para 3: a multigravid multiparous woman.

A *parturient* is a woman in labour, and a *puerpera* is a woman who has given birth to a child during the preceding 42 days.

A record should be made of all previous pregnancies, including previous miscarriages, and the duration of gestation in each pregnancy. In particular, it is important to note any previous antenatal complications, details of induction of labour, the duration of labour, the presentation and the method of delivery, as well as the birth weight and sex of each infant.

The condition of each infant at birth and the need for care in a special care baby unit should be noted. Similarly, details of complications during labour, as well as puerperium, such as postpartum haemorrhage, infections of the genital tract and urinary tract, deep vein thrombosis (DVT) and perineal trauma, should be enquired. It is vital to appreciate that these complications may have a recurrence risk and may influence the management of subsequent pregnancies; e.g. history of DVT requires thromboprophylaxis during the antenatal and postnatal periods.

Previous medical history

The effects of pre-existing medical conditions on pregnancy, as well as the effect of anatomical, biochemical, endocrine, metabolic and haematological changes associated with the physiological state of pregnancy on pre-existing medical conditions, should be considered.

The natural course of diabetes, renal disease, hypertension, cardiac disease, various endocrine disorders (e.g. thyrotoxicosis and Addison's disease) and infectious diseases (e.g. tuberculosis, HIV, syphilis and hepatitis A or B) may be altered by pregnancy. Conversely, they may adversely affect both maternal and perinatal outcome (see Chapter 9).

Family history

Most women will be aware of any significant family history of the common genetically based diseases, and it is not necessary to list all the possibilities to the mother, as it may increase her anxiety. A general enquiry as to whether there are any known inherited conditions in the family will be

sufficient, unless one partner (or both) is adopted and not aware of his/her family history.

Detailed and relevant information obtained with regard to demographics (e.g. maternal age; increased body mass index [BMI]); past obstetric, medical and surgical history (e.g. laparotomy, caesarean section, myomectomy); and family history will help in performing appropriate tests, as well as in making a care plan.

Examination

Examination during pregnancy involves general, systemic (cardiovascular system, respiratory system, general abdominal and, in specific circumstances, a neurological examination) and detailed obstetric (uterus and its contents) examinations (Table 6.2).

General and systemic examination

At the initial visit to the clinic, i.e. the booking visit, a complete physical examination should be performed to identify any physical problems that may be relevant to the antenatal care.

Height and weight are recorded at the first and all subsequent visits, and this will help in the calculation of BMI (BMI = weight in kg/height in m^2).

Pelvic examination

Routine pelvic examination to confirm pregnancy and gestation at booking is not indicated in settings where an ultrasound scan is freely available. If a routine cervical smear is due at the time of booking, this can usually be deferred until after the puerperium, as interpretation of cervical cytology is more difficult in pregnancy. Clinical assessment of the size and shape of the pelvis may be useful in specific circumstances such as a previous fractured pelvis, but not in routine practice. Hence, it is generally no longer carried out as part of the routine antenatal examinations.

A speculum examination in early pregnancy is indicated in the assessment of bleeding (see Chapter 18). Pelvic examination in later pregnancy is indicated for cervical assessment (see Chapter 11) and the diagnosis of labour and to confirm ruptured membranes (see Chapter 11). Digital vaginal examination is contraindicated in later pregnancy in cases of antepartum haemorrhage until placenta praevia can be excluded.

The role of vaginal examination in normal labour is discussed in Chapter 12.

Measuring blood pressure in pregnancy ABC

Blood pressure is recorded with the patient supine and in the left lateral supine position to avoid compression of the inferior vena cava by the gravid uterus (Fig. 6.2). If blood pressure is to be recorded in the sitting position, it should be recorded in the same position for all visits and on the same arm. The effect of posture on blood pressure has been noted in Chapter 3. Vena caval compression in late pregnancy may cause symptoms of syncope and nausea, and this is associated with postural hypotension, the condition being known as the *supine hypotensive syndrome*. If this is not recognized for a prolonged period, fetal compromise may occur secondary to a reduction in uteroplacental circulation.

Although in the past the diastolic pressure has always been taken as Korotkoff fourth sound, where the sound begins to fade, it is now agreed that where the fifth sound, i.e. the point at which the sound disappears, is clear, this should be used to represent the diastolic pressure. If the point at which the sound disappears cannot be identified because it continues towards zero, then the fourth sound should be used.

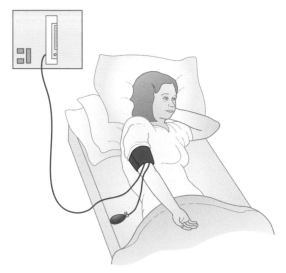

Fig. 6.2 Blood pressure recording standardized in the left lateral position.

Table 6.2 Examination in pregnancy

System	Change and explanation	Deviation from normal
Skin	**Face:** Many women develop a brownish pigmentation called *chloasma* over the forehead and cheeks, particularly where there is frequent exposure to sunlight (Fig. 6.3). The pigmentation fades after puerperium.	Chloasma (or melasma) can also be a symptom of Addison's disease, haemochromatosis or lupus and a side effect of light-sensitive drugs.

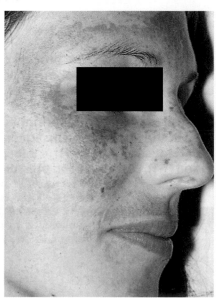

Fig. 6.3 Chloasma: facial pigmentation over the forehead and cheeks.

Table 6.2 Examination in pregnancy—cont'd

System	Change and explanation	Deviation from normal
	Abdomen: Examination of the abdomen commonly shows the presence of stretch marks, or *striae gravidarum* (Fig. 6.4). The scars are initially purplish in colour and appear in the lines of stress in the skin. These scars may also extend on to the thighs and buttocks and on to the breasts. In subsequent pregnancies, the scars adopt a silvery-white appearance. The linea alba often becomes pigmented and is then known as the *linea nigra*. This pigmentation often persists after the first pregnancy.	Stretch marks can also occur during rapid weight loss or weight gain and can also be found on other parts of the body. The hormone cortisone weakens the connective tissue; therefore increased production, e.g. Cushing's syndrome or higher intake of corticosteroid medications, can also present with stretch marks.

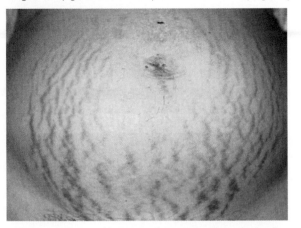

Fig. 6.4 Striae gravidarum on the anterior abdominal wall.

System	Change and explanation	Deviation from normal
Heart and lungs	**Heart:** Benign 'flow murmurs' due to the hyperdynamic circulation associated with normal pregnancy are common and are of no significance. These are generally soft systolic bruits heard over the apex of the heart, and occasionally a mammary souffle is heard, arising from the internal mammary vessels and audible in the second intercostal spaces. This will disappear with pressure from the stethoscope (Fig. 6.5).	Other cardiac murmurs can be signs of severe cardiac disease. If a murmur is heard in systole, it can indicate aortic or pulmonary stenosis or mitral or tricuspid regurgitation, whereas a murmur in diastole can be caused by mitral or tricuspid stenosis or aortic or pulmonary regurgitation. In these cases, cardiology review is necessary, as worsening of these conditions due to the cardiovascular changes in pregnancy can lead to heart failure.

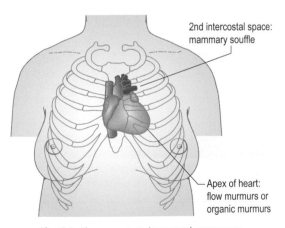

2nd intercostal space: mammary souffle

Apex of heart: flow murmurs or organic murmurs

Fig. 6.5 Flow murmurs in normal pregnancy.

System	Change and explanation	Deviation from normal
	Lungs: Examination of the respiratory system involves assessment of the rate of respiration and the use of any accessory muscles of respiration.	Gross lung pathology may adversely affect maternal and fetal outcome and should therefore be identified as early in the pregnancy as possible.

Continued

Table 6.2 Examination in pregnancy   cont'd

System	Change and explanation	Deviation from normal
Head and neck	**Mucosa:** The colour of the mucosal surfaces and the conjunctivae should be examined for pallor, as anaemia is a common complication of pregnancy.	Anaemia can also occur due to prolonged gastrointestinal bleeding, haemorrhoids and excessive menstrual bleeding (menorrhagia or dysmenorrhoea). It can be a sign of various haematological conditions as well.
	Teeth: The general state of dental hygiene should also be noted, as pregnancy is often associated with hypertrophic gingivitis and dental referral may be needed. Periodontitis and gingivitis can be associated with increased risk of infection and pre-term birth, although this is still debated in the literature.	Gingival hypertrophy can occur due to poor hygiene and inadequate diet. Inflammatory changes due to infections can have similar presentation. It can develop as a side effect of some medications, such as anti-convulsants, antihypertensives or immunosuppressants.
	Neck: Some degree of thyroid enlargement commonly occurs in pregnancy, but unless it is associated with other signs of thyroid disease, mild thyroid enlargement can generally be observed.	If signs of hyperthyroidism (diarrhoea, nervousness, hyperactivity, sweating, weight loss etc.) or hypothyroidism (tiredness, weight gain, increased cold sensitivity) appear, further investigations are needed.
Breasts	The breasts show characteristic signs during pregnancy, which include enlargement in size with increased vascularity, the development of Montgomery's tubercles and increased pigmentation of the areolae of the nipples (Fig. 6.6). 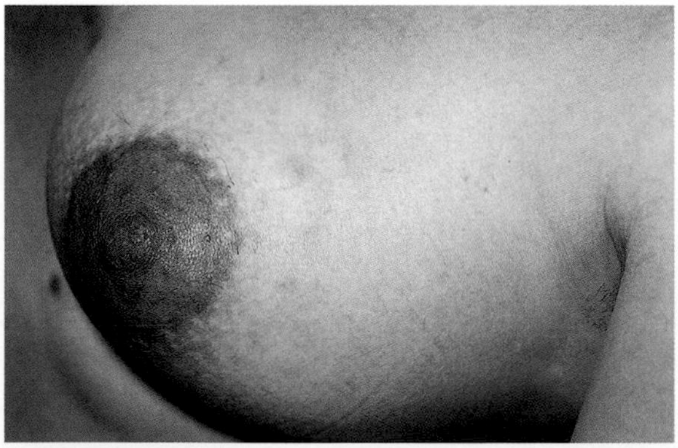 **Fig. 6.6** Physiological changes in the breast in early pregnancy. The areola becomes pigmented and Montgomery's tubercles develop.	Although routine breast examination is not indicated, it is important to ask about inversion of nipples, as this may give rise to difficulties during suckling, and to look for any pathology such as breast cysts or solid nodules in women who complain of any breast symptoms. Breast cancer during pregnancy is reportedly associated with rapid progression and poor prognosis. Hence, any complaint of a 'lump' in the breast should prompt a detailed breast examination.

Table 6.2 Examination in pregnancy—cont'd

System	Change and explanation	Deviation from normal
Abdomen	Hepatosplenomegaly should be excluded, as well as any evidence of renal enlargement. The uterus does not become palpable as an abdominal organ until 12 weeks' gestation.	Any other abnormal examination findings require further investigations. The diagnosis of appendicitis in pregnancy is difficult, as the growing uterus alters the anatomy; therefore extra caution is needed when examining a patient with abdominal pain.
Limbs, skeletal changes	**Limbs:** The legs should be examined for oedema and for varicose veins. They should also be examined for any evidence of shortening of the lower limbs, as this may give problems with gait as the abdomen expands. **Spine:** Posture also changes in pregnancy as the fetus grows and the maternal abdomen expands, with a tendency to develop some kyphosis and, in particular, to develop an increased lumbar lordosis as the upper part of the trunk is thrown backwards to compensate for the weight of the developing fetus (Fig. 6.7). This often results in the development of backache and sometimes gives rise to sciatic pain.	Other causes of oedema are liver, heart and kidney disease. Contraceptive pills, corticosteroids, malnutrition and prolonged immobility or standing can present with oedema. Other spinal deformities can be congenital, degenerative, idiopathic or caused by a disease (tumours, infections). They can interfere with labour as the pelvic diameters change in these conditions. The patient should be informed about her options for delivery.

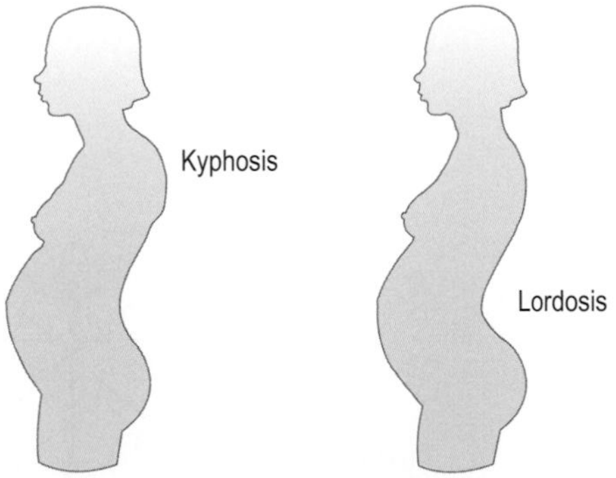

Fig. 6.7 Postural changes in pregnancy. With enlargement of the gravid uterus, there is an increased lumbar lordosis and a tendency to some degree of kyphosis.

The technique of pelvic examination in early pregnancy is the same as that for the non-pregnant woman and is described in Chapter 15.

The vulva should be examined to exclude any abnormal lesions and to assess the perineum in relation to any damage sustained in previous pregnancies. Varicosities of the vulva are common and may become worse during pregnancy.

The vaginal walls become more rugose in pregnancy as the stratified squamous epithelium thickens with an increase in the glycogen content of the epithelial cells.

There is also a marked increase in the vascularity of the paravaginal tissues so that the appearance of the vaginal walls becomes purplish-red. There is an increase in vaginal secretions, with increased vaginal transudation, increased shedding of epithelial cells and some contribution from enhanced production of cervical mucus.

The cervix becomes softened and shows signs of increased vascularity. Enlargement of the cervix is associated with an increase in vascularity, as well as oedema of the connective tissues and cellular hyperplasia and hypertrophy. The glandular content of the endocervix increases to occupy half the substance of the cervix and produces a thick plug of viscid cervical mucus that occludes the cervical os (Fig. 6.8).

Assessment of the bony pelvis

Routine antenatal clinical or radiological pelvimetry has not been shown to be of value in predicting the outcome of labour. However, it is important to assess the pelvis and fetus for possible disproportion when managing cases of delayed progress in labour. Clinical pelvimetry may be

of value where there has been previous trauma or abnormal development of the bony pelvis. Precise information about the various dimensions could be obtained by imaging.

The bony pelvis consists of the sacrum, the coccyx and two innominate bones. The pelvic area above the iliopectineal line is known as the *false pelvis*, and the area below the pelvic brim is the *true pelvis*. The latter is the important section in relation to childbearing and parturition. Thus, the wall of the true pelvis is formed by the sacrum posteriorly, the ischial bones and the sacrosciatic notches and ligaments laterally, and anteriorly by the pubic rami, the obturator fossae and membranes, the ascending rami of the ischial bones and the pubic rami (Fig. 6.9).

Clinical pelvimetry involves assessment of the pelvic inlet (sacral promontory), mid-cavity (pelvic side walls including the ischial spines, the interspinous diameter and the hollow of the sacrum) and the pelvic outlet (subpubic angle and the intertuberous diameter).

In a normal female or gynaecoid pelvis, because the sacrum is evenly curved, maximum space for the fetal head is provided in the pelvic mid-cavity. The sacrum should feel evenly curved.

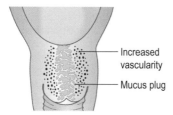

Fig. 6.8 Cervical changes in pregnancy include increased glandular content and a thick mucus plug.

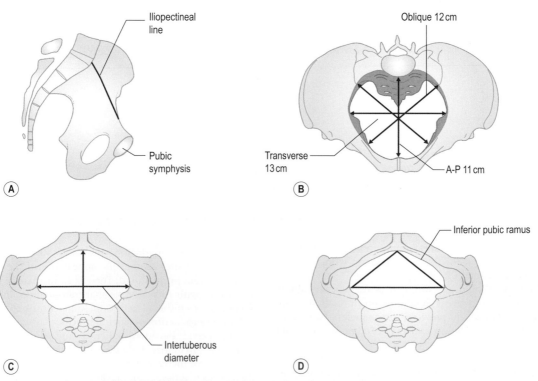

Fig. 6.9 (A) Inlet of the true pelvis is bounded by the sacral promontory, iliopectineal lines, pubic rami and pubic symphysis. (B) Dimensions of the inlet of the true pelvis. (C) Pelvic outlet bounded by the inferior pubic rami and the ischial tuberosities and the sacrosciatic ligaments. (D) The inferior pubic rami should form an angle of 90 degrees.

If the sacrum feels flat, then the pelvis may contract towards the pelvic outlet, as in the android or male-like pelvis, and may lead to impaction of the fetal head as it descends through the pelvis.

The planes of the pelvis

The shape and the dimensions of the true pelvis are best understood by consideration of the four planes of the pelvis.

Plane of the pelvic inlet. The plane of the pelvic inlet, or pelvic brim, is bounded posteriorly by the sacral promontory, laterally by the iliopectineal lines and anteriorly by the superior pubic rami and upper margin of the pubic symphysis. The plane is almost circular in the normal gynaecoid pelvis but is slightly larger transversely than anteroposteriorly.

The true conjugate or anteroposterior diameter of the pelvic inlet is the distance between the midpoint of the sacral promontory and the superior border of the pubic symphysis anteriorly (Fig. 6.10). The diameter measures approximately 11 cm. The shortest distance, and the one of greatest clinical significance, is the obstetric conjugate diameter. This is the distance between the midpoint of the sacral promontory and the nearest point on the posterior surface of the pubic symphysis.

It is not possible to measure either of these diameters by clinical examination; the only diameter at the pelvic inlet that is amenable to clinical assessment is the distance from the inferior margin of the pubic symphysis to the midpoint of the sacral promontory. This is known as the *diagonal conjugate diameter* and is approximately 1.5 cm greater than the obstetric diameter. In practical terms, it is not usually possible to reach the sacral promontory on clinical examination, and the highest point that can be palpated is the second or third piece of the sacrum. If the sacral promontory is easily palpable, the pelvic inlet is contracted (Fig. 6.11A).

Plane of greatest pelvic dimensions. The plane of greatest pelvic dimensions has little clinical significance and has an anteroposterior and transverse diameter of approximately 12.7 cm. The anteroposterior diameter extends from the midpoint of the posterior aspect of the pubic symphysis to the junction of the second and third pieces of the sacrum. The transverse diameter passes laterally through the middle of the acetabuli.

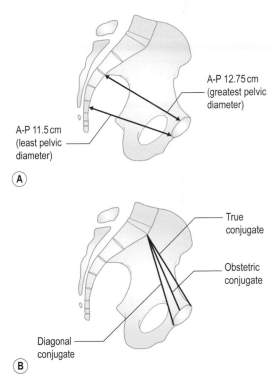

Fig. 6.10 (A) Anteroposterior (A-P) diameters of the mid-cavity and pelvic outlet. (B) Conjugate diameters of the pelvic inlet.

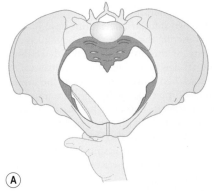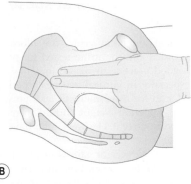

Fig. 6.11 (A) Clinical assessment of the ischial spines at the plane of least pelvic dimensions. (B) Assessment of the pelvic inlet.

The only indication of the shape of the pelvis at this level is the curvature of the sacrum and the shape of the sacrosciatic notch, which should subtend at an angle of 90 degrees. This normally allows the admission of two fingers along the sacrospinous ligaments, which extend from the ischial spines to the lateral aspects of the second and third pieces of the sacrum.

Plane of least pelvic dimensions. The plane of least pelvic dimensions represents the level at which impaction of the fetal head is most likely to occur. The anteroposterior diameter extends from the inferior margin of the pubic symphysis and transects the line drawn between the ischial spines. Both the transverse (interspinous) and the anteroposterior diameters can be assessed clinically, and the interspinous diameter is the narrowest space in the pelvis (10 cm). The ischial spines should be palpated to see if they are prominent and to make an estimate of the interspinous diameter (Fig. 6.11B).

Outlet of the pelvis

The outlet of the pelvis consists of two triangular planes. Anteriorly, the triangle is bounded by the area under the pubic arch, and this should normally subtend at an angle of 90 degrees. The transverse diameter is the distance between the ischial tuberosities, i.e. the intertuberous diameter, which is normally not less than 11 cm. The posterior triangle is formed anteriorly by the intertuberous diameter and posterolaterally by the tip of the sacrum and the sacrosciatic ligaments.

Clinically, the intertuberous diameter can be assessed by placing the knuckles of the clenched fist between the ischial tuberosities. The subpubic angle can be assessed by placing the index fingers of both hands along the inferior pubic rami or by inserting two fingers of the examining hand under the pubic arch.

Obstetric examination at subsequent routine visits

At all subsequent antenatal visits, the blood pressure should be recorded and the urine tested for protein and glucose. It is good practice to record maternal weight at each visit, especially in clinical settings where recourse to ultrasound scan for assessment of fetal growth is not freely available. Maternal weight should increase by an average of approximately 0.5 kg/week after the eighteenth week of gestation.

Rapid and excessive weight gain is nearly always associated with excessive fluid retention, and static weight or weight loss may indicate the failure of normal fetal growth. Excessive weight gain is often associated with signs of oedema, and this is most readily apparent in the face, the hands (where it may become difficult to remove rings), on the anterior abdominal wall and over the lower legs and ankles. 'Non-dependent' oedema over the sacral pad is rare in pregnancy and, if present, causes such as pre-eclampsia should be excluded.

Abdominal palpation

Palpation of the uterine fundus

The estimation of gestational age is the first step in examination of the abdomen in the pregnant woman. Several methods are employed to assess the size of the fetus.

The uterus first becomes palpable above the symphysis pubis at 12 weeks' gestation, and by 24 weeks' gestation it reaches the level of the umbilicus. At 36 weeks' gestation, the uterine fundus is palpable at the level of the xiphisternum and then tends to remain at this level until term or to fall slightly as the presenting part enters the pelvic brim.

All methods of clinical assessment of gestational age are subject to considerable inaccuracies, particularly in the early assessment related to the position of the umbilicus, and the fundal height will be affected by the presence of multiple fetuses, excessive amniotic fluid or, at the other extreme, the presence of a small fetus or oligohydramnios.

Measurement of symphysial–fundal height

Direct measurement of the girth, or the symphysial–fundal height, provides a more reliable method of assessing fetal growth and gestational age.

Using two standard deviations from the mean, it is possible to describe the tenth and ninetieth centile values. The sensitivity of this method for the detection of small for gestational age babies varies from 20% to 70% in different studies. Serial measurements by the same person plotted on customized growth charts are more likely to detect growth-restricted babies. The accuracy is considerably reduced as a random observation after 36 weeks' gestation. The predictive value is also lower for large-for-dates infants. However, the technique is simple and easily applicable and is particularly useful where other, more precise techniques are not available.

Measurement of symphysial–fundal height ABC

The ulnar border of the left hand is placed on the uterine fundus. The distance between the uterine fundus and the top of the pubic symphysis is measured in centimetres. To minimize observer bias, the distance is measured from the fundus to the superior edge of the symphysis pubis with the side of the tape measure with the centimetre measures facing downwards. The tape measure is then turned over to show the distance in centimetres. The mean fundal height measures approximately 20 cm at 20 weeks and increases by 1 cm/week so that at 36 weeks the fundal height will be 36 cm (Fig 6.12).

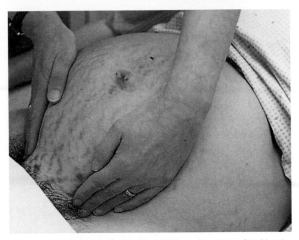

Fig. 6.13 Palpation of the presenting part and the fetal back.

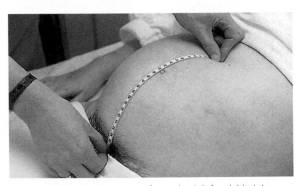

Fig. 6.12 Measurement of symphysial–fundal height.

Measurement of abdominal girth

Measurement of girth provides another method of assessment. The measurement of girth is made at the level of the maternal umbilicus. Assuming that the average non-pregnant girth is 60 cm, no significant increase will occur until 24 weeks' gestation. Thereafter the girth should increase by 2.5 cm weekly so that at full term the girth will be 100 cm.

If the non-pregnant girth is greater or smaller than 60 cm, then an appropriate allowance must be made. Thus, a woman with a 65-cm girth would have a measurement of 95 cm at 36 weeks' gestation.

Palpation of fetal parts

Fetal parts are not usually palpable before 24 weeks' gestation. When palpating the fetus, it must be remembered that the presence of amniotic fluid necessitates the use of 'dipping' movements with flexion of the fingers at the metacarpophalangeal joints. The purpose of palpation is to

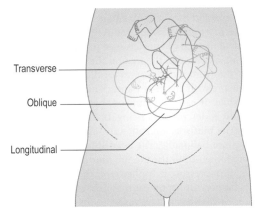

Transverse

Oblique

Longitudinal

Fig. 6.14 Fetal lie describes the relationship of the long axis of the fetus to the long axis of the uterus.

describe the relationship of the fetus to the maternal trunk and pelvis (Fig. 6.13).

Lie

The term *lie* describes the relationship of the long axis of the fetus to the long axis of the uterus (Fig. 6.14). Facing the feet of the mother, the examiner's left hand is placed along the left side of the maternal abdomen and the right hand on the right lateral aspect of the uterus. Systematic palpation towards the midline with the left and then the right hand will reveal either the firm resistance of the fetal back or the irregular features of the fetal limbs.

If the lie is *longitudinal*, the head or breech will be palpable over or in the pelvic inlet. If the lie is *oblique*, the long axis of the fetus lies at an angle of 45 degrees to the long axis

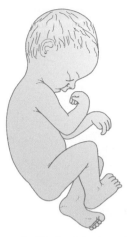

Fig. 6.15 The normal attitude of the fetus is one of flexion.

Table 6.3 Diameters of presentation		
Presenting part	Diameter	Size (cm)
Vertex	Suboccipitobregmatic	9.5
Brow	Verticomental	13.5
Face	Submentobregmatic	9.5
Deflexed vertex	Occipitofrontal	11.7

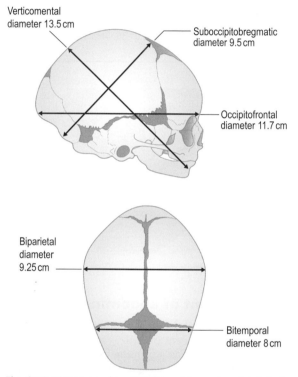

Fig. 6.16 Diameters of presentation of the mature fetal skull.

of the uterus and the presenting part will be palpable in the iliac fossa. In a *transverse* lie, the fetus lies at right angles to the mother and the poles of the fetus are palpable in the flanks.

Having ascertained the lie and the location of the fetal back, it is now important to feel for the head and breech by firm pressure with alternate hands. The head is hard, round and discrete. It can be 'bounced' between the examining hands and is described as being 'ballotable' in earlier gestations. The buttocks are softer and more diffuse, and the breech is not ballotable. The head should be sought in the lower abdomen or in the uterine fundus. Facing the mother's feet, firm pressure is applied over the presenting part. If the head is presenting, note is made as to whether it is easily palpable or whether it is necessary to apply deep pressure.

The normal attitude of the fetus is one of flexion (Fig. 6.15), but on occasions, as with the 'flying fetus', it may exhibit an attitude of extension.

Presentation

In a longitudinal lie, the presenting part may be the head (*cephalic*) or the breech (*podalic*). In a transverse lie, the presenting part is the shoulder.

Depending on the degree of flexion or deflexion, various parts of the head will present to the pelvic inlet. Where the head is well flexed, the presentation is the *vertex*, i.e. the area that lies between the anterior and posterior fontanelles anteroposteriorly and biparietal eminences laterally. If the head is completely extended, the face presents to the pelvic inlet (*face presentation*), and if it lies between these two attitudes, the brow presents (*brow presentation*). The brow is the area between the base of the nose and the anterior fontanelle. The diameter of presentation for the vertex is the suboccipitobregmatic diameter (Table 6.3, Fig. 6.16). If

the head is deflexed, the occipitofrontal diameter presents. With a brow presentation, the verticomental diameter presents to the pelvic inlet. Presentation and position can be accurately determined only by vaginal examination when the cervix has dilated and the suture lines and fontanelles can be palpated. This situation only really pertains when the mother is well established in labour.

Position

The position of the fetus is a description of the relationship of the denominator of the presenting part to the inlet of the maternal pelvis. It must not be confused with the presentation. It provides a further description of the

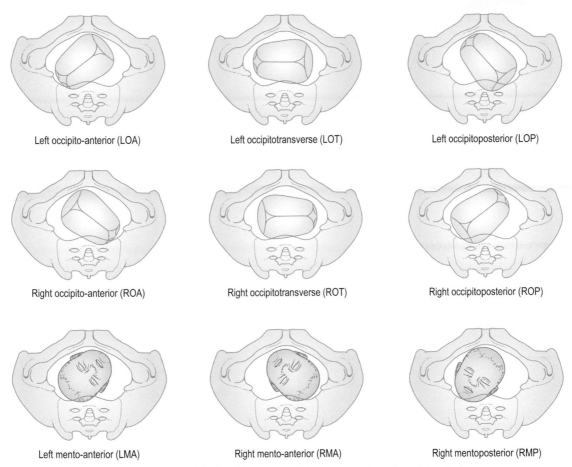

Left occipito-anterior (LOA)　　Left occipitotransverse (LOT)　　Left occipitoposterior (LOP)

Right occipito-anterior (ROA)　　Right occipitotransverse (ROT)　　Right occipitoposterior (ROP)

Left mento-anterior (LMA)　　Right mento-anterior (RMA)　　Right mentoposterior (RMP)

Fig. 6.17 Positions of the head in vertex and face presentations viewed from below.

relationship of the presenting part to the maternal pelvis and is of particular importance during parturition. The denominators for the various presentations are as follows:

Presentation	Denominator
Vertex	Occiput
Face	Chin (mentum)
Breech	Sacrum
Shoulder	Acromion

Thus, in a vertex presentation, six different positions are described (Fig. 6.17).

Viewed from below the pelvis, these include the right and left occipitotransverse positions as well as left and right anterior and posterior positions. Except in the advanced second stage, it is very rare for the head to be identified in a direct anterior or posterior position.

With a face presentation, the prefix *mento-* is included, and with a breech presentation the prefix is *sacro-*. No such description is given to a brow presentation, as there is no defined peripheral prominence to define as denominator. There is no mechanism of vaginal delivery in a brow presentation unless it is corrected.

The position can be determined from abdominal palpation by palpating the anterior shoulder of the fetus. If this is near the midline and easily palpable, the position is anterior. If it is not easily palpable and the limbs are prominent, the position is probably posterior.

However, the position of the presenting part can be most accurately determined by palpating the suture lines and fontanelles, or the breech presentation through the dilated cervix once labour has started.

The degree of flexion of the head can also be determined. On abdominal palpation, a deflexed or extended head tends to feel large, and the nuchal groove between the occiput and the fetal back is easily identified.

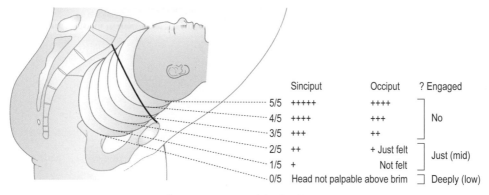

		Sinciput	Occiput	? Engaged
	5/5	+++++	++++	No
	4/5	++++	+++	
	3/5	+++	++	
	2/5	++	+ Just felt	Just (mid)
	1/5	+	Not felt	
	0/5	Head not palpable above brim		Deeply (low)

Fig. 6.18 Stations of the fetal head.

Station and engagement

The station of the head is described in fifths above the pelvic brim (Fig. 6.18). The head is *engage*d when the greatest transverse diameter (the biparietal diameter) has passed through the inlet of the true pelvis. The head that is engaged is usually fixed and only two-fifths palpable. It is usually difficult to feel abdominally.

> ❗ A small head may still be mobile even though it is engaged. A large head may be fixed in the pelvic brim and yet not be engaged. As a general rule, a head that is easily palpable abdominally is not engaged, whereas a head that is presenting and is deeply engaged is difficult to palpate.
>
> Where it is difficult to locate the head, this may either be because the head is under the maternal rib cage, as with a breech presentation, or because it is deeply engaged with 0/5'th of the head palpable or a rare case of anencephaly.
>
> Under these circumstances, a vaginal examination should be performed, as the leading part of the engaged head will be palpable at the level of the ischial spines.

Auscultation

Auscultation of the fetal heart rate is a routine part of the obstetric examination. It is now standard practice to use a

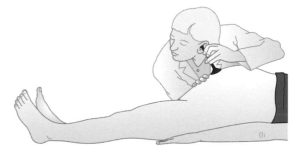

Fig. 6.19 Auscultation of the fetal heart.

hand-held Doppler ultrasound device that will produce an electronic signal to enable the heartbeat to be recognized and counted. If the transducer of an electronic fetal monitor is used, the fetal heart sounds should be confirmed with a Pinard fetal stethoscope (Fig. 6.19). The fetal heart sounds are best heard in late pregnancy below the level of the umbilicus over the anterior fetal shoulder (approximately halfway between the umbilicus and the anterosuperior iliac spine) or in the midline where there is a posterior position. With a breech presentation, the sound is best heard at the level of the umbilicus. The rate and rhythm of the heartbeat should be recorded.

Essential information

Maternal demographics

- Age, height and weight (BMI)
- Socioeconomic status, support at home
- History of smoking, substance misuse and alcohol-related or domestic violence
- Previous history of depression or attempted suicides
- Involvement with social care services

Obstetric history: present pregnancy

- Menstrual history (date of LMP, length and regularity of menstrual cycle, use of hormonal contraception prior to conception)
- Establish EDD using Naegele's rule (EDD = subtract 3 months/add 7 days to LMP or add 9 months and 7 days to LMP)

Essential information—cont'd

- Calculate the period of amenorrhoea from LMP to calculate the gestational age

Enquire about common symptoms associated with pregnancy

- Nausea and vomiting, frequency of micturition, excessive lassitude, breast tenderness
- Onset (quickening) and frequency of fetal movements

Enquire about symptoms that may be associated with abnormal pregnancy

- Painful swelling of feet or redness (DVT)
- Headaches, visual disturbances, epigastric pain or reduced urine output (pre-eclampsia)
- Vaginal bleeding (antepartum haemorrhage)
- Leakage of fluid (pre-labour rupture of membranes)

Previous obstetric history

- Previous pregnancy losses (miscarriages, ectopic pregnancies and terminations)
- Previous viable pregnancies, i.e. parity
- Stillbirths or neonatal deaths
- Method of delivery (spontaneous vaginal, assisted vaginal, failed assisted vaginal and abdominal)
- Gestational age, birth weight and sex of infants
- Previous antenatal or postnatal complications

Previous medical history

- Diabetes mellitus (gestational, insulin dependent, non-insulin dependent), cardiac disease, hypertension, renal disease, infectious disease such as HIV or hepatitis B or C

- DVT or pulmonary embolism
- Psychiatric illness

Examination

- General examination (pallor, cyanosis, icterus, teeth and nail beds) and systemic examination (cardiovascular system (CVS), respiratory system (RS), abdominal)
- Systolic flow murmurs are common; others would need full cardiological examination and investigations
- Examine breasts and nipples if clinically indicated

Speculum examination

- To exclude local causes of antepartum bleeding (cervical polyps, growths) and pre-labour rupture of membranes (based on the history)

Vaginal examination

- Clinical pelvimetry and to assess cervical dilatation and descent of the presenting part (to assess progress of labour)

Obstetric palpation

- Inspection (shape of the abdomen, linea nigra, striae gravidarum, surgical scars and fetal movements)
- Palpation (measure symphysial–fundal height, feel for presenting part, determine lie, position and engagement of the presenting part, amniotic fluid volume and estimated fetal weight)
- Auscultation of fetal heart

Chapter | 7 |

Normal pregnancy and antenatal care

Shaylee Iles

LEARNING OUTCOMES

After studying this chapter you should be able to:

Knowledge criteria

- Describe the aims and patterns of routine antenatal care
- List the key elements of pre-conceptual care
- Contrast the changing demographics of pregnancy
- Discuss the significance of previous obstetric history on planning antenatal care
- List the routine investigations used in antenatal care, including screening for fetal abnormality
- Discuss the risks of substance misuse in pregnancy
- Discuss the role of anti-D immunoprophylaxis

Clinical competencies

- Carry out a routine antenatal booking visit
- Provide antenatal education on general lifestyle advice in pregnancy

Professional skills and attitudes

- Consider the importance of the interaction between social and cultural factors and pregnancy
- Consider principles of safe prescribing in pregnancy

Aims and patterns of routine antenatal care

The concept that the reproductive outcomes of a woman might be improved by antenatal supervision is surprisingly recent and was first introduced in Edinburgh in 1911. In many societies, particularly in isolated and low-resource settings, antenatal care either is not available or, for social or religious reasons, is not used when it is available. Unfortunately, it is often least available in those communities where the need is greatest and where antenatal disorders, particularly those linked to malnutrition or over-nutrition, are most common.

The basic assumption is that pregnancy and birth are normal physiological events in which complications may, and do, arise at any stage. Antenatal care aims to detect, prevent or treat these adverse outcomes in order to ensure optimal health of the mother and fetus throughout pregnancy and in the puerperium. It also aims to prepare parents for the transition to parenting and care of the infant.

The ways by which these objectives are achieved will vary according to the initial health and history of the mother and are a combination of screening tests, educational and emotional support and monitoring of fetal growth and maternal health throughout the pregnancy.

In modern antenatal care, the timing of visits, particularly in the first 28 weeks of pregnancy, is closely geared to attendance for screening tests. In uncomplicated pregnancy, a reduction in the number of visits compared to the original suggested schedule of 4 weekly until 28 weeks, 2 weekly until 36 weeks and weekly thereafter has not been shown to adversely affect maternal or perinatal outcome, although maternal satisfaction may be reduced.

Antenatal care is provided through a variety of different mechanisms and may be provided by general practitioners, midwives and obstetricians, often in a pattern of shared care. Pregnancies that are considered to be high risk should receive a high proportion of their care by obstetricians or specialists in fetomaternal medicine. Risk stratification should be assessed at the earliest antenatal visits and care planned accordingly. Guidelines for consultation and referral, such as those produced by the Australian College of Midwives or the National Institute for Health and Clinical Excellence (NICE), can be a useful tool to assess risk and determine the most suitable model of care. Pregnancy risk and the most suitable care provider may alter during the course of pregnancy.

Pre-conceptual care and vitamin supplementation

Ideally, all women would present prior to conception to allow their health care professional to provide them with pre-pregnancy care and counselling. This role is often best provided by the woman's usual general practitioner. This appointment allows for an opportunity to undertake screening tests and provide advice regarding conception and early pregnancy care. Unfortunately, despite widely available contraception, approximately half of all conceptions are not planned.

Essential components of pre-conceptual care include the assessment of the need for immunization for rubella, varicella and pertussis. If the history of past vaccination or infection is uncertain, serology may be required. If serology is negative or immunization is due, this can then be provided. As these vaccines are live attenuated viral vaccines, it is recommended that the woman use adequate contraception to defer conception for 28 days following administration. Administration of the influenza vaccine on a seasonal basis to women who are intending to be or who are pregnant is also recommended due to the increased incidence of serious morbidity associated with influenza infection in pregnancy. This visit is also an ideal opportunity to undertake routine cervical cancer screening if due.

Dietary and vitamin supplementation advice should also be given at this time. It is recommended that all women take a folic acid supplement (400–500 µg daily) for at least 1 month prior to conception and the first 3 months of pregnancy as an effective means of reducing the incidence of neural tube defects. Certain risk groups may be recommended to take a higher dose (5 mg daily), such as those on anti-epileptic agents, obese women, diabetic women or women with a past history of neural tube defects. Iodine supplementation of 150 µg per day is also recommended in countries or regions where there is a dietary deficiency of iodine to aid in the development of the fetal brain. Consideration of screening for vitamin D deficiency in at-risk populations (including those with darker skin tones or who are always covered while outside) can be considered, with supplementation given if required.

Maternal medical conditions, including medications, can be reviewed and optimized at this time. This provides an opportunity to discuss the impact of pregnancy on the medical condition, as well as the impact of the medical condition on pregnancy. Medication may need to be altered or doses reduced where appropriate. Referral to specialist physician colleagues for treatment optimization may be appropriate.

Optimization of pre-conceptional health with advice on a nutritious diet and regular moderate exercise should also be provided at this time. Exploration and discussion around the use of licit and illicit substances should also be explored.

Changing demographics of pregnancy

Maternal age is an important determinant of outcome in obstetric services, with increased risk being associated with both extremes of maternal age. The median age of women giving birth in developed countries has continued to rise and currently sits at just over 30 years. Fertility rates for women over 40 have trebled since 1990 and now exceed the fertility rate for women under 20 years. Fertility in women under 25 (including amongst adolescent women) is now at the lowest rate since recording began in the UK in 1938. The tendency for women to delay childbearing until later in life is seen consistently across developed countries. The reasons for this are complex and due to a number of social, economic and educational factors. Fertility rates are highest in the 30–34 years age group.

Use of assisted reproductive technologies (ARTs) has increased along with the rise in median birthing age. Approximately 3.6% of babies born are conceptions assisted by ART in Australia and the UK. In addition, rates of multiple pregnancies have plateaued, currently around 1.6% of all mothers. The previous rapidly rising rates were largely due to the increases in ART and increasing maternal age. However, rates of multiples in ART pregnancy are declining due to the increased use of single-embryo transfer. The majority of multiple pregnancies remain due to spontaneous conceptions.

The absolute number of babies born to each woman continues to be low, with 75% of mothers giving birth to their first or second baby. The median age of first-time mothers also continues to rise and is currently around 28 years.

Women are active participants in antenatal care, with over 98% having at least one antenatal visit and 92% having five or more visits. Pre-term birth occurs in around 8.7% of all pregnancies, with more than 80% occurring between 32 and 36 weeks.

Rates of caesarean section as a proportion of births increase with increasing maternal age and with increasing body mass index (BMI).

The booking visit

The details of antenatal history and routine clinical examination are discussed in the preceding chapter. However, certain observations should be obtained at the first visit and it is preferable that these observations be made within the first 10 weeks of pregnancy. The measurement of maternal height and weight is important and has value in prediction of pregnancy outcomes. Women with a low BMI (less than 20, where BMI is estimated as weight (kg) divided by height (m^2)) are at an increased risk of fetal growth restriction and perinatal mortality. Women with a high BMI are recognized as being at increased antenatal, intrapartum and postnatal risk, with the risks beginning to rise from a BMI of 30.

The initial measurement of blood pressure should be taken as early as possible to determine the presence of pre-existing hypertension or as a reference point for hypertension detected at later gestations.

Consideration of past obstetric history, including mode of delivery

A record should be made of all previous pregnancies, including previous miscarriages and terminations, and the duration of gestation in each pregnancy. In particular, it is important to note any previous antenatal complications, details of onset of labour, the duration of labour, the presentation and the method of delivery and the birth weight and gender of each infant. The mode of delivery (spontaneous, assisted or caesarean section) has implications for the current birth and must be explored. Previous operation records should be sought if relevant to aid in appropriate counselling for this pregnancy.

The condition of each infant at birth and the need for care in a special care baby unit should be noted.

Complications of the puerperium, such as postpartum haemorrhage, extensive perineal trauma or wound breakdown, infections of the genital tract, deep vein thrombosis or difficulties with breast-feeding, may all be relevant to the current pregnancy.

Recommended routine screening tests

Beginning at the first visit, a number of screening tests are recommended. Some will be repeated later in the pregnancy. The omission of offering these tests will generally now be considered to be evidence of substandard practice, so they have medicolegal importance as well as clinical relevance. National evidence-based guidelines are available to guide the health care practitioner.

Haematological investigations
Full blood count

Anaemia is a common disorder in pregnancy and in most communities will be due to iron deficiency, either because of the depletion of iron stores or because of reduced iron intake. The majority of cases of pathological anaemia in pregnancy are due to iron deficiency. However, it may also less commonly be due to folate or vitamin B_{12} deficiency, haemoglobinopathies (sickle cell or thalassemia) or various parasitic infections.

A full blood count should be performed at the first visit and repeated at 28 and 34–36 weeks' gestation. Women who have deficient iron stores should be given oral supplements of iron starting early in pregnancy. Those women unable to tolerate oral iron supplements should be considered for iron infusion. Screening for haemoglobinopathies should be routinely offered to those racial groups where conditions such as thalassaemia and sickle cell disease are common.

Blood group and antibodies

Blood group should be determined in all pregnant women, and screening for red cell antibodies should be undertaken early in pregnancy. In Rhesus (Rh)-negative women, screening for Rh antibodies should be performed at the first visit (preferably in the first trimester) and then repeated at 28 weeks' gestation. ABO antibodies may also cause problems in the fetus and newborn, but no method is available to counter this problem.

The use of anti-D immunoglobulin

Around 15% of Caucasian women will be Rh negative and be at risk of developing anti-D antibodies during or immediately following pregnancy. The formation of anti-D antibodies may pose a risk to the wellbeing and even survival of a subsequent fetus due to the pre-formed antibodies crossing the placenta and attacking the red blood cells of an Rh-positive fetus. The effects on the fetus and newborn can be devastating and include fetal anaemia, hydrops, neonatal anaemia, jaundice, kernicterus or fetal death in utero. There is very strong evidence dating from the 1960s that postpartum administration of anti-D immunoglobulin (anti-D Ig) can dramatically reduce the incidence of this complication.

Until the past few years, anti-D Ig was given only to women with a sensitizing event in pregnancy or postnatally to women delivered of an Rh-positive infant. Given within 72 hours of birth, this dose reduces the risk of Rh isoimmunization to around 1.5%. Quantitation of the degree of fetomaternal haemorrhage and the need for further doses should be undertaken by flow cytometry (where available) or the Kleihauer-Betke test prior to administration of the first dose.

Sensitizing events include normal delivery, miscarriage, termination of pregnancy, ectopic pregnancy, invasive prenatal diagnosis, abdominal trauma, antepartum haemorrhage or external cephalic version. Sensitization

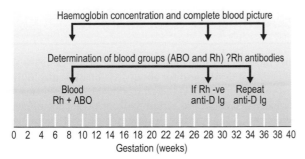

Fig. 7.1 Schedules for routine tests of haemoglobin estimation and detection and administration of Rh antibodies. *Ig*, Immunoglobulin; *Rh*, Rhesus.

during pregnancy can also occur without the woman being aware of such an event. Hence, now that anti-D Ig is readily available, it has become standard practice to give anti-D Ig prophylaxis at 28 and 34 weeks' gestation (Fig. 7.1). This will prevent maternal immunization by an Rh-positive fetus in all but 0.2% of Rh-negative women, in whom the infusion of cells from the fetus overwhelms the dose of antibody administered. This is in addition to the earlier noted indications.

Infection screening

Rubella

All girls are offered rubella vaccination between the ages of 11 and 14 years, often through a school-based vaccination programme. In pregnancy, around 2.5% of women in the Australian population are found to be seronegative. A greater proportion are found to have low levels of immunity. Around 50% of non-immune women will have been previously vaccinated. All seronegative and low-level seropositive women should be offered immunization in the immediate puerperium. Vaccination is performed with a live attenuated rubella virus vaccine and involves a single dose injected subcutaneously. Although there is no evidence to suggest any significant increase in abnormality rate in the babies in women who have conceived immediately before or following rubella vaccination, it is generally recommended that pregnancy be avoided for 1 month after vaccination. Non-immune women should be advised to avoid contact with infected individuals. Any clinically suspected infection should be investigated with paired sera, preferably with the original sample taken at the time of booking.

Syphilis

Routine screening for syphilis is recommended practice. Although relatively rare, the condition is treatable and has major neonatal sequelae if left untreated. Increasing rates

in some jurisdictions mean that testing at 28 and 36 weeks' gestation may also be recommended. A number of non-specific and specific tests exist, and advice should be sought from the local pathology laboratory as to availability.

Hepatitis

Universal screening for hepatitis B and C in pregnancy is recommended. Hepatitis B vaccination, as well as the administration of hepatitis B immunoglobulin (HBIG), is recommended for at-risk infants, and hepatitis B vaccination for all infants. Completion of the full vaccination schedule protects at-risk infants from hepatitis B infection in 90% of cases. Newer agents available to treat hepatitis C infection mean detection of this condition is an important public health measure. (see the chapter 9 on maternal medical conditions).

Human immunodeficiency virus

The basis of tests for the detection of HIV is the detection of HIV antibodies. A positive test should always be followed up with an HIV RNA test to determine the disease load and monitor treatment efficacy.

Seropositive mothers always have seropositive babies due to transplacental transmission of antibodies, but this may not indicate active infection in the baby. However, up to 45% of babies will have contracted HIV if active management programmes are not used. As treatment is highly effective in reducing transmission rates to less than 2%, there is a strong case for routine screening of all women. These strategies include caesarean section with any detectable viral load, avoidance of breast-feeding and antiretroviral therapy in both the antenatal and intrapartum period as well as for the newborn. (see the chapter 9 on maternal medical conditions).

Group B *Streptococcus*

Group B *Streptococcus* (GBS) is a gram-positive bacterium that is a common commensal carried in the gastrointestinal tract. It can be cultured from the vagina in up to 25% of women in pregnancy and may also be a cause of urinary tract infection. During vaginal delivery, there is a risk of transmission to the neonate. This risk is increased in pre-term delivery and prolonged rupture of membranes. Neonatal infection occurs in 1–2 per 1000 births and can result in overwhelming sepsis associated with significant morbidity and mortality. Ninety percent of infections present within the first days of life, but late presentations at up to 3 months of age can occur.

The organism can be detected on vaginal and rectal swabs and the rate of vertical transmission reduced by the use of intrapartum antibiotic treatment with intravenous penicillin. Screening for GBS using a low vaginal and peri-anal swab taken between 34 and 36 weeks is recommended by many centres but is not universal practice.

Urinary tract infection

Screening for asymptomatic bacteriuria is of proven benefit. The presence of pathogenic organisms in excess of 10,000 organisms/mL indicates significant bacteriuria. The incidence of ascending urinary tract infection, including acute pyelonephritis, is increased in pregnancy and is associated with increased pregnancy loss and pre-term birth, as well as maternal morbidity. Early treatment of asymptomatic bacteriuria reduces the incidence of such infections and thus improves maternal health.

Gestational diabetes mellitus

Gestational diabetes mellitus (GDM) is associated with an increased incidence of intrauterine fetal death, as well as intrapartum and neonatal complications. Screening programmes follow one of two pathways:

- Selection by history (Australasian Diabetes in Pregnancy Criteria: ADIPS):
  - Previous hyperglycaemia in pregnancy
  - Previously elevated blood glucose level
  - Ethnicity: Asian, Indian, Aboriginal, Torres Strait Islander, Pacific Islander, Maori, Middle Eastern, non-white African
  - Family history of diabetes mellitus (DM) (first-degree relative with DM or sister with GDM)
  - Previous macrosomic infant with a birth weight in excess of 4.5 kg or >90th centile
  - Obesity (pre-pregnancy BMI >30)
  - Polycystic ovarian syndrome (PCOS)
  - Maternal age >40 years
  - Medications: corticosteroids, anti-psychotics

  Under these circumstances, a full glucose tolerance test (GTT) should be performed using either a 75-g or 100-g loading dose of glucose. The test should be performed at the booking visit and again at 28 weeks' gestation unless diagnosed prior.

  Or

- Universal screening: The screening of all women at 26–28 weeks' gestation will identify more women with impaired glucose tolerance or diabetes than those screened by risk factors alone. The full GTT is done with criteria for diagnosis as outlined by the International Association of Diabetes in Pregnancy Study Groups (IADPSG).

Most jurisdictions who choose to only screen at-risk populations do so because of the practical difficulties and costs of screening the whole population, particularly in large maternity hospitals.

Screening for fetal anomaly

Structural fetal anomalies account for some 20–25% of all perinatal deaths and for about 15% of all deaths in the first year of life. There is therefore a strong case to be made for early detection and termination of pregnancy offered where this is appropriate. Common structural anomalies include those of the cardiac, craniospinal, renal and gastro-intestinal systems.

These anomalies are generally detectable by ultrasound scanning, and this will be discussed in the chapter on congenital abnormalities. This is most commonly done at the 18–22-week fetal anomaly ultrasound.

Aneuploidy and early structural assessment

Nuchal translucency and biochemical screening

The offer of screening for trisomy 21 (Down's syndrome) has become routine in most antenatal services. The logical consequence of such a programme is to offer invasive testing and then termination of pregnancy where there is evidence of aneuploidy. Although the value of the test is reduced if termination is not an option, a positive result can help parents prepare for the birth of an additional-needs child. Screening is by the use of biochemical and ultrasound tests. It is important that women understand that these are screening tests and therefore have their limitations. They will not detect every case, and high-risk results do not necessarily mean that the baby is affected. Despite the increased incidence of Down's syndrome in mothers over 35 years, screening on the basis of age alone will not detect most affected fetuses, and it is recommended to offer screening to all women. The major modality for screening for Down's syndrome is the use of ultrasound measurement of nuchal translucency, a measurement of fluid behind the fetal neck (see Chapter 10, Fig. 10.7). This is combined with maternal age and the results of biochemical tests to provide a risk for this fetus of trisomy 21, 13 and 18 (see Chapter 10). The sensitivity of this test for the detection of trisomy 21 is 95%.

Non-invasive prenatal testing (NIPT)

Since 2011, aneuploidy screening has become available on maternal blood, which detects the presence of fetal cell-free DNA. Able to be done from 10 weeks' gestation to allow for an adequate fetal fraction in the sample, the sensitivity for detection of trisomy 21 is over 99%, with marginally lower rates for trisomy 18 and 13. Sex chromosome identification allowing for gender determination is also reported. It is important to note that this is also a screening test, and confirmatory testing with invasive tests (such as chorionic villus sampling or amniocentesis) is required before clinical decision-making can occur. In most jurisdictions this is currently available as a privately funded test; however, it is anticipated that over the next few years, the cost–benefit analysis will result in governments deciding to fund this test as part of routine antenatal investigation. Other commercial applications of this test currently available include testing for other common genetic concerns such as cystic fibrosis (CF), spinal muscular atrophy (SMA) and fragile X. Full screening for trisomy of all chromosomes is also available. This is an area of rapid change, and it is anticipated that many other genetic conditions will be able to be tested with this technology over the short to medium term.

It is important to note that NIPT does not replace the structural assessment that is done with the ultrasound component of the nuchal translucency assessment, and hence if NIPT is chosen for aneuploidy screening, an early structural ultrasound (without measurement of the nuchal translucency) should also be recommended. This allows for multiple gestations and major structural malformations to be detected.

Schedules of routine antenatal care

Subsequent visits

Although the pattern of antenatal care will vary with circumstances and with the normality or otherwise of the pregnancy, a general pattern of visits will partly revolve around the demands of the screening procedures and the obstetric and medical history of the mother. The measurement of blood pressure is performed at all visits, and the measurement of symphysis/fundal height should be recorded, accepting that this observation has a limited capacity to detect fetal growth restriction. Serial ultrasound measurements would have a greater detection rate if performed at every visit, but this is not practicable or necessary for women who are not considered to be at high risk. A suggested regime for antenatal visits is listed in Table 7.1.

In general, where pregnancies have been accurately dated by early ultrasound so that the gestational age is certain, induction of labour after 41 weeks reduces the incidence of complications of placental insufficiency, such as meconium staining, intrapartum hypoxia and fetal compromise, and the risk of fetal and neonatal death. Rates of macrosomia

Table 7.1 Visits for antenatal care

8–12 weeks	Initial visit, confirmation of pregnancy, search for risk factors in maternal history. Cervical screening where indicated, advice on general health, smoking and diet. Discuss and organize screening procedures. Check maternal weight and give advice on recommended folic acid and iodine supplements. Dating scan if uncertainty exists.
11–14 weeks	Screening for trisomies with ± nuchal translucency scan and blood tests or NIPT and structural ultrasound if requested. Confirm booking arrangements. Offer dietary supplements of iron if any evidence of anaemia.
16 weeks	Check all blood results. Offer routine ultrasound anomaly scan to be performed between 18 and 20 weeks' gestation
20 weeks	Check ultrasound result, BP, fundal height.
24 weeks	BP, fundal height, fetal activity.
28 weeks	BP, fundal height, fetal activity, full blood count and antibody screen. Administer anti-D if Rh negative. Glucose tolerance test.
32 weeks	BP, fundal height, fetal activity and fetal growth scan where pattern of fetal growth is in doubt or low-lying placenta on anomaly scan
34 weeks	BP, fundal height, fetal activity, also second dose of anti-D for Rh-negative women, full blood count
36 weeks	BP, fundal height, fetal activity, group B *Streptococcus* vaginal and perianal swab determine presentation
38 weeks	BP, fundal height, fetal activity, maternal wellbeing
40 weeks	BP, fundal height, fetal activity, maternal wellbeing
41 weeks	BP, fundal height, fetal activity, assessment by vaginal examination as to cervical favourability, cardiotocograph, amniotic fluid index. Individualize care with regard to induction of labour and ongoing assessment.

BP, Blood pressure; *NIPT*, non-invasive prenatal testing.
Adapted from Kean L (2001) Routine antenatal management. Curr Obstet Gynaecol 11:63–69.

and major perineal trauma are also reduced. Meta-analysis suggests that there is reduction in caesarean deliveries with induction of labour after 41 weeks; however, instrumental births and intrapartum usage of analgesia are increased.

Antenatal education

An important and integral part of antenatal care is the education of the mother and her partner about pregnancy, childbirth and the care of the infant. This process should start before pregnancy as part of school education and should continue throughout pregnancy and the puerperium. There are various ways by which this can be achieved, but commonly, the needs are met by regular antenatal classes during the course of the pregnancy. It is preferable that those staff who are involved in general antenatal care and delivery be part of the team that provides intrapartum care to the woman so that the processes of care and education are seen as one entity (Table 7.2).

Table 7.2 General lifestyle advice in pregnancy	
Health behaviour	**Recommendation**
Nutrition	Eating the recommended number of daily servings of the five food groups and drinking plenty of water are important during pregnancy. Additional servings of the five food groups may contribute to healthy weight gain in women who are underweight, but these should be limited by women who are overweight or obese. Small to moderate amounts of caffeine are unlikely to harm the fetus.
Exercise	Low- to moderate-intensity physical activity during pregnancy has a range of benefits and is not associated with negative effects on the pregnancy or baby.
Smoking	Smoking and passive smoking can have negative effects on the pregnancy and the baby. Smoking cessation is strongly recommended.
Alcohol	Not drinking alcohol is the safest option for women who are pregnant.
Illicit substances	Illicit substances and non-medical use of medications (e.g. opioids) have negative effects on the pregnancy and the baby.

Adapted from Department of Health (2018) *Clinical Practice Guidelines: Pregnancy Care*. Canberra: Australian Government Department of Health, page 84.

Dietary advice

There can be no doubt about the importance of diet in pregnancy. At one extreme, gross malnutrition is known to result in intrauterine growth restriction, anaemia, prematurity and fetal malformation. Lesser degrees of malnutrition may also be associated with an increased incidence of fetal malformations, particularly neural tube defects, and it is therefore important to provide guidance on diet and to ensure that a diet of appropriate quality and quantity is maintained throughout pregnancy and the puerperium. However, in the developed world, the concerns of overnutrition and maternal obesity are much more frequently encountered. Of note, despite excessive caloric consumption, it is not uncommon for vitamin and mineral deficiencies to also be encountered in this population, largely due to choice of intake.

Clearly, there will be substantial variation in the nature of the diet depending on cultural factors and actual physical size, but general principles can be provided as advice to meet the needs of the mother and of the developing fetus.

Advice should be given early in pregnancy regarding *Listeria* risk and advice given to avoid high-risk foods such as soft cheeses, delicatessen meats, salad bars and soft-serve ice cream.

Energy intake

A total energy intake of 2000–2500 kcal/day is necessary during the last two trimesters of pregnancy because of the demands of both maternal and fetal metabolism. This requirement may increase to 3000 kcal in the puerperium in lactating women.

Protein

First-class protein is expensive in most countries, with some notable exceptions such as Argentina and Australia, and is therefore likely to be deficient in less developed nations. It is also likely to be deficient in the diet of those who choose to avoid meat and meat products. Animal protein is obtained from meat, poultry, fish, eggs and cheese. Vegetable protein occurs in nuts, lentils, beans and peas. An average of 60–80 g daily is desirable. Those women deriving their protein intake solely from vegetable sources are likely to need vitamin B_{12} supplementation. Iron-deficiency anaemia is also found more commonly in this group.

Fats

Fats provide an important component of a balanced diet. Essential fatty acids may play an important part in cellular growth and in preventing the development of hypertension during pregnancy. Fats are also an important source of energy and a source of fat-soluble vitamins, including vitamins A, D and K.

Animal fats are found in meat, eggs and dairy products and contain a high percentage of saturated fats. Vegetable fats, on the other hand, are important because they contain unsaturated fats such as linoleic and linolenic acids.

Carbohydrates

Carbohydrates are the primary source of energy for both mother and fetus and are therefore an essential dietary component during pregnancy. However, excessive carbohydrate consumption can result in excessive weight gain and fat accumulation, so a balanced dietary intake of carbohydrate is an essential. In particular, it should be remembered that there is a close correlation between maternal and fetal blood glucose levels and that glucose is the major source of energy for the fetus.

Minerals and vitamins

Other than folic acid and iodine, routine supplementation with iron and other vitamins should not be necessary during pregnancy. However, where there is evidence of dietary deficiency or in cases of multiple gestations, iron and vitamin supplements should be given from the first trimester onwards.

> Where deficiencies do arise, this is generally because of dietary choice rather than from economic pressures. This situation can be overcome by giving folic acid and pregnancy multivitamin supplements. In some urban environs, folate deficiency tends to be part of a pattern of malnutrition and should be anticipated in early pregnancy so that supplements of iron and folic acid can be given.

All women should be given advice at the booking visit regarding appropriate weight gain in pregnancy. Target weight gains depend on pre-pregnancy weight and make allowance for the weight of the fetus, amniotic fluid, placenta, uterus, blood volume and fat stores for breast-feeding.

Recommendations for ideal weight gain are found in Table 7.3.

Exercise in pregnancy

Pregnant women should be encouraged to undertake reasonable activity during pregnancy. This will be limited with advancing gestation by the physical restrictions imposed by the changes in abdominal size and by the balance restrictions imposed on the mother, but during early pregnancy there is no need to limit sporting activities beyond the

Table 7.3 U.S. Institute of Medicine (IOM) 2009 gestational weight gain targets

Pre-pregnancy BMI (kg/m²)	Recommended weight gain (kg)
<18.5	12.5–18.0
18.5–24.9	11.5–16
25.0–29.9	7.0–11.5
≥30.0	5.0–9.0

common-sense limits of avoiding excessive exertion and fatigue. There may be exceptions to this situation in women with a history of previous pregnancy losses. Swimming is a useful form of exercise, particularly in late pregnancy, when the water tends to support the enlarged maternal abdomen.

Substance use and misuse in pregnancy

Smoking

Smoking has an adverse effect on fetal growth and development and is therefore contraindicated in pregnancy. The mechanisms for these effects are as follows (Fig. 7.2):

- *The effect of carbon monoxide on the fetus.* Carbon monoxide has an affinity for haemoglobin 200 times greater than oxygen. Fresh air contains up to 0.5 ppm of carbon monoxide, but in cigarette smoke values as high as 60,000 ppm may be detected. Carbon monoxide shifts the oxygen dissociation curve to the left in both fetal and maternal haemoglobin. Maternal carbon monoxide saturation may rise to 8% in the mother and 7% in the fetus so that there is specific interference with oxygen transfer.
- *The effect of nicotine on the uteroplacental vasculature as a vasoconstrictor.* Animal studies on the effect of infusions of nicotine on cardiac output have shown that high-dose infusions produce a fall in cardiac output and uteroplacental blood flow. However, at levels up to five times greater than those seen in smokers, there are no measurable effects, and it is therefore unlikely that nicotine exerts any adverse effects by reducing uteroplacental blood flow.
- *The effect of smoking on placental structure.* Some changes are seen in the placental morphology. The trophoblastic basement membrane shows irregular thickening, and some of the fetal capillaries show reduced calibre. These changes are not consistent or gross and are not associated with any gross reduction in placental size. The morphological changes have not been demonstrated in those women subjected to passive smoking.

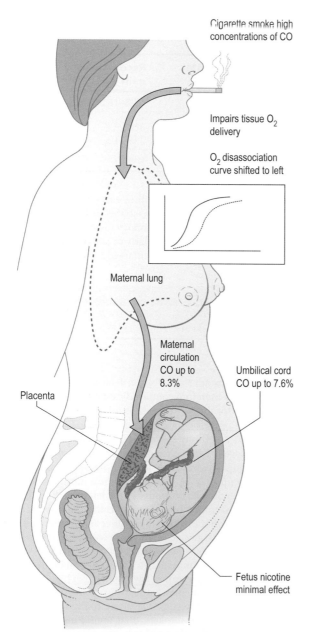

Fig. 7.2 The effects of smoking on the fetoplacental unit.

Women should be advised to stop smoking during pregnancy. The use of nicotine replacement therapy (patches) as a harm-minimization option for women who smoke and feel unable to quit can be considered.

> Paradoxically, there is a considerable volume of evidence to show that women who smoke in pregnancy have a substantially reduced chance of developing pre-eclampsia. However, if they do develop pre-eclampsia, there is a significantly increased risk of perinatal loss. ✔

Alcohol intake

Fetal alcohol syndrome (FAS) has been attributed to consumption of eight or more standard drinks per day. Features in the infant include growth restriction, various structural defects and, in particular, facial defects, multiple joint anomalies and cardiac defects. Women who drink alcohol at this rate often have concomitant vitamin and mineral deficiencies due to inadequate diet. Increasingly, there is awareness of fetal alcohol spectrum disorder (FASD), a range of neurodevelopmental and behavioural effects attributable to alcohol consumption in pregnancy in a dose-dependent manner. All women considering pregnancy, and during pregnancy, should be asked about consumption of alcohol and provided education on the potential for adverse effects on the fetus. Research is not clear as to what level of alcohol consumption is safe in pregnancy, so a recommendation to abstain from any consumption is the safest choice.

Illicit drug use

The common forms of illicit substance misuse that occur during pregnancy are from amphetamines, opioids, cocaine and marijuana. All of these drugs have adverse effects on both the mother and the fetus, including the adverse effects related to lifestyle and malnutrition.

Amphetamine use, especially crystal methamphetamine (Ice), has become the most significantly misused drug in pregnancy, paralleling increased use in wider society. Use in pregnancy is associated with an increased risk of miscarriage, pre-term birth, growth restriction, placental abruption, fetal death in utero and developmental anomalies. Referral to a drug dependency service for advice on cessation is recommended.

Opioid addiction is associated with an increased incidence of intrauterine growth restriction, perinatal death and pre-term labour. In addition to heroin, misuse of prescription opioids such as oxycodone and hydromorphone is causing increasing concern. Furthermore, many infants with intrauterine opioid exposure will suffer from neonatal withdrawal manifestations. The mother should be referred

- *The effect on perinatal mortality.* Smoking during pregnancy reduces the birth weight of the infant and reduces the crown–heel length. Perinatal mortality is increased as a direct effect of smoking, and this risk has been quantified at 20% for those women who smoke up to 20 cigarettes per day and 35% in excess of one packet per day.

to a drug dependence service for withdrawal of heroin and replacement with methadone or buprenorphine.

Cocaine usage may induce cardiac arrhythmias and central nervous system damage in mothers as well as placental abruption, fetal growth restriction and pre-term labour. Management of cocaine addiction is directed at withdrawing the drug.

Marijuana has no apparent adverse effect on pregnancy, although the active ingredient of 9-tetrahydrocannabinol has been shown to have teratogenic effects in animal studies. Consumption is usually associated with significant tobacco use, which has major detrimental effects as outlined earlier.

Coitus in pregnancy

There are no contraindications to coitus in normal pregnancies at any stage of gestation other than the physical difficulties imposed by changes in abdominal size. It is, however, sensible to avoid coitus where there is evidence of threatened miscarriage or a previous history of recurrent miscarriage. Because of the risk of introducing infection, it is also advisable to avoid coitus where there is evidence of pre-labour rupture of the membranes and where there is a history of antepartum haemorrhage. Women with a known placenta praevia are also advised to avoid intercourse.

Breast care

Breast-feeding should be encouraged in all women unless there are specific contraindications that would have adverse fetal or maternal consequences. Previous damage or surgery to the breasts or grossly inverted nipples may make breast-feeding difficult. There are also a small number of medications that are concentrated in breast milk and may be hazardous for the infant, in which case breast-feeding is contraindicated. In some maternal infections, such as HIV, breast-feeding is contraindicated. However, these circumstances are uncommon and, in most conditions, the mother should be advised of the benefits to both her child and herself of breast-feeding.

In the antenatal period, good personal hygiene, including breast care, should be encouraged. Colostrum may leak from the nipples, particularly in the third trimester, especially in multiparous women. The breasts should be supported with an appropriate maternity brassiere. Antenatal referral to a lactation consultant for women who have risk factors for potentially encountering difficulty with breast-feeding, such as previous difficulty or breast surgery, should be offered.

Social and cultural awareness

Pregnancy and childbirth form one part of the complexities of life for the women who present for antenatal care. Supportive and extensive discussion will enable health care practitioners to develop an understanding of the woman and the other aspects in her life, including social and cultural factors, which may have a profound impact on her pregnancy outcome. Different cultural beliefs and expectations, socioeconomic status and supports, competing life priorities and levels of education can all impact strongly on pregnancy outcome. Acknowledgement and respect of cultural diversity will assist in providing appropriate and timely antenatal and peripartum care to all women.

Safe prescribing in pregnancy

The use of prescription and over-the-counter medications, as well as complementary and alternative medications, is common. Some women will require ongoing treatment of pre-existing medical conditions, e.g. epilepsy or asthma. Some conditions may develop de novo in pregnancies that require therapy, e.g. gestational diabetes and thromboembolism. Simple analgesics, antipyretics, antihistamines and antiemetics are all commonly consumed. A discussion of the risks and benefits of individual medications is beyond the scope of this text. Extensive information is available in most drug formularies about the safety of categories of drugs in pregnancy and lactation. Reputable online resources such as www.motherisk.org are available around the clock and are often helpful. The safest course before prescribing in pregnancy is to always check. Many medications have been shown to have no adverse outcomes when used in pregnancy or lactation.

Essential Information

Basic aims of antenatal care

- To ensure optimal maternal health
- To detect and treat disorders to ensure a healthy mother and infant

Pre-conception care

- Immunization for rubella, varicella, pertussis and influenza as indicated
- Folic acid and iodine supplementation
- Optimization of maternal health

Changing demographics of pregnancy

- Increasing maternal age
- Increasing use of ART

Routine screening tests

- Haematological investigations to detect anaemia, and haemoglobinopathies in susceptible groups
- Blood group and antibodies; prevention of Rhesus disease

Infection screening

- Rubella, varicella, syphilis, hepatitis B and C, HIV, GBS

Screening for maternal disorders

- Diabetes
- Urinary tract infection

Testing for fetal anomalies

- Nuchal translucency
- NIPT
- Second-trimester ultrasound
- Invasive diagnostic testing

Antenatal education

- Dietary advice
- Exercise
- Substance use in pregnancy
  - Smoking
  - Alcohol
  - Illicit drugs
- Coitus

Chapter | 8 |

Obstetric disorders

Henry G. Murray

LEARNING OBJECTIVES

After studying this chapter you should be able to:

Knowledge criteria

- Describe the pathophysiology, aetiology and presentation of the major antenatal complications of pregnancy:
  - Hypertension in pregnancy
  - Antepartum haemorrhage and placenta accreta
  - Multiple pregnancy, breech presentation
  - Abnormal and unstable lie and prolonged pregnancy

Clinical competencies

- Plan initial investigations and management of these obstetric disorders
- Interpret the investigation results of scan, blood and urine tests performed in cases of obstetric disorders
- Explain to the mother and her partner the consequences of the obstetric disorder

Professional skills and attitudes

- Empathize with the woman and her family should an adverse event occur as a result of an obstetric disorder

Hypertensive disorders of pregnancy

Hypertensive disorders remain the commonest complication of pregnancy in the developed world and are consistently one of the main causes of maternal death. The incidence varies substantially in different countries and is influenced by a number of factors, including parity, ethnic group and dietary intake. In the UK, the condition occurs in 10–15% of all pregnancies, and 4–13% of the population will develop pre-eclampsia, i.e. hypertension with proteinuria. While most episodes of hypertension are specifically related to the pregnancy and will resolve when the pregnancy is completed, some women who suffer from other forms of hypertension, e.g. essential hypertension or that due to renal disease, will continue to have raised blood pressure (BP). These diseases may influence the outcome of the pregnancy, and the progress of the disease may be influenced by the pregnancy.

In its mildest form, hypertension alone arising in late pregnancy appears to be of minimal risk to mother or child.

In its most severe form, the condition is associated with placental abruption, convulsions, proteinuria, severe oedema and life-threatening hypertension, which may result in cerebral haemorrhage, renal and hepatic failure, as well as disseminated intravascular coagulopathy (DIC). This may lead to fetal and maternal death.

The association between convulsions and pregnancy was described in ancient Greek and Egyptian writings. The first description of eclampsia, with the occurrence of convulsions, hypertension and proteinuria, was given by Vasquez in 1897.

Definitions

Hypertension in pregnancy is defined as a systolic pressure above 140 mmHg or a diastolic pressure above 90 mmHg on two or more occasions at least 4 hours apart. Diastolic pressure is taken at the fifth Korotkoff sound. At times in pregnancy, there is no fifth sound; in these circumstances, it is necessary to use the fourth sound.

Some definitions of hypertension also include reference to a rise in systolic pressure of at least 30 mmHg or a

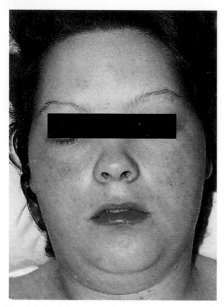

Fig. 8.1 Facial oedema in severe pre-eclampsia.

rise in diastolic pressure of at least 15 mmHg. There is no evidence that these women have adverse outcomes if the systolic BP remains less than 140 mmHg or diastolic less than 90 mmHg.

Proteinuria is defined as the presence of urinary protein in concentrations greater than 0.3 g/L in a 24-hour collection or in concentrations greater than 1 g/L on a random sample on two or more occasions at least 6 hours apart.

Oedema is defined as the development of pitting oedema or a weight gain in excess of 2.3 kg in a week. Oedema occurs in the limbs, particularly in the feet and ankles and in the fingers, or in the abdominal wall and face (Fig. 8.1). Oedema is very common in otherwise uncomplicated pregnancies. This is the least useful sign of hypertensive disease. It has therefore been dropped from many classifications of pregnancy-induced hypertension.

Classification

The various types of hypertension are classified as follows:
- **Gestational hypertension** is characterized by the new onset of hypertension without any features of pre-eclampsia after 20 weeks of pregnancy or within the first 24 hours postpartum. Although by definition the blood pressure should return to normal by 12 weeks after pregnancy; it usually returns to normal within 10 days after delivery.
- **Pre-eclampsia** is the development of hypertension with proteinuria after the twentieth week of gestation. It is more commonly a disorder of women in their first pregnancy.

- **Eclampsia** is defined as the development of convulsions secondary to pre-eclampsia in the mother.
- **Chronic hypertensive disease** is the condition in which hypertension has been present before pregnancy and may be due to various pathological causes.
- **Superimposed pre-eclampsia or eclampsia** is the development of pre-eclampsia in a woman with chronic hypertensive disease or renal disease.
- **Unclassified hypertension** includes those cases of hypertension arising in pregnancy on a random basis where there is insufficient information for classification.

> The critical factor that changes the prognosis for the mother and infant is the development of proteinuria. Those women who develop hypertension alone tend to have normal fetal growth with a good prognosis for the infant, whereas those who develop proteinuria have placental changes that are associated with intrauterine growth restriction and a poorer fetal prognosis. From a management point of view, the final diagnosis can only be made after the pregnancy has been completed, so the assumption must be made that any woman who develops hypertension must be considered to be at risk. **!**

Pathogenesis and pathology of pre-eclampsia and eclampsia

The exact nature of the pathogenesis of pre-eclampsia remains uncertain. Nearly every major system in the body is affected by the advanced manifestations of the condition. Therefore, every system that is studied appears to show changes without necessarily doing more than manifesting secondary effects.

The pathophysiology of the condition, as outlined in Figure 8.2, is characterized by the effects of:
- Arteriolar vasoconstriction, particularly in the vascular bed of the uterus, placenta and kidneys
- DIC

Blood pressure is determined by cardiac output (stroke volume × heart rate) and peripheral vascular resistance. Cardiac output increases substantially in normal pregnancy, but blood pressure normally falls in the mid-trimester. Thus, the most important regulatory factor is the loss of peripheral resistance that occurs in pregnancy. Without this effect, all pregnant women would presumably become hypertensive!

As sympathetic tone appears to remain unchanged, peripheral resistance is determined by the balance between humoral vasodilators and vasoconstrictors. In pregnancy, there is a specific loss of sensitivity to angiotensin II, which normally counters the effect of locally active vasodilator prostaglandins, resulting in systemic vasodilatation.

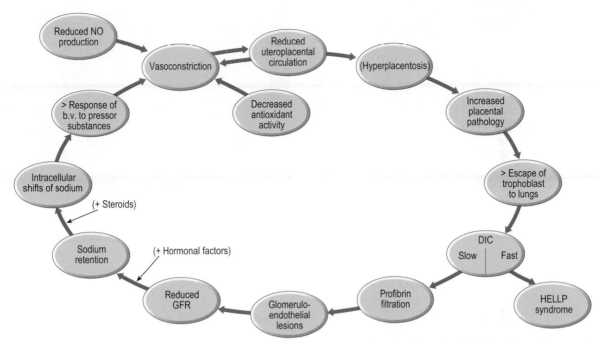

Fig. 8.2 The cycle of changes involved in the pathogenesis of pre-eclampsia. *b.v.,* Blood vessels; *DIC,* disseminated intravascular coagulation; *GFR,* glomerular filtration rate; *HELLP,* haemolysis–elevated liver enzymes–low platelets; *NO,* nitric oxide.

However, any factors that increase the activity of the renin–angiotensin system or reduce the activity of tissue prostaglandins will result in raising of the BP, thus countering the normal pregnancy changes.

Pre-eclamptic women appear to retain some sensitivity to infused angiotensin II, and there is evidence that platelet AII receptors are increased, all of which increases the chance of vasoconstriction and platelet aggregation.

Current evidence also suggests that pre-eclampsia is a disease of endothelial dysfunction. Nitric oxide (NO) or endothelial-derived relaxing factor (EDRF) is a potent vasodilator. In pre-eclampsia, NO synthesis is reduced, possibly because of an inhibition of NO synthetase activity.

A further area of consideration is the damaging effect of lipid peroxides on the endothelium. Normally, the production of antioxidants limits these effects, but in pre-eclampsia, antioxidant activity is decreased and endothelial damage occurs throughout the body, resulting in fluid loss from the intravascular space. All these changes occur in the second trimester long before a rise in BP is measurable in the mother.

Once vasoconstriction occurs in the placental bed, it results in placental damage and the consequent release of trophoblastic material into the peripheral circulation. This trophoblastic material is rich in thromboplastins, which precipitate variable degrees of DIC. This process gives rise to the pathological lesions, most notably in the kidney, liver and placental bed. The renal lesion results in sodium and water retention, with most of this fluid moving to the extracellular space due to vascular endothelial damage which permits fluid extravasation. In fact, the intravascular space is reduced in severe pre-eclampsia as plasma volume diminishes. At the same time, increased sodium retention results in increased vascular sensitivity to vasoconstrictor influences, which promotes further vasoconstriction and tissue damage in a vicious circle of events that may ultimately result in acute renal failure with tubular or cortical necrosis, hepatic failure with periportal necrosis, acute cardiac failure and pulmonary oedema, and even cerebral haemorrhage as BP becomes uncontrolled.

As the vasoconstriction progresses, the placenta becomes grossly infarcted, and this results in intrauterine growth restriction, increased risk of abruption and sometimes fetal death.

Why do some women develop pre-eclampsia and others do not? Is there a genetic predisposition in some women? The answer to this second question is almost certainly yes. Longitudinal studies in the United States, Iceland and Scotland have shown that the daughters of women who have suffered from pre-eclampsia or eclampsia have themselves a one in four chance of developing the disease, a risk that

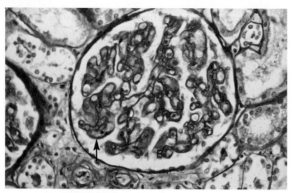

Fig. 8.3 Renal changes in pre-eclampsia include endothelial swelling (E), apparent avascularity of the glomerulus and fibrin deposition (arrow) under the basement membrane.

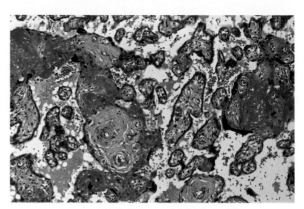

Fig. 8.4 Placental changes in pre-eclampsia include an increase in syncytial knots, proliferation of cytotrophoblast and thickening of trophoblastic basement membrane.

is 2.5 times higher than in the daughters-in-law of such women. The data suggest that a single recessive maternal gene is associated with pre-eclampsia. However, the data could also support a hypothetical model of dominant inheritance with partial penetrance. Although various gene loci have been proposed, further long-term studies are ongoing to try and identify the correct candidate gene. It is in fact unlikely that there is a single pre-eclampsia gene; it is probable that there are interactions between several genes, with external environmental factors enhancing this predisposition. These factors include autoimmune conditions, diseases that increase venous and arterial thromboembolic disease (thrombophilias) and the existence of underlying chronic renal disease or essential hypertension. Dietary intake may also be a factor.

The renal lesion

The renal lesion is, histologically, the most specific feature of pre-eclampsia (Fig. 8.3). The features are:
- Swelling and proliferation of endothelial cells to such a point that the capillary vessels are obstructed.
- Hypertrophy and hyperplasia of the intercapillary or mesangial cells.
- Fibrillary material (profibrin) deposition on the basement membrane and between and within the endothelial cells.

The characteristic appearance is therefore one of increased capillary cellularity and reduced vascularity. The lesion is found in 71% of primigravid women who develop pre-eclampsia but in only 29% of multiparous women. There is a much higher incidence of women with chronic renal disease in multiparous women.

The glomerular lesion is always associated with proteinuria and with reduced glomerular filtration resulting in a raised serum creatinine. Decreased renal blood flow and proximal tubular changes result in impaired uric acid secretion, leading to hyperuricaemia.

Placental pathology

Placental infarcts occur in normal pregnancy but are considerably more extensive in pre-eclampsia. The characteristic features in the placenta (Fig. 8.4) include:
- increased syncytial knots or sprouts
- increased loss of syncytium
- proliferation of cytotrophoblast
- thickening of the trophoblastic basement membrane
- villous necrosis

In the uteroplacental bed, the normal invasion of extravillous cytotrophoblast along the luminal surface of the maternal spiral arterioles does not occur beyond the deciduomyometrial junction, and there is apparent constriction of the vessels between the radial artery and the decidual portion (Fig. 8.5). These changes result in reduced uteroplacental blood flow and in placental hypoxia.

Disseminated intravascular coagulation

In severe pre-eclampsia and eclampsia, thrombosis can be seen in the capillary bed of many organs. Multiple platelet and fibrin thrombi can be identified in the brain. Similar changes are seen in the periportal zones of the liver and in the spleen and the adrenal cortex. Thrombocytopenia may occur in some cases, but in only 10% of eclamptic women does the platelet count fall below 100,000/mL. There is an increase in fibrin deposition and in circulating fibrin degradation products as a result of increased fibrin production and impaired fibrinolysis. There seems to be little doubt that while these changes are not the cause of pre-eclampsia, they do play an important role in the pathology of the disease.

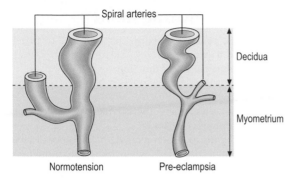

Fig. 8.5 Trophoblast invasion of the spiral arterioles results in dilatation of these vessels. This process is defective in pre-eclampsia.

Other associations with pregnancy hypertension

It has been postulated that pre-eclampsia may be due to an abnormality of the maternal host response to placentation. There is a lower incidence of pre-eclampsia in consanguineous marriages and an increased incidence of hypertension in first pregnancies of second marriages. Levels of human leukocyte antigen (HLA)-G are altered in pre-eclamptic women.

Indices of cell-mediated immune response have also been shown to be altered in severe pre-eclampsia. However, there are many other factors that operate independently from any potential immunological factors, such as race, climatic conditions and genetic or familial factors. One of these includes raised free fatty acids found in pre-eclampsia and their possible causative role in the increased incidence of pre-eclampsia in women with diabetes and obesity.

The HELLP syndrome

A severe manifestation of pre-eclampsia occurs in a variant known as the *HELLP syndrome*. In this syndrome, there is a triad of manifestations that include haemolysis (H), elevated levels of liver enzymes (EL) and a low platelet count (LP). This manifestation is an extension of the DIC causing the haemolysis and low platelets and the endothelial dysfunction/hypoxia in the liver resulting in the release of liver transaminases, especially the alanine aminotransferase (ALT).

The thrombocytopenia is often rapidly progressive and if left to become severe may result in haemorrhage into the brain and the liver. The syndrome demands intervention and immediate consideration of termination of the pregnancy after any treatable manifestations like hypertension are controlled.

Management of gestational hypertension and pre-eclampsia

The object of management is to prevent the development of eclampsia and to minimize the risks of the condition to both the mother and the fetus. The achievement of these objectives depends on careful scrutiny of the condition of both the mother and the fetus and timely intervention to terminate the pregnancy when the risks of continuation outweigh the risks of intervention.

Blood pressure measurement

A rise in BP is usually the first sign to be noted at the antenatal visit. BP should be recorded in a constant position at each visit, as it is posture dependent. The most comfortable position is seated, using a sphygmomanometer compatible with BP measurement in pregnancy and a cuff of an appropriate size applied to the right upper arm. Automated BP machines can be unreliable in measuring BP in pregnancy.

If the pressure is elevated, the measurement should be repeated after a short period of rest. If the BP remains elevated, then continuing close observation is essential. This may be achieved by hospital admission if significant pre-eclampsia is suspected, a visit to a 'day ward' for hypertension of uncertain significance or careful scrutiny at home by a visiting midwife or the family general practitioner for the possibility of white coat hypertension. The woman should be advised to rest. However, although bed rest improves renal blood flow and uteroplacental flow and commonly results in a diuresis and mild improvement in the BP, it has not been shown to improve overall outcomes in the mother or the fetus.

The development of more than 1+ proteinuria or a spot urinary protein/creatinine ratio of more than 30 mg/mmol is an absolute indication for close surveillance of the pregnancy, as this change constitutes the dividing line between minimal risk and significant risk to both mother and baby.

If the hypertension persists or worsens and the mother is at or close to term, the fetus should be delivered. If it is considered that the fetus would benefit from further time in utero and there is no maternal contraindication, treatment with antihypertensive drugs should be considered. It must be remembered that prolonging the pregnancy in pre-eclampsia is solely for the benefit of the fetus.

Antihypertensive drug therapy

In the presence of an acute hypertensive crisis, controlling the BP with medication is essential, but in the case of mild gestational hypertension and moderate pre-eclampsia, their role is more contentious. There is, however, convincing evidence that the treatment of mild or moderate chronic hypertension in pregnancy reduces the risk of developing severe hypertension and the need for hospital admission.

In women with gestational hypertension, treatment with antihypertensive drugs should be confined to those women who fail to respond to conservative management, including stopping work if that is possible. Early antihypertensive treatment possibly reduces the risk of progression to severe proteinuric hypertension. Management is based on the principle of minimizing both maternal and fetal morbidity and mortality. BPs of more than 170 mmHg systolic or 110 mmHg diastolic must be treated as a matter of urgency to lower the risk of intracerebral haemorrhage and eclampsia. Until recently it was believed that if BP stays above 160/100 mmHg, antihypertensive treatment is essential, as there is a risk of maternal cerebral haemorrhage. Data from the UK maternal death enquiry 2011 clearly show that treatment is warranted at levels above 150/100 mmHg.

The drugs most commonly used are:
- methyldopa (oral)
- hydralazine (oral and intravenous (IV))
- combined alpha- and beta-blockers such as labetalol (oral or IV)
- alpha-blocker such as prazosin (oral)
- calcium channel blockers such as nifedipine (oral)
  Note: Angiotensin-converting enzyme (ACE) inhibitors are contraindicated in pregnancy.

Where acute control is required, an IV bolus of hydralazine 5 mg or labetalol 20 mg should be administered. Oral medications can take a variable time to control BP.

Steroids: Where a woman is less than 34 weeks' gestation and her hypertensive disease is severe enough that early delivery is contemplated, betamethasone 11.4 mg intramuscularly (IM), two doses 12–24 hours apart. Should be given to minimize neonatal consequences of prematurity like respiratory distress syndrome (RDS), intraventricular haemorrhage and necrotizing enterocolitis.

Maternal investigations

The most important investigations for monitoring the mother are:
- The 4-hourly measurement of BP until such time that the BP has returned to normal.
- Regular urine checks for proteinuria. Initially, screening is done with dipsticks or spot urinary protein/creatinine ratio, but once proteinuria is established, 24-hour urine samples should be collected. Values in excess of 0.3 g/L over 24 hours are abnormal.
- Maternal serum screening for pre-eclampsia.

Laboratory investigations

- Full blood count with particular reference to platelet count and haemolysis.
- Tests for renal and liver function.
- Uric acid measurements: a useful indicator of progression in the disease.
- Clotting studies where there is severe pre-eclampsia and/or thrombocytopaenia.
- Catecholamine measurements in the presence of severe hypertension, particularly where there is no proteinuria, to rule out phaeochromocytoma.

Case study

Mrs F was pregnant with her first child after a long history of subfertility. She had been admitted to hospital before her pregnancy for tubal evaluation by dye laparoscopy, but at no time then or subsequently during her pregnancy had she shown any evidence of hypertension. At 32 weeks' gestation, she was admitted to hospital at 10 PM with acute headache and severe hypertension, with a BP reading of 220/140 mmHg. There was no proteinuria and no hyper-reflexia. There was no evidence of fetal growth restriction. Despite initial attempts to control her BP with intravenous hydralazine and labetalol, and despite delivery of the fetus, her hypertension remained severe and uncontrollable and she went into high-output cardiac failure and died at 7 AM the following morning. Autopsy revealed a large phaeochromocytoma in the right adrenal gland.

This is an extremely rare form of hypertension in pregnancy. It has an appalling prognosis unless it is detected early and the tumour removed. In this case, it presented late. All other antenatal recordings of BP had been normal. Although it would not have helped in this case as the BP readings were always normal, where hypertension is severe and presents early in pregnancy, it is always worth checking urinary catecholamines.

Fetoplacental investigations

Pre-eclampsia is an important cause of fetal growth restriction and perinatal death, and it is therefore essential to monitor fetal wellbeing using the following methods:
- Serial ultrasounds for:
  - **Measurements of fetal growth every 2 weeks.** Parameters measured are fetal biparietal diameter, head circumference, abdominal circumference and femur length.
  - **Measurements of liquor volume and fetal Doppler studies up to twice weekly.**
  - **Daily cardiotocography (CTG) in advanced cases close to requiring delivery.**

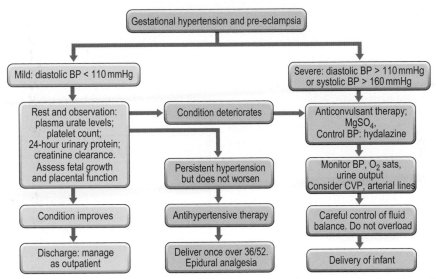

Fig. 8.6 Flow diagram of the management of gestational hypertension and pre-eclampsia. *BP*, Blood pressure; *CVP*, central venous pressure.

Doppler flow studies

- The use of serial Doppler waveform measurements in the fetus with every assessment of liquor is an essential part of assessment of the fetal wellbeing/oxygenation status. The resistance to flow in the umbilical artery is a measure of placental blood vessel integrity, with raised resistance being a measure of small-vessel disease. The fetal middle cerebral artery normally has a high resistance pattern, and a fall in resistance relates to vasodilatation and fetal hypoxia. Where the resistance in the umbilical vessels exceeds that in the middle cerebral vessels (cerebral/placental ratio (CPR) is less than 1), the fetus is at significant risk of morbidity associated with hypoxia. Consideration must be given to very close observation or delivery of these pregnancies, regardless of the fetal growth parameters, albeit that fetuses that are growth restricted from maternal pre-eclampsia are more likely to have an abnormal CPR than an appropriately grown fetus. At any time, absent or reverse flow in diastole in the umbilical artery of the fetus indicates severe vessel disease, with probable severe fetal compromise, and delivery of the fetus must be considered if the CTG is abnormal.
- As a single investigation, doppler ultrasound of maternal vessels after 14 weeks has not been shown to add to the ability to effectively treat maternal pre-eclampsia.
- **Antenatal CTG measured daily in admitted cases of pre-eclampsia:** CTG recordings are used in conjunction with Doppler assessment. The measurement of the antenatal CTG (fetal heart rate in relation to uterine activity) provides a useful tool in the detection of fetal wellbeing. A normal reactive trace is an assurance of a non-hypoxic fetus. A trace with recurrent decelerations and a loss of baseline variability is a strong indication of fetal metabolic acidaemia. Lesser anomalies on CTG trace can be over-interpreted, leading to an over-diagnosed fetal compromise. The CTG recording must therefore be interpreted with care.

A summary of the various management strategies for pregnancy-related hypertension is shown in Figure 8.6. This flow diagram shows the various pathways of progression and their management. An initial presentation of mild hypertension may improve with conservative management, or it may progress rapidly to the severe forms of pre-eclampsia and ultimately eclampsia.

Prevention of pre-eclampsia

There is no doubt that careful management and anticipation can largely prevent the occurrence of eclampsia, but preventing pre-eclampsia should be the gold standard of care.

The first opportunity to prevent pre-eclampsia is at the 12-week scan. In the mother, the finding of increased resistance in the uterine arteries at 12 weeks, along with a finding of maternal hypertension and low pregnancy-associated plasma protein – A (PAPP-A) and Placental Growth Factor (PlGF) levels, has been associated with poor pregnancy outcome, in particular early-onset pre-eclampsia (significant pre-eclampsia before 32 weeks). Treatment with aspirin 100–150 mg has been shown to improve the pregnancy outcome by delaying the need for fetal delivery to close to term.

There is some evidence that calcium supplements may reduce the risk of pre-eclampsia in the general population, but only in women who have dietary deficiency.

In women with essential hypertension and those with pre-eclampsia in previous pregnancies, aspirin has been shown to reduce the incidence of pre-eclampsia in subsequent pregnancies.

In women who have had severe pre-eclampsia in the previous pregnancy, a thrombophilia screen should be undertaken postnatally, as there is an incidence of underlying thrombotic tendencies that may also benefit from the use of low-molecular-weight heparin therapy in addition to aspirin in a subsequent pregnancy.

Symptoms of pre-eclampsia and eclampsia

Pre-eclampsia is commonly an asymptomatic condition. However, there are symptoms that must not be overlooked, and these include frontal headache, blurring of vision, sudden onset of vomiting and right epigastric pain. Of these symptoms, the most important is the development of epigastric pain – either during pregnancy or in the immediate puerperium (Fig. 8.7).

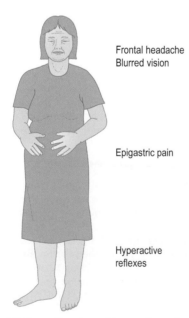

Frontal headache
Blurred vision

Epigastric pain

Hyperactive reflexes

Fig. 8.7 Presenting signs of impending eclampsia.

Where a woman presents with headache, markedly raised BP and hyperreflexia, and has blood testing confirming severe pre-eclampsia, delivery of the fetus must be considered. The initial treatment is to control the BP with IV medication and prevention of seizures with an infusion of magnesium sulphate 4 g IV over 20 minutes with 1 g/h until the risk of seizures has ceased 24 hours after delivery (see also Eclampsia later).

The occurrence of epigastric pain is commonly misdiagnosed or overlooked as a feature of severe pre-eclampsia and impending eclampsia. Occurring often in the late second or the early third trimester, an erroneous diagnosis of indigestion, heartburn or gallstones is sometimes made, and unless the BP is recorded and the urine checked for protein, the significance of the pain can be overlooked until the woman presents with seizures.

Induction of labour

In a pregnancy complicated by hypertensive disease, delivery of the fetus should be considered for the following maternal and/or fetal/placental reasons:
- maternal
  - gestation >37 weeks
  - uncontrollable BP
  - HELLP syndrome
  - rising liver dysfunction
  - falling platelets
  - falling haemoglobin due to haemolysis
  - deteriorating renal function (creatinine >90 mmol/L)
  - eclampsia
  - acute pulmonary oedema
- fetal/placental
  - fetal compromise on CTG tracing
  - absent or reversal of end diastolic flow in the umbilical artery
  - abnormal cerebro/placental ratio on Doppler scanning of the fetal vessels
  - no fetal growth over more than 2 weeks on ultrasound
  - placental abruption with fetal compromise

If the decision has been made to proceed to delivery, the choice will rest with either the induction of labour or delivery by caesarean section. This decision will be determined by the seriousness of the clinical situation. If there is time, antenatal steroids should be given for gestations of less than 34 weeks to minimize neonatal morbidity. In an extreme situation like eclampsia or severe fetal compromise, delivery should not be delayed in order to administer steroids. Similarly, where a fetus is to be delivered at a gestation of less than 30 weeks, a loading dose and infusion of magnesium sulphate should be considered in the hour before delivery by lower uterine segment caesarean section (LUSCS) or during an induced labour, as it provides neuroprotection for the neonatal brain. Where an infusion of magnesium sulphate is being used as prophylaxis against maternal seizures (eclampsia), this infusion acts to protect the neonatal brain and no further dosing is required.

If the cervix is unsuitable for surgical induction (Bishop score of less than 7), it can often be ripened by the introduction of a prostaglandin E preparation into the posterior fornix of the vagina or the use of a mechanical balloon catheter (Foley catheter) through the cervix.

If the cervix has a Bishop score of greater than 7, labour is induced by artificial rupture of membranes and oxytocin infusion (see Chapter 11).

Complications

Complications can be grouped as follows:
- fetal
  - growth restriction, hypoxia, death
- maternal
  - severe pre-eclampsia is associated with a fall in blood flow to various vital organs. If the mother is inadequately treated and/or the fetus is not delivered in a timely manner, complications include renal failure (raised creatinine/oliguria/anuria), hepatic failure, intrahepatic haemorrhage, seizures, DIC, adult RDS (ARDS), cerebral haemorrhage/infarction and heart failure
- placental
  - infarction, abruption

Eclampsia

The onset of convulsions in a pregnancy complicated by pre-eclampsia denotes the onset of eclampsia. Eclampsia is a preventable condition, and its occurrence often denotes a failure to recognize the early worsening signs of pre-eclampsia. Although it is more common in primigravid women, it can occur in any pregnancy during the antepartum, intrapartum or postpartum period. It carries serious risks of intrauterine death for the fetus and of maternal death from cerebral haemorrhage and/or renal and hepatic failure.

All cases must be managed in hospital and preferably in hospitals with appropriate intensive care facilities. Any woman admitted to hospital with convulsions during the course of pregnancy or who is admitted in a coma associated with hypertension should be considered to be suffering from eclampsia until proved otherwise.

Case study

Not all women admitted with seizures in pregnancy are eclamptic. Marilyn D was a single mother who was brought into an accident and emergency department by two friends with a statement that she had fitted on two occasions. She was booked for confinement at the same hospital, and her antenatal records showed that her pregnancy had so far been uncomplicated. She was 34 weeks pregnant, and on admission her BP was 140/90 mmHg. There was a trace of protein in the urine. She was brought into hospital on a Saturday night, and her friends stated that they had stopped the car on the way into hospital and laid Marilyn down on the pavement by the roadside because of the violence of her seizure.

After careful assessment of the BP that settled to 110/75 mmHg and normal biochemical testing, it was decided to proceed with observation, and within 24 hours, there were no further fits. Further discussion with Marilyn revealed that she had taken a mixture of illicit drugs, including amphetamines: a diagnosis that was suggested by one of the medical students!

Management of eclampsia

The three basic guidelines for management of eclampsia are:
- Control the fits.
- Control the BP.
- Deliver the infant.

Control of fits

In the past various drugs were used to control the fits:
- Eclamptic seizures are usually self-limiting. Acute management is to ensure patient safety and protect the airway.
- Magnesium sulphate is the drug of choice for the control of fits thereafter. The drug is effective in suppressing convulsions and inhibiting muscular activity. It also reduces platelet aggregation and minimizes the effects of DIC. Treatment is started with a bolus dose of 4 g given over 20 minutes. Thereafter blood levels of magnesium are maintained by giving a maintenance dose of 1 g/h. The blood level of magnesium should only be measured if there is significant renal failure or seizures recur. The therapeutic range is 2–4 mmol/L. A level of more than 5 mmol/L causes loss of patellar reflexes, and a value of more than 6 mmol/L causes respiratory depression. Magnesium sulphate can be given by intramuscular injection, but the injection is often painful and sometimes leads to abscess formation. The preferred route is therefore by IV administration.

> It is not always possible to monitor the blood levels of magnesium. It is, however, important to avoid toxic levels of magnesium, as they may result in complete respiratory arrest. Eclampsia is associated with hyper-reflexia and, on occasions, with clonus, so a guide to the levels of magnesium can be obtained by regular checks of the patellar reflexes. If patellar reflexes are absent, magnesium should be stopped. In the event of the suppression of respiration, the effects can be reversed by the administration of 10 mL of 10% calcium gluconate given intravenously over 2–3 minutes.

After the first seizure, it is important to ensure that further fits are prevented, BP is well controlled, fluid balance is strictly monitored, and urine output is maintained at 0.5–1.0 mL/kg/h. To this end, the patient should be managed jointly with staff in an intensive care/high-dependency unit. Constant nursing attendance is essential by staff accustomed to managing patients with airway problems. As a general principle, total fluid input should be restricted to 80–100 mL/h. If the urine flow falls to below 30 mL/h, a central venous pressure measurement should be considered. Fluid overload in these women may induce pulmonary oedema and ARDS with lethal consequences.

Control of blood pressure

It is essential to control the BP to minimize the risk of maternal cerebral haemorrhage. Hydralazine is a useful drug in acute management and is given intravenously as a 5-mg bolus over an interval of 5 minutes and repeated after 15 minutes if the BP is not controlled. If the mother is still pregnant, it is important not to drop the BP below a diastolic BP of 90 mmHg in order not to compromise the uterine/placental blood flow.

An alternative is to use IV labetalol, starting with a bolus of 20 mg followed by further doses of 40 mg and 80 mg to a total of 200 mg.

Subsequent BP control can be maintained with a continuous infusion of hydralazine at 5–40 mg/h or labetalol at 20–160 mg/h.

Epidural analgesia relieves the pain of labour and helps to control the BP by causing vasodilatation in the lower extremities. However, it is essential to perform clotting studies before inserting an epidural catheter because of the risk of causing bleeding into the epidural space if there is a coagulopathy.

Delivery of the infant

A diagnosis of severe pre-eclampsia/eclampsia indicates that the risk to both the mother and the infant of continuing the pregnancy will exceed the risk of delivery. Where the gestation is less than 26 weeks, serious neonatal morbidity associated with prematurity and an increased risk for the requirement of a classical caesarean section necessitates

that the decision to deliver includes consultation with neonatal and maternofetal medicine specialists.

It is essential to establish reasonable control of the BP before embarking on any procedures to expedite delivery, as the intervention itself may precipitate a hypertensive crisis.

If the cervix is sufficiently dilated and the conditions of the mother and the fetus allow, an artificial rupture of the membranes may be performed and labour induced with an oxytocin infusion. If this is not possible or the maternal or fetal condition is compromised, it is best to proceed to delivery by caesarean section, which requires early consultation with an anaesthetic colleague.

Management after delivery

The risks of eclampsia do not stop with delivery, and the management of pre-eclampsia and eclampsia continues for up to 7 days after delivery, although if a seizure occurs for the first time 48 hours after delivery, alternative diagnoses such as epilepsy or intracranial pathology such as cortical vein thrombosis must be considered. Up to 45% of eclamptic fits occur after delivery, including 12% after 48 hours.

The following points of management should be observed:

- Maintain the patient in a quiet environment under constant observation.
- Maintain appropriate levels of pain relief. If the mother has been treated with magnesium sulphate, continue the infusion for 24 hours after the last fit or until a diuresis is seen.
- Continue antihypertensive therapy until the BP has returned to normal. This will usually involve transferring to oral medication, and although there is usually significant improvement after the first week, hypertension may persist for the next 6 weeks.

Case study

Mrs T was a 28-year-old primigravida and the wife of one of the junior medical staff. Her pregnancy was uneventful until 37 weeks, when she developed hypertension and was admitted to hospital for bed rest. Her BP stayed around 140/90 and there was a trace of protein in the urine. At 38 weeks' gestation, labour was induced and she had a normal delivery of a healthy male infant. The following day she was fully mobile but complained to the midwifery staff that she had a frontal headache and indigestion, with epigastric discomfort. She was given paracetamol and an antacid, but the symptoms persisted. Her hypertension also persisted, with the highest reading being 145/98 mmHg. Later that day she had a seizure. Unfortunately, she fell against the side of her bed and fractured her zygoma. Although she had not had a fit before delivery, it is important to remember that symptoms of severe pre-eclampsia in a postnatal woman are as significant after delivery as they are antenatally.

- Strict fluid balance charts should be kept and BP and urine output observed on an hourly basis during the day and 2-hourly at night. Biochemical and haematological indices should be made on a daily basis until the values have stabilized or started to return to normal.

Although most mothers who have suffered from preeclampsia or eclampsia will completely recover and return to normal, it is important to review all such women at 6 weeks after delivery. If the hypertension or proteinuria persists at this stage, they should be investigated for other factors such as underlying renal disease. Women should also be investigated for the possibility of an autoimmune, thrombophilic or antiphospholipid cause of her disease. Long term, women with severe pregnancy-induced hypertension have been found to have a higher rate of hypertension and cardiovascular disease later in life.

Antepartum haemorrhage

The definition of antepartum haemorrhage varies from country to country. The World Health Organization (WHO) definition, accepted by many countries including the UK, is haemorrhage from the vagina after the twenty-fourth week of gestation. In other countries, including Australia, the defined gestation is 20 weeks; however, a few use a 28-week definition. The factors that cause antepartum haemorrhage may be present before 20 weeks, but the distinction between a threatened miscarriage and an antepartum haemorrhage is based on whether the fetus is considered potentially viable at the time of the bleed. Antepartum bleeding remains a significant cause of perinatal and maternal morbidity and mortality.

Vaginal bleeding may be due to:
- haemorrhage from the placental site and uterus: placenta praevia, placental abruption, uterine rupture
- lesions of the lower genital tract: heavy show/onset of labour (bleed from cervical epithelium), cervical ectropion/carcinoma, cervicitis, polyps, vulval varices, trauma and infection
- bleeding from fetal vessels, including vasa praevia (very rare)

The rate of antepartum haemorrhage is generally increased in women who smoke or who have a lower socio-economic status. The rate therefore varies from 2% to 5% depending upon the population studied. For any woman admitted with bleeding, the cause is often not immediately obvious. In any large obstetric unit, the diagnoses after admission are approximately:
- unclassified/uncertain cause: 50%
- placenta praevia: 30%
- placental abruption: 20%
- vasa praevia (rare)

Placenta praevia

The placenta is said to be praevia when all or part of the placenta implants in the lower uterine segment and therefore lies beside or in front of the presenting part of the fetus (Fig. 8.8).

Incidence

Approximately 1% of all pregnancies are complicated by clinical evidence of a placenta praevia. Unlike the incidence of placental abruption, which varies according to social and nutritional factors, the incidence of placenta praevia is remarkably constant.

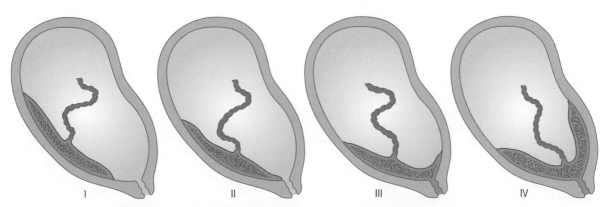

Fig. 8.8 The placental siting for placenta praevia. Grade I, II, III and IV, respectively.

Placenta praevia is more common in multiparous women, in the presence of multiple pregnancy and where there has been one or more previous caesarean sections.

Aetiology

Placenta praevia is presumed to be due to a delay in implantation of the blastocyst so that implantation occurs in the lower part of the uterus.

Classification

Placenta praevia is diagnosed using ultrasound. Given that the lower segment forms at 24–28 weeks of pregnancy, a diagnosis of placenta praevia cannot be made before that gestation. If a placenta is detected to be within 2 cm of the cervix before 24 weeks, it is called 'low lying', with 95% of such placentas ending well clear of the cervix after the lower segment develops.

There are numerous classifications of placenta praevia. The classification that affords the best anatomical description and clinical information is based on grades. Grade I is defined as a placenta with the lower edge implanted on the lower segment but not to or over the internal cervical os; grade II is when the lower edge of the placenta reaches the internal os, but the bulk of the placenta is in the upper uterine segment; grade III is determined when the placenta is covering the cervical os, but some placental tissue is also seen attached to the upper uterine segment; and grade IV is determined when all the placenta is in the lower segment with the central portion of the placenta over the cervical os (see Fig. 8.8). Women with a grade I or grade II placenta on the anterior wall of the uterus will commonly achieve a normal vaginal delivery without excess blood loss. A posterior grade II placenta praevia, where the placental mass is in front of the maternal sacrum, prevents the descent of the fetal head into the pelvis, and along with a grade III and IV placenta praevia, it will necessitate delivery by caesarean section, either urgently if labour or significant bleeding commences pre-term or electively at or near term.

Bleeding in placenta praevia results from separation of the placenta as the formation of the lower segment occurs and the cervix effaces. This blood loss occurs from the venous sinuses in the wall of the lower uterine segment. Bleeding may be profuse and/or relentless, so fetal delivery may be required to ensure maternal wellbeing. If the blood loss is controlled but the separation of the placenta is significant, fetal compromise may result, which will be detected on the CTG tracing, and delivery will be required for fetal reasons. Very occasionally, fetal blood loss may occur at the time of maternal bleeding if the placenta is disrupted. This will result in anomalies on the CTG record allowing for a timely delivery. For these reasons, close fetal monitoring must be undertaken during any bleeding.

Where the fetal condition and the maternal condition are stable and the bleeding settles, delivery is delayed at least to 35 weeks, but until 37–38 weeks if possible.

Symptoms and signs

The main symptom of placenta praevia is painless vaginal bleeding. There may sometimes be lower abdominal discomfort where there are minor degrees of associated placental separation (abruption).

The signs of placenta praevia are:
- vaginal bleeding
- malpresentation of the fetus
- normal uterine tone

The bleeding is unpredictable and may vary from minor – common with the initial bleed – to massive and life-endangering haemorrhage.

Case study

Jane T was admitted to hospital at 28 weeks' gestation with a painless vaginal haemorrhage of approximately 100 mL in her first pregnancy. The presenting part was high but central, and the uterine tone was soft. A diagnosis of a grade III anterior placenta praevia was made on ultrasound, and the fetus showed no sign of compromise. Given the site of the placenta and the risk of a further and more substantial bleed, Jane was advised to stay in hospital under observation until delivery. The bleeding settled, and at 32 weeks' gestation, she asked to go home to marry her partner. As this necessitated a 1-hour flight, she was strongly advised against this action so her partner flew to Janet instead, and the wedding was arranged in a church close to the hospital. At the wedding, Janet had a further substantial bleed as she walked down the aisle and was rushed back into hospital. On admission the bleeding was found to be settling and the fetus was not compromised. Given the gestation was less than 35 weeks, management was to observe and attempt to prolong the gestation to improve neonatal outcome. At 35 weeks' gestation Janet had a massive haemorrhage in the ward to the extent that blood soaked her bed linen and flowed over the side of the bed. The resident staff inserted two IV lines and she was rushed to theatre. She was shocked and hypotensive, and it was extremely difficult to maintain her BP. The fetal heart showed hypoxic decelerations and finally a bradycardia associated with poor placental perfusion. A 'crash section' was performed, and the diagnosis of grade III placenta praevia was confirmed. A healthy male infant was delivered. Janet was resuscitated with over 10 units of blood and blood product. Had Janet been at home at the time of the bleed, it is possible that neither she nor her baby would have survived.

Diagnosis

Clinical findings

Painless bleeding occurs suddenly and tends to be recurrent. If labour starts and the cervix dilates, profuse haemorrhage may occur. Where there is a grade I anterior or lateral placental praevia, the bleeding may be less profuse. As labour is establishing, it may be safe to rupture the fetal membranes, which may assist the descent of the head and slow the blood loss even further. If it is safe, the labour can be allowed to progress to a vaginal delivery.

Abdominal examination

- **Displacement of the presenting part:** The finding of painless vaginal bleeding with a high central presenting part, a transverse or an oblique lie strongly suggests the possibility of placenta praevia. Although a speculum examination may be undertaken by a skilled obstetrician in these cases to check the amount of the blood loss in the vagina and that it is not of vaginal origin, a digital vaginal examination must not be undertaken until an ultrasound has been performed. A digital examination may disrupt the placenta and cause excessive bleeding.
- **Normal uterine tone:** Unlike with abruption, the uterine muscle tone is usually normal and the fetal parts are easy to palpate.

Diagnostic procedures

- **Ultrasound scanning:** Transabdominal and, for posterior placentas, transvaginal ultrasound are used to localize the placenta where there is a suggestion of placenta praevia. Anteriorly, the bladder provides an important landmark for the lower segment, and diagnosis is more accurate. When the placenta is on the posterior wall, the sacral promontory is used to define the lower segment; however, if this cannot be seen with transabdominal scanning, a transvaginal scan is used to determine the distance from the cervical os to the lower margin of the placenta. Localization of the placental site in early pregnancy may result in an inaccurate diagnosis, as development of the lower segment will lead to an apparent upwards displacement of the placenta by 30 weeks.
- **Magnetic resonance imaging:** This is used when the placenta is implanted on the lower uterine segment over an old caesarean scar. It may help to determine whether the placental tissue has migrated through the scar (placenta percreta) or even into the bladder tissue, although ultrasound is a better modality of imaging in this situation – see the Placenta accreta spectrum section.

Management

When antepartum haemorrhage of any type occurs, the diagnosis of placenta praevia should be suspected and hospital admission advised. An IV line should be established and the mother resuscitated as necessary after blood has been taken for full blood count and cross-match. A CTG should be performed to determine fetal status. A cause for the bleeding should be sought by ultrasound imaging, remembering that in up to 50% of cases of antepartum haemorrhage no obvious cause will be seen. In the acute setting, in the absence of an ultrasound diagnosis, a vaginal examination on a woman who has suffered an antepartum haemorrhage should be performed only in an operating theatre which is prepared for an emergency caesarean section and with cross-matched blood readily available.

There is only one indication for performing a vaginal examination:
- When there is serious doubt about the diagnosis due to inadequate ultrasound facilities, labour appears to have commenced and bleeding has settled. The patient can be taken to theatre by a very senior obstetrician. First the examination has to be by digital palpation through the vaginal fornices to feel whether the presenting part can be felt easily. If there is difficulty in palpating the fetal head and/ or a boggy mass is felt, then it is likely that that boggy mass is placenta that is low lying. If the presenting part is easily felt via the fornices suggesting that there is no placenta in the lower segment, careful digital examination through the cervix can occur with the intention of rupturing the membranes to induce labour.

Conservative management of placenta praevia should always be considered in the pre-term situation and where the bleeding is not life threatening. This involves keeping the mother in hospital with cross-matched blood until fetal maturity is adequate and then delivering the child by caesarean section depending on the grade of placenta praevia. After any bleed, the mother should be treated by oral iron or iron infusion where necessary so that an adequate haemoglobin concentration is maintained. As with any antepartum haemorrhage, anti-D immunoglobulin needs to be given if the mother is Rhesus negative. To ascertain the dose required, blood is taken for the Kleihauer-Betke test to determine the extent of any fetomaternal transfusion.

Postpartum haemorrhage is also a hazard of the antenatal low-lying placenta, as contraction of the lower segment is less effective than contraction of the upper segment, leaving bleeding from the venous sinuses uncontrolled.

There is an increased risk of placenta accreta/increta/ percreta (placenta accreta spectrum) where, in the situation of placenta praevia, placental implantation occurs over the site of a previous uterine scar.

Placenta accreta spectrum

Placenta accreta spectrum is the term used to describe the condition where the placenta is abnormally adherent to the uterine wall. The term includes placenta accreta (placenta attached to the myometrium and not the decidua), placenta increta (placental invasion into the myometrium) and placenta percreta (placental invasion through the uterine wall and into the serosa and surrounding structures). The abnormal invasion is due to an absence of the normal decidual basalis at the time of trophoblast attachment. The absence of the decidual layer is found over scars associated with previous uterine trauma or surgery such as caesarean section, endometrial ablation, myomectomy, uterine artery embolization as a treatment for fibroids, dilatation and curettage or manual removal of placenta.

The primary issue with placenta accreta spectrum disorder is that the placenta does not separate from the uterine wall in the third stage of labour, and blood vessels feeding the placental bed can bleed – at times profusely. Placenta accreta spectrum in the upper segment of the uterus is usually diagnosed when a manual removal of the placenta is attempted for retained placenta in the third stage of labour. Bleeding at this time can usually be controlled with the use of oxytocic drugs with or without the use of an intrauterine balloon catheter. Occasionally bleeding is not controlled and a surgical procedure like a B Lynch suture or, if that

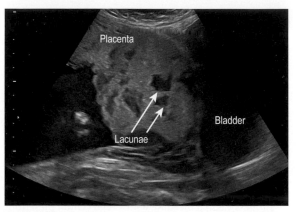

Fig. 8.9 Ultrasound picture of a placenta praevia accreta showing presence of placental lacunae.

Case study

Mrs J is 30-year-old woman in her third pregnancy. Her two previous pregnancies were delivered by uncomplicated caesarean sections for obstructed labour on both occasions. In this pregnancy, she had a normal 12-week scan. The 20-week scan reported the presence of a low-lying anterior placenta which covered the cervical os and the presumed site of the uterine scar. At 24 weeks, she had an ultrasound scan that confirmed the signs of placenta accreta: multiple hypoechoic areas in the placenta overlying the scar, which represent vascular lacunae, and a loss of the uterine serosa/maternal bladder interface (Fig. 8.9) and maternal vessels passing from the bladder to the uterine margin.

Delivery was planned for 35 weeks, which is best to minimize pathology for both mother and fetus. A multidisciplinary meeting was held to plan surgery, which included:

- Obstetricians
- Gynaecology oncology specialist
- Vascular surgeon
- Anaesthetists
- Urologists – to place ureteric stents into the ureters, given the probable involvement of the placenta invasion into the bladder and the pelvic sidewall
- Interventional radiology – to discuss the benefits or otherwise of internal iliac artery balloons to help stem blood loss from the surgical site

The blood bank was alerted about the case 48 hours before the procedure, and blood was cross-matched and the mother was administered steroids to promote fetal lung maturation.

The mother was fully counselled and consented for a caesar-

ean section. She was told the baby would be delivered through a classical caesarean incision and after delivery the placenta would be visualized. If obvious percreta was not seen and the placenta appeared to separate normally, it would be removed and haemostasis achieved if possible. If the placenta did not separate at all and there was no bleeding, the possibility of leaving it in situ, completing the operation and then removing the placenta at a later date was discussed; however, this scenario is associated with delayed bleeding and possible sepsis. The third scenario explained was that if at operation the percreta was obvious on opening the abdomen and after delivery of the baby, a hysterectomy would be performed with highly trained surgeons, such as a gynaecology oncologist, given the abnormal blood vessels feeding the placental site. The use of internal iliac balloons was not discussed due to the lack of strong evidence they are of benefit.

At operation, ureteric stents were put in place to aid the identification of the ureters at surgery. On opening the abdomen, a major degree of placenta accreta was diagnosed, the baby was delivered through a classical caesarean section incision, the uterine incision was closed to restore haemostasis and a difficult hysterectomy was performed. A cell saver was used to try to minimize the need for transfusion; however, the invasion of the placenta into the pelvic tissue resulted in the loss of 7 L of blood. Blood replacement with blood products to maintain clotting was transfused to the point that the maternal haemoglobin after operation was 87 g/L. Following delivery, the mother was debriefed and given counselling support. Mother was discharged on day 5, and baby was discharged after 10 days due to prematurity and slow feeding issues.

fails, a hysterectomy is required. The antenatal detection of an upper-segment placenta accreta spectrum disorder is uncommon, as the area of the accreta is usually small.

The placenta praevia accreta, where there is a placenta praevia and the placenta is abnormally attached over the area of a previous caesarean section scar, is one of the most lethal conditions in obstetrics. In this condition, the trophoblast grows into the scar tissue and may invade the serosa or the overlying bladder. Where the accreta involves more than a small section of the scar, massive haemorrhage may occur at delivery.

Abruptio placentae

Abruptio placentae or accidental haemorrhage is defined as haemorrhage resulting from premature separation of the placenta. The term *accidental* implies separation as the result of trauma, but most cases do not involve trauma and occur spontaneously.

Aetiology

The incidence of placental abruption varies from 0.6% to 7.0%, with the rate depending on the population studied. It occurs more frequently under conditions of social deprivation in association with dietary deficiencies, especially folate deficiency, and tobacco use. It is also associated with hypertensive disease, maternal thrombophilia, fetal growth restriction and a male fetus. Although motor vehicle accidents, falls, serious domestic violence and blows to the abdomen in later pregnancy are commonly associated with placental separation, trauma is a relatively uncommon cause. In the majority of cases, no specific predisposing factor can be identified for a particular episode. There is a high recurrence rate both within a pregnancy if delivery is not required with the first episode and in subsequent pregnancies.

The main fetal effect is a high perinatal mortality rate. In one study of 7.5 million pregnancies in the United States, the incidence of placental abruption has been recorded as 6.5/1000 births with a perinatal mortality in associated cases of 119/1000 births. Fetal prognosis is worst with maternal tobacco use.

Whatever factors predispose to placental abruption, they are well established before the abruption occurs.

Case study

Mandy, a 23-year-old primigravida, was admitted to hospital at 35 weeks' gestation with a complaint that she had developed severe abdominal pain followed by substantial vaginal bleeding. On examination, she was restless and in obvious pain. Her BP was 150/90 mmHg, and the uterus was rigid and tender. Her pulse rate was 100 beats/min, and she looked pale and tense. The uterine fundus was palpable at the level of the xiphisternum. The fetal lie was longitudinal, with the head presenting. The fetal heartbeat could not be detected, and the diagnosis of intrauterine fetal death was made using ultrasound. An IV line was established and blood cross-matched as a matter of urgency. Mandy was given pain relief, and her blood picture and clotting profile were examined. Vaginal examination showed that the cervix was effaced and 3 cm dilated and the membranes were bulging through the os. A forewater rupture was performed and blood-stained amniotic fluid was released. Labour ensued, and Mandy was delivered 3 hours later of a stillborn male infant. A large amount of clot was delivered with the placenta, and some 50% of the placenta appeared to have been avulsed from the uterine wall.

Clinical types and presentation

Although three types of abruption have been described, i.e. revealed, concealed or mixed (Fig. 8.10), this classification is not clinically helpful. Commonly the classification is made after delivery when the concealed clot is discovered.

Unlike placenta praevia, placental abruption presents with pain, vaginal bleeding of variable amounts and increased uterine activity.

Haemorrhage

Abruption involves separation of the placenta from the uterine wall and subsequent haemorrhage. The amount of haemorrhage revealed will depend on the site of the abruption. A bleed from the lower edge of the placenta will pass more easily through the cervical os than a bleed from the upper margin. Blood within the uterus causes an increase in the resting tone of the uterus and possibly the onset of contractions. The increased tone and blood clot may make palpation of the fetus and auscultation of the fetal heart difficult. The retained blood clot may also lead to abnormal consumption of maternal clotting factors and profuse bleeding.

It is important to realize that any pregnant woman presenting after 20 weeks with the sudden onset of abdominal pain and/or uterine contractions with or without significant bleeding may have suffered a placental abruption. Urgent assessment of the mother's BP, pulse and oxygenation is warranted, as she may have a large concealed bleed. If her pulse rate is above the measure of her systolic BP, e.g. pulse is 110 beats per minute and systolic BP is 80 mmHg, she could have lost 1 L or more of blood. If she bleeds further, she will become shocked with the development of marked tachycardia, hypotension and oliguria. She requires IV fluids, blood for full blood count and cross-matching, fetal CTG and/or ultrasound assessment of fetal welfare and placental status and possible visualization of blood in the uterus. Unfortunately, the visualization of fresh bleeding in the uterus can be difficult with ultrasound, so an abruption management should be based on clinical findings.

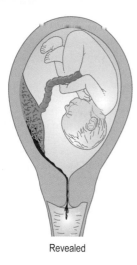
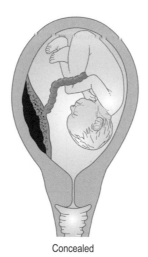
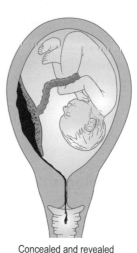

Revealed   Concealed   Concealed and revealed

Fig. 8.10 Types of placental abruption.

In some severe cases, haemorrhage penetrates through the uterine wall and the uterus appears bruised. This is described as a *Couvelaire uterus*. On clinical examination, the uterus will be tense and hard and the uterine fundus will be higher than is normal for the gestational age. With this severe form of abruption, the mother will often be in labour and in approximately 30% of cases the fetal heart sounds will be absent and the fetus will be stillborn.

The prognosis for the fetus in any abruption is dependent on the extent of placental separation and is inversely proportional to the interval between onset of the abruption and delivery of the baby. This means that early assessment and delivery in cases with fetal compromise are essential.

Clinical assessment/differential diagnosis

The diagnosis of abruption is made on the history of vaginal bleeding, abdominal pain, increased uterine tone and, commonly, the presence of a longitudinal lie of the fetus. The condition of the mother may be worse than the revealed blood would indicate. This must be distinguished from placenta praevia, where the haemorrhage is painless, the fetal lie is unstable with the uterus having a normal tone and an amount of blood loss that relates to maternal condition. Occasionally, however, some manifestations of placental abruption may arise where there is a low-lying placenta. In other words, placental abruption can arise where there is low placental implantation and, on these occasions, the diagnosis can only really be clarified by an ultrasound scan localizing the site of the placenta.

The diagnosis of abruption should also be differentiated from other acute emergencies such as acute hydramnios, where the uterus is enlarged, tender and tense but there is no haemorrhage. Other acute abdominal emergencies such

as perforated ulcer, volvulus of the bowel and strangulated inguinal hernia may simulate concealed placental abruption, but these problems are rare during pregnancy.

Management

The patient must be admitted to hospital and the diagnosis established on the basis of the history, examination findings (Fig. 8.11) and ultrasound findings. In pre-term pregnancy, mild cases (mother stable and CTG normal) may be treated conservatively. An ultrasound examination should be used to assess fetal growth and wellbeing, and the placental site should be localized to confirm the diagnosis. If the fetus is pre-term, the aim of management is to prolong the pregnancy if the maternal and fetal conditions allow. Conditions that are associated with abruption, e.g. hypertension, should be managed appropriately. If the haemorrhage is severe, resuscitation of the mother is the first prerequisite, following which fetal condition can be addressed.

It is often difficult to assess the amount of blood loss accurately, and IV infusion should be started with normal saline, Hartmann's solution or blood substitutes until blood is cross-matched and transfusion can be commenced. A urinary catheter is essential to monitor the urine output.

If the fetus is alive and close to term and there are no clinical signs of fetal compromise, or if the fetus is dead, induction of labour is performed as soon as possible and, where necessary, uterine activity is stimulated with an oxytocin infusion. Where the fetus is alive, the fetal heart should be monitored and caesarean section should be performed if signs of fetal compromise develop. If induction is not possible because the cervix is closed and maternal condition is unstable due to ongoing bleeding, or a maternal coagulopathy develops, delivery should be effected by caesarean section with senior

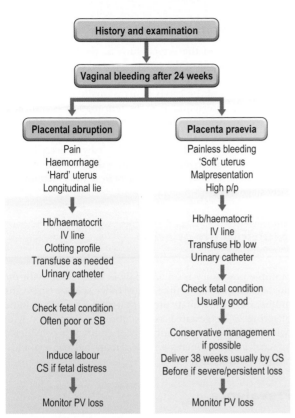

Fig. 8.11 Differential diagnosis and management of antepartum haemorrhage. *CS,* Caesarean section; *IV,* intravenous; *Hb,* Haemoglobin concentration; *p/p,* Presenting part; *PV,* per vaginum; *SB,* still birth.

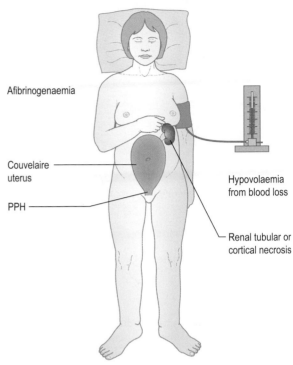

Fig. 8.12 Complications of placental abruption. *PPH,* Postpartum haemorrhage.

obstetric and anaesthetic staff present, whether or not the fetus is alive. Pain relief is achieved by the use of opiates. Epidural anaesthesia should not be used until a clotting screen is available and is seen to be normal.

If the fetus is pre-term and maternal and fetal conditions are stable, the mother should be admitted and monitored until all signs of bleeding and pain have settled. The mother may be discharged home 48 hours after blood loss has ceased and so long as any predisposing factors like hypertension have been adequately treated. Most units subsequently will induce labour at 37–38 weeks if the pregnancy remains stable.

Complications

The complications of placental abruption are summarized in Figure 8.12.

Afibrinogenaemia

Afibrinogenaemia occurs when the clot from a severe placental abruption causes the release of thromboplastin into the maternal circulation. This in turn may lead to DIC and the consumption of coagulation factors, including platelets, with the development of hypofibrinogenaemia or afibrinogenaemia. The condition may be treated by the infusion of fresh frozen plasma, platelet transfusion and fibrinogen transfusion after delivering the fetus. It may lead to abnormal bleeding at operative delivery or uncontrolled postpartum haemorrhage unless the clotting defect has been corrected. Given that replacing products with the placenta in place may worsen the maternal clotting status through the rapid production of fibrin degradation products, replacement should be timed to be given after the placenta has been delivered at caesarean section.

Renal tubular or cortical necrosis

This is a complication of undertreated hypovolaemia and DIC. A careful assessment of urinary output is essential. Anuria in a pregnant woman must be urgently and aggressively managed. If it is not, it may, on occasion, necessitate haemodialysis or peritoneal dialysis.

Other causes of antepartum haemorrhage

These are summarized in Figure 8.13.

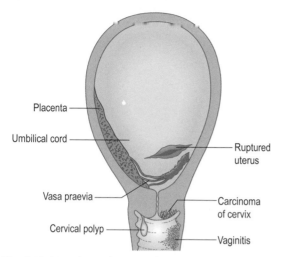

Placenta

Umbilical cord

Vasa praevia

Cervical polyp

Ruptured uterus

Carcinoma of cervix

Vaginitis

Fig. 8.13 Non-placental causes of antepartum haemorrhage.

Vasa praevia

Vasa praevia is a very rare condition where one of the branches of the fetal umbilical vessels lies in the membranes and across the cervical os. This occurs when there is a membranous insertion of the cord and the vessels course through the membranes to the placenta, or if there is succenturiate lobe of the placenta and the vessels in the membrane connect the main placental mass and the separate lobe. Rupture of the membranes over the cervical os may cause a tear in the vessels, which will result in the rapid exsanguination of the fetus. Vasa praevia can be diagnosed with colour Doppler ultrasound at the fetal anatomy scan.

Unexplained antepartum haemorrhage

In almost 50% of cases of women presenting with vaginal bleeding in pregnancy, it is not possible to make a definite diagnosis of abruption or placenta praevia.

Where the bleeding is confirmed to be coming from the uterine cavity, it is proposed that the cause is bleeding from the edge of the placenta. Whatever the cause, there is a significant increase in perinatal mortality, and it is therefore important to monitor placental function and fetal growth for the rest of the pregnancy. The pregnancy should not be allowed to proceed beyond term.

Vaginal infections

Vaginal moniliasis or trichomoniasis may cause blood-stained discharge and, once the diagnosis is established, should be treated with the appropriate therapy.

Cervical lesions

Benign lesions of the cervix, such as cervical polyps, are treated by removal of the polyp. Cervical erosions are best left untreated.

Carcinoma of the cervix is occasionally found in pregnancy. If the pregnancy is early, termination is indicated followed by staging of the cancer and definitive therapy. If the diagnosis is made late in pregnancy, the diagnosis should be established by biopsy, the baby delivered when mature and the lesion treated according to the staging, including caesarean section and radical hysterectomy for early-stage disease.

Multiple pregnancy

Multiple pregnancy is an anomaly in the human with the single-cavity uterus, unlike many other species where the mother has a bicornuate uterus that allows for two or more offspring to be gestated as the norm. A pregnancy with twins, triplets or higher numbers of embryos is considered high risk given the increased risk of maternal and fetal morbidity and mortality.

Prevalence

The prevalence of multiple pregnancies varies with race and the use of assisted reproductive techniques. The prevalence of natural twinning is highest in Central Africa, where there are up to 30 twin sets (60 twins) per 1000 live births, and lowest in Latin America and Southeast Asia, where there are only 6–10 twin sets per 1000 live births. North America and Europe have intermediate rates of 5–13 twin sets per 1000 live births. Between 1985 and 2005 the rates of twins more than doubled due to reproductive technologies. The twins resulted from ovulation induction and the replacement of more than one fertilized embryo in the in vitro fertilization (IVF) cycle. Given the risks of multiple pregnancy, the technique of replacing multiple embryos to enhance the conception rate has been abandoned, resulting in a fall in the rates of twins.

The natural prevalence of triplet pregnancy rate appears to have increased over the past 30 years. In 1985, the rate in the UK was 10.2/100,000, but in 2002–2006, the rate was close to 25/100,000. The cause of this rise is unclear. Higher multiple births such as quadruplets and quintuplets are commonly associated with the use of fertility drugs, but if one excludes this cause, figures for England and Wales suggest a pregnancy rate of 1.7/1,000,000 maternities.

The highest naturally occurring multiple pregnancy recorded so far is nonuplets.

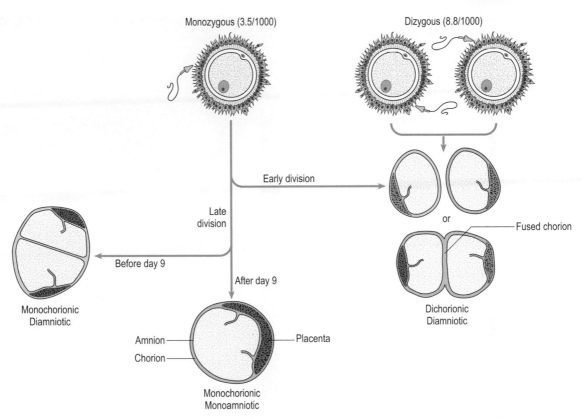

Fig. 8.14 Types of twinning, indicating the structure of the membranes and placentae. Note that twins of different sexes are always dizygous and those with a single chorion are always monozygous. Dichorionic twins of the same sex can be monozygous or dizygous.

Types of twinning and determination of chorionicity

Any multiple pregnancy may result from the release of one or more ova at the time of ovulation.

Monozygotic multiple pregnancy

If a single ova results in a multiple pregnancy, the embryos are called *monozygotic*, with alternative names of *uniovular* and *identical*. Both babies will have the same gender. The rate of monozygotic twins is approximately 1/280 pregnancies, is unaffected by race and is increased by reproductive technology for unknown reasons. The zygote divides some time after conception (Fig. 8.14). If the split postconceptually occurs at:

0–4 days there will be two embryos, two amnions and two chorions (as for dizygotic twins): 25–30%

4–8 days there will be two embryos, two amnions and one chorion: 65–70%

9–12 days there will be two embryos, one amnion and one chorion: 1–2%

13+ days there will be conjoined twins, one amnion and one chorion: <1%

Given that the embryo splits under some unknown influence, monozygotic multiple pregnancy is considered to be an anomaly of reproduction. Occasionally the embryo splits into three, resulting in monozygotic triplets. In the case of triplets, the splitting may occur at the same time or sequentially, resulting in conjoined twins with a separate singleton pregnancy all within one chorion!

The determination of monozygocity is undertaken at an early ultrasound scan, preferably before 14 weeks. A pregnancy where the zygote splits after 4 days will show a single thin membrane (monochorionic diamniotic) or no membrane (monochorionic monoamniotic) separating the two embryos and a single placental mass. If the split in the embryo was in the first 4 days, there may be two separate placental masses or a single mass with a membrane that is easier to visualize on ultrasound and which has a twin peak sign where the membrane and the placenta intersect. This appearance is the same as that for diamniotic dichorionic twins where there is a single placental mass. Early determination of zygosity is important, as it allows the caregiver to plan the management of the pregnancy. Genetic assessment of amniotic fluid, chorionic villous samples or postnatally obtained cord blood can be used to confirm zygosity. These techniques are seldom used in the face of modern ultrasound technology.

Dizygotic twins

These come from the separate fertilization of separate ova by different sperm. In 50% of such pregnancies the fetuses are male–female, with 25% being male–male and 25% being female–female. All will have either two separate placentas on ultrasound or a single placenta with a thick membrane with a 'twin peak' sign. The presence of a lambda (chorion in between membranes) or T (absence of chorion in between membranes) sign at the site of membrane insertion of the placenta in the first trimester is valuable in that it allows for the determination of whether a set of twins is monochorionic diamniotic or dichorionic diamniotic (Fig. 8.15). Monochorionic diamniotic twins are higher risk, as they may have placental vascular anastomosis, which may give rise to complications of twin-to-twin transfusion and its consequent sequelae. They also have a higher rate of fetal anomaly.

The rate of dizygotic twins varies with:
- *Familial factors:* The familial tendency is apparent in dizygotic twinning, but this appears to be on the maternal side only. In a study of records at Salt Lake City, the twinning rates of women who were themselves dizygotic twins was 17.1/1000 maternities compared with 11.6/1000 maternities for the general population, but the rate for males who were themselves dizygotic twins was only 7.9/1000 maternities.
- *Parity and maternal age:* Studies in Aberdeen have shown that the rate increases from 10.4/1000 in primigravidae to 15.3/1000 in the para 4+ group. There is also a small increase in twinning in older mothers.
- *Ovulation induction:* Multiple pregnancy is common following the use of drugs to induce ovulation. It is important to note that the use of gonadotrophin therapy can result in twins, triplets or even higher-order pregnancies. To some degree, this can be avoided by monitoring ovarian follicular development and withholding the injection of human chorionic gonadotrophin (which causes ovulation) if excessive numbers of follicles develop. The use of fertility drugs accounts for 10–15% of all multiple pregnancies and has therefore significantly altered the incidence of multiple pregnancy.

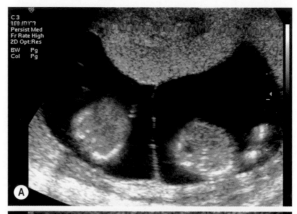

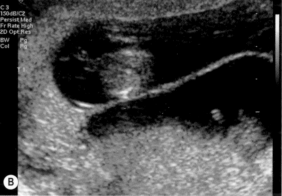

Fig. 8.15 Ultrasound figure demonstrating (A) T and (B) lambda sign.

As mentioned earlier, the risk of multiple pregnancy as a result of IVF has decreased with the limitation of the number of embryos transferred.

Complications of twin pregnancy

The normal processes of maternal physiological adaptation to pregnancy are exaggerated in the presence of twins (or a higher-order pregnancy). Total weight gain is, on average, 3.5 kg greater than in singleton pregnancy. There is an increase in red cell mass as in singleton pregnancies. However, this does not match the expansion in plasma volume that exceeds that of a singleton pregnancy by 17% at term, and a relative anaemia develops. The use of haemoglobin estimation to determine iron deficiency is therefore flawed, and serum ferritin should be used. Compared with singleton pregnancies, maternal cardiac output was greater by 20% because of an increase in stroke volume by 15% and heart rate by 3.5%.

It is thus to be expected that the increased strain put on the mother by carrying more than one fetus will result in a higher incidence of complications (Table 8.1).

Table 8.1 Risks associated with twin pregnancies

Obstetric complication	Risk*
Anaemia	×2
Pre-eclampsia	×3
Eclampsia	×4
Antepartum haemorrhage	×2
Postpartum haemorrhage	×2
Fetal growth restriction	×3
pre-term delivery	×6
Caesarean section	×2

*Approximate risk compared with singleton pregnancies.

Table 8.2 Rates of pre-term delivery by fetal number

Number of fetuses	<28 weeks
Singleton	0.7%
Twins	4.4%
Triplets	21.8%

Complications unrelated to zygosity

Nausea and vomiting
Early onset of nausea and vomiting is often the sign that points to a twin pregnancy before ultrasound confirmation. The incidence of vomiting in twins is significantly higher compared with that of singletons.

Anaemia
Twins are associated with extra metabolic demands on the mother. At a minimum, all mothers should consider iron and folate supplements throughout gestation.

Miscarriage
Resorption of a fetus between 6 and 10 weeks occurs in over 15% of twin pregnancies and is referred to as the *vanishing twin syndrome*. The incidence of threatened and actual miscarriage is higher in twins. Evidence from Aberdeen has shown that threatened miscarriage occurs in 26% of twin pregnancies and 20% of singleton pregnancies, and missed miscarriage between 10 and 14 weeks is twice that of singletons.

Antepartum haemorrhage
The incidence of antepartum haemorrhage as a result of abruption and placenta praevia doubles in twin pregnancies.

Pre-eclampsia
There is an increased incidence of gestational hypertension, pre-eclampsia and eclampsia in twin pregnancies. The rate in primigravidae is five times that of singletons, and in multigravidae, the rate is ten times that of women with singleton pregnancies.

Intrauterine growth restriction (IUGR)
In 20% of twins, one fetus is significantly smaller than the other as defined by a difference in the abdominal circumference of more than 20%. Given that this difference is impossible to detect clinically, regular ultrasound screening of growth and fetal wellbeing in twin pregnancies is mandatory.

Pre-term labour
The occurrence of pre-term labour is the most important complication of twin pregnancy (Table 8.2). The onset of labour before 37 weeks' gestation occurs in over 40% of twin pregnancies. The phenomenon appears to be associated with overdistension of the uterus associated with the presence of more than one fetus and is further increased if the amniotic fluid volume is increased.

Complications related to zygosity
Monozygotic twins have a higher perinatal mortality rate than dizygotic twins. This is due to a higher incidence of congenital abnormalities, pre-term delivery and abnormalities of placental vasculature including the twin–twin (fetofetal) transfusion syndrome.

Twin-to-twin transfusion syndrome (TTTS)
This syndrome arises in 10–15% of all monochorionic diamniotic twin pregnancies. In this condition, one fetus (the donor) transfuses the other (the recipient) through interlinked vascular channels in the placenta. Presentation occurs in the second trimester. The donor twin is oliguric and growth-restricted with oligohydramnios, and the recipient fetus exhibits polyhydramnios and is at risk of cardiomegaly and hydrops fetalis.

Without treatment, the perinatal mortality in significant TTTS exceeds 80%. Treatment options include serial amniocenteses to remove fluid from around the recipient twin, selective feticide or laser ablation, via a fetoscope, of the communicating vessels. Laser treatment has survival rates of 49–67%. If one twin dies in utero before laser treatment, the other twin also often dies as a result of acute haemodynamic changes.

Monoamniotic and conjoined twinning
Monoamnionicity occurs in 1% of monochorionic twins, and cord entanglement by 22 weeks is a common complication, such that survival rates are as low as 50%.

Conjoined twinning occurs in 1.3/100,000 births, with fusion occurring at different sites on the bodies of the fetuses. Whether any set of twins can be successfully separated and the outlook for a normal life after birth depend on the site of fusion, which is determined with tertiary-level ultrasound and magnetic resonance imaging (MRI) by 18–20 weeks' gestation. Where there is a major cardiovascular connection or a shared essential organ (heart, brain), perinatal death of at least one twin at separation is almost certain.

Prenatal diagnosis

The risk of structural abnormalities such as anencephaly and congenital heart defects is increased in multiple pregnancies, particularly with monozygotic babies. Determination of chorionicity, prenatal diagnosis and assessment for impending TTTS is particularly important and can be performed at the 12-week scan. Whereas an increase in the nuchal translucency in a dichorionic twin is more likely associated with a fetal anomaly/aneuploidy, a raised nuchal translucency in one of a monochorionic twin pair is often a warning of possible TTTS, given both twins have the same genetic makeup. Screening for abnormalities presents particular difficulties because of the need to differentiate between the two sacs, and all such screening should be referred to a specialist obstetric scanning centre.

> ! The missed diagnosis of twins and other multiple pregnancies was relatively common before the advent of modern ultrasound screening techniques and still occurs where such facilities are not available on a routine basis. Although the initial clinical diagnosis of twins was always made in the past on the basis of an abnormally enlarged uterus, such assessments were notoriously inaccurate. The real danger of undiagnosed twins is that oxytocic drugs are administered after delivery of the first twin, leading to entrapment of the second twin. This situation cannot be reversed even with the use of tocolytic drugs and often results in the death of or damage to the second twin. If there is any suspicion of undiagnosed twins and ultrasound is not available, do not give oxytocic drugs; palpate the maternal abdomen immediately after delivery of the first twin to ensure there is not a second baby still in the uterus.

Management of twin pregnancy

Multiple pregnancies exhibit every type of complication at a greater frequency than occurs in singleton pregnancy. Early diagnosis is therefore essential and provides a convincing argument for routine early-pregnancy ultrasound scanning (Fig. 8.16).

The commonest clinical sign of twin pregnancy is the greater size of the uterus, which is easier to detect in early,

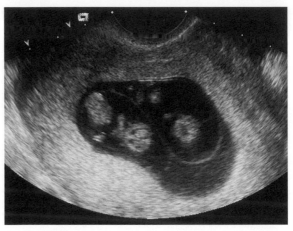

Fig. 8.16 Ultrasound scan of twins early in pregnancy. (Reproduced with permission from Leonard PC (2018) Building a Medical Vocabulary: With Spanish Translations, 10th edn. Elsevier, St Louis.)

rather than late, pregnancy. There are, of course, other reasons why the uterus may be abnormally enlarged, such as hydramnios and uterine fibroids.

Treatment of any antenatal complication is the same as in singleton pregnancies, but remember that the onset of complications, particularly pre-term labour and pre-eclampsia, tends to be earlier and of greater severity. Routine hospital admission from 28 weeks' gestation for bed rest has been advocated in the past, but clinical trials have failed to demonstrate efficacy. However, careful antenatal supervision and ultrasound examinations to detect fetal growth anomaly or TTTS should be undertaken 2 to 4-weekly. It is important that women with multiple pregnancies are booked for confinement where complications can be readily treated.

IUGR is common and, if detected, early induction of labour should be considered. The overall incidence of IUGR in one or both twins is 29%, involving 42% of monochorionic twins and 25% of dichorionic twins.

Management of labour and delivery

Delivery poses many difficulties in twin pregnancy because of the variety and complexity of presentations and because the second twin is at significantly greater risk from asphyxia due to placental separation and cord prolapse.

Presentation at delivery

There are a number of permutations for presentation in twin pregnancy at delivery, which are partly influenced by the management of the second twin. Rounded-up figures for these presentations are shown in Figure 8.17.

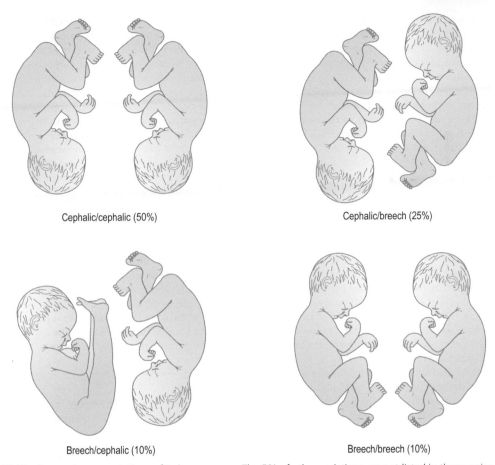

Cephalic/cephalic (50%) Cephalic/breech (25%)

Breech/cephalic (10%) Breech/breech (10%)

Fig. 8.17 The four major presentations of twin pregnancy. The 5% of other variations are not listed in these major groups.

By far the commonest presentation is cephalic (twin 1)/cephalic (twin 2) (50%), followed by cephalic/breech (25%), breech/cephalic (10%) and breech/breech (10%). The remaining 5% consist of cephalic/transverse, transverse/cephalic, breech/transverse, transverse/breech and transverse/transverse.

Method of delivery

A decision about the method of delivery should preferably be made before the onset of labour.

Caesarean section
The recent term twin trial looking at the safest way to deliver twins has shown that there is no indication for the routine delivery of twins by caesarean section when the first twin is presenting by the vertex. Delivery by elective caesarean section is indicated for the same reasons that exist for singleton pregnancies. However, the threshold for intervention is generally lower. Where an additional complication to the twinning exists, such as a previous caesarean scar, a long history of subfertility, severe pre-eclampsia or diabetes mellitus, most obstetricians will opt for elective caesarean section. Pre-term labour between 28 and 34 weeks' gestation is an indication for caesarean delivery to ensure the safe delivery of the second twin, as is malpresentation of the first twin. Furthermore, the presentation does have an important part to play in deciding the best method of delivery. Caesarean section rates for twins increased in the UK from 28% in 1980–1985 to 42% in 1995–1996, and in general, very few obstetricians now advise vaginal delivery for twin breech presentation or for a breech presentation of the first twin for fear of locked twins.

Vaginal delivery
When labour is allowed to proceed normally, it is advisable to establish an IV line at an early stage. Labour normally lasts the same length of time as a singleton labour.

115

Continuous fetal monitoring is advised to ensure the wellbeing of both babies. The first twin can be monitored on the CTG machine either with a scalp electrode or by abdominal ultrasound transducer, with the second being monitored by ultrasound. It is important to ensure that both fetal heart rates are being accurately monitored by ensuring the two recordings differ. When the first twin is delivered, the lie and presentation of the second twin must be immediately checked and the fetal heart rate recorded. If the lie of the second twin is not longitudinal, an experienced assistant at delivery should perform an external cephalic version (ECV) to stabilize the fetus either as a breech or cephalic presentation.

For delivery of the second twin, the membranes should be left intact until the presenting part is well into the pelvis and cord prolapse excluded. If the uterus does not contract within a few minutes, an oxytocin infusion should be started. If fetal heart rate anomalies occur, then delivery should be expedited by forceps delivery or breech extraction. For this reason, many obstetricians prefer an epidural anaesthetic to be placed in labour. Under very exceptional circumstances, it may be necessary to deliver the second twin by caesarean section. It is important to use oxytocic agents after the delivery of the second twin, as there is an increased risk of postpartum haemorrhage.

Not all obstetricians advocate immediate stimulation of the uterus after delivery of the first twin. It is reasonable to wait for the spontaneous onset of further contractions without further intervention if the fetal heart rate is normal. However, because of the ever-present risk of placental separation and intrauterine asphyxia in the second twin, an upper limit of 30 minutes between the two deliveries is generally accepted as reasonable practice. The delivery of an asphyxiated second twin after a long birth interval will always lead to the question as to why intervention did not take place at an earlier stage.

Higher-order multiple births such as triplets or quadruplets are now delivered by caesarean section. In these pregnancies, the onset of labour is often pre-term, the birth weights are low and the presentations uncertain.

Complications of labour

There are several complications of labour, some of which are associated with malpresentation. Babies may become obstructed, particularly where there is a transverse lie which is, in fact, an indication for delivery by caesarean section. If caesarean section is performed in the presence of an obstructed transverse lie, it may on occasions be preferable to make a vertical incision in the lower and upper segment rather than a transverse incision because of the possibility of extension of the lower segment incision into the uterine vessels and the broad ligaments, resulting in profuse haemorrhage.

As noted earlier, the vaginal delivery of twins requires the attendance of experienced practitioners. Once the first twin has been delivered, the attendant stabilizes the lie of the second twin via abdominal palpation to ensure it is longitudinal. An oxytocin infusion may then be needed to ensure the uterus contracts to cause the baby to descend into the pelvis. The fetal heart is auscultated throughout this process to ensure fetal welfare. If the baby presents by the vertex, the membranes are ruptured once the head is in the pelvis. If the baby is breech, in the absence of spontaneous descent, the attendant may need to hold the fetal foot after placing a hand into the uterus, rupture the membranes with a contraction and guide the foot and breech into the pelvis to effect delivery (if possible, the foot can be grasped with intact membranes to avoid cord prolapse). As this can be uncomfortable, as noted earlier, many attendants prefer, if the mother is agreeable, to have an epidural cannula in place during the labour of a twin pregnancy so adequate analgesia can be administered if the second stage becomes complicated. Very occasionally, after the delivery of the first twin, the placentae separate and attempt to deliver before the second baby. In this event, or in the event that the second baby cannot be delivered easily, a caesarean section must be urgently performed.

Case study

A 22-year-old woman in her first pregnancy with twins presented at 37 weeks' gestation in spontaneous labour. The presentation of both babies was cephalic. An epidural catheter was sited for analgesia, and labour progressed uneventfully, with the first twin delivering spontaneously. The presentation of the second twin was confirmed as cephalic with a longitudinal lie. As the presenting part was still above the pelvic brim, an oxytocin infusion was commenced to maintain uterine contractions, and the membranes were left intact awaiting descent of the presenting part. Shortly afterwards, external monitoring of the fetal heartbeat showed a bradycardia of 60 beats/min. Delivery of the second twin was expedited by reaching inside the uterus with the membranes still intact (internal podalic version), locating the feet of the fetus and rotating the fetus to the breech presentation before rupturing the membranes and delivering the infant by breech extraction.

Locked twins

This is a very rare complication, where the first twin is a breech presentation and the second is cephalic. Clinically, as the first twin descends during the delivery, the twins lock chin to chin. The condition is usually not recognized until delivery of part of the first twin has occurred and its survival is unlikely unless an urgent caesarean section is organized.

Twins where ultrasound reveals the first is presenting by the breech and the second by the vertex are often delivered by elective caesarean section.

Conjoined twins

The union of twins results from the incomplete division of the embryo after formation. Union may occur at any site but commonly is head-to-head or thorax-to-thorax. The antenatal assessment of the twins with tertiary-level ultrasound before 20 weeks allows for the prognosis to be determined and whether surgical separation may be attempted postnatally.

If the union is recognized by ultrasound before the onset of labour, then the twins should be delivered by caesarean section. If the abnormality is not recognized before the onset of labour, then the labour will usually obstruct.

Perinatal mortality

Approximately 10% of all perinatal mortality is associated with multiple pregnancies. Compared with a singleton pregnancy, the mortality rate increases with the number of fetuses: twins ×4 (monochorionicity ×8, with the second twin vs. first twin ×1.5); triplets ×8.

The commonest cause of death in both twins is prematurity. Over 50% of twins and 90% of triplets deliver before 37 weeks. Second-born twins are more likely to die from intrapartum asphyxia with separation of the placenta following delivery of the first twin, or where cord prolapse occurs in association with a malpresentation or a high presenting part when the membranes are ruptured.

Perinatal mortality rates for multiple pregnancy vary with access to high-level obstetric care, especially with monochorionic pregnancies. Overall, perinatal mortality rates in a multiple pregnancy in 2010 in Australia were 32.5, 52 and 231/1000 live and stillbirths for twins, triplets and higher multiple births, respectively. In comparison with singleton births of like gestational age, twins have a relative risk for low-birth-weight infants (<2.5 kg) of 4.3.

Perhaps of greater concern is the fact that the risk of producing a child with cerebral palsy is 8 times greater in twins and 47 times greater in triplets compared with singleton pregnancies.

Prolonged pregnancy

The terms *prolonged pregnancy*, *post-dates pregnancy* and *post-term pregnancy* are all used to describe any pregnancy that exceeds 294 days from the first day of the last menstrual period in a woman with a regular 28-day cycle.

Box 8.1 Post-maturity syndrome

Clinical features

- Dry, peeling and cracked skin, particularly on the hands and feet
- Absence of vernix caseosa and lanugo (fine hair)
- Loss of subcutaneous fat
- Meconium staining of the skin

Complications

- Increased perinatal mortality
- Intrapartum fetal distress
- Increased operative delivery rate
- Meconium aspiration

The term *post-maturity* refers to the condition of the infant and has characteristic features (Box 8.1). These are all indicators of intrauterine malnutrition and may therefore occur at any stage of the pregnancy if there is placental dysfunction. Post-maturity is often associated with oligohydramnios, an increased incidence of meconium in the amniotic fluid, and an increased risk of intrauterine aspiration of meconium-stained fluid into the fetal lungs. It is found in 2% of pregnancies at 41 weeks and up to 5% of pregnancies at 42 weeks. Unexpected stillbirth in such prolonged pregnancies is a particular tragedy for the mother, and she and her carer will always live with the knowledge that the child would almost certainly have survived had action to deliver the baby been taken earlier.

The accurate diagnosis of prolonged pregnancy varies with the method of dating. On the basis of the date of the last menstrual period, the incidence is about 10%, but by using accurate ultrasound dating in the first trimester this figure can be reduced to 1%. This provides a strong case for routine ultrasound dating in early pregnancy.

Aetiology

Prolonged pregnancy can be considered one end of the spectrum of normal pregnancy. However, the condition may be familial and is sometimes associated with abnormalities of the fetal adrenal–pituitary axis, as in anencephaly.

Management

Evidence in many large studies suggests an increase in perinatal mortality after 39 weeks that necessitates a close appraisal of every pregnancy at term to ensure continuation beyond 40 weeks is safe for the fetus. To do this, many units employ a postdate service where women present between 40 and 41 weeks for a CTG and amniotic fluid index (AFI) assessment. Those with a low AFI, taken as less than 5 cm, die at increased risk of post-maturity syndrome and fetal hypoxic morbidity. They are offered induction after counselling. For those with normal liquor and CTG, large studies have shown that whether a woman is induced at 41–42 weeks or whether the labour is allowed to start spontaneously, the caesarean section rates are the same. Many units will therefore have a policy of offering induction to all women by 41+5 weeks. Those women who decline induction need careful monitoring with frequent CTG and liquor volume assessment until delivery. Management in this form has resulted in reported fetal morbidity of close to zero.

Labour management

Should the decision be made to induce labour, this may in itself prove difficult, as the cervix is often unfavourable, with a Bishop's score of less than 3. In these circumstances, cervical preparation with prostaglandins or mechanical methods should be attempted. If this fails and the infant is large, it may on occasions be preferable to deliver the child by elective caesarean section.

Careful observation during labour is mandatory, as these are high-risk pregnancies.

Breech presentation

The incidence of breech presentation depends on the gestational age at the time of onset of labour. At 32 weeks, the incidence is 16%, falling to 7% at 36 weeks and 3–5% at term. Thus it is clear that the fetus normally corrects its own presentation, and attempts to correct the presentation before 37 weeks are generally unnecessary.

Types of breech presentation

The breech may present in one of three ways (Fig. 8.18):
- **Frank breech:** The legs lie extended along the fetal trunk and are flexed at the hips and extended at the knees. The buttocks will present at the pelvic inlet. This presentation is also known as an *extended breech*.
- **Flexed breech:** The legs are flexed at the hips and the knees with the fetus sitting on its legs so that both feet present to the pelvic inlet.
- **Knee or footling presentation:** One or both of the lower limbs of the fetus are flexed and breech of the baby is above the maternal pelvis so that a part of the fetal lower limb (usually feet) descends through the cervix into the vagina.

The position of the breech is defined using the fetal sacrum as the denominator. At the onset of labour, the breech enters the brim of the true pelvis with the bitrochanteric diameter (less than 10 cm) being the diameter of

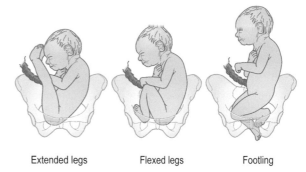

Extended legs   Flexed legs   Footling

Fig. 8.18 Types of breech presentation.

descent. This diameter is slightly smaller than the biparietal diameter in the full-term fetus. The type of breech presentation has a significant impact on the risk of vaginal breech delivery. The more irregular the presenting part, the greater the risk of a prolapsed cord or limb. A foot pressing into the vagina below the cervix may stimulate the mother to bear down before the cervix is fully dilated, which leads to entrapment of the head in the cervix (see Fig. 8.18).

Causation and hazards of breech presentation

Breech presentation is common before 37 weeks' gestation, but most infants will turn spontaneously before term (as previously discussed). Breech presentation may, however, be associated with factors such as multiple pregnancy, congenital abnormalities of the maternal uterus, fetal malformation, fetal hypotonia secondary to medication use and placental location, either placenta praevia or cornual implantation.

There is also evidence to suggest that persistent breech presentation may be associated with the inability of the fetus to kick itself around from breech to vertex and that there may therefore be some neurological impairment of the lower limbs (Box 8.2).

> **!** There is a higher incidence of neurological impairment in breech babies even when delivered by caesarean section, although the overall risk is still less than 1%.

Delivery by the breech carries some specific hazards to the infant compared with normal vertex presentation, particularly in pre-term infants and in infants with a birth weight in excess of 4 kg:
- There is an increased risk of cord compression and cord prolapse because of the irregular nature of the presenting part. This is particularly the case where the legs are flexed or there is a footling presentation.

- Entrapment of the head behind the cervix is a particular risk with the pre-term infant, in whom the bitrochanteric diameter of the breech is significantly smaller than the biparietal diameter of the head. This means that the trunk may deliver through an incompletely dilated cervix, resulting in entrapment of the larger head. If the delivery is significantly delayed, the child may be asphyxiated and either die or suffer brain damage.
- The fetal skull does not have time to mould during delivery and therefore, in both pre-term and term infants, there is a significant risk of intracranial haemorrhage.
- Trauma to viscera may occur during the delivery process, with rupture of the spleen or gut if the obstetrician handles the fetal abdomen.

Management

Antenatal management

Because of the risks to the fetus of breech birth, the best option is to avoid vaginal breech delivery through accurate diagnosis and performance of ECV.

External cephalic version

Indication
Breech presentation persisting after 36 weeks' gestation.

Contraindications
ECV should not be attempted where there is a history of antepartum haemorrhage, where there is placenta praevia, where there is a significant nuchal cord, where the CTG is abnormal, where there is a previous uterine scar or where the pregnancy is multiple. It is also pointless to turn the infant if the intention is to deliver the child by elective caesarean section for some other indication.

Technique
The mother rests supine with the upper body slightly tilted down. The presentation of the fetus and placental position are confirmed by ultrasound. The fetal heart rate is checked, preferably with a small strip of CTG. A tocolytic agent (oral nifedipine or subcutaneous terbutaline SC terbutaline) is given to relax the uterus, as this improves the success rate (Fig. 8.19).

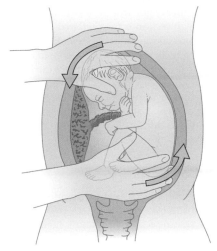

Fig. 8.19 External cephalic version: pressure is applied in the opposite direction to the two fetal poles.

The breech is disimpacted from the pelvic brim and shifted to the lower abdomen, and the fetus is gently rotated, keeping the head flexed. The fetal heart rate should be checked during the procedure.

It is essential not to use excessive force and, if there is evidence of fetal bradycardia, the fetus should be returned to the original presentation if the version is not past the halfway point and the fetus monitored with continuous CTG. Anti-D should be administered to the patient who has Rhesus-negative blood group.

Complications

The risks of the procedure are cord entanglement, placental abruption and rupture of the membranes. Persistent fetal bradycardia occurs in approximately 1%, and this may necessitate urgent delivery by caesarean section. There is some evidence to suggest that even where external version is successful, the section rate is higher than normal due to dystocia and fetal compromise. ECV is successful in up to 50% of cases in the best hands.

Where a breech presentation persists near term, the mother should be counselled about her delivery options (see later). If she wishes to consider a vaginal breech delivery, it is important to consider issues that may impede that delivery, like the size and shape of the maternal pelvis and a macrosomic fetus.

Although the size and shape of the maternal pelvis can be assessed by pelvic examination or formally using MRI, neither technique has been shown to be accurate in determining the possible success of a breech delivery.

Fetal size can be assessed by ultrasound. If the fetal gestational age is less than 32 weeks and more than 28 weeks, the birth weight will be less than 2 kg, and delivery by caesarean section is the preferred option. If, later in pregnancy, the fetal weight is assessed to be in excess of 3.8 kg, then delivery by section is the preferred option, but it must be remembered that such estimates can be unreliable. Other contraindications for breech delivery are where there is fetal anomaly, a footing breech, a deflexed fetal head, a low-lying placenta, abnormal fetal welfare tests or an acute maternal condition like placental abruption/severe pre-eclampsia.

Method of delivery

In 2000, the term breech trial was published, which suggested that the delivery of the breech-presenting fetus was safest by caesarean section. As a result, many units now no longer perform vaginal delivery of the breech. Since that time, considerable literature has shown that the trial had methodological issues and the conclusions may not have been justified. Some units therefore reintroduced vaginal breech delivery as a safe option in selected cases (see earlier), where obstetricians with the appropriate expertise for assisting delivery are available and the mother is keen to pursue this option.

Vaginal breech delivery

The first stage of labour should be no different from labour in a vertex presentation. Epidural analgesia is the preferred method of pain relief but is not essential. The woman should be advised to attend hospital as soon as contractions commence or the membranes rupture, and vaginal examination should be performed on admission to exclude cord presentation or prolapsed cord. The presence of meconium-stained liquor has exactly the same significance as with a vertex presentation except in the second stage of labour, when descent of the breech will often result in the passage of meconium.

Technique

When the cervix is fully dilated and the presenting part is low in the pelvis, the mother is encouraged to bear down with her contractions until the fetal buttocks and anus come on view (Fig. 8.20). To minimize soft tissue resistance, an episiotomy should be considered under either local or epidural anaesthesia, unless the pelvic floor is already lax and offers little resistance. The legs are then lifted out of the vagina by flexing the fetal hip and knees. The baby is then expelled with maternal pushing, with the obstetrician only touching the upper thighs and then only to ensure that the fetal back remains anterior. Once the trunk has delivered as far as the scapula, the arms can usually be easily delivered one at a time by sliding the fingers over the shoulder and sweeping them downwards

across the fetal head. If the arms are extended and pose difficulty in delivering, the body of the fetus is rotated by holding the baby's pelvis until the posterior arm comes under the symphysis pubis. The arm can then be delivered by flexing at the elbow and the shoulders. The procedure is repeated by rotating the body to deliver the other arm (Loveset's manoeuvre). The trunk is then allowed to remain suspended for about 30 seconds to allow the head to enter the pelvis and then the legs are grasped and swung upwards through an arc of 180 degrees until the child's mouth comes into view. At this point, the baby may spontaneously deliver; however, a number of techniques, including the use of forceps, can be used to ensure the safe delivery of the head. The time taken for the delivery from the legs to the head should be no more than 4 minutes to ensure neonatal wellbeing.

After the baby is delivered, the cord is then clamped and divided and the third stage is completed in the usual way.

The essence of good breech delivery is that progress should be continuous and handling of the fetus must be minimal and as gentle as possible.

Possible complications occur with poor technique and allowing the mother to push before full dilatation of the cervix.

Caesarean section

Delivery by caesarean section is indicated if the estimated birth weight is greater than 3.8 kg, for footling presentations or where the head is deflexed on ultrasound, where there is no obstetrician with available expertise in vaginal breech delivery or where there is an additional complication such as severe pre-eclampsia, fetal growth restriction, placental abruption, placenta praevia or a previous caesarean section. If the birth weight is calculated to be less than 700 g, the perinatal outcome both in terms of mortality and morbidity is poor irrespective of the method of delivery therefore.

Although there has been no large randomized trial of caesarean section for very-low-birth-weight infants, descriptive studies in some very large series show some improved outcome where the infant is delivered in this way. Caesarean section is currently the method of choice for delivery of very-low-birth-weight infants presenting as a breech.

Normally, the technique used is LUSCS. However, with a pre-term infant, the lower segment may not have formed, and, under these circumstances, the preferred method is a midline incision through that part of the lower segment that is formed; a classical (upper uterine longitudinal) incision may on occasions be the incision of choice. In very-low-birth-weight infants, the buttocks and trunk are substantially narrower than the head, and entrapment of

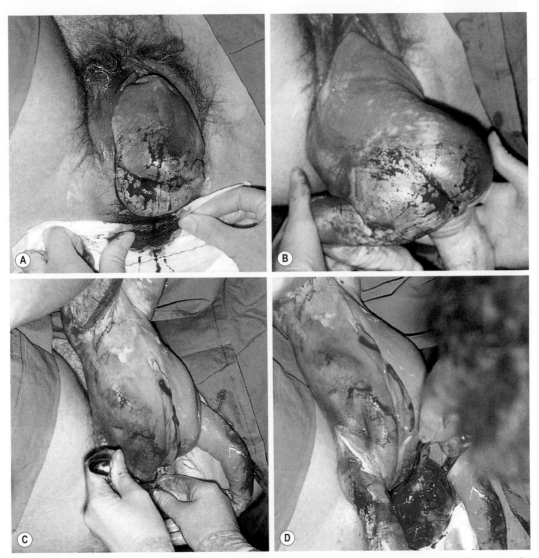

Fig. 8.20 Breech presentation. (A) Buttock on view. (B) Trunk expelled. (C) and (D) Forceps applied to aftercoming head.

the head may occur at the time of delivery through the uterine incision unless an adequate incision is made.

Unstable lie, transverse lie and shoulder presentation

An unstable lie is one that is constantly changing. It is commonly associated with multiparity, where the maternal abdominal wall is lax, low placental implantation or uterine anomalies such as a bicornuate uterus, uterine fibroids and polyhydramnios.

Complications

If an unstable lie resulting in a transverse lie persists until the onset of labour, it may result in prolapse of the cord or a shoulder presentation and a prolapsed arm or a compound presentation when both an arm and a leg may present (Fig. 8.21).

Management

No action is necessary in an unstable lie until 37 weeks' gestation unless the labour starts spontaneously. It is important to look for an explanation by ultrasound scan for

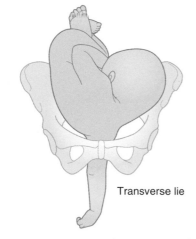

Transverse lie

Shoulder presentation

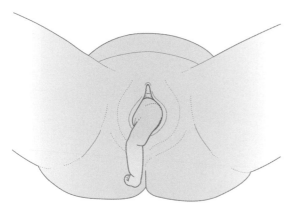

Anterior arm presentation

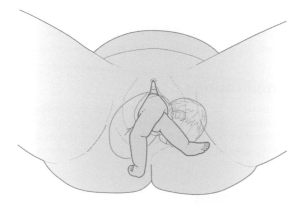

Anterior arm and leg presentation

Fig. 8.21 Prolapse of the arm into the vagina, sometimes resulting in a shoulder presentation.

> **Box 8.3 Management of unstable lie**
>
> - Exclude causes that are fixed
> - Hospitalization at 37 weeks
> - Stabilizing induction at term
> - Be prepared for cord prolapse

placental localization, the presence of any pelvic tumours (fibroids/low-lying placenta/ovarian cyst in the pouch of Douglas) and the presence of fetal abnormalities. However, it must be remembered that, in most cases, no obvious cause is found.

After 37 weeks, in the absence of any cause, an attempt should be made to correct the lie by ECV. It is advisable to admit the mother to hospital by 39 weeks' gestation if the unstable lie persists in case spontaneous rupture of the membranes occurs accompanied by a prolapse of the cord. Admission will allow for rapid delivery by caesarean section.

Assuming that no specific factor such as a low-lying placenta can be identified, the approach may take one of three courses:

- Keep the mother in hospital and await spontaneous correction of the lie, or correct the lie as labour starts spontaneously.
- Stabilize induction, performed by first correcting the lie to a cephalic presentation and then rupturing the membranes as the head approaches the pelvic brim assisted by gentle suprapubic pressure, followed by oxytocin infusion.
- Delivery by caesarean section at term.

If there are any other complicating factors, it may on occasions be advisable to deliver the mother at term by planned elective section (Box 8.3).

If the mother arrives in established labour with a shoulder presentation or prolapsed arm, no attempt should be made to correct the presentation or to deliver the child vaginally; delivery should be effected by caesarean section. Sometimes, if the arm is wedged into the pelvis, it may be safer to deliver the child through a classic or midline upper segment incision rather than through a lower segment incision as, in these cases, there may be little lower segment formed.

Essential information

Hypertension in pregnancy

- Commonest complication of pregnancy in the most developed countries
- Gestational hypertension – hypertension alone after 20 weeks or within 24 hours of delivery in a previously normotensive woman
- Pre-eclampsia – hypertension and proteinuria after 20 weeks
- Eclampsia – pre-eclampsia plus convulsions, up to 48 hours after delivery
- Pathogenesis of pre-eclampsia uncertain – increase in angiotensin II receptors, endothelial dysfunction, decreased antioxidants all contribute
- Management of pre-eclampsia
  - Bed rest
  - Antihypertensive drug therapy
- Management of eclampsia
  - Control of fits
  - Control of BP
  - Deliver infant by induction of labour or caesarean section

Antepartum haemorrhage

- Vaginal bleeding after 24 weeks

Placenta praevia

- Lower segment implantation
- Incidence 1%
- Classification – marginal, central and lateral
- Diagnosis – painless loss, unstable lie, soft uterus
- Diagnosis confirmed by ultrasound or MRI
- Diagnosis – rule out placenta accreta spectrum if mother has a caesarean section scar
- Management – conservative until 37 weeks unless placenta accreta spectrum
- Hospital admission for all major degrees
- Blood held – cross-matched
- Caesarean section unless grade 1
- Prognosis for the fetus – good
- Rule out placenta accreta spectrum if there is a previous caesarean scar

Placenta accreta spectrum

- Abnormally adherent placenta usually onto a previous caesarean scar
- Diagnosis made by 28 weeks' gestation
- Care at high-risk centre
- Anticipate massive blood loss at delivery
- Deliver by 35 weeks
- Commonly requires hysterectomy after delivery of the fetus

Placental abruption

- Incidence 0.6–7%
- Diagnosis – uterus hypertonic, tender
- Normal fetal lie
- Commonly associated with maternal hypertension
- Management – replace blood loss
  - Check for DIC
  - Deliver the infant if abruption severe
  - Prognosis for fetus poor
- Maternal complications
  - Afibrinogenaemia
  - Renal tubular necrosis

Other causes

- Cervical and vaginal lesions
- Vasa praevia

Prevalence of multiple pregnancy

- Monozygous twin rates constant
- Dizygous rates increasing

Prolonged pregnancy

- Is associated with increase in perinatal mortality
- Is associated with increased incidence of meconium
- Management options are
  - Routine induction after 41 weeks
  - Increased monitoring

Breech presentation

- Occurs in 3% of pregnancies at term
- Associated with
  - Pre-term delivery
  - Multiple pregnancy
  - Fetal abnormality
  - Placenta praevia
  - Uterine abnormalities
- ECV at 37 weeks
- Elective caesarean section
- Criteria for vaginal delivery are
  - Fetal weight more than 1.5 kg, less than 4 kg
  - Flexed or frank breech
  - Flexed head

Unstable lie

- Associated with
  - High parity
  - Polyhydramnios
  - Uterine anomalies
  - Low-lying placenta

Chapter | 9 |

Maternal medicine

Suzanne V. F. Wallace and David James

LEARNING OUTCOMES

After studying this chapter you should be able to:

Knowledge criteria

- Describe the aetiology, risk factors, risks and management of:
  - Anaemia in pregnancy
  - Gestational diabetes
  - Infections in pregnancy
  - Thromboembolic disease in pregnancy
  - Liver disease
- Contrast the clinical presentation and management of pre-existing medical conditions in pregnancy, including:
  - Diabetes
  - Obesity
  - Thrombophilias
  - Epilepsy
  - Thyroid disease
  - Cardiac disease
  - Respiratory disease
  - Renal disease
  - Haemoglobinopathies
- Discuss the role of pre-conceptual counselling for women with pre-existing illness and the risks and modifications required to continue drug treatment during pregnancy

Clinical competencies

- Explain to the mother the causes and plan the management of minor complaints of pregnancy, including:
  - Abdominal pain
  - Heartburn
  - Constipation
  - Backache
  - Syncope
  - Varicosities
  - Carpal tunnel syndrome

Introduction

Maternal medicine encompasses the spectrum of medical conditions a woman can present with in pregnancy. Some of these may pre-date pregnancy and others may develop during pregnancy. Currently in the UK, with improvements in other areas of obstetric care, most maternal deaths are now caused by medical conditions. In the most recent edition of the *UK and Ireland Confidential Enquiries into Maternal Deaths and Morbidity 2013–15*, venous thromboembolism was responsible for maternal death in 1.13 per 100,000 maternities, whilst cardiac disease was responsible for maternal death in 2.34 per 100,000 maternities.

There are an increasing number of women with medical conditions in pregnancy. Women with significant pre-existing medical conditions that in the past may have led to voluntary or involuntary infertility (for example, cystic fibrosis (CF)) are now becoming pregnant in increasing numbers. In addition, more women are older when embarking on pregnancy and have more acquired problems such as obesity and hypertension.

Whether a woman is known to have a medical condition prior to pregnancy or develops one within pregnancy, the key to successful management is to have a framework to ensure that all the implications of the condition are considered (Fig. 9.1). This enables robust pregnancy plans to be made whether a disease is common or rare.

> Multidisciplinary and multi-professional team-working are also essential elements in caring for these women.

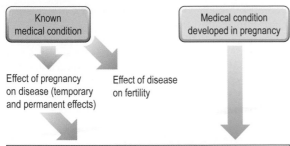

Effect of disease on pregnancy		
	Maternal risks/complications	Fetal/neonatal risks/complications
First trimester		
Second trimester		
Third trimester		
Labour		
Delivery		
Postnatal		
Medication issues		

Fig. 9.1 Framework for medical disorders in pregnancy.

Minor complaints of pregnancy

Minor complaints of pregnancy, by definition, do not cause significant medical problems. However, minor medical complaints are often not perceived as minor by the women affected and can have considerable impact on a woman's quality of life in pregnancy. In addition, many of the symptoms of minor conditions of pregnancy are the same as those of significant pathological diseases that need to be excluded. Symptoms frequently relate to physiological adaptations of the body to pregnancy, and women should be reassured (once pathology has been excluded) that these symptoms represent normal pregnancy changes.

Abdominal pain

Abdominal pain or discomfort is common in pregnancy and is usually transient and physiological. However, it is important to identify cases where there may be a pathological cause. ✔️

The physiological causes include:
- stretching of the abdominal ligaments and muscles
- Braxton Hicks ('practice') contractions

- pressure of the gravid uterus on the abdominal contents
- constipation

It is important to differentiate physiological abdominal pain from pathological causes in women with severe, atypical or recurrent pain. These include:
- early pregnancy problems such as ectopic pregnancy and miscarriage
- gynaecological causes such as ovarian torsion
- urinary tract infection
- surgical causes such as appendicitis and pancreatitis
- later obstetric causes such as placental abruption and labour

Social causes, particularly domestic abuse, should be considered in women who present with recurrent episodes of abdominal pain where organic pathology has been excluded.

Once a pathological cause has been excluded, reassurance is often a successful management option and analgesics are rarely required.

Heartburn

Gastro-oesophageal reflux is more likely to occur in pregnancy because of delayed gastric emptying, reduced lower oesophageal sphincter pressure and raised intragastric pressure. It affects up to 80% of pregnant women, particularly in the third trimester. The differential diagnoses are:
- other causes of chest pain such as angina, myocardial infarction and muscular pain
- causes of upper abdominal pain that can mimic reflux, for example, pre-eclampsia, acute fatty liver of pregnancy (AFLP) and gallstones

Conservative management includes dietary advice to avoid spicy and acidic foods and to avoid eating just prior to bed. Symptoms can be improved by changing sleeping position to a more upright posture. If conservative measures are not successful, antacids are safe in pregnancy and can be used at any time. Histamine-receptor blockers, such as ranitidine, and proton pump inhibitors have a good safety profile in pregnancy and can be used if antacids alone are insufficient to improve symptoms.

Constipation

Constipation is postulated to be more common in pregnancy because of both elevated progesterone levels slowing colonic motility and the pressure of the uterus on the rectum. It is particularly common in the first trimester. It can be exacerbated by oral iron supplements, frequently taken in pregnancy.

Women should be advised to increase their fluid and dietary fibre intake. Most osmotic and stimulant laxatives are safe in pregnancy and can be considered if conservative management is unsuccessful. Rarely, severe constipation can be a cause of unstable lie in late pregnancy by preventing the fetal head from descending into the pelvis.

Backache

Backache is a very common pregnancy complaint, especially as pregnancy advances. The commonest cause is a combination of pressure from the gravid uterus causing an exaggerated lumbar lordosis and a hormonal effect on the supporting soft tissues. Differential diagnoses include urinary tract infection, pyelonephritis and early labour.

Physiotherapy review can help by advising on posture and appropriate stretches and exercises. Simple analgesics may be required. Whilst paracetamol and codeine formulations are safe in pregnancy, aspirin and non-steroidal anti-inflammatory medication should be avoided. One disadvantage of codeine is that it can cause constipation.

Syncope

Physiological vasodilatation from the effects of progesterone on the vascular smooth muscle causes a pooling of blood in dependent areas, causing postural hypotension that can lead to syncope. Later in pregnancy, caval compression from the gravid uterus can occur (from around 20 weeks' gestation), reducing further the venous return to the heart and precipitating hypotension. Whilst syncope in pregnancy is usually benign, if it is recurrent anaemia, hypoglycaemia, dehydration and arrhythmias should be excluded.

Women should be advised to sit for a while prior to standing when getting up from a lying position and to avoid prolonged standing; later in pregnancy, lying supine should be avoided to reduce caval compression and supine hypotension. Dehydration should be avoided.

Varicosities

Varicosities in the legs or vulva may worsen or appear de novo because of a combination of pressure on the pelvic veins from the gravid uterus reducing venous return from lower limb veins and the progestogenic effect on relaxing the vascular smooth muscle. Their appearance is usually diagnostic but if painful then thrombophlebitis and deep vein thrombosis (DVT) should be excluded.

Elevating the legs while sitting or lying may improve symptoms. The use of compression stockings can both alleviate symptoms and reduce the risk of venous thromboembolism from stasis in the dilated veins. If severe varicosities are present and there are other risk factors for venous thromboembolism, heparin prophylaxis may need to be considered.

Carpal tunnel syndrome

Fluid retention occurs in pregnancy due to increased capillary permeability. This can cause or worsen carpal tunnel syndrome through compression of the median nerve as it travels through the carpal tunnel.

Wrist splints that reduce wrist flexion are usually the mainstay of treatment in the majority of cases. In severe cases steroid injections are occasionally required and can be given in pregnancy. Surgical release of the carpal tunnel ligament is rarely required with pregnancy-related carpal tunnel syndrome, as most resolve post-pregnancy.

Pelvic girdle dysfunction (symphyseal pelvic dysfunction, SPD)

Raised levels of relaxin in pregnancy increase joint mobility to allow expansion of the pelvic ring for birth. However, in some women, this effect can be exaggerated and cause discomfort either at the symphysis, the hip or at other points around the pelvis; this usually worsens with increasing gestation. Women often describe characteristic pain on walking or standing with tenderness over the pelvic ring. Urinary tract infection should be excluded with anterior pain.

Physiotherapists will advise on exercises to improve stability, techniques for minimizing symptoms during daily activities and positions for birth. A pelvic girdle support may improve symptoms. As with back pain, simple analgesics can be used. The problem usually resolves after pregnancy.

Medical problems arising in pregnancy

Anaemia

Anaemia commonly occurs in pregnancy. While in many developed countries it is mild and quickly and easily treated, resulting in minimal complications, in some countries, it is severe and a major contributor to maternal death.

Aetiology

Pregnancy causes many changes in the haematological system, including an increase in both plasma volume and red cell mass; the former is greater than the latter, with the result that a 'physiological anaemia' often occurs. There is an increased iron and folate demand to facilitate both the increase in red cell mass and fetal requirements, which is not always met by maternal diet. Iron-deficiency anaemia is thus a common condition encountered in pregnancy, particularly in the third trimester. Table 9.1 shows the changes in haemoglobin and red cell parameters in normal pregnancy.

Table 9.1 Haemoglobin and red cell indices (mean and calculated 2.5th–97.5th percentile reference ranges)

Red cell indices	Gestation			
	18 weeks	32 weeks	39 weeks	8 weeks postpartum
Haemoglobin (Hb) g/L	119 (106–133)	119 (104–135)	125 (109–142)	133 (119–148)
Red cell count × 10¹²/L	3.93 (3.43–4.49)	3.86 (3.38–4.43)	4.05 (3.54–4.64)	4.44 (3.93–5.00)
Mean cell volume (MCV) fL	89 (83–96)	91 (85–97)	91 (84–98)	88 (82–94)
Mean cell haemoglobin (MCH) pg	30 (27–33)	30 (28–33)	30 (28–33)	30 (27–32)
Mean cell haemoglobin concentration (MCH) g/dL	34 (33–36)	34 (33–36)	34 (33–36)	34 (33–36)
Haematocrit	0.35 (0.31–0.39)	0.35 (0.31–0.40)	0.37 (0.32–0.42)	0.39 (0.35–0.44)

Reproduced with permission from Shepard, MJ, Richards VA, Berkowitz RL, et al. (1982) An evaluation of two equations for predicting fetal weight by ultrasound. Am J Obstet Gynecol 142:47–54. © 1982 Elsevier.

Risk factors

Pre-pregnancy risk factors are those associated with chronic anaemia:

- iron deficiency secondary to poor diet
- menorrhagia
- short interval between pregnancies
- presence of anaemic conditions, such as sickle cell disease, thalassaemia and haemolytic anaemia

Risk factors within pregnancy include multiple pregnancy due to the increased iron demand in multiple pregnancy scenarios.

Clinical features and diagnosis

Anaemia is often identified as the result of routine full blood count measurements. Some women will present with symptoms such as shortness of breath and lethargy. There is a variation in normal haemoglobin levels in pregnancy and a gradual fall as pregnancy progresses. Anaemia can be diagnosed with a haemoglobin level less than 100 g/L in the first trimester and less than 105 g/L in the second and third trimesters.

Implications for pregnancy

Iron-deficiency anaemia mainly affects the mother. With mild anaemia, the fetus is usually unaffected despite the reduced oxygen-carrying capacity of the mother. However, the baby is more likely to have iron deficiency in the first year of life because of a lack of development of fetal iron stores in utero. With severe anaemia, there is an increased risk of pre-term birth and low birth weight and possibly greater blood loss at delivery.

The implications to the mother in all trimesters are the risk of developing symptomatic anaemia that can cause fatigue, reduced work performance and an increase in susceptibility to infections. If anaemia persists to the time of delivery, there will be a lack of reserve if significant blood loss occurs. There is a strong association between severe anaemia and maternal mortality. The risk of requiring blood transfusions peripartum is also raised.

Management

Prompt recognition and treatment of developing anaemia optimize a woman's haemoglobin levels in pregnancy and reduce the risk of commencing labour anaemic.

 Although most anaemia in pregnancy is secondary to iron deficiency, consideration should be given as to whether there is an underlying anaemia condition or if folate deficiency could also be involved.

If there is clinical suspicion that iron deficiency is not the cause of the anaemia or if a woman has failed to respond to iron supplementation, then the iron status should be assessed by either ferritin or zinc protoporphyrin levels, folate measured and haemoglobin electrophoresis performed to exclude haemoglobinopathies. Oral iron supplementation is recommended as first-line treatment. This is better absorbed if taken with ascorbic acid (for example, orange juice) and if tea and coffee are avoided at the time of ingestion. Dietary advice should also be given. Compliance with iron supplementation is often poor due to the side effects of constipation and gastric irritation. If iron is either not tolerated or if improvements in haemoglobin are not seen despite iron therapy, then parenteral iron can be considered. Sometimes a blood transfusion is considered if the anaemia is severe and it is diagnosed close to delivery.

Adequate continued postnatal treatment is essential to reduce the risk of a woman entering a further pregnancy anaemic.

B_{12} deficiency is extremely rare in pregnancy, but if it is diagnosed, treatment is with oral or parenteral B_{12} supplementation.

Prophylaxis

Routine iron supplementation (usually combined with folic acid) throughout pregnancy may reduce the risk of iron deficiency. This is currently not a routine recommendation in the UK due to the lack of evidence of improved outcomes. In some other countries where iron deficiency is common, this is standard practice.

Gestational diabetes

Gestational diabetes is an increasingly common antenatal condition occurring in up to 9% of all pregnancies in Western countries. However, the prevalence is much higher in at-risk populations (e.g. Asian or obese women).

Aetiology

Pregnancy induces a diabetogenic state. This is predominantly because of increased resistance to the actions of insulin due to the placental production of the anti-insulin hormones (human placental lactogen, glucagon and cortisol), though the increased production of maternal glucocorticoids and thyroid hormones during pregnancy also contributes to this. In response, the maternal pancreas must increase its production of insulin to combat this. In some women this is not achieved, and gestational diabetes is the result.

Risk factors

Risk factors are the same as those for type 2 diabetes and are listed in Box 9.1. This list is taken from the NICE Clinical Guideline 'Diabetes in pregnancy' (2008, amended 2015). The guideline only recommends that some of the risk factors be used for screening in practice. The presence of one or more of these risk factors should lead to the offer of a 75-g oral glucose tolerance test (OGTT). However, many clinicians feel that the presence of any risk factor, rather than a subset, should trigger the offer of an OGTT.

Clinical features and diagnosis

Gestational diabetes may be asymptomatic. As such, a screening programme needs to be in place that can either be universal or selective. Most units prefer a selective approach for practical and financial reasons. Selective screening is offered

---

> ### Box 9.1 **Women at increased risk of glucose intolerance in pregnancy**
>
> - Previous macrosomic infant (more than 4.5 kg or above)*
> - Previous gestational diabetes*
> - First-degree relative with diabetes*
> - Obesity (BMI more than 30 kg/m²)*
> - Specific ethnic family origin with a high prevalence of diabetes*:
>   - South Asian (specifically women whose country of family origin is India, Pakistan or Bangladesh)
>   - Black Caribbean
>   - Middle Eastern (specifically women whose country of family origin is Saudi Arabia, United Arab Emirates, Iraq, Jordan, Syria, Oman, Qatar, Kuwait, Lebanon or Egypt)
> - Macrosomia in current pregnancy (variably defined in different studies, e.g. fetal abdominal circumference measured with ultrasound >90th centile, or fetal weight estimated using formulae based on ultrasound measurements)
> - Glycosuria ≥1+ on more than one occasion or ≥2+ on one occasion
> - Previous unexpected perinatal death
> - History of polycystic ovary syndrome
> - Polyhydramnios
> - Fasting blood glucose (FBG) more than 6.0 mmol/L or random blood glucose more than 7.0 mmol/L
>
> ---
>
> *Risk factors in bold are those that the NICE Clinical Guideline recommends should be used for screening in practice during pregnancy in the form of a 75-g oral glucose tolerance test.
> From National Institutes for Health and Clinical Excellence (2008, amended and updated 2015). *Diabetes in pregnancy: Management of diabetes and its complications from pre-conception to the postnatal period*. NICE Publication Guideline NG 63.

---

to the at-risk groups listed in Box 9.1. As described earlier, screening is by a 75-g OGTT at 28 weeks, or if very high risk, early in the second trimester and then repeated at 28 weeks (if normal at the first test). In the OGTT, a fasting glucose level is first measured, then a 75-g loading dose of glucose is given and a further glucose level taken at 2 hours post–sugar load. There is an ongoing debate as to the levels of glucose at which gestational diabetes should be diagnosed. Table 9.2 indicates the two most commonly used diagnostic criteria.

Implications for pregnancy

Gestational diabetes is predominantly a disease of the third and sometimes second trimester (Table 9.3). In the mother, the presence of gestational diabetes increases the risk of recurrent infections and of pre-eclampsia developing. For the fetus, there is increased risk of polyhydramnios

Table 9.2 Diagnostic criteria for gestational diabetes using a 75-g oral glucose tolerance test

Diagnostic criteria		Normal fasting value (venous plasma glucose)	Normal 2-hour value (venous plasma glucose)
WHO 1999[a]	One or more abnormal values required	<7.0 mmol/L	<7.8 mmol/L
IADPSG[b]	One or more abnormal values required	<5.1 mmol/L	<8.5 mmol/L

IADPSG, International Association of Diabetes and Pregnancy Study Groups; *WHO*, World Health Organization.
In a given population, use of the IADPSG criteria results in more diagnoses of 'gestational diabetes' than using the WHO criteria.
[a]World Health Organization. *Definition, Diagnosis and Classification of Diabetes Mellitus and Its Complications: Report of a WHO Consultation. Part 1: Diagnosis and Classification of Diabetes Mellitus.* Geneva, World Health Organization, 1999.
[b]Metzger BE, Gabbe SG, Persson B, et al. (2010) International association of diabetes and pregnancy study groups recommendations on the diagnosis and classification of hyperglycemia in pregnancy. Diabetes Care 33:676–682.

Table 9.3 Effect of gestational diabetes on pregnancy

	Maternal risks/complications	Fetal/neonatal risks/complications
First trimester	–	–
Second trimester Third trimester	Pre-eclampsia Recurrent infections	Macrosomia Polyhydramnios Stillbirth
Labour	Induction of labour Poor progress in labour	
Delivery	Instrumental birth Traumatic delivery Caesarean section	Shoulder dystocia
Postnatal		Neonatal hypoglycaemia Neonatal unit admission Respiratory distress syndrome Jaundice
Longer term	Type 2 diabetes later in life	Obesity and diabetes in childhood and later life

and macrosomia, with the latter being related to the degree of glucose control. There is an increased risk of stillbirth. Considering birth, women with gestational diabetes are more likely to have an induction of labour. If vaginal birth occurs, shoulder dystocia, an instrumental birth and extended perineal tears are more common. Women with diabetes are more likely to have a caesarean section. Babies are more likely to need admission to the neonatal unit. They are at increased risk of neonatal hypoglycaemia due to the relative over-activity of the fetal pancreas in utero. This is less likely to occur if maternal blood sugars are well controlled around the time of birth. Maternal glucose readily crosses the placenta, whilst insulin does not.

Remember that glucose crosses the placenta readily and that maternal hyperglycaemia results in elevated blood glucose levels in the fetus. Insulin, on the other hand, does not pass across the placenta, and therefore the fetus is entirely dependent on the supply of its own insulin production for the regulation of its blood sugar levels.

Whilst for the majority of women gestational diabetes will resolve post-pregnancy, in some women, this diagnosis is the unmasking of type 2 diabetes and diabetic care will need to continue.

Women who have had gestational diabetes remain at higher risk of developing type 2 diabetes later in life. These women should have some form of regular screening, such as annually, to exclude diabetes.

For the babies, fetal programming effects increase the risk of obesity and diabetes in later childhood.

Management

Multidisciplinary teams consisting of obstetricians, diabetic physicians, diabetic specialist nurses and midwives and dieticians should manage diabetes in pregnancy.

Antenatally, the aim is to reduce the risk of complications by achieving good glucose control. Initially, this is by dietary measures aiming to avoid large fluctuations in glucose levels: consuming increased amounts of low-glycaemic-index carbohydrate and lean protein and avoiding high-glycaemic-index carbohydrate foods. If this is unsuccessful then medication can be used. Metformin and glibenclamide are increasingly used in pregnancy and may reduce the need for insulin, but a number of women with gestational diabetes will need insulin to optimize control. The aim is that pre-prandial/fasting capillary glucose levels should be between 4.0 and 6.0 mmol/L and that the 2-hour post-prandial value should be between 6.0 and 8.0 mmol/L. Randomized controlled trial evidence has demonstrated that treatment of gestational diabetes with the aim of achieving normoglycaemia in the woman improves outcomes. Serial growth scans are advised to alert to increasing macrosomia.

Vigilance should be maintained for the development of pre-eclampsia.

Delivery at term is recommended to reduce the risk of stillbirth. This may need to be brought forward depending on the degree of diabetic control, the presence of macrosomia or if other conditions have arisen, such as pre-eclampsia. If pre-term delivery is considered, antenatal corticosteroids should be considered to reduce the likelihood and severity of respiratory distress in the newborn. The corticosteroids may necessitate a short-term increase in diabetic treatment to keep blood glucose values in the normal range. In labour, blood glucose should be regularly measured and hyperglycaemia treated to reduce the risk of neonatal hypoglycaemia. The fetus should be continuously monitored. Diabetic therapy can be discontinued with the delivery of the placenta. The baby will need blood glucose measurements to look for hypoglycaemia, and feeding

should be commenced early to assist the baby in maintaining its sugar level.

Postnatally, all diabetic treatment should be discontinued and capillary glucose testing continued. In the majority of women, these values will be normal, indicating that this was genuine gestational diabetes. If they remain elevated, then there is a suspicion of type 2 diabetes and referral to a diabetic team is indicated. Women should be advised of the long-term implications of gestational diabetes and the need for regular screening by, for example, an annual OGTT by their general practitioner. Advice on reducing other lifestyle risks associated with diabetes may also be appropriate.

Infections acquired in pregnancy

Women will encounter infections in pregnancy just as they would outside of pregnancy. However, the relative immunosuppressive conditions of pregnancy can affect the way the body responds to the infection.

Risk factors

Pregnant women with small children or who work with children are more likely to come across many infectious conditions.

Implications on pregnancy and management

The implications on pregnancy and management vary depending on the specific infection. Once more, it is vital to consider both the impact on the mother and the fetus. The impact on the fetus can change when the same infection is contracted at different gestations.

Chicken pox

Chicken pox is a highly infectious childhood illness caused by *Varicella zoster* virus; it has significant implications on both the mother and fetus. Pregnant women are particularly at risk of developing a varicella pneumonia that has a high maternal and fetal mortality rate. If acquired early in pregnancy, there is a 1–2% risk to the fetus of congenital varicella syndrome (eye defects, limb hypoplasia and neurological abnormalities). If acquired near term there is a risk of neonatal varicella that has a significant mortality risk.

If a non-immune pregnant woman is exposed to chicken pox, she can be offered zoster immunoglobulin to reduce the risk of infection. If a woman becomes infected, acyclovir should be given to reduce the risk of maternal complications. Ultrasound imaging can screen for congenital varicella syndrome. With infection at term, delivery should ideally be delayed to allow time for passive transfer of antibodies to the fetus. Care should be taken to avoid contact with other non-immune pregnant women.

Parvovirus B19

Infection with parvovirus B19 is also known as *erythema infectiosum*, *fifth disease* or *slapped cheek syndrome*. A common childhood illness, maternal symptoms can include fever, rash and arthropathy, but often effects are minimal. In contrast, there are potentially significant fetal effects as parvovirus infects rapidly dividing cells and can cause miscarriage in early pregnancy and fetal anaemia and heart failure ('fetal hydrops') later in pregnancy.

Management includes the use of simple analgesics and antipyretic agents for the maternal symptoms and avoidance of contact with other pregnant women. If the infection is contracted after 20 weeks, serial Doppler ultrasound scanning of the blood flow in the fetal middle cerebral artery can detect fetal anaemia (blood flow increased) that may need to be treated with in utero blood transfusions.

Influenza H1N1

Influenza H1N1 caused a worldwide pandemic infection in 2009 and 2010 and is now one of the predominant seasonal influenza virus strains. Pregnant women present with fever and cough similar to non-pregnant individuals. However, pregnant women are at greater risks of complications such as respiratory failure and secondary bacterial infections and have a significantly higher risk of dying than non-pregnant individuals. In addition, implications include an increased risk of pre-term birth, stillbirth and neonatal death.

Management includes treatment with antiviral agents, such as oseltamivir or zanamivir, and respiratory support if necessary. All pregnant women should be advised to be immunized against H1N1.

Human immunodeficiency virus infection

HIV is a virus that weakens the immune system, and over time AIDS may develop. HIV also increases the risk of catching other infections and developing cancers. However, people with HIV infection may be asymptomatic for many years. The number of people living with HIV worldwide is increasing, and a significant proportion of these are women of reproductive age. With advancing disease, highly active antiretroviral therapy (HAART) has been shown to reduce morbidity and mortality from HIV infection.

Implications of pregnancy for the disease
Pregnancy does not appear to accelerate the course of HIV infection or increase the chance of AIDS developing.

Implications of the disease for pregnancy
The main concern in pregnancy is the high risk of vertical transmission (up to 45%) of HIV from mother to baby without medical intervention. This can occur transplacentally in the antenatal period, during vaginal birth and postnatally through breast-feeding. The risk is highest in advanced disease, at seroconversion and with high viral loads. In women who do not breast-feed, transmission rates fall to less than 25%. With medical intervention in the form of multiple antiretroviral therapy, it is possible to reduce vertical transmission further to less than 2%.

In addition there are increased risks of miscarriage, fetal growth restriction, prematurity and stillbirth in women with advanced HIV disease.

Some women will already be on HAART prior to pregnancy, and this should be reviewed to consider the safety of individual medications in pregnancy. Many women will be treatment naïve.

Women who are taking HAART and have viral loads less than 400 copies/mL can deliver vaginally, as there is a very low risk of vertical transmission. However, those who are not taking HAART and/or have viral loads of ≥400 copies/mL or more should be advised to have a caesarean section to reduce the risk of vertical transmission.

There is some evidence that the hormonal effects of the pregnancy may increase the risk of toxicity of antiretroviral therapy in the woman, especially the nucleoside reverse transcriptase inhibitors. Side effects reported have included lactic acidosis, hepatic failure and even maternal death. In addition, some antiretroviral agents are thought to be teratogenic and should be avoided in pregnancy.

Screening
Although many women will know they have HIV when they become pregnant, some women will be unaware that they are HIV positive due to the long asymptomatic stage of the condition. In view of this, the high vertical transmission rate and the efficacy of intervention, many countries now advocate screening in pregnancy. This is usually performed early in pregnancy, but in high-risk women it may be appropriate to offer repeat testing later in pregnancy. Women should be fully counselled about the reason for screening for HIV and the improvements in outcome that can be achieved if HIV is diagnosed.

Management

> Women with HIV who become pregnant should be managed jointly by a specialist obstetrician and HIV physician. Input from the paediatric team should occur antenatally to discuss neonatal screening and treatment.

Women should be regularly assessed clinically and with blood measurements of viral load and CD4 count.

The initial package of care for women with HIV in pregnancy involves anti-HIV medication, caesarean section and avoiding breast-feeding. The use of anti-HIV drugs in pregnancy has been shown to reduce the risk of vertical transmission. Some women will already be taking HAART for their own health needs, and this should continue, provided the agents have not been reported to have any toxic effects in the woman or teratogenicity in the fetus. In treatment-naïve women, anti-HIV medication should commence in the second trimester and continue until birth. Regimes used include zidovudine monotherapy and HAART (nucleotide analogues and protease inhibitors appear relatively safe; non-nucleoside reverse transcriptase inhibitors should be avoided). However, HAART is the recommended treatment of choice. Whilst caesarean section is still advocated for women with non-suppressed disease, women with a viral load of <400 copies/mL who have taken HAART in pregnancy can now opt for vaginal birth without increasing transmission. Invasive procedures should be avoided in pregnancy and labour, for example, amniocentesis, the use of fetal scalp electrodes and fetal scalp blood sampling.

Neonatal screening for HIV infection commences at birth and continues until 12 weeks. Babies require neonatal antiretroviral treatment as post-exposure prophylaxis for several weeks. Women should be strongly advised not to breast-feed.

Confidentiality is an issue for some women with HIV whose families may not know their status. Women should be reassured that confidentiality can and will be maintained despite the increased medical intervention.

Acute viral hepatitis

Seven hepatitis viruses have been identified, the most common being hepatitis A, B and C. All can present similarly with general malaise, nausea, vomiting and pyrexia together with hepatic dysfunction; however, with hepatitis B and C, a significant proportion can be asymptomatic (up to 80% of women with hepatitis C). Hepatitis A is spread by the faeco-oral route, while B and C are transmitted by a blood-borne route. They can be differentiated by serological tests. Hepatitis A is usually cleared after the initial infection; hepatitis B can be cleared, can persist as a carrier state or can lead to chronic infection; and hepatitis C commonly leads to chronic infection and a long-term risk of cirrhosis and liver failure.

The incidence of hepatitis in pregnancy has a wide geographical variation. In the UK, 1–4% of women will be infected with hepatitis B or C.

Pregnancy does not usually change the course of an acute hepatitis infection. A small number of chronic hepatitis B carriers may suffer a reactivation of the disease state during pregnancy. There is some evidence that pregnancy in women with hepatitis C may cause acceleration of the disease progression.

Hepatitis usually does not impact on the pregnancy itself. In women who have a severe acute infection during pregnancy, there is an increase in the incidence of spontaneous pre-term labour. The main concern is the risk of transmission to the neonate. With hepatitis A, this can happen if acute infection occurs in the last couple of weeks before delivery. With chronic hepatitis B and C, carriage transmission can occur perinatally. In women with chronic hepatitis C, vertical transmission will occur in 1 in 20 births.

Management in pregnancy relates to prevention, identification and reduction of the risk of vertical transmission. The risk of hepatitis A infection can be reduced by hygiene measures and consideration of immunization for women in areas of endemic hepatitis A infection. Vaccination is not contraindicated during pregnancy. Women at risk of hepatitis B and C should be counselled regarding risk-taking behaviour (particularly intravenous drug use). Hepatitis B immunization can be offered before and during pregnancy; however, there is currently no effective immunization against hepatitis C.

Women can be screened for hepatitis B and C in pregnancy. This may be universal or selective screening based on a woman's history. Identification antenatally is important to reduce vertical transmission. In women with hepatitis C, co-infection with HIV should be excluded.

Vertical transmission of hepatitis B and C is not reduced by either caesarean delivery or avoidance of breast-feeding. Thus vaginal delivery is advocated (unless there are other obstetric indications for caesarean delivery) but with avoidance of interventions that may increase blood contact, such as fetal scalp electrode siting or fetal blood samples. Babies of mothers with hepatitis B can be treated with hepatitis B immunoglobulin and early hepatitis B immunization, which reduces transmission rates to 5–10%. There are limited options to reduce transmission rates with hepatitis C, but early identification of infected neonates ensures adequate follow-up for the risk of chronic liver disease.

Tuberculosis

Tuberculosis (TB) remains a world health issue with at least 8 million new cases per year and up to 2 million deaths. Although the developed world has low rates of infection, higher rates are found in refugees and travellers to and from endemic areas. TB and HIV are synergistic. HIV is one of the commonest triggers for TB reactivation, and TB is responsible for about 25% of the deaths in people with HIV. The two main proven risks to the fetus are the use of certain anti-tuberculous drugs and if the mother has severe respiratory illness with sustained hypoxia. *Mycobacterium tuberculosis* rarely crosses the placenta. The risks to the woman from untreated TB are the same as in non-pregnant patients. Tuberculin testing should be undertaken routinely in high-risk areas and specifically if the disease is suspected in a patient. Chest X-ray and sputum culture should be performed in those who test positive. If the diagnosis is confirmed, then multiple therapy, as in the non-pregnant patient, is indicated. Women with proven TB should also be screened for HIV. Streptomycin is the only drug that is absolutely contraindicated in pregnancy because of the risk of fetal ototoxicity.

Malaria

Malaria occurs in over 200 million people per year and results in more than 1 million deaths annually. It is a common complication of pregnancy in those countries where the disease is endemic. Pregnancy appears to increase the likelihood of infection. Women who live in endemic areas also show an increased prevalence of the severe forms of the disease. The severity of disease is related to the species of parasite, the level of parasitaemia and the immune status of the individual. *Plasmodium falciparum* is the most virulent of the organisms, as it attacks all forms of the erythrocyte. The parasite grows in the placenta, and placental malaria occurs in anywhere between 15% and 60% of cases. Congenital malaria is rare in infants born to mothers who have immunity, as protective immunoglobulin G (IgG) crosses the placenta.

The main risk of acute malaria to the woman is severe anaemia and its consequences. In the fetus, acute malaria is associated with an increased likelihood of growth restriction, miscarriage, pre-term birth, congenital infection and perinatal death.

Mothers travelling to endemic areas should take prophylaxis or, preferably, not go to the area until the pregnancy is completed. They should also be advised to keep their skin covered and to use insecticides to minimize the risk of being bitten by mosquitoes.

Drug treatment of an acute attack will depend on the nature of the infection. Prophylaxis is given in the form of chloroquine phosphate at a dose of 300 mg each week, starting 1 week before travel and continuing for 4 weeks after leaving the area. Where chloroquine-resistant strains exist, a combination of chloroquine and pyrimethamine with sulfadoxine can be used or proguanil and mefloquine. These drugs need to be taken with a folic acid supplement. Although chloroquine can cause retinal and cochleovestibular damage in high doses in both the mother and the fetus, it has never been shown to be associated with an increased incidence of birth defects where it has been taken for prophylaxis.

Rubella infection

Rubella (German measles or 'third disease') is an exanthematous disease caused by a single-stranded RNA virus acquired via respiratory droplet exposure. After a 2- to 3-week incubation period, symptomatic patients develop a rash, fever, arthralgias and lymphadenopathy. Fifty to seventy-five percent of infected patients manifest clinical features. Severe complications such as encephalitis and bleeding diathesis are rare.

Rubella infection is usually a mild illness in adults and children. However, fetal infection can be severe. Congenital rubella syndrome (CRS) may produce transient abnormalities (e.g. purpura, splenomegaly, jaundice, meningoencephalitis and thrombocytopenia) or permanent abnormalities (e.g. cataracts, glaucoma, heart disease, deafness, microcephaly and mental retardation). Long-term sequelae reported include diabetes, thyroid abnormalities, precocious puberty and progressive rubella pan-encephalitis. Defects involving virtually every organ have been reported.

The rate of fetal infection is highest at 11 weeks and >36 weeks. However, the overall rate of congenital defects is greatest in the first trimester (90%) and declines steadily in the second and third trimesters.

The introduction of rubella vaccine has dramatically reduced the incidence of CRS. The problem should be prevented by childhood vaccination as part of the measles, mumps and rubella (MMR) programme backed up by vaccination programmes for girls in their early teens. However, sporadic cases still occur, especially in women who have not been vaccinated. Thus, ideally women should check their serological status before they conceive and, if negative, they should be offered vaccination. Though the advice is to avoid conception for at least 28 days after vaccination, there is no evidence that vaccination in pregnancy has any effect on the fetus and is not an indication for termination.

In many countries, rubella immunity (indicated by positive serum IgG) status is checked at the first clinic visit for all women. However, in the UK this practice stopped in 2016 because of the low population prevalence of rubella. If a rubella-immune woman is exposed to infection, the absence of the acute marker (serum IgM) by 3 weeks after exposure confirms that she has not been infected and can be reassured. However, if a rubella-susceptible woman is exposed, it is first important to confirm the diagnosis in the index case. The management thereafter will depend on whether the woman develops infection (diagnosed by becoming IgM positive), the stage of pregnancy and the woman's wishes.

Zika virus infection

Zika virus is a mosquito-borne flavivirus transmitted by *Aedes aegypti* mosquitoes, which also transmits dengue and chikungunya virus. The mosquitoes are found throughout much of Africa, Asia, the Americas and the Pacific Islands. There has been a rapid spread of the virus and associated illness in humans since 2015, although the first outbreak was reported in 2007. Consequently, there is still much about the virus and its effects that is not understood.

In 2017, a joint RCOG/RCM/PHE/HPS clinical guideline, 'Zika Virus Infection and Pregnancy', was published to help health care professionals.

The majority of cases of Zika virus are acquired from infected mosquito bites; however, a few cases of sexual transmission and some through blood transfusions have been reported. Most people (80%) infected with Zika virus have no symptoms. If symptoms do develop, these generally occur 3–12 days following the exposure. Those with symptoms have a mild, short-lived (2- to 7-day) illness comprising rash, pruritus, fever, headache, arthralgia, myalgia, conjunctivitis and lower back pain. These symptoms are similar to those of dengue fever and chikungunya, and patients should be tested for all three organisms. Pregnant women are not more vulnerable to infection, nor do they have a more serious illness. Serious complications in an adult from Zika virus infection are rare, although an increase in triggering of Guillain–Barré syndrome has been reported. Zika virus can be detected by polymerase chain reaction (PCR) of blood within 1 week of symptoms developing. This usually is performed at a national specialist laboratory. Testing of asymptomatic women is generally not recommended unless there are suspected fetal complications (see later).

The main concerns in pregnancy are the fetal implications of Zika virus infection. Some cases of maternal-fetal transmission have been reported.

Following a systematic review of the literature up to 30 May 2016, the World Health Organization (WHO) concluded that Zika virus infection during pregnancy is a cause of congenital brain abnormalities. Abnormalities associated with congenital Zika virus syndrome (CZVS) include a variety of cranial abnormalities (including microcephaly with brain atrophy, cerebral calcification, ventriculomegaly, periventricular cysts, microphthalmia) and extra-cranial abnormalities (including fetal growth restriction, oligohydramnios, talipes). The reported risk of CZVS in Zika-positive pregnancies has varied widely (6–46%). It is not clear whether the risk of maternal–fetal transmission is greater in the symptomatic woman. In women with no evidence of cranial abnormalities on ultrasound scan, it is at present unclear if a positive result predicts a subsequent fetal abnormality or what proportion of neonates born after infection will have symptomatic disease.

No specific antiviral therapy is available for Zika virus infection. Treatment is generally supportive involving rest, fluids, analgesics and antipyretics. In a pregnant woman with laboratory evidence of Zika virus in her serum or amniotic fluid, the options should be discussed in detail with a specialist in fetal medicine and a neonatal specialist. Some women choose to terminate the pregnancy even if there are no fetal abnormalities on ultrasound examination. Others will opt for continuing the pregnancy and having serial ultrasound scans to monitor fetal anatomy and growth through the rest of the pregnancy.

Whilst viable virus has been detected in breast milk, there is currently no evidence that Zika virus can be transmitted to babies through breast milk, and mothers are advised that there is no contraindication to breast-feeding. There is currently no vaccine or drug available to prevent Zika virus infection. It is recommended that pregnant women postpone non-essential travel to areas with high risk of Zika virus transmission until after pregnancy and consider the same for areas with moderate risk of Zika virus transmission. If pregnant women travel to high- or moderate-risk areas, they should take all necessary bite-prevention measures (light-coloured, loose-fitting clothes that cover as much exposed skin as possible, DEET-based insect repellents and sleeping/resting under a mosquito net) and be monitored and/or tested on their return. It is also recommended that women avoid becoming pregnant by using effective contraception while travelling in an area with high or moderate risk of Zika virus transmission and for at least up to 6 months on her return.

Testing of asymptomatic pregnant women is not recommended in the absence of ultrasound-identified fetal microcephaly or other related intracranial abnormalities, but serial fetal ultrasound is recommended.

Acute pyelonephritis and urinary tract infections

Asymptomatic bacteriuria occurs in 2–10% of all sexually active women. When pregnant, 12–30% of this group of women will develop pyelonephritis from ascending infection due to structural and immune changes to the renal tract. If the bacteriuria is treated with antibiotics, the risk of later development of acute ascending urinary tract infection can be minimized. Nevertheless, approximately 1% of all pregnancies are complicated by an episode of acute pyelonephritis. The common organism is *Escherichia coli*, and this should be treated aggressively with antibiotics according to known sensitivity. Most community-acquired infections are usually sensitive to amoxicillin or cefuroxime. Additional treatment with fluid replacement, pain relief and bed rest may also be of benefit. Pyelonephritis in pregnancy must not be underestimated, as over 15% of women will develop a bacteraemia, with a small proportion of these progressing to septic shock and/or pre-term labour.

Thromboembolic disease

Venous thromboembolism (VTE) is one of the leading causes of maternal mortality in the developed world. VTE is around 10 times more common in pregnancy than when not pregnant.

Aetiology

Pregnancy is a prothrombotic state. Coagulation factors increase, endogenous anticoagulants decrease and fibrinolysis is suppressed. These effects commence in the first trimester and last until a few weeks following birth. In addition venous stasis occurs in the lower limbs from compression on the pelvic vessels, further exacerbating the problem.

Risk factors

Risk factors can pre-date pregnancy, can occur as a result of obstetric conditions or can be transient. They include:

* pre-existing risk factors:
  * a personal or family history of VTE
  * thrombophilias, obesity, cigarette smoking, some medical conditions (such as sickle cell disease), gross varicose veins and increased maternal age
* transient risk factors:
  * episodes of immobility and dehydration
  * ovarian hyperstimulation
  * surgical procedures
* obstetric risk factors:
  * multiple pregnancy
  * pre-eclampsia
  * operative delivery

Clinical features and diagnosis

VTE presents as in non-pregnant individuals: DVT with swelling and tenderness of a leg and pulmonary embolism (PE) with respiratory symptoms (shortness of breath and pleuritic chest pain) or collapse. In pregnancy, DVT is more likely to occur on the left (90%) due to compression of the left common iliac vein by the right common iliac artery and ovarian artery (the vein is not crossed on the right). The majority of DVTs in pregnancy occur in the iliofemoral veins, so lower limb symptoms may not be as obvious. Clots in the iliofemoral veins are more likely to embolize than those in the calf.

D-Dimer measurements are of limited help in pregnancy; although the negative predictive value is high, a positive result does not help to establish a diagnosis, as it can increase with the physiological changes in the coagulation system that occur in pregnancy.

Radiological investigations should be performed as in non-pregnant individuals. Doppler ultrasound of the lower limb veins or magnetic resonance imaging (MRI) of the pelvic veins should be performed to assess for DVT. Spiral artery computed tomography (CT) or venous perfusion scanning are used to diagnose PE. Although care must be taken when undertaking radiological examinations in pregnancy because of the radiation risk to the fetus, ultimately if an investigation needs to be done to establish a diagnosis, it should be done.

Implications for pregnancy

Antenatally, if VTE is adequately treated, there are minimal direct effects to mother or fetus. If a woman in pregnancy has a PE that is untreated, then there is a 30% risk of maternal death. However, if the woman receives prompt and appropriate treatment, that mortality risk reduces to 3–8%. There are additional risks from the medications used to treat VTE (see later). Postnatally, the risk remains high, and therapy will need to continue for a number of weeks.

Management

All women should have an individual risk assessment undertaken for VTE in pregnancy. Depending on the risk score, a plan for thromboprophylaxis can be made to reduce the risk of thrombosis occurring. For women with low risk, this may not require additional measures; for some women, postnatal prophylaxis may be required, and for those at highest risk antenatal prophylaxis may be recommended with graduated elastic compression stockings and low-molecular-weight heparin (LMWH). In this last scenario, thromboprophylaxis should be started as early as possible in pregnancy.

> **!** If acute VTE is suspected in pregnancy, prompt management is vital, and heparin therapy should be commenced empirically whilst awaiting investigations.

If a DVT or PE is excluded on subsequent diagnostic testing (see earlier), then the heparin can be discontinued.

LMWH has been used extensively in pregnancy, as it does not cross the placenta and has a good safety profile. In contrast, warfarin crosses the placenta and is associated with an embryopathy if used in the first trimester and with fetal intracranial bleeding when used in the third trimester. Most women with VTE can be adequately managed on LMWH, so warfarin is rarely needed in this scenario. On most occasions, heparin therapy can be temporarily stopped around the time of birth to reduce the risk of postpartum haemorrhage and to enable regional anaesthesia to be given if required (LMWH use is associated with epidural haematoma). Simple measures such as avoiding dehydration and using graduated elastic compression stockings should also be employed.

Postnatally, women traditionally continue on heparin prophylaxis or treatment for 6 weeks. If an acute venous thromboembolic event has occurred in this pregnancy, it is likely that heparin prophylaxis will be needed in future pregnancies. Women should also be advised to avoid oestrogen-containing contraceptives.

Liver disease

Obstetric cholestasis

Aetiology

The exact aetiology of obstetric cholestasis is uncertain; however, there appears to be a genetic predisposition to sensitivity to oestrogen, which causes abnormalities in liver function. In addition, it has been speculated that hormonal, environmental and dietary factors are involved.

Risk factors

Certain ethnicities (South American, South Asian and northern European) and a past history of obstetric cholestasis are the predominant risk factors for obstetric cholestasis.

Clinical features and diagnosis

Obstetric cholestasis presents with intense itching, especially on the palms of the hands and soles of the feet in the second or third trimester. There is rarely a rash associated with the itching, but excoriation marks are frequently present. Rarely, pale stools, dark urine and jaundice are noted. The diagnosis is confirmed by a rise in bile acids and/or raised liver transaminases where other pathology (autoimmune disease, gallstones and viral infection) has been excluded.

Some women experience similar symptoms when taking the combined oral contraceptive pill or in the second half of the menstrual cycle.

Implications for pregnancy

Antenatally, the pruritus can be debilitating, giving minimal rest, especially at night. The impact on other liver functions can result in a prolongation of blood clotting time. For the fetus, there is a small increase in the risk of stillbirth. The risk of pre-term birth is higher, but this is predominantly due to early induction of labour. The implications for labour and delivery are minimal, but meconium is more likely to be passed in pre-term fetuses with obstetric cholestasis.

Obstetric cholestasis has a high recurrence rate (over 90%) in future pregnancies.

Management

The pruritus of obstetric cholestasis can be difficult to treat. Topical emollients are safe for use in pregnancy but provide little symptomatic relief. Antihistamines are sometimes used for their sedative ability but have little impact on the itch itself. Ursodeoxycholic acid has been shown to improve both pruritus and liver function, but long-term safety data are lacking. In spite of this, it is the mainstay of antenatal treatment. In view of the potential risk of clotting abnormalities, oral water-soluble vitamin K supplementation can be used, particularly for those women whose clotting tests suggest an abnormality.

The best way to monitor the fetus antenatally has not yet been established. Methods such as serial growth ultrasound scans and cardiotocographs (CTGs) that can detect problems with placental function are not predictive of at-risk fetuses in obstetric cholestasis. Consequently, delivery once fetal maturation is reached is often recommended to reduce the small risk of late stillbirth.

Postnatally, women are usually advised to avoid oestrogen-containing contraceptives, which can precipitate a recurrence of symptoms.

Acute fatty liver of pregnancy

Aetiology

AFLP is a rare but serious condition of pregnancy. The aetiology is uncertain, but it shares many characteristics with severe pre-eclampsia and HELLP syndrome (haemolysis, raised liver enzymes and a low platelet count) and is postulated to be a variant of pre-eclampsia. There has been a recent suggestion of an association of the condition with a recessively inherited fatty oxidation disorder in some cases.

Risk factors

First pregnancy, multiple pregnancy and obesity are all risk factors.

Clinical features and diagnosis

AFLP usually presents in the third trimester with non-specific symptoms of nausea, vomiting, abdominal pain and general malaise. Jaundice may also be present, and women can rapidly deteriorate with liver failure, renal impairment and coagulopathy. Liver and renal function tests are usually abnormal, and hypoglycaemia may be present.

Implications for pregnancy

The condition is associated with high maternal and fetal mortality. Maternal death occurs secondary to hepatic encephalopathy, haemorrhage and disseminated intravascular coagulation.

Management

Women with a history of AFLP in a previous pregnancy should be reminded of the symptoms and given an emergency contact number to use if they recur; liver function monitoring and testing for proteinuria should be undertaken regularly.

Management must be multidisciplinary with support from critical care professionals. Initial management is supportive to correct the abnormalities present (electrolyte imbalance, hypoglycaemia and coagulopathy). Once the woman is stable, delivery should be expedited. Dialysis may be necessary postnatally; rarely, liver transplantation is required.

Information regarding recurrence rates is sparse given the rarity of the condition but is suggestive of an increased chance of recurrence.

Pre-existing medical conditions and pregnancy

An increasing number of women are now entering pregnancy with pre-existing medical conditions. Ideally, these women should be offered pre-conceptual counselling to allow the implications of pregnancy with their specific medical condition to be discussed and a plan put in place. This may involve deferring pregnancy until a specific target in the disease management is met. However, this opportunity is frequently missed.

Renal disease in pregnancy

Pregnancies complicated by chronic renal disease are rare (0.15%); however, they are associated with a significant risk of adverse maternal and fetal outcomes. In the majority of cases, the risks and management relate to the degree of renal impairment and not to the underlying cause of the renal disease.

Implications of pregnancy on the disease

In women with chronic renal disease, pregnancy can cause a deterioration of renal function. Mostly this will recover after the end of the pregnancy, but for some women this will lead to a permanent reduction in renal functioning and a shorter time to end-stage renal failure. The likelihood of renal deterioration depends on baseline creatinine as shown in Table 9.4.

Implications of the disease on pregnancy

Renal disease is associated with increased risks of pre-eclampsia, growth restriction, pre-term birth and a caesarean birth. The risks of an adverse outcome are related to the degree of renal impairment, the presence of hypertension and the presence of proteinuria. Most women with mild renal impairment will have good outcomes.

Management

Women with chronic renal disease should ideally be seen for pre-pregnancy counselling to discuss the implications of a potential pregnancy so that informed decisions can be made. For some women, the risk of deterioration to end-stage renal failure and a requirement for dialysis will be too great to undertake a pregnancy.

Pregnant women with renal disease should be offered care in multidisciplinary clinics that include an obstetrician and a renal or obstetric physician. Initial review should involve assessment of baseline renal function, blood pressure and proteinuria. Low-dose aspirin (75 mg) from 12 weeks until delivery should be offered to reduce the risk of pre-eclampsia. Women already on antihypertensive treatment may need their medications reviewed to ensure that they are safe for use in pregnancy. Careful surveillance of blood pressure, renal function and for urinary tract infection is required throughout pregnancy. Growth scans should be arranged in the third trimester to assess fetal growth. For women with proteinuria, prophylactic LMWH should be considered to reduce the risk of VTE. All women are at increased risk of urinary tract infections; women with chronic renal disease and the presence of more than one confirmed urinary tract infection may benefit from the use of long-term prophylactic antibiotics.

Special circumstances

In addition to the general considerations, some renal conditions need further plans. For example, polycystic kidney disease is an autosomal-dominant condition, so women affected by this condition should be counselled about the inheritance risk to their baby.

Women with renal transplants generally do very well in pregnancy. Conception should be avoided (for up to 12 months in some guidelines) in the immediate post-transplant

Table 9.4 Maternal renal function and chronic renal disease in pregnancy

	Serum creatinine (mmol/L)	Loss of >25% renal function in pregnancy (%)	Deterioration of renal function postpartum (%)
Mild renal impairment	<125	2	0
Moderate renal impairment	124–168	40	20
Severe renal impairment	>177	70	50

Data from Williams D, Davidson J. (2008) Chronic kidney disease in pregnancy. Br Med J 336:211–215.

period, when risks of rejection are highest and anti-rejection medications are being stabilized. Many immunosuppressive drugs are safe for use in pregnancy, but pre-pregnancy counselling is important to allow time for change in medications in those cases where teratogenicity is a risk.

Renal calculi

Symptomatic renal stone disease is no more common in pregnancy than in the non-pregnant state. Ultrasound is the first-line investigation for diagnosis but it has low positive predictive value (60%). MRI is more accurate and is considered to be safe in pregnancy. However, women with renal calculi have an increased frequency of urinary tract infections, and such infections should be treated for longer than isolated urinary tract infections in women without renal stones. Fluid loading, alkalinization of the urine and pain relief with conservative management should be the first line of management, as this will tend to prevent the precipitation of uric acid and cystine stones. The majority (>80%) of stones pass spontaneously with conservative measures. In cases not responding to this approach, stenting has been performed successfully. However, in the absence of comprehensive data concerning safety, extracorporeal lithotripsy is contraindicated in pregnancy.

Diabetes mellitus

Diabetes is one of the commonest pre-existing medical conditions women are seen with in pregnancy. The incidence of pregnant women with pre-existing diabetes is around 0.4%. The majority of these have type 1 diabetes; however, with changes in population demographics there are an increasing number of women with type 2 diabetes. Women with type 2 diabetes tend to be older, be more obese and have more unplanned pregnancies than women with type 1 diabetes. Rates of complications in pregnancy are similar in both groups of women.

Implications of pregnancy on the disease

- The anti-insulin effects of placental hormones result in a larger insulin requirement in pregnancy. Women have to increase their insulin requirements up to threefold to combat this. These changes revert to the pre-pregnancy state within hours of birth.
- Vomiting in early pregnancy can complicate diet and medication balance.
- Pregnancy can reduce the 'warning signs' of hypoglycaemia.
- In women with complications of diabetes, such as retinopathy and nephropathy, pregnancy can accelerate the progress of these complications.

Implications of the disease on pregnancy (Table 9.5)

Many of the complications seen with gestational diabetes are also seen with women with pre-existing diabetes. However, there are additional complications related to abnormal

Table 9.5 Risks of pre-existing diabetes in pregnancy

	Maternal concerns	Fetal/neonatal concerns
First trimester	Increased insulin requirements	Miscarriage Fetal abnormality
Second trimester Third trimester	Pre-eclampsia Recurrent infections Worsening retinopathy if vascular disease	Macrosomia Polyhydramnios Stillbirth Growth restriction
Labour	Induction of labour Poor progress in labour	Pre-term delivery
Delivery	Instrumental birth Birth trauma Caesarean section	Shoulder dystocia
Postnatal	Return to pre-pregnancy control within hours of birth	Neonatal hypoglycaemia Neonatal unit admission Respiratory distress syndrome Jaundice
Longer term	–	Diabetes in childhood (2–3% if mother has type 1; 10–15% if mother has type 2)

glucose homeostasis in the periconception period and in the first trimester, as well as complications related to long-standing underlying vascular disease in women with pre-existing disease.

There is an increased risk of congenital abnormality in women with pre-existing diabetes, particularly neural tube defects and congenital heart disease. The likelihood of this occurring is related to the level of glycaemic control periconceptionally and in early pregnancy. Women with an HbA1c above 10% have up to a 25% chance of a fetal abnormality. Women are at an increased risk of fetal loss throughout pregnancy, which again is related to glycaemic control.

Although fetal macrosomia is the most common fetal growth pattern in diabetes, in women with pre-existing vascular disease and those who develop early pre-eclampsia, fetal growth restriction can be a problem.

Women with hypertension and/or diabetic nephropathy are at high risk of developing pre-eclampsia (approximately 30%).

Management

 Pre-conception counselling for women with pre-existing diabetes enables them to be informed about pregnancy and diabetes.

Pre-conception counselling also allows women to consider the best time to try to conceive. As many of the complications of diabetes relate to the level of glycaemic control, the aim is to get the HbA1c less than 6.1% before conception. If this is achieved, the complication rate of pregnancy in women with diabetes is not much greater than the normal population. Medications can be reviewed. Insulins, both traditional and the newer agents, have been shown to be safe in pregnancy. Metformin is usually continued, but other oral hypoglycaemic agents are usually stopped. Consequently, many women with type 2 diabetes will require insulin in pregnancy. However, some of the medications used to treat the complications of diabetes are not safe. For example, angiotensin-converting enzyme (ACE) inhibitors used in the treatment of diabetic nephropathy should be stopped in pregnancy. Women with diabetes should take a higher periconceptual dose of folic acid (5 mg/d rather than the normal 400 µg/d) in view of the increased risk of neural tube defects.

Multidisciplinary team-working is key in managing women with diabetes. Obstetric diabetes clinics will often consist of an obstetrician, endocrinologist, diabetes specialist nurse, dietician and specialist midwife. Women will be seen regularly throughout pregnancy by this team.

The metabolic goal during pregnancy is to maintain blood glucose as close to the normal non-diabetic range as possible while avoiding severe hypoglycaemia. This involves increasing capillary blood glucose monitoring and tightening control more than is usual outside of pregnancy. The target levels are the same as given in the section on gestational diabetes (see earlier). Because women are encouraged to keep glucose control tight, they can experience unpleasant attacks of hypoglycaemia. Various measures (oral glucose preparations and/or intramuscular (IM) glucagon) need to be in place to deal with this complication.

Fetal assessment for abnormalities involves combined testing for chromosomal problems (if the mother wishes) in the first trimester and a routine anatomy scan at 20 weeks. Additional scanning to look at cardiac anatomy is sometimes recommended in view of the increased risk of congenital cardiac disease. Regular serial growth scans can detect both macrosomia and fetal growth restriction.

For maternal wellbeing, low-dose aspirin from the second trimester can reduce the risk of pre-eclampsia developing. In women with vascular disease, care should be taken to keep blood pressure well controlled to reduce the risk of disease deterioration. All women with pre-existing diabetes should have an ophthalmic assessment in each trimester for evidence of development of worsening of diabetic retinopathy.

Women with diabetes should give birth in a hospital with neonatal facilities. Delivery plans will depend on the stability of diabetes in pregnancy, fetal size and maternal and fetal wellbeing; however, delivery at around 38–39 weeks is usually recommended. Vaginal birth is often planned, but caesarean section rates are high in this group of women. If the estimated fetal birth weight is 4.5 kg or more, many recommend an elective caesarean section. The fetus should be monitored continuously in labour. Vigilance for shoulder dystocia secondary to fetal macrosomia is required with a vaginal delivery. The neonates are at risk of neonatal hypoglycaemia. This risk can be reduced by strict glycaemic control in labour, and a sliding-scale infusion of insulin–dextrose is often required to achieve this control in women with pre-existing diabetes.

Postnatally, women return to pre-pregnancy treatment regimens as soon as they are delivered and eating and drinking.

Thyroid disease in pregnancy

Thyroid disorders of various types complicate approximately 2–5% of pregnancies. Increased oestrogen in normal pregnancy leads to an increase in thyroid-binding globulin that necessitates an increased production of thyroid hormone to maintain free T_4 and T_3 levels. These changes, along with a fall in iodine levels in the maternal plasma due to increased renal loss, result in an enlargement of the thyroid gland of 10–20%. A fall in the thyroid-stimulating hormone (TSH) levels is also a feature of the first half of pregnancy, which may be explained by thyroid stimulatory effects of human chorionic gonadotrophin.

Hypothyroidism

Hypothyroidism is the commonest thyroid problem to occur in pregnancy and complicates up to 5% of pregnancies. Most cases have a basis in **autoimmune diseases,** where autoantibodies like thyroid peroxidase and those associated with Hashimoto's disease cause gland destruction and fibrosis. Hypothyroidism may also be **iatrogenic** as the consequence of thyroidectomy, radio-iodine ablation or excessive doses of antithyroid drugs.

Implications of pregnancy on the disease
There are few effects of pregnancy on hypothyroidism. An increase in replacement therapy is usually required.

Implications of the disease on pregnancy
Maternal and fetal outcomes are worse with overt hypothyroidism. The most serious but rare consequence of untreated hypothyroidism is myxoedema coma (comprising hypothermia, bradycardia, reduced reflexes and altered consciousness together with hyponatraemia, hypoglycaemia, hypoxia and hypercapnia). It is a medical emergency with a 20% mortality rate, requiring supportive therapy and thyroid replacement. More commonly, there are increased risks of spontaneous abortion, pre-eclampsia, pregnancy-induced hypertension, postpartum haemorrhage and low birth weight. However, some recent studies have questioned the association with hypertensive disease in pregnancy. There is a risk of a slight reduction in IQ in the infant but no increased risk in congenital malformations. With adequate replacement, pregnancy outcomes are excellent.

Management
Thyroid function testing in these women should be performed every trimester using pregnancy-specific reference ranges, and replacement should be adjusted as T_4 levels fall due to the increase in maternal extracellular fluid levels. The diagnosis of inadequate treatment/hypothyroidism in the mother is made by a raised level of TSH.

Where hypothyroidism is secondary to treatment for maternal hyperthyroidism, neonatal surveillance for neonatal thyroid dysfunction, itself secondary to transplacental transmission of TSH receptor antibodies, should be undertaken.

Iodine deficiency in many countries is endemic. Untreated, it is associated with poor fetal outcomes from miscarriage, stillbirth, neonatal death and congenital abnormalities, including cretinism. All pregnant women should be encouraged to ensure an adequate iodine intake in pregnancy, if necessary through supplementation. Where the mother is receiving adequate replacement therapy, the outcome for the infant is normal.

Hyperthyroidism

Hyperthyroidism occurs in approximately 0.2% of pregnancies, 95% of which are due to Graves' disease. Diagnosis is made by the finding of elevated T_4 and T_3 levels associated with a lowered TSH level.

Implications of pregnancy on the disease
Pregnancy is usually associated with an increased requirement for thyroxine. Women being treated for hyperthyroidism often need less treatment in pregnancy; however, postpartum flares are common. Untreated thyrotoxicosis can result in a thyroid crisis and heart failure in pregnancy with a 25% mortality rate.

Implications of the disease on pregnancy
Uncontrolled hyperthyroidism is associated with higher rates of pre-eclampsia, fetal growth restriction, prematurity, stillbirths and thyrotoxicosis in the fetus.

Neonatal thyrotoxicosis occurs in 1% of babies. This is transient and due to the transfer of TSH receptor antibodies across the placenta.

Management
Thyroid function testing should be carried out every 4–6 weeks and therapy adjusted accordingly. Pregnancy-specific ranges for thyroid function tests should be used. Most antithyroid medications are safe in pregnancy, but specialist advice from an endocrinologist should be sought.

Serial growth measurements and ultrasound examination for fetal goitre, together with regular assessment of fetal heart rate (looking for fetal tachycardia as a marker of fetal hyperthyroidism), are advisable.

Adjustment of maternal thyroid medication will be necessary after delivery. A prolonged postnatal hospital stay may be required to assess the neonate for signs of thyrotoxicosis.

Obesity

The impact of obesity in pregnancy is increasing. Prevalence is dependent on the population served, though a national survey in the UK in 2009 found that in 9.3 per 100,000 maternities women had a body mass index (BMI) of more than 50 (UK Obesity Surveillance System). Women with obesity often feel stigmatized; however, obesity is associated with significant medical problems in pregnancy that must be addressed. Obese women are more likely to suffer with co-morbidities such as hypertension, sleep apnoea, diabetes and cardiovascular disease, all of which can increase further the risks of pregnancy.

Implications of pregnancy on obesity

The optimum weight gain in pregnancy has not been established. However, in obese women, it is prudent to minimize weight gain during the antenatal period.

Implications of obesity on pregnancy (Table 9.6)

Antenatally, obesity is associated with number of maternal and fetal complications. In the first trimester, the risk of miscarriage and congenital abnormality (especially neural tube defects) is increased, although the aetiology of this has not been established. Throughout pregnancy, there is an increased risk of VTE. Later in pregnancy, obese women are more likely to develop pre-eclampsia and gestational diabetes. In addition, many minor complications of pregnancy such as gastro-oesophageal reflux and pelvic girdle dysfunction are more likely to occur in women with a raised BMI.

Obesity is associated with fetal macrosomia; however, maternal adiposity can have significant impact on the ability to accurately determine fetal size, both clinically and using ultrasound. There is an increased risk of stillbirth and neonatal death. In the long term, children of obese mothers are more likely to have childhood obesity and juvenile diabetes.

Obese women are more likely to have an induction of labour, to have poor progress in labour and to have a caesarean section. This higher rate of caesarean births in obese

women is thought to be secondary to a combination of fetal macrosomia, co-morbid conditions and the hormonal effect of adipose tissue on labour.

The risks of caesarean section, both anaesthetic and obstetric, are higher in women with a higher BMI. If vaginal birth is achieved, shoulder dystocia and extended perineal tears are more frequent. There is a higher risk of postpartum haemorrhage.

Management

Ideally, pre-conceptual counselling would allow women to defer pregnancy until a nearer normal BMI is achieved, but this rarely occurs.

Women with obesity should have hospital-based care because of the associated risks in pregnancy and at birth. Support from a dietician should be offered with the aim of achieving a healthier diet rather than weight reduction. Folic acid should be taken until 12 weeks. Some authorities recommend a higher dose (5 mg) in view of the increased risk of neural tube defects, but evidence for this is lacking. A thorough assessment for other risk factors for pre-eclampsia and VTE should be performed. Based on this, aspirin to reduce the risk of pre-eclampsia or as thromboprophylaxis to reduce the risk of VTE may be appropriate. An OGTT to screen for gestational diabetes should be offered in the late second trimester.

The efficacy of routine ultrasound screening for anomalies is reduced in obese women because of poor visualization. Furthermore, although clinical assessments of

Table 9.6 Risks of obesity in pregnancy

	Maternal risks/complications	Fetal/neonatal risks/complications
First trimester	Venous thromboembolism	Miscarriage Fetal abnormality
Second trimester Third trimester	Pre-eclampsia Gestational diabetes Venous thromboembolism	Macrosomia Stillbirth Difficulty in performing fetal assessment
Labour	Induction of labour Poor progress in labour	–
Delivery	Instrumental birth Caesarean section Traumatic birth (vaginal and caesarean births) Anaesthetic complications (difficulties with intubation or epidural insertion)	Shoulder dystocia
Postnatal	Postpartum haemorrhage Venous thromboembolism	Neonatal unit admission Neonatal death
Longer term	–	Childhood obesity Juvenile diabetes

fetal growth are limited by maternal habitus, there is little evidence that ultrasound provides a more accurate assessment, again because of poor visualization.

In view of the potential complications of labour and birth, obese women should deliver in a hospital unit. If there are no other contraindications to vaginal birth, this should be the planned method.

Thrombophilia

Thrombophilia can be inherited or acquired. Inherited thrombophilias are found in approximately 15% of the Caucasian population, the most common being factor V Leiden and the prothrombin (factor 2) gene mutation. Less common inherited conditions are deficiencies of proteins C, S and anti-thrombin. The most common acquired thrombophilia is antiphospholipid syndrome (APS) that is associated with number of adverse outcomes in pregnancy. Other acquired conditions are paroxysmal nocturnal haemoglobinuria and essential thrombocytopenia. Thrombophilias are responsible for 20–50% of venous thromboembolic events in pregnancy.

Implications of pregnancy on the disease

Pregnancy is a prothrombotic state, and as such women with thrombophilia are at particular risk of VTE during this time. Different thrombophilias are associated with differing levels of risk of clotting, and management must be individualized accordingly.

Implications of the disease on pregnancy

Thrombophilias (both inherited and acquired) are known to be associated with obstetric problems in addition to their risks of VTE. For example, in women with factor V Leiden, associations with fetal loss, pre-eclampsia, placental abruption and in utero growth restriction have all been described. Adverse pregnancy outcomes, including recurrent miscarriage, fetal death and premature birth secondary to placental disease, form part of the definition of APS.

Screening

Screening for thrombophilias should be considered in women with a personal or family history of VTE and women with a poor obstetric history such as recurrent miscarriage, stillbirth, early-onset pre-eclampsia and abruption. However, screening tests performed in pregnancy can be difficult to interpret because of the normal changes in the haemopoietic system. Ideally, these should be performed either postnatally after an adverse event (allowing time for resolution of pregnancy changes to occur) or in the setting of pre-conceptual counselling.

Management

Women with thrombophilia should be ideally seen in a combined obstetric–haematology clinic. Input from a haematologist is key when planning care for the large spectrum of disorders with their varying risks of thrombosis and pregnancy-related morbidity. A full assessment of all risk factors for VTE in addition to the thrombophilia will allow decisions about the appropriate prophylaxis to be made: whether this be antenatal and/or postnatal LMWH or avoiding dehydration and the use of graduated compression stockings.

As previously discussed, LMWH is safe for use in pregnancy, but care should be taken to plan for reducing or briefly stopping its use around the time of birth to minimize the risks of bleeding and ensure that a woman has the full range of analgesic options available to her. In terms of the other obstetric risks of thrombophilias, except for APS, it is unclear if treatment with aspirin or heparin improves pregnancy outcome. However, for women with APS, there is some evidence that the use of aspirin (and possibly heparin) does reduce the incidence of pregnancy complications.

> Surveillance during the pregnancy should include vigilance for thrombosis and stroke, pre-eclampsia and serial assessment of fetal growth and umbilical artery Doppler recordings.

Epilepsy

Epilepsy affects approximately 1 in 100 of the obstetric population.

Implications of pregnancy on the disease

The effect of pregnancy on epilepsy is variable. Usually the seizure frequency is unchanged, but a minority of women will have increased seizures. This is thought to be due to several factors, including non-compliance with medication, stress and sleep deprivation and lower anticonvulsant drug levels secondary to haemodilution.

> Often anti-epileptic drug levels fall in pregnancy and rise in puerperium, so drug doses may need to be altered to maintain seizure control.

There is a suggestion that the risk of sudden unexplained death in epilepsy is increased in pregnancy. However, again this may relate to non-compliance with medication rather than an underlying pregnancy effect.

Implications of disease on pregnancy

Different anti-epileptic medications have different effects on the fetus. Sodium valproate appears to have the greatest risk and should be avoided if possible in women of reproductive age.

In women with epilepsy, there is a higher risk of congenital abnormalities (3% compared with 1–2% in the general population); this risk is increased further if a woman is taking anti-epileptic drugs (4–9%). The main abnormalities are neural tube defects and heart abnormalities.

Other fetal risks that are increased include the perinatal death rate, in utero growth restriction and more subtle long-term neurodevelopmental effects. Tonic-clonic seizures and, in particular, status epilepticus contribute to the increased risk of fetal death. These fetal risks are increased further when more than one anti-epileptic drug is being taken. Carbamazepine, levetiracetam and lamotrigine are considered the safest anti-epileptic drugs for use in pregnancy. Some anticonvulsant medications induce vitamin K deficiency that can lead to an increased risk of haemorrhagic disease of the newborn.

The probability of having a child with epilepsy is increased if either parent has epilepsy, approximately 4–5%, but increases to up to 20% if both parents are affected.

Management

Ideally women with epilepsy should be seen preconceptually for counselling about their risks in pregnancy and to review their medications. Medications may need to be altered, and sometimes it is appropriate to advise delaying pregnancy until a 'safer' drug regimen is established. Women should be advised not to abruptly stop their medication because of fears about the fetus, and it should be emphasized that the risk of uncontrolled epilepsy is greater than the risks of the medications being taken. The overall aim before and during pregnancy is to be on the fewest medications at the lowest dose commensurate with the epilepsy remaining controlled. A higher 5-mg dose of folic acid is recommended periconceptually and in the first trimester due to the increased risk of neural tube defects.

Women should be managed by a multidisciplinary team with the aim of avoiding seizures in pregnancy. Combined screening for chromosomal disorders and anatomy scanning can be performed as normal. Serial growth scans may be required, particularly if a woman is on more than one medication. If anti-epileptic medication that induces vitamin K deficiency is being taken, vitamin K can be given to the mother in the last few weeks of pregnancy, and the baby can receive IM vitamin K just after birth to reduce the risk of haemorrhagic disease of the newborn.

Although women worry about seizures occurring in labour, given the associated tiredness and stress, this is uncommon, but giving birth in a hospital unit is advisable.

Women with epilepsy should be given advice antenatally and after birth regarding safe practices when looking after their newborn, such as not bathing the baby on their own and changing the baby on the floor rather than a high changing table.

Breast-feeding is safe for women on most anti-epileptic medications.

Migraine

Headaches are common in pregnancy. The most common are migraine and those due to tension. New-onset headaches, especially those associated with focal or abnormal neurological signs, impaired intellect and pain that impairs sleep, need specialist assessment.

In women who suffer migraine before pregnancy, the frequency of attacks drops by 50–80% during pregnancy, especially in the third trimester, but increases again in the puerperium. If an attack does occur, the initial treatment comprises simple analgesia, avoidance of light, bed rest and various coping mechanisms. If these simple measures do not work and the migraine is persistent, then more potent analgesics, beta-blockers and/or tricyclic antidepressants have all been used with success. The ergot derivatives often used as prophylaxis/treatment outside pregnancy are contraindicated in pregnancy due to their vasoconstrictive effects.

Cardiac disease

There has been a large increase in cardiac disease in pregnancy in recent years. The overall prevalence of chronic cardiac disease complicating pregnancy in the United States currently is 1.4%. Although some of this is explained by women who themselves have had congenital heart disease now having children, the majority are acquired. Cardiac disease is now the main cause of indirect maternal death in the UK and the United States. A multitude of cardiac conditions can be encountered in pregnancy, including valvular lesions, congenital heart disease, cardiomyopathies, arrhythmias and ischaemic heart disease.

Implications of pregnancy on the disease

Pregnancy puts a great strain on the maternal cardiovascular system. The associated rise in cardiac output can result in deterioration of some conditions, such as aortic stenosis, as these women have a fixed cardiac output. In other conditions, such as regurgitant lesions, pregnancy can be well tolerated.

Many symptoms of cardiac disease are also symptoms of pregnancy, such as breathlessness, palpitations and syncope; cardiovascular signs are also mimicked by pregnancy (bounding pulse, systolic murmur), and as a result it can be

143

difficult to diagnose a new cardiac condition or deterioration in a known cardiac condition.

Depending on the underlying heart condition, women can be at risk in pregnancy for the following conditions:

- congestive cardiac failure
- worsening hypoxia
- arrhythmias and sudden death
- bacterial endocarditis
- VTE
- angina and myocardial infarction
- aortic dissection

Implications of the disease on pregnancy

Again, the implications of cardiac disease on pregnancy will depend on the specific cardiac problem. However, increased risks include pre-eclampsia, intrauterine growth restriction, pre-term birth and fetal loss. Some medications taken in these conditions, such as ACE inhibitors and warfarin, are teratogenic, and their use will need to be reviewed as to whether there is a suitable alternative or if, on balance, the medication should be continued. In women with congenital heart disease, there is an increased risk of the condition in their children of up to 5%.

Management

Multidisciplinary management between obstetricians, cardiologists and obstetric anaesthetists should ideally start at the pre-conception phase with a careful discussion of the potential risks for the woman and the fetus. For some women with poor cardiac functional status, pregnancy may not be advisable. The risk of maternal death can be extremely high in some conditions; for example, in women with Eisenmenger's syndrome, maternal death rates of 40–50% are described. If a woman does decide to undertake pregnancy, it is important to optimize her medical status before she conceives.

Although the New York Heart Association (NYHA) classification provides some information about possible prognosis (Box 9.2), care plans should be individualized. Antenatally, stressors such as anaemia and infection should be minimized. Medication may need to be altered in some women, and anticoagulation may also be required. Fetal surveillance should include serial growth scans and Doppler measurements, as well as screening for cardiac defects. Maternal surveillance may involve regular echocardiograms.

Labour is a problematic time, and attempts should be made to minimize pain and ensure fluid balance is diligently maintained. The haemodynamic changes that occur in the immediate postpartum period mean that this is often the riskiest time for women with cardiac disease, and careful surveillance and joint management by the obstetric, cardiac and anaesthetic teams are vital.

> ### Box 9.2 New York Heart Association classification
>
> **Grade 1:** Normal exercise tolerance
> **Grade 2:** Breathless on moderate exertion
> **Grade 3:** Breathless on less-than-moderate exertion
> **Grade 4:** Breathless at rest without significant activity
>
> #### Class I
>
> No limitations on physical activity; ordinary physical activity does not cause undue fatigue, palpitation, dyspnoea or angina pain
>
> #### Class II
>
> Slight limitation on physical activity; ordinary physical activity results in fatigue, palpitation, dyspnoea or angina pain
>
> #### Class III
>
> Marked limitation on physical activity; less-than-ordinary activity causes fatigue, palpitation, dyspnoea or angina pain
>
> #### Class IV
>
> Inability to perform any physical activity without discomfort; symptoms of cardiac insufficiency or angina syndrome may be present, even at rest; any physical activity increases discomfort

---

Respiratory disorders

Respiratory disease, predominantly asthma, is common in pregnancy. As with the assessment of cardiac disease, differentiating physiological changes from pathological ones can be difficult as women experience a sense of breathlessness (dyspnoea) that increases from early pregnancy to peak at 30 weeks.

Asthma

Asthma is an increasingly common disorder and can be expected to affect 5–10% of pregnant women.

Implications of pregnancy on the disease

The effect of pregnancy on asthma is not predictable, although approximately one-third of women will improve, one-third will get worse and one-third stay the same. Approximately 10% of women with asthma will have an acute exacerbation in pregnancy.

Implications of the disease on pregnancy

Women with well-controlled asthma have good pregnancy outcomes, and there are no established adverse effects of well-controlled asthma on pregnancy. In contrast, women with poorly controlled asthma or those with severe exacerbations in pregnancy are at increased risk of fetal growth restriction, premature birth and pre-eclampsia.

Management

Baseline peak flow measurements should be taken at the start of pregnancy. Women should be encouraged to continue their asthma medication, as a significant number of exacerbations are caused by cessation of medication due to concerns about the possible effects on the fetus. Most asthma medications are safe in pregnancy (including steroid therapy), although there is less information about some of the newer therapies. The management of acute exacerbations of asthma is the same in pregnancy as in non-pregnant asthmatics.

Cystic fibrosis

Although CF is ultimately a fatal disease, the life expectancy of someone with CF has markedly increased in the last 30 years due to early diagnosis and improvements in treatment. The incidence of CF is 0.05–0.1% of births in Caucasian populations in which 5% of adults carry the recessive gene. The increased life expectancy has provided opportunities for women with CF to consider pregnancy. As a result, women with CF account for 0.4–0.8% of pregnancies in United States and UK, with up to 80% achieving a live birth.

Implications of pregnancy on the disease

Although pregnancy can be tolerated well, many women do experience difficulties as the effects on lung function can be unpredictable and maintaining adequate nutrition can be problematic. The risks of pregnancy relate to the degree of pulmonary dysfunction and associated pulmonary hypertension. In women with initial poor lung function (FEV_1 <50%), significant decline can occur in pregnancy that may be irreversible.

Implications of the disease on pregnancy

As an autosomal-recessive condition, there is a risk of transmission of the disease to the infant. Prenatal diagnosis can be offered. There is an increased risk of gestational diabetes due to fibrosis in the pancreas. Around one-third of babies of women with CF will be born pre-term. Fetal growth restriction may be an issue in those with poor nutritional status.

Management

Ideally pregnancies should be planned and pre-pregnancy advice sought. This involves genetic counselling, the optimization of treatment of lung and gastrointestinal function and an assessment for pulmonary hypertension. Significantly raised pulmonary pressures are associated with a high maternal mortality, and pregnancy should be avoided.

High-dose folate (5 mg/day) should be taken periconceptually to reduce the risk of fetal anomaly.

Multidisciplinary care is essential, including obstetricians, respiratory physicians and obstetric anaesthetists. Pulmonary function tests should be performed at the start of pregnancy and repeated according to symptoms. Nutritional support is mandatory, and specialist dieticians should be able to advise on the necessary supplements. Chest infections should be treated promptly.

Women should be screened for gestational diabetes with an OGTT. Fetal growth should be monitored, and vigilance for pre-term labour should be maintained.

Delivery should occur in a setting with access to high-dependency care and respiratory care if needed. Caesarean section under regional analgesia may be needed for severe respiratory compromise.

Autoimmune disease

Autoimmune disease is five times more common in women than men. Systemic lupus erythematosus (SLE), scleroderma, APS and autoimmune thyroid disorders (discussed earlier) all can have an effect on placental function and result in miscarriage, fetal growth restriction, early-onset severe pre-eclampsia, thrombosis and fetal death. Some autoimmune conditions, such as rheumatoid arthritis and Crohn's disease, improve in the altered steroid environment of pregnancy, but there is a serious increased risk of relapse during the puerperium.

Systemic lupus erythematosus

SLE is a multisystem disorder characterized by periods of relapse and remission. The diagnosis of SLE is dependent on the serological finding of the antinuclear antibody (ANA) in the serum and at least 4 of 11 other clinical or laboratory criteria published by the American Rheumatology Association, including rash, renal impairment, arthritis and thrombocytopenia.

Implications of pregnancy on the disease

There is some evidence that relapses occur more frequently in pregnancy, and there certainly is an increase in 'flares' or exacerbations in the postnatal period. About 75% of patients have renal disease. Women with an exacerbation of lupus nephritis are at risk of deterioration in their renal function that may be irreversible during pregnancy (see the previous section on chronic renal diseases).

Implications of the disease on pregnancy

Women with SLE are at increased risk of early miscarriage, stillbirth, early-onset pre-eclampsia, fetal growth restriction and pre-term birth. The likelihood of these occurring is increased if they have renal involvement or if they also have APS.

Women, especially those with APS alongside their SLE, are at increased risk of VTE.

Infants are at risk of neonatal lupus and congenital heart block.

Management

Women should be managed by a multidisciplinary team with the opportunity for pre-pregnancy counselling. Outcomes are better if pregnancy is avoided until at least 6 months after a 'flare'.

Women should be advised to take low-dose aspirin to reduce the risk of pre-eclampsia, and LMWH should be used in addition where APS co-exists.

The disease should be monitored by symptom review and regular assessment of disease markers, especially renal function and antiphospholipid antibodies. Immunosuppression can be continued in women with severe lupus, although the agents used may need to be changed if teratogenic.

Labour is usually induced at 37–38 weeks to avoid late-pregnancy thrombotic complications.

Haemoglobinopathies

Sickle cell syndromes

These genetic disorders involve abnormalities in haemoglobin synthesis resulting in abnormal S haemoglobin being produced. The disease spectrum can range from the relatively asymptomatic sickle cell trait, where women are heterozygous for the sickle gene, to homozygous sickle cell disease, where women can have regular sickle cell crises. Although there is a strong link with certain ethnicities, especially those from sub-Saharan Africa and the Middle East, sickle cell syndromes are now seen throughout the world.

Implications of pregnancy on the disease

Pregnancy complications such as nausea and vomiting, anaemia and infection can all increase the likelihood of a sickle cell crisis occurring in women with sickle cell disease, and so pregnancy can result in an increased frequency of crises.

Implications of the disease on pregnancy

The genetic implications of the sickle cell syndromes depend on the status of the partner, and so early partner testing is recommended. Depending on the result of this, women may need input from the genetics team to determine if they wish to proceed with prenatal diagnosis.

Women with the sickle cell trait generally do well in pregnancy, although anaemia and infections can be a problem. In contrast, sickle cell disease is associated with significant obstetric complications, including increased risks of miscarriage, pre-term birth, fetal growth restriction and perinatal mortality. There are also increased maternal risks of VTE, antepartum haemorrhage and pre-eclampsia.

Management

Pre-pregnancy women and their partners should be counselled about the risks for pregnancy. They should also be advised against conception until the disease management is optimized.

Joint care between obstetricians and haematologists is advised. Women whose partners also carry the sickle gene can be offered prenatal diagnosis if desired. All women with sickle cell syndromes should be advised to take a higher dose (5 mg) of folic acid to reduce the risk of neural tube defects, as their haemolytic anaemia increases their risk of folate deficiency. In women with sickle cell disease, low-dose aspirin should be considered to reduce the risk of pre-eclampsia and prophylactic antibiotics to reduce the risks of infection. Serial growth scans should be performed to look for evidence of growth problems. Anaemia can worsen during pregnancy, and blood transfusions may be required to maintain an adequate haemoglobin level. If crises occur, they should be treated promptly to reduce the risk to the fetus.

During pregnancy and labour, dehydration should be avoided, and the need for VTE prophylaxis should be regularly assessed depending on the presence of other risk factors.

The thalassaemias

These disorders are associated with a reduction in the rate of production of the alpha- and beta-globin chains of haemoglobin. In alpha-thalassaemia, the degree of impairment depends on the number of alpha-globin genes absent, with one absent causing minimal symptoms and four being incompatible with life. Most of the women with alpha-thalassaemia who become pregnant will have one or two alpha genes missing and will have mild anaemia. In beta-thalassaemia individuals can be homozygous or heterozygous, resulting again in a spectrum of symptomatology. Women with homozygous beta-thalassaemia rarely become pregnant; however, women with heterozygous beta-thalassaemia have minimal symptoms and no impairment to pregnancy.

Implications of pregnancy on the disease

Pregnancy can cause a significant worsening of the mild anaemia seen in many women with thalassaemias.

Implications of the disease on pregnancy and management

The main implication of the thalassaemias on pregnancy is the risk of inheriting the thalassaemia genes. Partner testing will identify women who are at risk of carrying a homozygous fetus, who can then be referred for prenatal testing. Problematic anaemia may need to be treated with transfusions in pregnancy. Iron therapy must be used cautiously, as women are at risk of iron overload. Fetal growth should be monitored because of the risk of fetal growth restriction.

Conclusions

It is essential to have a framework for considering the implications of medical conditions in pregnancy on both the woman and the fetus. Such conditions now are responsible for an increasing number of maternal deaths, and adequate understanding is essential if this trend is to be reversed.

Essential information

Minor complaints in pregnancy

- These are usually due to physiological changes in pregnancy, but it is important to ensure there is not a pathological cause

Anaemia

- In the UK, this is defined as a haemoglobin level <11 g/dL (some use <10.5 g/dL), especially towards the start of the third trimester
- Usually caused by:
  - Inadequate intake of dietary iron
  - Impaired absorption of iron (gastric achlorhydria, malnutrition, chronic diarrhoea, hookworm)
- Investigations – Mean Corpuscular Volume (MCV), Mean Corpuscular Haemoglobin Concentration (MCHC), serum iron and iron-binding, ferritin, folate and vitamin B; others if cause still obscure
- Management, usually with oral iron/folic acid

Diabetes

- Classified as type 1, type 2 or gestational
- Needs strict management, with the aim of keeping capillary glucose in the non-diabetic range
- Management by diet and insulin (type 1); diet, oral hypoglycaemic agents ± insulin (type 2); diet ± oral hypoglycaemic agents ± insulin (gestational diabetes)

Infections acquired in pregnancy

- Some infections in pregnancy can adversely affect the mother and the fetus, though not always equally seriously
- Vertical transmission of HIV can be reduced to a minimum by antiretroviral therapy during pregnancy. If virus is detectable at the end of pregnancy, elective delivery by caesarean section is recommended.
- The main management strategy in women with hepatitis, A, B or C is to implement a variety of measures to prevent vertical transmission, though an elective caesarean section does not appear to help this.

- The main risk of TB in pregnancy is on the health of the woman. Placental transfer is rare. Streptomycin is the only anti-tuberculous drug that is contraindicated.
- Asymptomatic and symptomatic bacteriuria are common infections in pregnancy, and prompt recognition and treatment are necessary to prevent progression to pyelonephritis.
- Some infections can be prevented by prior immunization (such as rubella), and some can be treated effectively during pregnancy. For others (such as Zika virus infection), there is no effective treatment, and avoidance of contracting the infection during pregnancy is the best approach.

Thromboembolism

- This is one of the major causes of maternal deaths.
- A previous history of the condition and hereditary conditions with increased coagulability increase the risk.
- Every mother should be assessed in the antenatal period, during labour and postpartum for the possible risk, and prophylactic measures (especially using LMWH) should be undertaken.
- If a DVT or PE is suspected clinically, full anticoagulation should be commenced until the results of the investigations are available. If the diagnosis is not confirmed, the treatment is stopped.

Liver disease

- Obstetric cholestasis is of uncertain aetiology.
- It produces intense itching of the woman's palms and soles of the feet.
- It is associated with an increased risk of fetal death, and elective delivery at 37–38 weeks is often advocated to lessen that risk.

Renal disease

- Moderate–severe chronic renal disease usually worsens during pregnancy and may not improve after delivery.

Essential information—cont'd

- Renal disease causes increased rates of intrauterine growth restriction, pre-term delivery and perinatal loss.
- Multidisciplinary management is necessary to optimize the outcome for the woman and fetus.

Thyroid disease

- Hypothyroidism is most commonly due to autoimmune disease or iatrogenic (post-thyroidectomy). Iodine deficiency is less common. Raised levels of TSH are diagnostic, and the effectiveness of thyroxine treatment should be monitored with TSH levels.
- Hyperthyroidism in pregnancy is usually due to Graves' disease. It can cause low birth weight and premature labour and birth. Treatment is with anti-thyroid drugs.

Obesity

- Ideally obese women should defer pregnancy until they reach their optimal BMI.
- Obese women should have hospital-based care because of the increased risks.
- Screening should be undertaken for gestational diabetes and excessive fetal growth.
- Special preparation is necessary for a caesarean section (e.g. a large operating table).

Epilepsy

- A minority of women have an increase in seizure frequency in pregnancy.
- All anti-epileptic drugs have been reported to be teratogenic, with sodium valproate appearing to have the greatest risk. However, the hazards of epilepsy exceed the risks of treatment.
- The main priority in pregnancy is to prevent seizures with the fewest drugs and at the lowest effective dose.

Cardiac disease

- The risks for the woman and fetus vary with the diagnosis.
- The NYHA classification gives an indication as to the severity of the cardiac disease in the woman, though some of the symptoms of cardiac disease are also normal physiological complaints in pregnancy.
- Surveillance and management should be by a multidisciplinary team and individualized.

Respiratory disease

- Asthma
  - This is common in pregnancy and is not commonly exacerbated by the pregnancy.
  - Some symptoms are normal complaints in pregnancy.
  - Baseline peak flow measurements should be taken at the start of pregnancy.
  - Treatment for both acute attacks and ongoing maintenance is the same as for non-pregnant individuals and is considered safe.
- Cystic fibrosis
  - Though an uncommon condition, it is associated with increased risk for the woman and fetus.
  - Surveillance and management should be by a multidisciplinary team and individualized.

Chapter | 10 |

Congenital abnormalities and assessment of fetal wellbeing

David James and Suzanne V. F. Wallace

LEARNING OUTCOMES

After studying this chapter you should be able to:

Knowledge criteria

- Describe the common structural abnormalities resulting from abnormal development
- List the risk factors for the common fetal abnormalities
- Compare the diagnostic tests for fetal abnormality
- Describe the role of ultrasound scanning in pregnancy in screening, diagnosis and assessment of fetal abnormalities and in assessing fetal growth and health
- Describe the aetiology, risk factors and management of Rhesus isoimmunization

Clinical competencies

- Interpret the results of investigations of fetal wellbeing
- Plan the investigation and management of the small for gestational age baby

Professional skills and attitudes

- Reflect on the impact on a family of a diagnosis of fetal abnormality

Congenital abnormalities

Fetal abnormality is found in:
- over 50% of conceptions
- about 70% of miscarriages
- 15% of deaths between 20 weeks' gestation and 1 year postnatal
- 1–2% of births, including major and minor anomalies (a major abnormality is an abnormality or abnormalities that result in the death of the baby or severe disability)
- 8% of special needs register/disabled children

The overall incidence of congenital abnormalities in the UK has fallen over the past three decades due to the introduction of screening programmes in pregnancy, the resultant greater success at diagnosis during pregnancy and parents opting to terminate a pregnancy once a severe abnormality has been diagnosed.

The commonest four groups of congenital abnormalities are neural tube defects (3–7/1000), congenital cardiac defects (6/1000), Down's syndrome (1.5/1000) and cleft lip/palate (1.5/1000) (Table 10.1).

Neural tube defects

Neural tube defects are the commonest of the major congenital abnormalities and include anencephaly, microcephaly, spina bifida with or without myelomeningocele, encephalocele, holoprosencephaly and hydranencephaly (Fig. 10.1). The incidence is approximately 1/200, and the chance of having an affected child after one previous abnormal child is 1/20.

Commonly cases are identified by ultrasound (US) screening in the early second trimester. Where there is an open neural tube, maternal serum alpha-fetoprotein (MSAFP) levels are raised. US assessment for other abnormalities should be undertaken and karyotyping offered if they are found.

Multidisciplinary counselling and care are recommended. Infants with anencephaly or microcephaly do not usually survive. Many die during labour and the remainder

Table 10.1 Major congenital abnormalities

Abnormality	Approximate incidence (per 1000 births)
Neural tube defects	3–7
Congenital heart disease	6
Down's syndrome	1.5
Cleft lip/palate	1.5
Talipes	1–2
Abnormalities of limbs	1–2
Deafness	0.8
Blindness	0.2
Others, including urinary tract anomalies	2
Total	**15–30**

Reproduced with permission from James DK, Weiner CP, Gonik B, Crowther CA, Robson SC, eds (2011) High Risk Pregnancy: Management Options, 4th edn. Saunders Elsevier, St Louis.

within the first week of life. Infants with open neural tube defects often survive, particularly where it is possible to cover the lesion surgically with skin after birth. However, the defect may result in paraplegia and bowel and bladder incontinence and the need for repeated further surgery. The child often has normal intelligence and has insight, being particularly aware of the problems posed for the parents. Closed lesions generally do not cause problems and may escape detection until after birth.

Permission for postmortem should be sought with abortuses, stillbirths or neonatal deaths to exclude other abnormalities.

There is good evidence that pre- and periconceptual folic acid supplementation (400 μg/day) reduces the incidence of this condition. Once a woman is pregnant, the major effort is directed toward screening techniques that enable recognition of the abnormality and the offer of a termination of the pregnancy where there is a lethal abnormality.

Folic acid dietary supplementation is indicated both before and during pregnancy in those women who have experienced a pregnancy complicated by a neural tube defect. In these cases, a higher dose of folic acid prophylaxis (5 mg/day) is recommended.

Fetal surgery for open neural tube defects has been undertaken but should be considered experimental at present.

Congenital cardiac defects

The likelihood of a pregnant woman having a fetus with a congenital cardiac defect is about 0.6%. Some of these infants present with intrauterine growth restriction and oligohydramnios, but in many cases the condition is only recognized and diagnosed after birth. With improvements in real-time US imaging, recognition of many cardiac defects has become possible. However, early recognition is essential if any action is to be taken. Screening is performed by US. Most centres would undertake nuchal translucency scanning in the first trimester (around 11 weeks) and a four-chamber view of the fetal heart in the second trimester (at 18–20 weeks) (Fig. 10.2). In addition, some centres are looking at blood flow in the ductus venosus and across the tricuspid valve at 11 weeks and the left and right outflow tracts at 18–20 weeks to try and identify more abnormalities. Despite this screening, even in the best centres less than 50% of congenital heart defects are currently identified prenatally.

The most common defects are ventricular and atrial septal defects, pulmonary and aortic stenosis, coarctation and transpositions of the great vessels, including the tetralogy of Fallot. These lesions can generally now be recognized on the four-chamber views recorded during detailed 18- to 20-week-gestation scans.

Once an abnormality is identified, management comprises further diagnostic US examination to establish the extent of the defect and whether there are any other fetal abnormalities (this may include karyotyping) and multidisciplinary counselling and care. In some cases where the prognosis is poor, the parents may opt for a termination of pregnancy. In other cases, delivery should occur in a centre with full neonatal cardiological services, including cardiac surgery.

Defects of the abdominal wall

Defects of the abdominal wall can be diagnosed by US imaging. US screening in the second trimester (18–20 weeks) in the best centres detects over 95% of cases. They include **gastroschisis** (Fig. 10.3A) and **exomphalos** (Fig. 10.3B). In both cases, the bowel extrudes outside the abdominal cavity. The main differences between the two are that a gastroschisis is a defect that is separate from the umbilical cord (usually 2–3 cm below and to the right), does not have a peritoneal covering and is usually an isolated problem. In contrast, an exomphalos is essentially a large hernia of the umbilical cord with a peritoneal covering and an increased risk of an underlying chromosomal abnormality, especially trisomy 18.

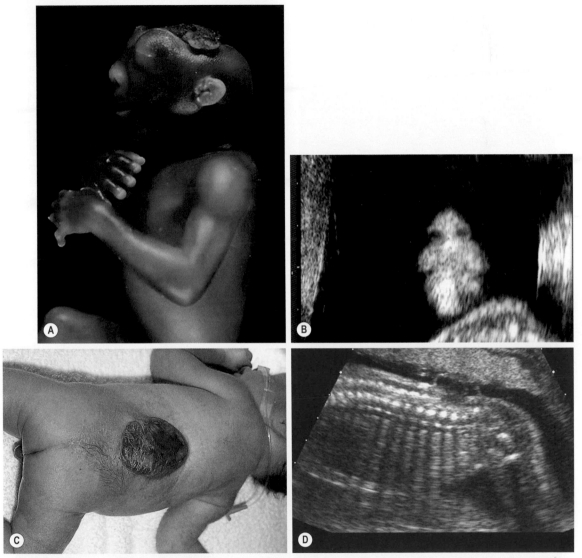

Fig. 10.1 Two common abnormalities of the central nervous system. (A) Anencephaly in a newborn. (B) Mid-trimester ultrasound image of anencephaly (face visualized but no cranium). (C) Spina bifida with open neural tube defect. (D) Mid-trimester ultrasound image of spina bifida. (A Courtesy Ed Uthman, MD. https://commons.wikimedia.org/w/index.php?curid=1405306. C Reproduced with permission from Lissauer T, Carroll W (2018) Illustrated Textbook of Paediatrics, 5th edn. Elsevier.)

If a gastroschisis is diagnosed, the parents can be told the prognosis is very good. Multidisciplinary care is needed. Delivery can be vaginal and should take place in a hospital with neonatal surgical facilities. All babies will require neonatal surgery to correct the defect; however, over 90% will survive.

In contrast, exomphalos has a very poor prognosis. Apart from the association with chromosomal abnormality, there is an increased risk (over 60%) of co-existent structural defects, especially cardiac. Further careful detailed US examination of the fetus should be undertaken once the diagnosis is made and karyotyping offered. Multidisciplinary care is advisable. If the parents opt to continue with the pregnancy rather than have a termination of pregnancy, this should take place in a unit with comprehensive neonatal facilities, including surgery.

Chromosomal abnormalities

Chromosomal abnormalities are common, with an estimated incidence of at least 7.5% of all conceptions.

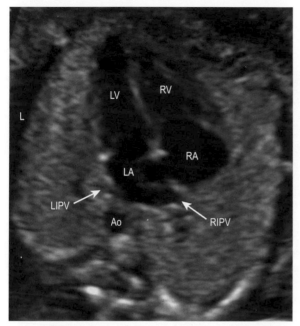

Fig. 10.2 Four-chamber ultrasound view of the fetal heart. *Ao*, Aorta; *L*, Left; *LA*, Left atrium; *LIPV*, Left interstitial pulmonary vein; *LV*, Left ventricle; *RA*, Right atrium; *RIPV*, Right interstitial pulmonary vein; *RA*, Right atrium.

However, many of these result in a miscarriage, and the liveborn incidence is much less than that, at about 0.6%. Chromosomal abnormalities can be identified from culturing and karyotyping fetal/placental cells in the amniotic fluid or from the chorionic plate. The chromosomal abnormalities include both structural and numerical abnormalities of the karyotype. The commonest abnormality is that associated with trisomy 21, or Down's syndrome (DS). In this condition, in at least 92% of cases the chromosomal abnormality is that each cell has three rather than two number 21 chromosomes (about 8% of cases are translocations – see later). This condition is discussed further later. The next most common are abnormalities of the sex chromosomes (Klinefelter's syndrome with one extra sex chromosome in the form of two X-chromosomes and one Y-chromosome; Triple-X syndrome with an extra sex chromosome in the form of three X-chromosomes; and Turner's syndrome with one only one sex chromosome, an X-chromosome), followed by trisomies 13 and 18 (Patau and Edwards syndromes, respectively).

Down's syndrome

DS is characterized by the typical abnormal facial features (Fig. 10.4), learning disability of varying degrees of severity and congenital heart disease. The karyotype includes an additional chromosome in group 21 ('trisomy 21'; Fig. 10.5). The incidence overall is 1.5/1000 births. However, the chance increases with advancing maternal age (see later). The underlying reason is thought to be an increased frequency of non-disjunction at meiosis.

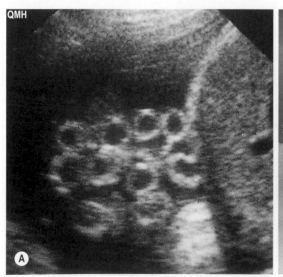

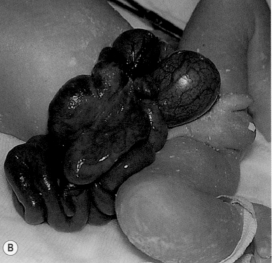

Fig. 10.3 (A) Gastroschisis – bowel contained within peritoneal sac. (B) Exomphalos – bowel extrusion. (Reproduced with permission from Lissauer T & Carroll W (2018) Illustrated Textbook of Paediatrics, 5th edition, Elsevier.)

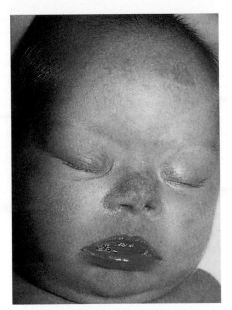

Fig. 10.4 Facial appearance of infant with Down's syndrome.

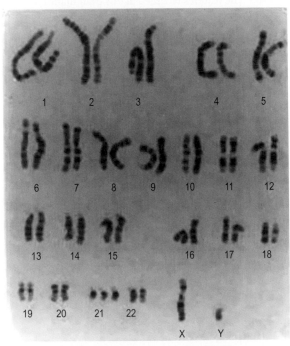

Fig. 10.5 Trisomy 21 karyotype (male).

About 6–8% of affected infants have the disease as a result of a translocation and the extra 21 chromosome carried on to another chromosome, usually in group 13–15.

The mother or the father will usually be a carrier of a balanced translocation.

Assessing fetal normality

Screening

Screening in this context is the process whereby women with a higher chance of fetal abnormality are identified in the general population. This screening is undertaken using identification of clinical risk factors, US and biochemical testing of maternal serum. Clinical risk factors can be identified throughout pregnancy, though the options for management are different depending on the gestational age. US and biochemical screening are offered to women in the first half of pregnancy. Ideally women should be offered a combined screening test (using US and biochemistry) for aneuploidy towards the end of the first trimester and a detailed US scan at about 20 weeks. The early scan also allows gestational age to be confirmed. If a woman presents too late for the first-trimester aneuploidy screening, then she should be offered a biochemical screening test at about 16 weeks.

Clinical risk factors: early pregnancy

These include:
- maternal age and risk of aneuploidy especially DS (Tables 10.2 and 10.3).
- maternal drug ingestion:
  - anticonvulsant drugs (e.g. phenytoin, carbamazepine and sodium valproate) can produce defects of the central nervous system, especially neural tube defects.
  - cytotoxic agents used in cancer therapy or for immunosuppression with organ transplantation are associated with an increased risk of fetal growth restriction.
  - warfarin is teratogenic when used in the first trimester and can produce a fetal bleeding disorder when used later in pregnancy.
- previous history of fetal abnormality:
  - if, for example, a woman has had a DS baby in the past, she has a greater chance of recurrence than the likelihood given by her age alone.
  - however, not all fetal abnormalities are associated with a greater risk of recurrence in a subsequent pregnancy.
- maternal disease (see Chapter 9), including:
  - diabetes: the reported risks of fetal abnormality vary between 3% and 8%. This figure is reduced significantly if the diabetes is well controlled before and during the first trimester and the woman takes periconceptual folic acid.

Table 10.2 The chance of having a pregnancy affected by Down's syndrome according to maternal age at the time of birth

Maternal age at delivery (years)	Chance of Down's syndrome
15	1:1578
20	1:1528
25	1:1351
30	1:909
31	1:796
32	1:683
33	1:574
34	1:474
35	1:384
36	1:307
37	1:242
38	1:189
39	1:146
40	1:112
41	1:85
42	1:65
43	1:49
44	1:37
45	1:28
46	1:21
47	1:15
48	1:11
49	1:8
50	1:6

Reproduced with permission from James DK, Weiner CP, Gonik B, Crowther CA, Robson SC, eds (2011) High Risk Pregnancy: Management Options, 4th edn. Saunders Elsevier, St Louis.

- congenital cardiac disease: a woman who has a congenital cardiac defect has a 1–2% risk of a cardiac abnormality in her fetus.

Clinical risk factors: late pregnancy

The following are risk factors associated with a higher likelihood of fetal abnormality:
- persistent breech presentation or abnormal lie in late pregnancy

- vaginal bleeding; however, the majority of pregnant women with vaginal bleeding in pregnancy do not have a fetal abnormality
- abnormal fetal movements, both increased and decreased, though for women to be aware of this perhaps subtle difference, they usually must have had a normal pregnancy previously, which they can use as a reference
- abnormal amniotic fluid volume: both polyhydramnios (which is commonly associated with abnormalities of the gastrointestinal system, especially obstruction) and oligohydramnios (which is commonly associated with obstructive abnormalities of the renal tract, such as urethral valves or renal agenesis)
- growth restriction, though most fetuses that are growth restricted do not have an abnormality

Ultrasound

Most pregnant women in the UK present for their first visit to a health professional in the first trimester. This means that they can be offered two US scans in the first half of pregnancy.

The first scan ideally is performed between 11w+0d and 13w+6d. The features recorded at this examination are:
- Confirmation of the location of pregnancy (i.e. that it is in the uterus).
- Confirmation of fetal viability by the demonstration of cardiac activity.
- Establishing the number of fetuses. If there are twins, then the chorionicity should be determined by identifying either the 'lambda sign' (dichorionic) or 'T-sign' (monochorionic) (Fig. 10.6).
- Assessment of gestational age by measurement of crown–rump length (CRL) (see Chapter X).

If the woman wishes to have screening for fetal abnormality, she can have:
- Measurement of fetal nuchal translucency (NT) (Fig. 10.7) as part of the 'combined testing' programme (see next section).
- Fetal anatomical screening for malformations. Not all major structural anomalies are easily detectable at this gestation. Those that are include anencephaly, holoprosencephaly and major abdominal wall defects.

The second US scan is offered to women when they are between 18 and 20 weeks. Most are undertaken at 20 weeks. The features recorded at this examination are:
- Confirmation of fetal viability.
- Establishing the number of fetuses.
- Measurement of fetal biometry (head and abdominal circumferences, biparietal diameter (BPD) and femur length). From these, the gestational age can be established or confirmed. Most centres use the BPD only for this, though some use a combination of measurements.
- Assessment of amniotic fluid volume.

Table 10.3 Chromosomal abnormalities by maternal age at the time of amniocentesis performed at 16 weeks' gestation (expressed as rate per 1000)

Maternal age (years)	Trisomy 21	Trisomy 18	Trisomy 13	XXY	All chromosomal anomalies
35	3.9	0.5	0.2	0.5	8.7
36	5.0	0.7	0.3	0.6	10.1
37	6.4	1.0	0.4	0.8	12.2
38	8.1	1.4	0.5	1.1	14.8
39	10.4	2.0	0.8	1.4	18.4
40	13.3	2.8	1.1	1.8	23.0
41	16.9	3.9	1.5	2.4	29.0
42	21.6	5.5	2.1	3.1	37.0
43	27.4	7.6		4.1	45.0
44	34.8			5.4	50.0
45	44.2			7.0	62.0
46	55.9			9.1	77.0
47	70.4			11.9	96.0

- Assessment of placental location and cord insertion.
- Offering the woman an anatomical survey which seeks to confirm a normal appearance in a number of organ systems listed next. The success at identifying structural abnormalities in these systems at about 20 weeks varies, and the approximate rates of detection with US reported in 2009 are:
  - All major malformations – 37%
  - Central nervous system – 84%
  - Exomphalos and gastroschisis – 80%
  - Respiratory – 75%
  - Major cardiac abnormalities – 63% (all cardiac abnormalities have a detection rate of <50%)
  - Genitalia – 58%
  - Diaphragmatic hernia – 38%
  - Gastrointestinal – 31%
  - Kidneys and urinary tract – 31%
  - Musculoskeletal – 26%
  - Facial clefts – 22%

Biochemistry

Women should be offered combined fetal aneuploidy screening between $11w^{+0d}$ and $13w^{+6d}$. In most centres, this comprises a risk estimate for trisomy 21 based on NT measurement (increased in trisomy 21), maternal age (increased chance of trisomy 21 with higher age) and maternal serum markers (free β-human chorionic gonadotrophin (β-hCG), which is higher with trisomy 21, and pregnancy-associated plasma protein A (PAPP-A), which is lower with trisomy 21). For each of these three parameters, the likelihood of a trisomy 21 fetus, given the background risk from the woman's age, is calculated against a database of over 200,000 pregnancies with known fetal trisomy 21 status. The three likelihood ratios can be merged into a single risk for the individual woman. Using a risk cut-off of 1:150 for trisomy 21, this screening approach has a detection rate of 90%, for a 5% false-positive rate.

This combined testing also identifies over 90% of other chromosomal abnormalities, including trisomies 18 and 13, Turner's syndrome and triploidy. Increased NT with a normal karyotype is at increased risk for major cardiac defects as well as other structural anomalies, rare genetic syndromes and other unfavourable outcomes.

If the NT and/or the combined testing indicates a high risk, more detailed ultrasonic examination of the fetus should be undertaken and karyotyping offered.

If the NT is raised but the karyotype is normal and the 11^{+0} to 13^{+6} week anomaly scan is apparently normal, it is advisable to repeat the anomaly scan at 14–16 weeks and again at 20–22 weeks to exclude anomalies. Detection rates for fetal anomalies are dependent on the organ system involved, sonographer experience and the mother's body mass index (BMI).

Whilst aneuploidy screening is best performed by combined screening in the first trimester (see earlier), when this has not taken place, women should be offered an alternative combination screening test at 14–17 weeks comprising

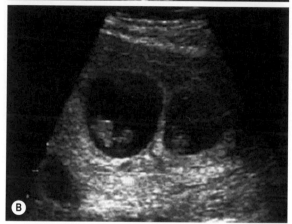

Fig. 10.6 Chorionicity. (A) Monochorionic twins (T-sign). (B) Dichorionic twins (lambda sign). (Reproduced with permission from Dodd JM, Grivell RM, Crowther CA (2011) Multiple pregnancy. In: James DK, Weiner CP, Gonik B, Crowther CA, Robson SC, eds. High Risk Pregnancy: Management Options, 4th edn. Saunders Elsevier, St Louis.)

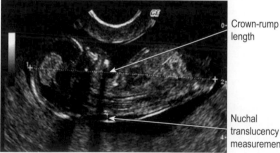

Crown–rump length

Nuchal translucency measurement

Fig. 10.7 Nuchal translucency (NT) measurement (undertaken when crown–rump length (CRL) = 45–84 mm). NT measurement: strict sagittal view appropriate for CRL, appropriate magnification (>70% image), away from the amnion, neutral position of the fetal head, biggest of three to five measurements.

maternal age and the 'quadruple test' (β-hCG, unconjugated oestriol (uE3), MSAFP and inhibin-A). Again, individual likelihood ratios for a trisomy 21 fetus are calculated for each (given the background risk from the woman's age) and combined into a single risk estimate. This second-trimester screening test does not 'perform' as well as the first-trimester test, having a detection rate (using a 1:150 risk threshold) of 65%, for a 5% false-positive rate. If the combined risk is raised, women should be offered karyotyping.

The recommendation from the UK National Screening Committee is that a trisomy 21 risk of greater than 1:150 indicates a 'high' risk and that further assessment in the form of chorionic villus sampling (CVS) in the first trimester or amniocentesis in the second trimester should be discussed with the woman and her partner. In practice, many prefer to present the risk estimate to the woman and allow her to make her own decision. For example, a woman aged 40 years who has a trisomy 21 risk of 1 in 130 from a quadruple test undertaken at 16 weeks may consider that to be an acceptable risk compared to her background age risk of 1:75 at that stage of pregnancy (see Table 10.3), especially when there is a risk of 1:100 of losing the pregnancy from an amniocentesis (see later). Conversely, a woman aged 20 years with a background risk of delivering a baby with trisomy 21 of over 1:1500 (see Table 10.2) may consider a 1:180 risk estimate in the first trimester to be too high and might want an invasive test (CVS, see later).

Non-invasive prenatal testing and diagnosis (NIPT and NIPD)

NIPT and NIPD allow women to have prenatal testing using a peripheral maternal blood sample.

These techniques are starting to be incorporated into clinical practice, though the degree they are used varies. They work on the basis that small quantities of fetal DNA derived from placental tissue circulate as cell-free fetal DNA (cffDNA) in the maternal plasma during pregnancy. Techniques have been developed to extract and analyze this cffDNA. The cffDNA is cleared from the maternal circulation within the first hour after birth, so it is specific to a woman's current pregnancy.

NIPT for aneuploidy is well established and can be used as a screening test for DS, Edwards syndrome, Patau syndrome and Turner's syndrome. The technology identifies approximately 98% of cases of DS, with a false-positive rate of less than 0.5%. It is less sensitive for Edwards syndrome (trisomy 18) and Patau syndrome (trisomy 13), with lower detection rates. However, NIPT is still a screening test, and when a positive result is obtained, an invasive diagnostic testing (by CVS or amniocentesis) is required to confirm the diagnosis. Its value is that it has a low false-positive rate and therefore has the potential to reduce the number of invasive diagnostic tests and pregnancy losses resulting from them.

In the United States, NIPT is recommended where women have an increased prior risk of aneuploidy (either because of their age or combined aneuploidy screening as described earlier). However, it is not used for routine primary screening in low-risk populations. In the UK, the way in which these tests are used varies; however, national guidance is anticipated.

In clinical practice, NIPD is currently offered:

- To determine the sex of a baby when the mother is known to be a carrier of a serious X-linked condition. An invasive diagnostic procedure will only be necessary if the fetus is male.
- To aid in the management of pregnancies at risk of the autosomal-recessive condition congenital adrenal hyperplasia. Dexamethasone may be given to women carrying affected female fetuses who are at risk of virilization.
- To determine the fetal genotype in Rhesus disease and some other red cell antibody disorders.

Finally, these techniques are not an alternative to invasive testing when a fetal structural abnormality is identified on US scan.

Counselling in advance of US and biochemical testing

Before a woman participates in any screening programme aimed at detecting fetal abnormalities, it is imperative that she has appropriate pre-test counselling. This should cover the following:

- emphasizing that the great majority of newborn babies are normal and that only a very small minority have an abnormality
- ensuring an understanding of the condition(s) that might be detected with the screening programme
- understanding:
  - the limitations of the screening programme, including the chances of missing an abnormality
  - what a 'normal' or 'negative' screening test means
  - what an 'abnormal' or 'positive' screening test means
  - what are the practical options if the screening test is 'abnormal' or 'positive'

Management options with an 'abnormal' or 'positive' test

Further counselling

Women (with their partner) with an abnormal/positive test should be seen as soon as possible by a health professional with the appropriate expertise and training for ongoing counselling and management. This will either be an obstetrician with a special interest in fetal problems or a fetal medicine subspecialist. The priority is for the woman and her partner to have non-directive counselling covering:

- what they have been told
- what they think the abnormal/positive test means

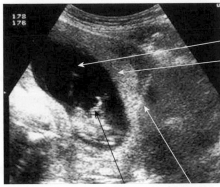

Fig. 10.8 Chorionic villus sampling (ultrasound visualization is mandatory and undertaken in a similar way to that shown for amniocentesis; see Fig 10.9A).

- what the abnormal/positive test actually means
- what the options are

Further assessment

It may be appropriate for the couple to consider further assessment in the form of:

- For women with an increased risk of a chromosomal abnormality, an invasive test such as a chorionic villus biopsy/sampling (Fig. 10.8) if the woman presents in the first trimester or an amniocentesis (Fig. 10.9) if the woman presents in the second trimester. Before undertaking the procedure, the woman should be informed that it is undertaken aseptically and will provide information about chromosome number and structure but that it carries a risk of miscarriage (about 1%).
- For women suspected to have a structural fetal abnormality, further imaging to clarify the diagnosis either in the form of further US examinations after 1–2 weeks (to allow for fetal growth and better visualization of fetal anatomy) or a magnetic resonance imaging (MRI) scan (especially useful with abnormalities of the central nervous system). If the anatomical appearances suggest that the fetus has a chromosomal abnormality, a CVS (which is more accurately termed *placental biopsy* at this stage of pregnancy) or amniocentesis could be offered.

Options for pregnancy

Once a fetal abnormality is diagnosed with a high chance of death or serious disability, after counselling, the parents may feel that they do not wish to continue with the pregnancy and opt for a termination. However, faced with the same facts, other parents may decide to continue with the

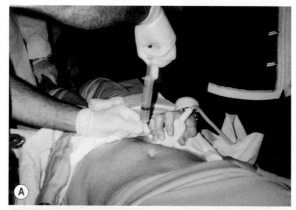

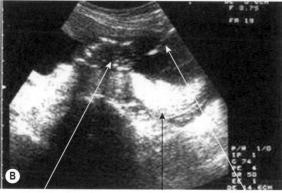

| Fetus (transverse section) | Posterior placenta | Needle in amniotic fluid |

Fig. 10.9 Amniocentesis. (A) Simultaneous ultrasound (US) visualization. (B) US image with needle *(arrows)*. (A Reproduced with permission from Chabner D-E. (2017) The Language of Medicine, 11th edn. Elsevier, St Louis.)

pregnancy. The decision is for the parents to make and no one else, hence the need for 'non-directive' counselling.

Possible interventions

With some fetal abnormalities, a woman and her partner may be offered interventions aimed at improving or ameliorating the fetal condition. Examples include:

- Maternally administered anti-arrhythmic drugs to treat fetal cardiac arrhythmias.
- Insertion of a vesicoamniotic drain into the fetal bladder to by-pass urethral obstruction in cases of urethral valves to prevent further renal back-pressure and damage.

Surveillance in pregnancy

All women who decide to continue with the pregnancy with a fetal abnormality will need to be seen regularly for support and counselling by a small number of health professionals who are aware of the diagnosis. In specific cases, there will be a need to undertake regular US examinations to assess whether complications of the abnormality are developing and warrant intervention (see earlier).

Delivery issues

Delivery issues may include:

- In advance of the delivery deciding on the place of birth based on the baby's likely need of resources after birth, e.g. neonatal intensive care or surgery, and arranging for the relevant neonatal medical professionals to meet the parents.
- Arranging elective delivery if it is considered desirable that the baby would benefit from delivery during the working day and week when full neonatal resources are available.
- With some fetal abnormalities, it is preferable to avoid a vaginal birth, e.g. where there may be a greater risk of fetal trauma, such as in a case of fetal hydrocephalus.

Assessing the health of a normally formed fetus

Screening for fetal health

> In contrast to the screening offered to pregnant women to assess their risk of fetal abnormality, what is offered to identify the unhealthy fetus is limited.

It relies initially on identification of clinical risk factors associated with a greater risk of fetal compromise. Women with no risk factors for fetal compromise ('low risk') have:

- Maternal vigilance for fetal activity over the second half of pregnancy.
- Fundal height measurement at every antenatal clinic visit. This involves measuring the distance between the maternal symphysis pubis and uterine fundus (see Fig. 6.12). The reverse blank side of tape measure uppermost and the distance (in cm) is read after it has been determined by turning the tape measure over. The normal range between 16 and 36 weeks is gestational age in weeks ±3 cm. Thus at 32 weeks the normal range is 32 ± 3 cm.
- Auscultation of the fetal heart at every antenatal clinic visit. This is undertaken either using a Pinard stethoscope (Fig. 10.10A) or a handheld Doppler US device (Fig. 10.10B). In routine practice, the rate is not recorded but just a note that the fetal heart is beating. Thus, abnormalities of the fetal baseline heart rate may be missed.

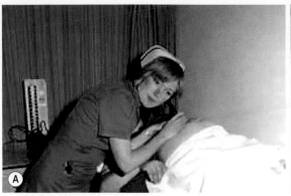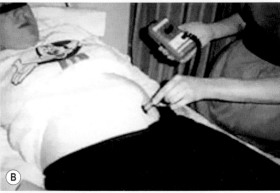

Fig. 10.10 Auscultation of the fetal heart (the aim is to place the stethoscope/transducer as close to the fetal heart as possible. If the fetal back is anterior, the best site is over the left fetal scapula. If the fetal back is posterior, the best site is around the maternal umbilicus. (A) Using the Pinard stethoscope; (B) using a handheld Doppler ultrasound recording device.

Women with risk factors ('high risk') have customized surveillance that is determined by the presumed underlying pathophysiological process. The more common examples are shown in Table 10.4.

Surveillance of fetal health in at-risk pregnancies

Based on the clinical risk assessment screening (see earlier), an individualized programme of fetal surveillance will be offered to 'at-risk' women during their pregnancy. The most commonly used methods are discussed here.

Fetal Doppler recordings

Fetal Doppler recordings are currently the best tools for fetal assessment in 'at-risk' pregnancies in the absence of fetal abnormality.

Doppler recordings of blood flow in the umbilical artery (UA)

This investigation has been shown to significantly improve fetal outcome in high-risk pregnancies. Figure 10.11A shows a normal recording.

Figure 10.11B shows an example of 'absent end-diastolic flow' (AEDV). The commonest explanation is an increase in placental vascular resistance ('downstream' from the point of recording), which is typical of umbilical placental vascular disease (UPVD). The prognosis for the fetus with AEDV is worse, with growth restriction, hypoxia and death all being commoner. However, the risk is not usually immediate, and management options include continued close surveillance with biophysical testing until a viable gestational age is reached or the biophysical testing is abnormal. If this abnormality occurs at 34 weeks or beyond, most would offer the

woman elective pre-term delivery (with pre-delivery maternal steroids to enhance fetal lung maturation) rather than continuing the pregnancy and the possibility of fetal death. The appearance of AEDV is preceded by the gradual reduction in the diastolic recording (and associated increase in 'systolic to diastolic (S/D) ratio'). A raised S/D ratio can be considered a milder and earlier stage of the same pathology with the same risk of eventual adverse outcome.

Figure 10.11C shows an example of 'reversed diastolic flow'. This is an even more ominous feature and is associated with a much higher chance of imminent fetal death. Management will depend on gestational age. If the pregnancy is at 26 weeks or more, elective pre-term delivery (with the attendant risks of prematurity) compared with continuing the pregnancy (and the high risk of fetal death) must be discussed with the parents. If the pregnancy is less than 26 weeks, the discussions are more difficult and the parents may opt for no intervention.

Doppler recordings of blood flow in the fetal middle cerebral artery (MCA) (Fig. 10.12)

An abnormal flow pattern in the UA Doppler may be associated with redistribution of blood flow in the fetus to allow better oxygenation to vital organs such as the brain and heart, leading to the 'brain-sparing' effect. This is demonstrated by a reduced resistance to blood flow in the MCA and an increase in systolic values. This is the reason for asymmetrical fetal growth restriction (FGR) being associated with UPVD in late pregnancy where head growth can remain normal whilst growth of the rest of the body can be restricted (see later).

The MCA also can be used as a non-invasive method of assessing the degree of fetal anaemia. This is most commonly used in women with Rhesus disease (where the women are Rhesus-negative and they are producing anti-D antibodies that can cross the placenta causing a haemolytic anaemia in a Rhesus-positive fetus). In those cases, US evidence of fetal

Table 10.4 Risk factors for fetal compromise

Type of risk	Risk factor/problem	Presumed pathophysiology	Surveillance
Specific	Maternal vascular disease, e.g. hypertension (pre-existing, severe pregnancy-induced hypertension, pre-eclampsia), antiphospholipid or lupus antibodies, renal impairment	Uteroplacental vascular disease (UPVD), i.e. poor blood flow to and within the placenta with associated reduced gaseous and nutritional transfer	Maternal vigilance for fetal movements Umbilical artery (UA) Doppler recordings; if this is abnormal, record middle cerebral artery (MCA) and ductus venosus (DV) Doppler US monitoring of fetal growth Biophysical assessment if any of these not normal
	Maternal diabetes, especially if associated with vascular disease	The pathophysiology of fetal risk is uncertain	The same package of surveillance is used as in women with UPVD, but it is less effective at predicting fetal death
	Twins	Main risks are: **For all twins:** fetal growth restriction from UPVD **For monochorionic twins (in addition):** the twin–twin transfusion syndrome (TTTS), i.e. shared placental circulation with risk of one fetus being the 'donor' and the other being the 'recipient'	For fetal growth restriction: • Fetal surveillance as in women at risk of UPVD (see earlier) For TTTS, monitoring of monochorionic twins to look for signs of TTTS: • Amniotic fluid volume (AFV) raised in one twin (recipient) and reduced in the other (donor) • Absence of urine in fetal bladders • Abnormal umbilical artery Doppler recording in either fetus
	Isoimmunization due to Rhesus antibodies	Transplacental passage of maternal antibodies (anti-D or Kell or Duffy) causing severe fetal anaemia	With severe fetal anaemia, the fetal MCA Doppler recording of blood flow is raised and confirmed by fetal blood sampling (FBS)
Non-specific major risk factors	Previous fetal death Previous fetal growth restriction Mother or father was small for gestational age when born PAPP-A <0.4 MoM (a first-trimester biochemical aneuploidy screening test) Maternal perception of reduced fetal movements Vaginal bleeding Abdominal pain Others: maternal age >40 yr, smoking >10/day, cocaine use	A variety of pathologies result in fetal death, fetal growth restriction, reduced movements, vaginal bleed and abdominal pain. Unless the cause is known, the normal approach initially is to assume it is UPVD	Fetal surveillance as in women at risk of UPVD (see earlier) In women with reduced fetal movement (FM), ongoing surveillance is only needed where the FM does not return to normal In women with vaginal bleeding or abdominal pain, ongoing surveillance is needed only where the symptoms persist
	Abnormal uterine size and/or growth (larger or smaller than normal) identified from abnormal symphysiofundal height charts/graphs	Many cases of clinically suspected abnormal fetal growth are not confirmed with US. If confirmed, a variety of pathologies result in fetal growth restriction. Unless cause is known, the normal approach is to assume it is UPVD	If abnormal fetal size/growth confirmed with US fetal assessment as in women at risk of UPVD (see earlier)

Table 10.4 Risk factors for fetal compromise—cont'd

Type of risk	Risk factor/problem	Presumed pathophysiology	Surveillance
Non-specific minor risk factors; three or more are considered an indication for uterine artery Doppler at 20–24 wk	Maternal age 35–39 Nulliparity BMI <20 or 30 or more Smoking </=10/day Invitro fertilization (IVF) single-ton pregnancy Previous pre-eclampsia	These are minor risk factors for fetal growth restriction presumed to be due to UPVD	Uterine artery Doppler at 20–24 wk – if abnormal for detailed US fetal assessment as in women at risk of UPVD (see earlier)

anaemia allows optimization of the timing of invasive fetal testing and fetal blood transfusion (Fig. 10.13).

Doppler recordings of blood flow in the fetal ductus venosus (DV) (Fig. 10.14)

This redistribution of blood flow within the fetus in association with UPVD is reflected in higher resistance in venous circulation due to an increasing afterload of the right heart and increasing intraventricular pressure caused by hypoxia of the fetal myocardium correlating with fetal acidosis. The most commonly used venous Doppler is the DV, which is a four-phase waveform that is important in regulating distribution of oxygen and nutrition. The 'a' wave, synonymous with atrial contraction of the fetal heart, is the common parameter used for monitoring in FGR. As FGR progresses, the rising cardiac afterload reduces forward venous flow during right atrial contraction, causing the 'a' wave to become progressively deeper. A reversed 'a' wave signifies heart failure and cardiac decompensation. The umbilical vein should have a constant velocity of flow to the fetus. In a compromised fetus, there may be retrograde pulsatility in the umbilical vein, which is commonly seen at the same degree of compromise when there is reversed 'a' wave in the DV. These findings are pre-terminal, indicating a need for immediate delivery.

Doppler recordings of blood flow in the maternal uterine artery (Fig. 10.15)

Uterine artery Doppler is a biophysical marker of placental function. Impaired placentation with abnormal blood-flow velocity and resistance in the placental vessels (indicated by a rise in the ratio of S/D values and/or 'notching' in the uterine artery waveform) in the first and second trimesters is associated with maternal fetal complications such as early-onset pre-eclampsia and FGR. In screening for fetuses at risk of growth restriction, the Royal College of Obstetricians and Gynaecologists (RCOG) is a professional association based in London. Its members, including people with and without medical degrees, work in the field of obstetrics and gynaecology, that is, pregnancy, childbirth and female sexual and reproductive health. The college has over 16,000 members in over 100 countries with nearly 50% of those residing outside the British Isles. In 2014, the RCOG recommended that in high-risk populations UA Doppler recordings at 20–24 weeks of pregnancy have a moderate predictive value for a severely small for gestational age (SGA) neonate. Women who are identified to have risk factors for delivery of an SGA neonate should be offered uterine artery Doppler. Women with an abnormal uterine artery Doppler at 20–24 weeks should be referred for serial US measurement of fetal size and assessment of wellbeing, with UA Doppler commencing at 26–28 weeks.

Fetal growth

Fetal growth is best documented in pregnancy using serial US measurements of head (HC) and abdominal (AC) circumferences.

Small fetuses

Three patterns of suboptimal fetal growth are recognized. Once the AC is on or below the lowest centile, the fetus is termed *small-for-dates*.

Figure 10.16A illustrates a constitutionally small fetus. Genetic factors contribute to this pattern. Typically, the mother will be short and/or of Asian ethnicity. If multiparous, her previous baby(ies) may have been small. Whilst this fetus is not at such a high risk of complications as in the pathologically small fetus (see later), those risks are still greater compared to a normally grown fetus.

Figure 10.16B and C represents fetal growth patterns that are due to a pathological cause. They represent different points on the spectrum of FGR. The asymmetrical type tends to occur later in pregnancy and is more commonly associated with conditions such as UPVD in the last trimester, whereas the symmetrical type tends to represent a pathological insult that operated from an early point in

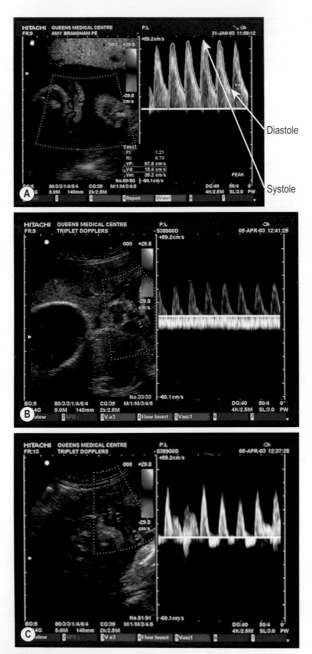

Fig. 10.11 Doppler ultrasound (US) recording of umbilical artery blood flow. (A) Normal. Note: The left US image shows the umbilical artery (UA) with red and blue colours indicating blood flow. The right US image is the Doppler recording taken from that UA. The peak of the wave represents the peak of the systolic phase and the trough the diastolic phase of the fetal cardiac cycle, respectively. In the normal fetoplacental circulation, there is always forward flow even when the heart is not contracting because there is a low resistance to flow within the placental circulation. (B) Abnormal – absent end diastolic flow. Note: There is no forward flow during diastole for most of the cardiac cycles. (C) Abnormal – reversed diastolic flow. Note: There is forward flow of blood in the UA during systole but the direction of flow reverses in diastole.

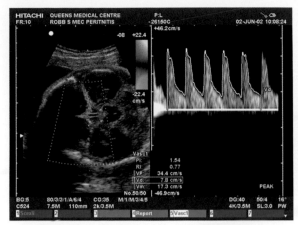

Fig. 10.12 Normal fetal middle cerebral artery Doppler waveforms.

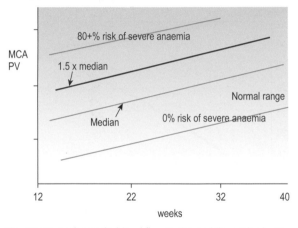

Fig. 10.13 Peak systolic blood flow in the middle cerebral artery as a predictor of fetal anaemia. Green lines indicate the normal range and median values; the solid red line indicates the threshold for the [1.5 × median] value. In cases of fetal haemolytic disease, fetuses with values below that line do not have severe anaemia, whilst those fetuses with values above the line have an 80% risk of severe anaemia requiring intrauterine transfusion. *MCA*, Middle cerebral artery; *PV*, peak velocity.

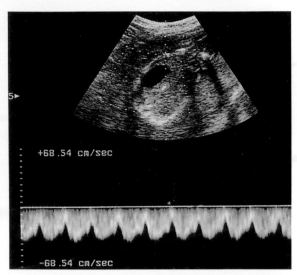

Fig. 10.14 Normal fetal ductus venosus Doppler waveforms.

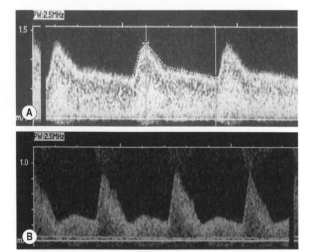

Fig. 10.15 Maternal uterine artery Doppler waveforms. The upper image (A) shows a normal uterine artery wave form with high-volume diastolic flow indicating successful trophoblastic implantation. The lower image (B) shows an abnormal uterine artery wave form with low-volume diastolic flow, with notching indicating unsuccessful trophoblastic implantation with increased placental resistance. (Reproduced with permission from Baschat AA (2011) Fetal growth disorders. In: James DK, Weiner CP, Gonik B, Crowther CA, Robson SC, eds. High Risk Pregnancy: Management Options, 4th edn, Saunders Elsevier, St Louis.)

pregnancy, e.g. fetal abnormality and severe early-onset pre-eclampsia. Both are associated with a higher risk of fetal death and hypoxia, pre-term delivery and placental bleeding.

Big fetuses

In an analogous way to small fetuses, large fetuses can either be:

- Constitutionally large ('large-for-dates') with the HC and AC growth trajectories both following the top centile line. Typically, the woman would be tall and/or of Afro-Caribbean ethnicity.

- Pathologically large ('macrosomia') with the HC growth trajectory following a centile in the normal range but the AC growth trajectory demonstrates accelerated growth upwards across centiles. This pattern of growth is most commonly seen in fetuses of diabetic women.

163

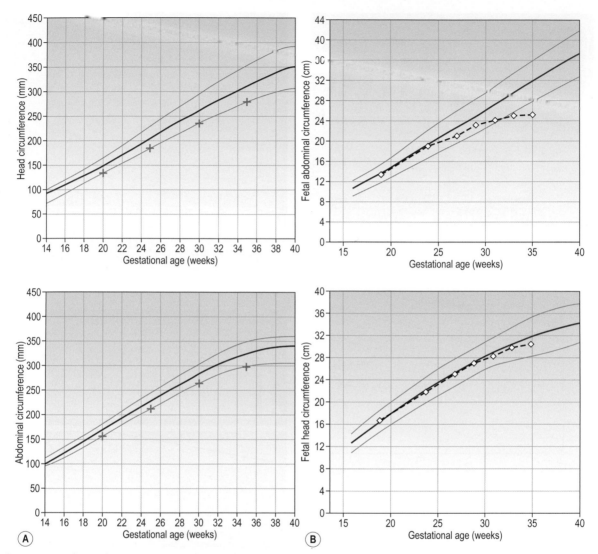

Fig. 10.16 Fetal growth patterns detected using ultrasound. (A) Constitutionally small fetus. Note: Both head circumference (HC) and abdominal circumference (AC) follow the lowest growth trajectories. (B) Asymmetrically small fetus. Note: The HC follows a normal trajectory, whilst the AC crosses trajectories and eventually falls outside the normal range. The lower and upper blue lines are the 5th and 95th growth centiles respectively and the red line is the 50th growth centile for the normal population.

Amniotic fluid volume (AFV)

The most accurate estimate of AFV is with US. Two methods are used:

- Single deepest pocket (the normal range is 2–8 cm).
- Amniotic fluid index (AFI), which is the sum of the depths of the pools of amniotic fluid in each of the four quadrants of the uterus (top right and left and bottom right and left). Figure 10.17 shows the normal range of the AFI during pregnancy.

Causes of reduced and increased amniotic fluid are discussed in Chapter X.

Biophysical measurements

The behaviour of a fetus is a useful indicator of his or her immediate wellbeing. With most fetal pathologies, these parameters are affected relatively late in the process. The five observations used in practice are:

- Fetal heart rate (FHR): this is recorded with a cardiotocograph (CTG) (as in labour). The maximum recording time is 40 minutes and in that time, there should be at least two accelerations of the FHR by 15 beats/min or more and lasting for at least 15 seconds. The patterns of heart rate change are similar to those described in labour

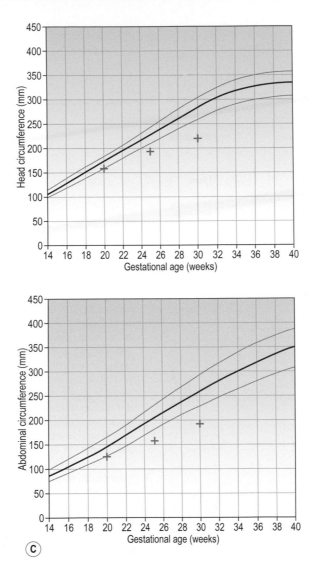

Fig. 10.16, cont'd. (C) Symmetrically small fetus. Note: Both HC and AC fall away from the normal growth trajectories. Such head growth compromise carries a greater likelihood of developmental delay in childhood.

(see Chapter 11), with the difference that uterine activity is minimal and more emphasis is therefore placed on the interpretation of baseline heart rate. An example of a normal antenatal CTG is shown in Figure 10.18. This shows a baseline variability of more than 5 beats/min with accelerations and no decelerations. Figure 10.19 shows a normal baseline rate but reduced baseline variability.

- Fetal movements: there should be at least three separate/discreet movements in 40 minutes of fetal observation with US.
- Fetal tone: at least one of these fetal movements should demonstrate a full 90-degree flexion–extension–flexion cycle.
- Fetal breathing: there should be a sustained 30-second period of regular fetal breathing movements during the 40-minute observation period.
- AFV: there should be at least one vertical pool measuring between 2 and 8 cm.

The use of all five parameters in combination is called *the biophysical profile* or *biophysical score* (BPP or BPS). A normal response is for the fetus to exhibit at least four of these parameters in a period of up to 40 minutes (they may be seen in a much shorter period). The original BPS was recorded over 30 minutes but that did not take account of the possibility of normal fetal 'sleep', which can last up to 40 minutes and during which no movements, accelerations

165

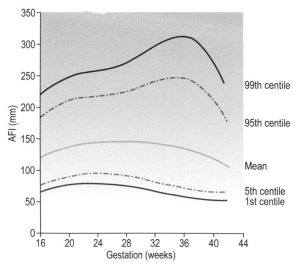

Fig. 10.17 Amniotic fluid index.

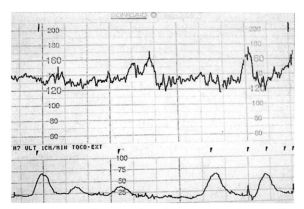

Fig. 10.18 Normal antenatal cardiotocograph. The recording shows a baseline variability of >5 beats/min and episodes of accelerations.

or breathing may be seen, hence the change to an observation window of 40 minutes.

Interventions

For non-specific risk

When a theoretic risk to the fetus is proven to be real by fetal surveillance, the only three interventions of value are:
- Elective delivery: if the risk is identified at 34 or more weeks, there is usually no reason to delay the delivery. Where the risk is identified before 34 weeks, the management is determined by the assessment of immediate

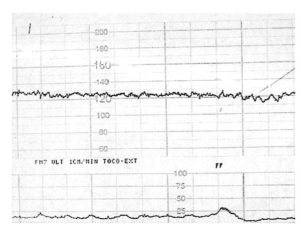

Fig. 10.19 Antenatal cardiotocograph showing a normal heart rate but reduced baseline variability.

risk of fetal death. Thus, if the BPS or CTG (acute measures of health) are abnormal and/or there is reversed end diastolic flow in the UA, then delivery without delay is discussed with the parents. Where there is no abnormality in these parameters, continued close monitoring could continue to 'gain' time in the pregnancy and allow the maternal administration of steroids.
- Steroids administered to a woman before pre-term birth: if it is clear that elective pre-term delivery is likely to occur in an at-risk pregnancy but only the chronic measures of fetal health are abnormal, e.g. suboptimal growth and absent UA Doppler diastolic recordings, the woman would be advised to have a course of betamethasone.
- Magnesium sulphate administered to woman before pre-term birth: pre-term birth is associated with an increased risk of brain injury in the newborn and subsequent neurodevelopmental disability. The injury can be in the form of one or more of the following: diffuse white matter injury, intraventricular and/or intraparenchymal haemorrhage and cystic and periventricular leukomalacia. The gestation when newborns are most susceptible is between 24 and 34 weeks. However, prenatal administration of magnesium sulphate to extremely pre-term infants (especially before 30 weeks) has been shown to have neuroprotective effects. The detailed mechanisms for this neuroprotective effect of magnesium sulphate are unknown.

For specific risk

These are relatively uncommon and include:
- maternal drugs for fetal cardiac arrhythmias
- intrauterine blood transfusion for fetuses with severe Rhesus isoimmunization
- laser ablation of placental vascular communications in twin-to-twin transfusion syndrome

Conclusions

- Most, though not all, fetuses with structural or chromosomal abnormality are identified during pregnancy with current screening programmes.
- In normally formed fetuses, once risk is identified, both specific and non-specific, the current methods of surveillance coupled with the judicious use of maternal steroid administration and elective delivery are effective in the sense that most fetuses identified to be 'at risk' will not die in utero.
- In normally formed fetuses that are apparently at no risk, the current method of routine surveillance during pregnancy (maternal perception of fetal movements, fundal height measurement and auscultation of the fetal heart) is limited and does not identify all fetuses that are genuinely at risk.

Essential information

Congenital abnormalities

- Fetal abnormality is found in:
  - over 50% of conceptions
  - about 70% of miscarriages
  - 15% of deaths between 20 weeks and 1 year postnatal
  - 1–2% of births, including major and minor anomalies
  - 8% of special needs register/disabled children
- The overall UK incidence has fallen over the past 30 years due to:
  - Introduction of screening programmes in pregnancy
  - Greater success at diagnosis during pregnancy
  - Parents choosing pregnancy termination
- The commonest four groups of defects are
  - Neural tube defects (3–7/1000 births)
  - Congenital cardiac defects (6/1000 births)
  - Down's syndrome (1.5/1000 births)
  - Cleft lip/palate (1.5/1000 births)
- Screening for fetal abnormality can be undertaken
  - Clinically in early pregnancy (including maternal age, certain drugs, previous abnormal baby, diabetes)
  - Clinically in late pregnancy (including abnormal uterine size, abnormal fetal movements, abnormal fetal lie)
  - Using US (including measurement of NT at the end of the first trimester and an anatomical survey at 20 weeks)
  - Biochemically (measurement of biochemical markers which in combination with NT measurement estimate chromosomal abnormality risk)
  - Balanced pre-test counselling is important with US and biochemical screening
- Options following non-directive counselling with an abnormal/positive screening test include
  - Further assessment (such as repeat US scan after an interval, amniocentesis or CVS to establish the felt karyotype, other imaging including MRI)
  - Specific interventions (such as anti-arrhythmic drugs, drainage of fetal fluid collections)
  - Termination of pregnancy

- Continuation of pregnancy with ongoing surveillance and specific plans for timing, mode and place of delivery

Assessing the health of a normally formed fetus

- Surveillance of fetal health in a low-risk pregnancy comprises
  - Maternal vigilance for fetal activity in the latter half of pregnancy
  - Fundal height measurement and charting
  - Auscultation of the fetal heart
- Surveillance of fetal health in a high-risk pregnancy comprises
  - Tests used will depend on the presumed underlying pathophysiology (such as maternal uterine artery Doppler, fetal Dopplers (UA, MCA and DV blood flow) and fetal growth for suspected UPVD and Doppler recordings of MCA blood flow if fetal anaemia is a risk)
  - The majority of fetuses, including those where there is uncertainty about the pathophysiology, will have combined serial measurements of
    - Fetal Doppler recordings (UA, MCA and DV blood flow)
    - Fetal growth (especially HC and AC)
    - Amniotic fluid volume
    - Biophysical parameters (FHR, movements, tone and breathing)
- Interventions
  - Non-specific or unknown pathophysiology
- Elective delivery – the timing, depending on the degree of fetal risk
- Maternal administration of steroids if a pre-term delivery is planned
  - Specific or known pathophysiology (rare)
  - Maternal anti-arrhythmic drugs for fetal cardiac arrhythmias
  - Fetal blood transfusion(s) for severe fetal anaemia
  - Laser ablation of placental vascular anastamoses with twin–twin transfusion syndrome

Chapter | 11 |

Management of labour

Sabaratnam Arulkumaran

LEARNING OUTCOMES

After studying this chapter you should be able to:

Knowledge criteria

- Describe the mechanisms, diagnosis and management of normal and abnormal labour
- Describe the methods of induction and augmentation of labour, including the indications, contraindications and complications
- Describe the aetiology and management of cord prolapse
- Discuss the impact and management of pre-term labour, pre-labour rupture of membranes and precipitate labour
- Summarize the methods of assessment of fetal wellbeing used in labour, e.g. meconium, fetal heart rate monitoring and fetal scalp blood sampling
- Explain the options available for pain relief and anaesthesia in labour

Clinical competencies

- Participate in the management of normal labour
- Interpret the results of fetal heart rate monitoring in labour
- Assess the progress of labour, including the use of partograms, and explain the findings to the labouring woman

Professional skills and attitudes

- Demonstrate respect for cultural and religious differences in attitudes to childbirth
- Demonstrate empathy by effective communication and providing reassurance to women in labour
- Demonstrate awareness of importance of multi-professional working in the care of women in labour (communicate findings and management plans with midwives and doctors)

Labour, or *parturition*, is the process whereby the products of conception are expelled from the uterine cavity after the twenty-fourth week of gestation. About 93–94% deliver at term, i.e. between 37 and 42 weeks, while about 7–8% develop pre-term labour and deliver pre-term from 24 to 37 weeks. *Pre-term labour* is defined as labour occurring before the commencement of the thirty-seventh week of gestation. Prior to 24 weeks, this process results in a pre-viable fetus and is termed *miscarriage*. *Prolonged labour* is defined as labour lasting more than 24 hours in a primigravida and 16 hours in a multigravida. Prolonged labour is associated with increased fetal and maternal morbidity and mortality.

Stages of labour

The early preparation (pre-labour phase) goes on for days and weeks, while the onset of painful uterine contractions and delivery is shorter and the process is called *parturition* or *labour*. The cervix ripens by becoming softer, shorter and dilated, which takes a greater speed with onset of uterine contractions.

For purposes of clinical management, the 'observed' labour, which is a continuum, is divided into three stages:

- **The first stage** commences with the onset of regular painful contractions and cervical changes until it reaches full dilatation and the cervix is no longer palpable. The first stage is divided into an early slow latent phase when the cervix becomes effaced and shortens from 3 cm in length and dilates up to 5 cm. Following recent studies, the latent phase has been defined to continue to 5 cm, and an active phase when the cervix dilates from 5 cm to full dilatation or 10 cm. The evidence comes from recent studies that have described rates of cervical dilatation in a large number of nulliparous and multiparous women admitted in spontaneous labour. Median time in nullipara for cervical change of 3–4 cm was 1.8 hours, 4–5 cm was

1.3 hours, 5–6 cm was 0.8 hours, 6–7 cm was 0.6 hours, 7–8 cm was 0.5 hours, 8–9 cm was 0.5 hours and 9–10 cm was 0.5 hours. Based on this, one could state that the active phase starts from 5 cm cervical dilatation.

- **The second stage** is the duration from full cervical dilatation to delivery of the fetus. This is subdivided into a pelvic or passive phase, when the head descends in the pelvis, and an active or perineal phase, when the mother gets a stronger urge to push and the fetus is delivered with the force of the uterine contractions and the maternal bearing-down effort.
- **The third stage** is the duration from the delivery of the newborn to delivery of the placenta and membranes.

Onset of labour

It is often difficult to be certain of the exact time of onset of labour because contractions may be irregular and may start and stop with no cervical change, i.e. 'false labour'. The duration of labour for management purposes is based on the observed progress of the contractions and cervical changes along with the descent of the head. This concept may have to be judged based on the place of practice, as in some remote areas a mother may be brought in after a day of labour with no progress. Her general condition and findings of the maternal and fetal conditions should dictate management. In the rare cases of cervical stenosis that can occur after surgery to the cervix, normal contractions of labour may produce thinning of the cervix without cervical dilatation.

The clinical signs of the onset of labour are:

- Regular, painful uterine contractions that increase in frequency, duration and intensity that produce progressive cervical effacement and dilatation and descent of the fetal presenting part.
- The passage of blood-stained mucus from the cervix, called the *show*, is associated with but is not on its own an indicator of the onset of labour.
- Similarly, rupture of the fetal membranes can be at the onset of labour, but this is variable and may occur without uterine contractions. If the latent period between rupture of membranes (ROM) to onset of painful uterine contractions is greater than 4 hours, it is called *pre-labour rupture of membranes (PROM)*, and this can occur at term or in the pre-term period, when it is called *pre-term pre-labour rupture of membranes (PPROM)*.

> Labour is one of the commonest clinical conditions, and yet the diagnosis may need time and sequential vaginal examination to assess cervical changes unless the mother is admitted in advanced labour.
>
> Accurate diagnosis of labour is important to avoid unnecessary interventions such as artificial rupture of membranes (ARM) or the use of oxytocin infusion.

Initiation of labour

The onset of labour involves progesterone withdrawal and an increase in oestrogen and prostaglandin action. The mechanisms that regulate these changes are unresolved but are likely to involve placental production of the peptide hormone corticotrophin-releasing hormone (CRH).

During pregnancy, painless irregular uterine activity is present. It is minimal in early pregnancy and greater with advancing gestation. A cascade of events is regulated and controlled by the feto-placental unit. At the end of gestation, there is gradual downregulation of those factors that keep the uterus and cervix quiescent and an upregulation of pro-contractile influences.

Placental development across gestation leads to an exponential increase in the number of syncytiotrophoblast nuclei in which transcription of the *CRH* gene occurs. This maturational process leads to an exponential increase in the levels of maternal and fetal plasma CRH. The CRH has direct actions on the placenta to increase oestrogen synthesis and reduce progesterone synthesis. In the fetus, the CRH directly stimulates the fetal zone of the adrenal gland to produce dehydroepiandrosterone (DHEA), the precursor of placental oestrogen synthesis. CRH also stimulates the synthesis of prostaglandins by the membranes. The fall in progesterone and increase in oestrogens and prostaglandins lead to increases in connexin 43 that promote connectivity of uterine myocytes and change uterine myocyte electrical excitability, which in turn lead to increases in generalized uterine contractions:

- The uterine myocytes contract and shorten, unlike the process in striated muscle, where cells contract but then return to their pre-contraction length.
- Ion channels within the myometrium influence the influx of calcium ions into the myocytes and promote contraction of the myometrial cells.
- Other hormones produced in the placenta directly or indirectly influence myometrial contractility (e.g. relaxin, activin A, follistatin, human chorionic gonadotrophin (hCG) and CRH) by influencing the production of cyclic adenosine monophosphate (cAMP) that causes relaxation of myometrial cells.

The integrity of the cervix is essential to retain the products of conception. It contains myocytes and fibroblasts, and towards term becomes soft and stretchable due to an increase in leucocyte infiltration and a decrease in the amount of collagen with the increase in proteolytic enzyme activity. Increased production of hyaluronic acid reduces the affinity of fibronectin for collagen. The affinity of hyaluronic acid for water causes the cervix to become soft and stretchable, i.e. ripening of the cervix.

Reduced cervical resistance (i.e. release of the brakes in a car) and increasing frequency, duration and strength of uterine contractions (i.e. accelerator of the car) are needed for the progress of labour. The first stage of labour that starts from onset of painful uterine contractions to full dilatation is divided into a slow latent phase when the cervix becomes shorter, i.e. effaced and dilated to 5 cm (an average of 6–8 hours in nulliparae and 4–6 hours in a multiparae) and an active phase of labour when the cervix dilates at an average of 1 cm per hour from 5 cm to full cervical dilatation.

Uterine activity in labour: the powers

The uterus exhibits infrequent, low-intensity contractions throughout pregnancy. As full term approaches, uterine activity increases in frequency, duration and strength of contractions. By palpation or external tocography one can identify the frequency and duration of contractions, but intrauterine pressure catheters are needed to assess the strength of contractions. It is likely that labour would be established if two contractions each lasting for >20 seconds are observed in 10 minutes in a regular manner. Normal resting tonus in labour starts at around 10–20 mmHg and increases slightly during labour (Fig. 11.1). Contractions increase in intensity with progress of labour, which in some ways is characterized by the increasing duration of contractions. The World Health Organization (WHO) recommends contraction recording on the partograph based on the frequency and duration of contractions.

> ! In late pregnancy, strong contractions can sometimes be palpated that do not produce cervical dilatation, and hence do not constitute true labour.

Progressive uterine contractions cause effacement and dilatation of the cervix as the result of shortening of myometrial fibres in the upper uterine segment and stretching and thinning of the lower uterine segment (Fig. 11.2). This process is known as *retraction*. The lower segment becomes elongated and thinned as labour progresses, and the junction between the upper and lower segment rises in the abdomen. Where labour becomes obstructed, the junction of the upper and lower segments may become visible at the level of the umbilicus; this is known as a *retraction ring* (also known as *Bandl's ring*).

A pacemaker for the uterus has never been demonstrated by anatomical, pharmacological, electrical or physiological studies. The electrical contraction impulse starts in one

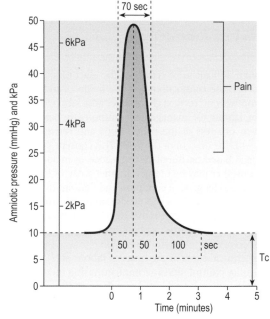

Fig. 11.1 Uterine contractions reach pressures of 50 mmHg (6.5 kPa) with first stage of labour. Contractions become painful when amniotic pressure exceeds 25 mmHg (3.2 kPa).

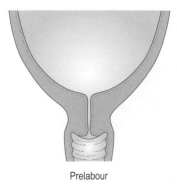

Prelabour

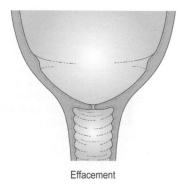

Effacement

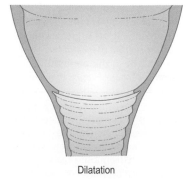

Dilatation

Fig. 11.2 Effacement and dilatation of the cervix in labour with formation of the lower uterine segment.

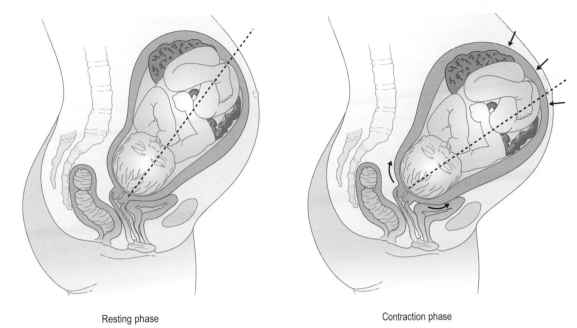

| Resting phase | Contraction phase |

Fig. 11.3 Change in direction of the fetal and uterine axis during contractions in labour.

or the other uterine fundal region and spreads downwards through the myometrium. Contractions are stronger and last longer in the fundus and upper segment than in the lower segment. This *fundal dominance* is essential for progressive effacement and dilatation of the cervix. As the uterus and the round ligaments contract, the axis of the uterus straightens and pulls the longitudinal axis of the fetus towards the anterior abdominal wall in line with the inlet of the true pelvis.

The realignment of the uterine axis promotes descent of the presenting part as the fetus is pushed directly downwards into the pelvic cavity (Fig. 11.3).

The passages

The shape and structure of the bony pelvis have already been described (see Chapter 1). The size and shape of the pelvis vary from woman to woman. Not all women have a gynaecoid pelvis; some may have a platypelloid, anthropoid or android pelvis, thus influencing the outcome of labour. Softening of the sacroiliac ligaments and the pubic symphysis allows expansion of the pelvic cavity, and this feature, along with the dynamic changes of the head diameter brought about by flexion, rotation and moulding, facilitates normal progress and spontaneous vaginal delivery.

The soft tissues of the pelvis are more distensible than in the non-pregnant state. Substantial distension of the pelvic floor and vaginal orifice occurs during the descent

and birth of the head. The distensible nature of the pelvic soft tissues, vagina and perineum helps to reduce the risk of tearing of the perineum and vaginal walls during descent and birth of the head.

The mechanism of labour

The pelvic inlet offers a larger lateral than an anteroposterior diameter. This promotes the head to normally engage in the pelvis in the transverse position. The passage of the head and trunk through the pelvis follows a well-defined pattern because the upper pelvic strait is transverse, the middle pelvic strait is circular and the outer pelvic strait is anteroposterior. The fetal head presents by the vertex in 95% of the cases, and hence is called *normal presentation*. With the vertex presentation, the head is well flexed in 90% of the cases and the head rotates to an occipito-anterior position and presents the shortest diameters, i.e. anteroposterior suboccipitobregmatic (9.5 cm) and lateral biparietal (9.5 cm) diameters; hence, the occipitoanterior position where the occiput is in the anterior half of the pelvis is called the *normal position*. A deflexed or extended head presents as an occipitoposterior or transverse position and with further extension as a brow or face presentation. Labour with an occipitoposterior position is prolonged as a larger anteroposterior diameter of occipitobregmatic or occipitofrontal diameter (11.5 cm) presents to the pelvis.

171

With the brow presentation, entry of the head into the pelvic brim is difficult, as it presents the largest anteroposterior mentovertical diameter (13.5 cm). The brow presentation can flex to a vertex or extend to a face presentation. If there is no progress of cervical dilatation, the baby is best delivered by caesarean section in a term brow presentation.

The process of normal labour therefore involves the adaptation of the fetal head to the various segments and diameters of the maternal pelvis, and the following processes occur (Fig. 11.4):

1. **Descent** occurs throughout labour and is both a feature and a prerequisite for the birth of the baby. Engagement of the head normally occurs before the onset of labour in most primigravid women but may not occur until labour is well established in a multipara. Descent of the head provides a measure of the progress of labour.

2. **Flexion** of the head occurs as it descends and meets the medially and forward-sloping pelvic floor, bringing the chin into contact with the fetal thorax. Flexion produces a smaller diameter of presentation, changing from the occipitofrontal diameter, when the head is deflexed, to the suboccipitobregmatic diameter, when the head is fully flexed.

3. **Internal rotation:** The head rotates as it reaches the pelvic floor, and the occiput normally rotates anteriorly from the lateral position towards the pubic symphysis. This is due to the force of contractions being transmitted via the fetal spine to the head at the point the spine meets the skull, which is more posterior and due to the medially and forward-sloping pelvic floor. Occasionally, it rotates posteriorly towards the hollow of the sacrum, and the head may then deliver as a face-to-pubis delivery.

4. **Extension:** The acutely flexed head descends to distend the pelvic floor and the vulva, and the base of the occiput meets the inferior rami of the pubis. The head now extends until it is delivered. Maximal distension of the perineum and introitus occurs just prior to the final expulsion of the head, a process that is known as *crowning* when the head is seen at the introitus but does not recede in between contractions.

5. **Restitution:** Following delivery of the head, it rotates back to be in line with its normal relationship to the fetal shoulders. The direction of the occiput following restitution points to the position of the vertex before the delivery.

6. **External rotation:** When the shoulders reach the pelvic floor, they rotate into the anteroposterior diameter of the pelvis. This is accompanied by rotation of the fetal head so that the face looks laterally at the maternal thigh.

7. **Delivery of the shoulders:** Final expulsion of the trunk occurs following delivery of the shoulders. The anterior shoulder is delivered first by traction posteriorly on the

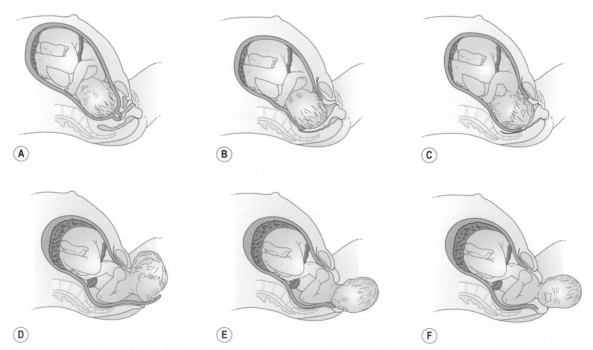

(A) (B) (C)

(D) (E) (F)

Fig. 11.4 The mechanisms of normal labour involve (A) descent of the presenting part; (B) flexion of the head; (C) internal rotation; (D) distension of the perineum and extension of the fetal head; (E) delivery of the head; (F) delivery of the shoulders.

fetal head so that the shoulder emerges under the pubic arch. The posterior shoulder is delivered by lifting the head anteriorly over the perineum, and this is followed by rapid delivery of the remainder of the trunk and the lower limbs.

The occiput normally rotates anteriorly, but if it rotates posteriorly, it deflexes and presents a larger diameter to the pelvic cavity. As a result, the second stage may be prolonged and the damage to the perineum and vagina is increased.

The third stage of labour

The third stage of labour starts with the completed expulsion of the baby and ends with the delivery of the placenta and membranes (Fig. 11.5).

Once the baby is delivered, the uterine muscle contracts, shearing off the placenta and pushing it into the lower segment and the vault of the vagina.

The classic signs of placental separation include trickling of bright blood, lengthening of the umbilical cord and elevation of the uterine fundus within the abdominal cavity. The uterine fundus becomes firm to hard and smaller and rounded instead of being broad and globular and sits on top of the placenta as it descends into the lower segment.

The duration of placental separation may be compressed using oxytocic drugs administered at the delivery of the anterior shoulder.

As the placenta is expelled, it is accompanied by the fetal membranes, although the membranes often become torn and may require additional traction by using a sponge forceps to grasp them. Uterine exploration is rarely needed to complete their removal. The completeness of the placenta and membranes should be recorded after checking the cord, placenta and membranes from the amniotic as well as the chorionic sides.

The whole process lasts between 5 and 10 minutes. If the placenta is not expelled within 30 minutes, a diagnosis of retained placenta is made and the third stage considered abnormal.

Most complications of labour and delivery such as postpartum haemorrhage, pelvic or perineal haematoma and any deterioration of the maternal or newborn condition take place within the first few hours of delivery and hence in most settings the mother and baby are closely examined with periodic observations in the delivery unit for up to 2 hours before the mother and baby are sent to the postnatal ward. The observations are continued for 6 hours if the mother is to be discharged home from the delivery unit.

Pain in labour

Contractions in labour are invariably associated with pain, particularly as they increase in strength, frequency and duration with progress of labour. The cause of pain is uncertain, but it may be due to compression of nerve fibres in the cervical zone or to hypoxia of compressed muscle cells. Pain is felt in the lower abdomen and as lumbar backache when the intrauterine pressure exceeds 25 mmHg.

The management of normal labour

The primary aim of intrapartum care is to deliver a healthy baby to a healthy mother. The preparation of the mother for the process of parturition begins well before the onset of labour. It is important for the mother and her partner to understand what happens during the various stages of labour. Strategies to deal with pain in labour, including mental preparation with controlled respiration, should be introduced during antenatal classes, as well as educating the mother about the regulation of expulsive efforts during the second stage of labour.

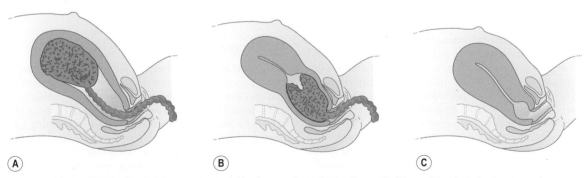

(A) (B) (C)

Fig. 11.5 The normal third stage: (A) separation of the placenta from the uterine wall; (B) expulsion into the lower uterine segment and upper vagina; (C) complete expulsion of the placenta and membranes from the genital tract.

Antenatal classes should also include instructions about neonatal care and breast-feeding, although this is a process that requires reinforcement in the postdelivery period.

The mother should be advised to come into hospital, or to call the midwife in the event of a home birth, when contractions are at regular 10- to 15-minute intervals, when there is a show or when the membranes rupture. If the mother is in early labour, she should be encouraged to take a shower and to empty her bowels and bladder. Shaving of the pubic hair or abdomen is no longer considered necessary and is likely to cause abrasions with some bleeding that may become the nidus for bacterial proliferation and subsequent infection.

The home birth rate in the UK is about 2–3%, but it is common practice to organize 'domino' (domiciliary in and out) deliveries, whereby the mother is discharged home 6 hours after delivery, provided that the delivery is uncomplicated.

Examination at the commencement of labour

On admission, the following examination should be performed:

- **Full general examination**, including temperature, pulse, respiration, blood pressure (BP) and state of hydration; the urine should be tested for glucose, ketone bodies and protein.
- **Obstetrical examination of the abdomen:** Inspection is followed by palpation to determine the fetal lie, presentation and position and the station of the presenting part by estimating fifths of head palpable. Auscultation of the fetal heartbeat is by a stethoscope or by using a Doptone device, which enables the mother and her partner to hear.
- **Vaginal examination** in labour should be performed only after cleansing of the vulva and introitus and using an aseptic technique with sterile gloves and an antiseptic cream. Once the examination is started, the fingers should not be withdrawn from the vagina until the examination is completed. Care should be taken to deflect the thumb away from the clitoral and vestibular area. The following factors should be noted:
- The position, consistency, effacement and dilatation of the cervix
- Whether the membranes are intact or ruptured and, if ruptured, the colour and quantity of the amniotic fluid
- The fetal presentation (e.g. vertex, breech) and position (e.g. left occipito anterior (LOA), right occipito anterior (ROA), right occipito posterior (ROP), etc.) of the presenting part and its relationship to the level of the ischial spines (e.g. station –1 or +1, etc.).
- In vertex presentation, the degree of caput (soft tissue scalp swelling), moulding (0, +1, +2 and +3) and synclitism (sagittal suture bisects the pelvis) should be noted.
- Assessment of the bony pelvis at the upper, middle and lower pelvic strait and the pelvic outlet.

General principles of the management of the first stage of labour

The guiding principles of management are:
- Observation of the progress of labour and intervention if it is slow
- Monitoring the fetal and maternal condition
- Pain relief during labour and emotional support for the mother
- Adequate hydration and nutrition throughout labour

Observation: the use of the partogram

The introduction of graphic records of progress of cervical dilatation and descent of the head was a major advance in the management of labour. It enables the early recognition of a labour that is non-progressive. The partogram (Fig. 11.6) is a single sheet of paper on which there is a graphic representation of progress in labour. On the same sheet, other observations related to labour can be recorded. There are sections to enter the frequency and duration of contractions, fetal heart rate (FHR), colour of liquor, caput and moulding, station or descent of the head, maternal heart rate, BP and temperature. The partogram should be started as soon as the mother is admitted to the delivery suite, and this is recorded as zero time, regardless of the time at which contractions started. However, the point of entry on the partogram depends on a vaginal assessment at the time of admission to the delivery suite. The value of this type of record system is that it draws attention visually to any aberration from normal progress in labour.

The use of partograms at an applied level was first introduced in remote obstetric units in Africa, where recognition that progress in labour is becoming abnormal enables early transfer to specialist units before serious obstruction occurs.

This has led to a major reduction in maternal mortality due to avoidance of uterine rupture, sepsis and postpartum haemorrhage and reduction in severe morbidity of vesico or recto vaginal fistula. Earlier recognition of obstructed labours and immediate attention by caesarean delivery where indicated prevents such tragedies.

Fetal condition

The FHR is auscultated every 15 minutes for a duration of 1 minute soon after a contraction in the first stage of labour and after every 5 minutes or after every other contraction for a duration of 1 minute in the second stage of labour. Counting for 15 seconds and multiplying by 4 or counting for 30 seconds and multiplying by 2 lead to error in the FHR observation. The FHR is charted as beats/min in the designated space in the partogram, and decelerations of heart rate that are heard soon after contractions are recorded by an arrow down to the lowest heart rate recorded on the partogram.

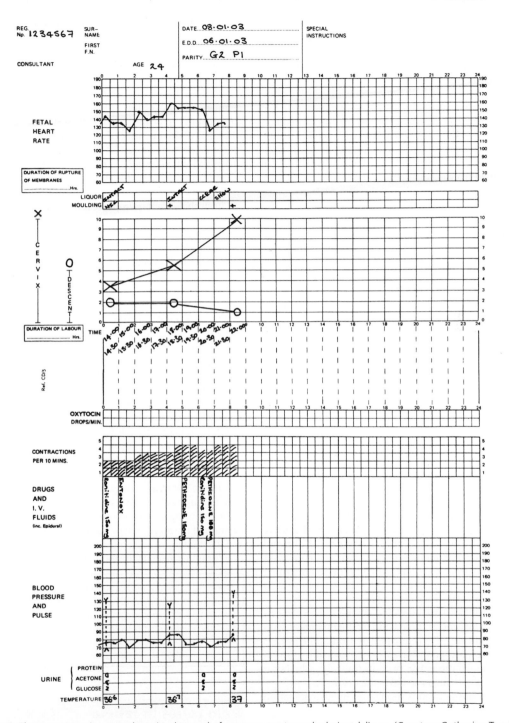

Fig. 11.6 The partogram is a complete visual record of measurements made during delivery. (Courtesy Catherine Tamizian.)

These records are an adjunct to the actual recording of auscultated FHR in the notes and/or electronic fetal monitoring (EFM) by continuous cardiotocography (CTG).

The time of ROM, the nature of the amniotic fluid, i.e. whether it is clear or meconium stained, and quantity are also recorded. Moulding of the fetal head and the presence of caput are also noted, as they provide an indicator of cephalopelvic disproportion. The suture lines meeting is moulding +, over-riding but reducible with gentle pressure is ++ and overriding and not reducible with gentle pressure is +++. The soft tissue swelling of the scalp called *caput* is also marked from + to +++ but is based on the relative impression formed by the clinician.

Progress in labour

Progress in labour is measured by assessing the rate of cervical dilatation and descent of the presenting part. The progress is assessed by vaginal examination on admission and every 3 to 4 hours afterwards during the first stage of labour. Cervical dilatation is plotted in centimetres along the scale of 0–10 of the cervicograph. The cervix is expected to efface and dilate from 0 to 5 cm (latent phase) in 6–8 hours in a multipara and 8–10 hours in a nullipara, followed by approximately 1 cm per hour from 5 to 10 cm dilatation (active phase) in nulli and multipara, although multipara tend to dilate faster. The expected progress recorded on the chart at a rate of 1 cm per hour from admission dilatation in the active phase of labour is called the *alert line*, which helps to identify those who are progressing slowly. A line 2 hours parallel with the alert line called the *action line* can be drawn to decide on when to actively intervene with artificial ROM or oxytocin infusion to augment labour in the absence of malpresentation, disproportion or concern for fetal condition.

If the progress of cervical dilatation lags more than 2 hours behind the expected rate of dilatation, it will cut the action line, indicating the poor progress in the active phase of labour. The UK National Institute for Health and Clinical Excellence guidelines suggest that when encountered with slow progress of <1 cm in 3 hours with no other changes such as cervical effacement or descent of the head in the presence of ruptured membranes, cephalopelvic disproportion should be excluded and labour augmented first by artificial ROM, and if there is no or slow progress, with an oxytocin infusion. Descent of the station of the head is charted on the partogram based on the palpable portion of the head above the pelvic brim in fifths, i.e. whether it needs 5, 4, 3, 2 or 1 finger to cover the head.

The station of the head is plotted on the 0–5 gradation of the partogram.

Descent is also recorded by assessing the level of the presenting part in centimetres above or below the level of the ischial spines and marked as –1, –2 and –3 when it is above the spines and +1, +2 and +3 if it is below the spines.

The nature and frequency of the uterine contractions are recorded on the chart by shading in the number of contractions per 10 minutes. Dotted squares indicate contractions of less than 20 seconds' duration, cross-hatched squares are contractions between 20 and 40 seconds' duration, while contractions lasting longer than 40 seconds are shown by complete shading of the squares. Frequency and duration of contractions can be measured by clinical palpation or external tocography. The intensity of contractions cannot be assessed by the degree of pain felt by the mother or by palpating the uterus abdominally and can only be determined by intrauterine pressure catheters. However, intrauterine catheters are not used routinely in the management of labour because their use has been shown not to improve the outcome.

Fluid and nutrition during labour

In most maternity units in the developed world, caesarean section rates now exceed 20%. The issue of what can be taken by mouth therefore becomes particularly important. If there is a likelihood that the mother will need operative delivery under general anaesthesia, then it is clearly important to avoid oral intake at any significant level during the first stage of labour. Delayed gastric emptying may result in vomiting and inhalation of vomitus if general anaesthesia for operative delivery is needed. On the other hand, most operative deliveries are now achieved under regional anaesthesia, and therefore there is a case for giving some fluids and light nutrition orally if labour is progressing normally and a vaginal delivery can be anticipated. Recent clinical trials have suggested little concern with feeding the mother with soft, easily digestible, solid nutrition in addition to fluids. Intravenous (IV) fluid replacement should be considered after 6 hours in labour if delivery is not imminent. The major cause of acidosis and ketosis is dehydration, and urine should be checked for ketones in addition to sugar and protein whenever the mother passes urine. Administration of normal saline or Hartmann's solution is preferred, and the fluid input and output should be monitored so not to over- or under-hydrate the mother.

> The classic signs of dehydration in labour include tachycardia, mild pyrexia and loss of tissue turgor. Remember that labour can be hard physical work and that the environmental temperature of delivery rooms is often raised to meet the needs of the baby rather than the mother, leading to considerable insensible fluid loss.

Pain relief in labour

A number of strategies are used in labour for the relief of pain, and these should be discussed with the pregnant mother in the antenatal period. Essentially, these techniques are aimed at reducing the level of pain experienced in labour whilst invoking minimal risk for the mother and baby.

The level of pain experienced in labour varies widely – some experience very little, whilst others suffer from abdominal and back pain of increasing intensity throughout their labour. Thus, any programme for pain relief must be tailored to the needs of the individual. The caregiver may be able to advise the best mode of pain relief based on whether the mother is nulliparous or multiparous, the current cervical dilatation, the rate of progress of labour and the extent to which the mother is feeling the pain. The mode of pain relief is best decided by the mother based on the advice given. Often this may result in a combination of methods, starting from the least to most effective method to alleviate her pain. The only technique that can provide complete pain relief is epidural analgesia.

Narcotic analgesia

Pethidine has traditionally been the most widely used narcotic agent but has been replaced in many centres in the UK and Australia by morphine. The common side effects for all the opiates are nausea and vomiting in the mother and respiratory depression in the baby. The effect on the neonate is particularly important when the drug is given within 2 hours of delivery. Opiates are often administered with anti-emetics to reduce nausea.

Remifentanil is used in some centres, as this is an ultra-short-acting opioid that produces superior analgesia to pethidine and has less of an effect on neonatal respiration.

Because some mothers are unsuitable for regional analgesia, e.g. those on anticonvulsants, opiates are likely to continue to play a significant role in pain relief in labour.

Inhalational analgesia

These agents are used in early labour until the mother switches to much stronger analgesics. It is best for short-term pain relief in the late first and second stage of labour. The most widely used agent is Entonox, which is a 50/50 mixture of nitrous oxide and oxygen. The gas is self-administered to avoid overdosing when they drop the mask off and is inhaled as soon as the contraction starts. Entonox is the most widely used analgesic in labour in the UK and provides sufficient pain relief for the majority.

Nitrous oxide has been shown to have adverse effects on birth attendants if exposure is prolonged; these effects include decreased fertility, bone marrow changes and neurological changes. Forced air change every 6–10 hours is effective in reducing the nitrous oxide levels and should be mandatory in all delivery rooms.

Non-pharmacological methods

Transcutaneous electrical nerve stimulation (TENS) involves the placement of two pairs of TENS electrodes on the back on each side of the vertebral column at the levels of T10–L1 and S2–S4. Currents of 0–40 mA are applied at a frequency of 40–150 Hz. This can be effective in early labour but is often inadequate by itself in late labour. For the technique to be effective, antenatal training of the mother is essential.

Other non-invasive methods include acupuncture, subcutaneous sterile water injections, massage and relaxation techniques, the effectiveness of which is debated.

Regional analgesia

Epidural analgesia is the most effective and widely used form of regional analgesia. It provides complete relief of pain in 95% of labouring women.

The procedure may be instituted at any time and does not interfere with uterine contractility. It may reduce the desire to bear down in the second stage of labour due to lack of pressure sensation at the perineum and reduced uterine activity due to loss of 'Ferguson's reflex', which is an increased uterine activity due to reflex release of oxytocin due to the presenting part stretching the cervix and upper vagina.

A fine catheter is introduced into the lumbar epidural space, and a local anaesthetic agent such as bupivacaine is injected (Fig. 11.7). The addition of an opioid to the local

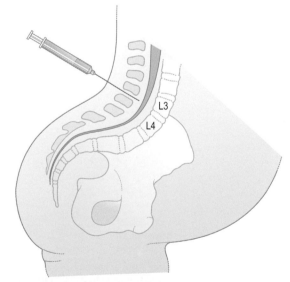

Fig. 11.7 Epidural anaesthesia is induced by injection of local anaesthetic agents into the lumbar epidural space.

anaesthetic greatly reduces the dose requirement of bupivacaine, thus sparing the motor fibres to the lower limbs and reducing the classic complications of hypotension and abnormal FHR.

The procedure involves:

- Insertion of an IV cannula and preloading with no more than 500 mL of saline or Hartmann's solution.
- Insertion of the epidural cannula at the L3–L4 interspace and injection of the local anaesthetic agent at the minimum dose required for effective pain relief.
- Monitoring BP, pulse rate and FHR and adjusting maternal posture to achieve the desired analgesic effect.

The complications of epidural analgesia include:

- Hypotension: this can be avoided by preloading and the use of low-dose anaesthetic agents and opioid solutions.
- Accidental dural puncture: occurs in fewer than 1% of epidurals.
- Postdural headache: about 70% of mothers will develop a headache if a 16- or 18-gauge needle is used. A postdural headache that persists for more than 24 hours should be treated with an epidural blood patch.

Contraindications to regional anaesthesia include:

- maternal refusal
- coagulopathy
- local or systemic infection
- uncorrected hypovolaemia
- inadequate or inexperienced staff or facilities

> Many women set out in labour without requesting any form of pain relief. However, as labour progresses, the realization that labour can be painful will change the requirements of the mother. It is therefore essential to have an epidural service that can be readily available so that the labour is not too far advanced before the epidural can become established.

Other forms of regional anaesthesia

Spinal anaesthesia is commonly used for operative delivery, particularly as a single-shot procedure. It is not used for control of pain in labour because of the superior safety of epidural analgesia and the ability to top up with suitable doses or as continuous infusion to get pain relief over a long period. Often a 'spinal–epidural' combination is used for caesarean section, with the spinal providing quick and effective anaesthesia whilst the epidural can be continued over the next 24 hours for good pain relief.

Paracervical blockade involves the infiltration of local anaesthetic agents into the paracervical tissues. This is rarely used for obstetric procedures and has the greater chance of side effects to the fetus should it enter a vessel.

Pudendal nerve blockade involves infiltration around the pudendal nerve as it leaves the pudendal canal and the inferior haemorrhoidal nerve (Fig. 11.8). It was a widely used form of local anaesthesia for operative vaginal

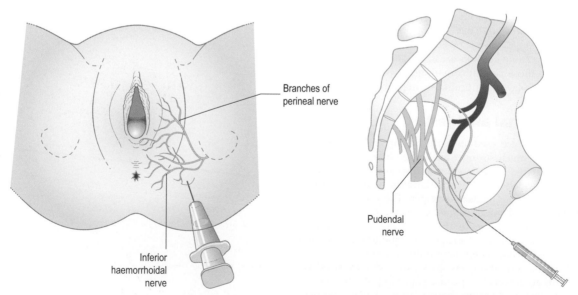

Fig. 11.8 Pudendal nerve blockade is achieved by injection of local anaesthetic around the pudendal nerve at the level of the ischial spine. Additional infiltration is used to block branches of the inferior haemorrhoidal and perineal nerves.

deliveries in the past but is now less frequently used, as it has been replaced by epidural anaesthesia.

Infiltration directly into the perineal tissues over the episiotomy site is still widely used for the repair of perineal wounds. Great care must be taken to avoid direct IV injection of the drug at the time of local infiltration. Toxic symptoms such as cardiac arrhythmias and convulsions may result from accidental injection of the anaesthetic drug, especially with larger dosages.

Posture in labour

Some women prefer to remain ambulant or to sit in a chair during the first stage of labour. However, most women prefer to lie down as labour advances into the second stage, although some will prefer to squat to use the forces of gravity to help expel the baby. In the past, women who had epidural anaesthesia had to remain supine because of temporary motor impairment. This has been overcome using low-dose anaesthesia combined with opiates. With such mixed epidurals, women can move about and often ambulate.

Water births

Some mothers prefer immersion in a water bath for pain relief. Flotation improves support of the pregnant uterus. Most women prefer to deliver outside water. There is a possibility of the baby inhaling the bath water with the first breath, which can cause problems to the baby if the bath is contaminated with maternal faeces. The temperature of the bath must be regularly checked, and the mother should not be left alone in the water bath.

Fetal monitoring

Changes in the FHR or the passage of new meconium-stained liquor (fetal bowel motion) may suggest possibility of fetal hypoxia. These signs can occur in normal labour but more so in high-risk pregnancies and need to be studied to determine the fetal condition, if necessary, with the adjunct use of fetal scalp blood sampling (FBS). Diminution of fetal movements (FMs) on admission may indicate fetal jeopardy, and cessation of movements may indicate death and hence enquiry about FM should be made on admission in labour.

Intermittent auscultation

The FHR is monitored every 15 minutes for a period of 1 minute soon after a contraction using a handheld Doppler ultrasound transducer or Pinard fetal stethoscope in the first stage of labour. In the second stage, the FHR is auscultated every 5 minutes or soon after every other contraction. Contractions are monitored by manual palpation over a period of 10 minutes to determine the frequency and duration. The frequency of intermittent auscultation (IA) was recommended on the basis that there was no difference in fetal and neonatal outcome in randomized studies that compared IA every 15 minutes for 1 minute after a contraction in the first stage and every 5 minutes in the second stage with EFM. Ideal auscultation practice should be listening and recording the baseline FHR on admission (cross-checked against the maternal pulse rate) followed by auscultation with the FMs to demonstrate an acceleration and soon after a contraction to confirm that there are no decelerations. Technological advances have made it possible for a hand-held Doptone to display the digital FHR and convert the information to produce a CTG on a light-emitting diode (LED) screen, which can be seen, stored within the device and reviewed later if the need arises (Fig. 11.9).

The clinical guidelines for the use of EFM have been produced by the National Institute for Health and Clinical Excellence in the UK, Australia and New Zealand College of Obstetricians and Gynaecologists and by similar bodies in the United States and Canada, as well as by the International Federation of Gynaecologists and Obstetricians (FIGO). They have great similarities and minor differences that are unlikely to influence clinical outcome. Admission CTG or routine CTG using electronic monitoring is not recommended for women classified as low risk. However, the woman's wishes should be respected after appropriate counselling. This may be that the woman wishes or not the use of admission CTG or continuous CTG. The specific indications for continuous EFM are listed in Table 11.1.

Fetal cardiotocography

EFM enables continuous monitoring of the FHR and the frequency and duration of uterine contractions. The heart rate of the fetus is usually calculated using a Doppler ultrasound transducer, which is applied externally to the maternal abdomen. The signals that are detected are those of cardiac movement, and what is measured is the time interval between cardiac cycles. Traditionally, this is converted to heart rate. The heart rate can also be measured from the RR wave intervals obtained from the fetal electrocardiogram (ECG) by direct application of an electrode to the presenting part.

Uterine activity is recorded either with a pressure transducer applied over the anterior abdominal wall between the fundus and the umbilicus or by inserting a fluid-filled catheter or a pressure sensor into the uterine cavity through the cervical canal (Fig. 11.10). External tocography gives an accurate measurement of the frequency and duration but

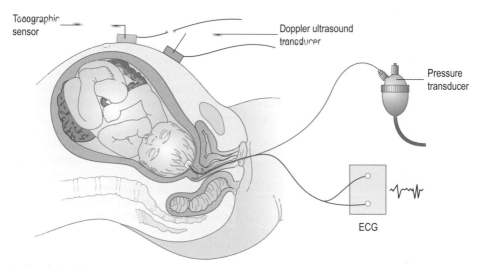

Fig. 11.9 Monitoring during labour. Contractions are recorded by intrauterine and extrauterine tocography; the fetal heart rate is recorded externally by Doppler ultrasonography or by direct application of an ECG electrode to the presenting part.

only relative information of intrauterine pressure. Accurate measurements of pressure need an intrauterine catheter or transducer, and this is not used as a routine in most centres due to lack of evidence of its clinical benefit.

Baseline heart rate

The definition of normality in the pattern of the FHR is easier than defining what is abnormal. The normal heart rate varies between 110 and 160 beats/min (Fig. 11.11). A rate faster than 160 is defined as *fetal tachycardia*, and a rate less than 110 is *fetal bradycardia*.

Table 11.1 Indications for the use of continuous electronic fetal monitoring

Maternal	Fetal
Previous caesarean section	Fetal growth restriction
Pre-eclampsia	Prematurity
Post-term pregnancy	Oligohydramnios
Prolonged rupture of the membranes	Abnormal Doppler artery velocimetry
Induced labour	Multiple pregnancy
Diabetes	Meconium-stained liquor
Antepartum haemorrhage	Breech presentation
Other maternal medical diseases	

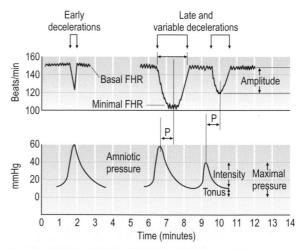

Fig. 11.10 Patterns of fetal heart rate change and amniotic pressure change in labour. *FHR*, Fetal heart rate.

Baseline variability

The heart rate exhibits variations from the baseline, which is known as *baseline variability*. Although there is variability on a beat-to-beat basis, the standard fetal monitor averages 3–5 beats and records it as baseline variability on the standard CTG. Hence, we term it as *baseline variability* rather than beat-to-beat variation, which is possible with computerized systems. The paper speed, whether it is 1 cm, 2 cm or 3 cm/min, will affect the appearance of the baseline variability. Baseline variability is a record of the oscillations in heart rate around the baseline rate and normally varies between 5 and 25 beats/min. Baseline variability is due to the millisecond-to-millisecond reaction of the sympathetic

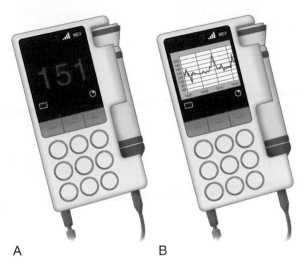

A   **B**

Fig.11.11 (A) Doptone showing digital display. (B) Doptone showing a CTG display.

and parasympathetic activity on the heart and reflects the integrity of the autonomic nervous system. It is reduced during the fetal sleep phase. Hypoxia, infection and medication can reduce baseline variability. An FHR with a variability of less than 5 beats/min for >90 minutes is abnormal and may indicate fetal jeopardy.

Transient changes in fetal heart rate (Tables 11.2 and 11.3)

Accelerations

Accelerations are defined as transient abrupt increases in heart rate of more than 15 beats/min for more than 15 seconds and are associated with FMs. Accelerations reflect the activity of the somatic nervous system and are a reassuring sign of a fetus that is not hypoxic.

Decelerations

Decelerations are defined as decreases in heart rate of more than 15 beats/min for more than 15 seconds. These are

Table 11.2 Classification of fetal heart rate trace features

Description	Feature		
	Baseline (beats/min)	Baseline variability (beats/min)	Decelerations
Reassuring	110–160	5–25	None or early Variable decelerations with no concerning characteristics* for less than 90 minutes
Non-reassuring	100–109† OR 161–180	Fewer than 5 for 30–50 minutes OR More than 25 for 15–20 minutes	Variable decelerations with no concerning characteristics* for 90 minutes or more OR Variable decelerations with any concerning characteristics* in up to 50% of contractions for 30 minutes or more OR Variable decelerations with concerning characteristics* in over 50% of contractions for less than 30 minutes OR Late decelerations in over 50% of contractions for less than 30 minutes, with no maternal or fetal clinical risk factors such as vaginal bleeding or significant meconium
Abnormal	Below 100 OR Above 180	Fewer than 5 for more than 50 minutes OR More than 25 for more than 25 minutes OR Sinusoidal	Variable decelerations with any concerning characteristics* in over 50% of contractions for 30 minutes (or less if any maternal or fetal clinical risk factors (see earlier)) OR Late deceleration for 30 minutes (or less if any maternal or fetal clinical risk factors) OR Acute bradycardia or a single prolonged deceleration lasting 3 minutes or more

*Regard the following as concerning characteristics of variable decelerations: lasting more than 60 seconds; reduced baseline variability within the deceleration; failure to return to baseline; biphasic (W) shape; no shouldering.
†Although a baseline fetal heart rate between 100 and 109 beats/minute is a non-reassuring feature, continue usual care if there is normal baseline variability and no variable or late decelerations.
Reproduced with permission from NICE (2017) Intrapartum Care: NICE guideline CG190, February 2017.

defined by their relationship to uterine contractions or by the pathophysiological mechanism that causes them. Some patterns of change are generally considered to have clinical significance in relation to hypoxia.

Early or head compression decelerations

These decelerations are synchronous with uterine contractions. There is a gradual fall and rise of the FHR. The nadir occurs at the peak of the contraction, and the decrease in heart rate is generally less than 40 beats/min. These decelerations are generally due to head compression and are physiological. Hence, they are seen in the late first and second stages of labour.

Late or placental insufficiency decelerations

The onset of the slowing of heart rate occurs >20 seconds after the contraction commences and does not return to the normal baseline rate until after the contraction is completed.

Late decelerations are due to placental insufficiency, and with repeated such decelerations, rise in the baseline rate and reduction in baseline variability may be indicative of fetal hypoxia.

Variable or cord compression decelerations

Variable decelerations vary in timing, shape and amplitude – hence their name. They have an initial slight transitory rise in the baseline rate followed by a precipitous fall followed by a quick recovery to the normal baseline rate and slightly beyond. The slight increase just before the sudden decline and the slight increase in the recovery is termed *shouldering*. The heart rate usually falls by more than 40 beats/min and is due to cord compression, which varies with each contraction, giving rise to variable shapes, sizes and timing of decelerations, and are considered non-reassuring features in a CTG trace. Increase in the depth and duration of the decelerations, reduction of interdeceleration intervals, rise in baseline rate and reduction in baseline variability suggest worsening hypoxia. Additional changes to simple variable decelerations in the form of slow recovery to baseline rate or a combined, i.e. variable followed immediately by late decelerations are called *atypical variable decelerations* or variable decelerations with 'concerning features' and are abnormal features.

> **!**
>
> The interpretation of the CTG now forms a major focus for litigation in cases of cerebral palsy and mental handicap. It is essential that where EFM is employed, any birth attendant responsible for intrapartum care should understand how to interpret the CTG and be able to take appropriate action. The actions taken are nursing the mother in the left lateral position or an alternative position, hydration and stopping oxytocin infusion if she was on this medication. If significant abnormality of heart rate persists, a fetal blood sample for acid–base status or operative delivery may be needed. This decision is also influenced by parity, cervical dilatation, rate of progress of labour and clinical risk factors.

The fetal electrocardiogram

The fetal ECG can be recorded from scalp electrodes or by the placement of maternal abdominal electrodes. For ECG waveform analysis a scalp electrode and a maternal skin reference electrode are necessary. Some units use computerized analysis of the ST waveform with the use of special equipment (STAN, Neoventa Ltd., Sweden) along with FHR

Table 11.3 Definition of normal, suspicious and pathological fetal heart rate (FHR) traces and recommended actions (NICE (2017) Intrapartum Care: NICE guideline CG190, February 2017)

Category	Definition	Action
Normal	An FHR trace in which all four features are classified as reassuring	Continue intermittent or continuous monitoring as indicated by risk factors.
Suspicious	An FHR trace with one feature classified as non-reassuring and the remaining features classified as reassuring	Exclude factors indicating need for immediate delivery (cord prolapse, uterine rupture, abruption). Treat dehydration, hyperstimulation, hypotension and change position. Continue CTG.
Pathological	An FHR trace with two or more features classified as non-reassuring or one or more classified as abnormal	Exclude factors indicating need for immediate delivery (cord prolapse, uterine rupture, abruption). Treat dehydration, hyperstimulation and change position. Deliver if prolonged bradycardia. Either obtain further information on fetal status by fetal blood scalp sampling or deliver.

to detect hypoxia (Fig. 11.12). Even with ST waveform analysis, manual interpretation of CTG is needed for clinical decision-making.

Fetal acid–base balance

Where abnormalities of FHR occur in labour, they may provide an indication of fetal acidosis, but to confirm these findings, the fetal acid–base status should be examined.

Fetal blood is obtained directly from the scalp through an amnioscope. The instrument is inserted through the cervix, which must be at least 2 cm dilated. The mother is requested to lie in the lateral position. The latter is preferable to a dorsal or lithotomy position, as it will avoid the risk of inducing supine hypotension. A small stab incision is made in the fetal scalp, and blood is collected into a heparinized capillary tube. The sample is then analyzed in a blood gas analyzer.

Normal pH lies between 7.25 and 7.35. A pH between 7.20 and 7.25 in the first stage of labour indicates mild acidosis, and sampling should be repeated within the next 30 minutes. If it is <7.20, delivery is recommended unless spontaneous delivery is imminent. If there is sufficient sample, a full blood gas analysis should be performed, as a raised Pco_2 with a normal base excess may indicate a respiratory acidosis that may correct itself if the posture of the mother is changed. The degree of metabolic acidosis in the fetus may also be assessed from fetal scalp blood by measuring lactate levels. This generally requires smaller blood volumes (5 µL) to measure and can be done using portable handheld devices. The exact values/cut-off used to determine the need for clinical action vary according to the normal values established using the device used.

Pre-term delivery

Delivery from 24 completed weeks (in the UK) up to 36 weeks and 6 days is considered a pre-term birth. The incidence varies from country to country and even within different ethnic and socioeconomic groups in the same country. The literature suggests an incidence of 6–12%. Of this, nearly 75% are between 34 and 37 weeks, and generally these infants suffer few short- or long-term complications. The high standards of perinatal care in well-resourced countries can care for babies with good intact survival at even less than 32 weeks or any infant with a birth weight more than 1500 g. Of those born at less than 32 weeks' gestation, about a third follow pre-labour ROM, a third are due to spontaneous pre-term labour and the remaining third are due to iatrogenic intervention where delivery is indicated for a medical or obstetric condition such as pre-eclampsia, antepartum haemorrhage or intrauterine growth restriction.

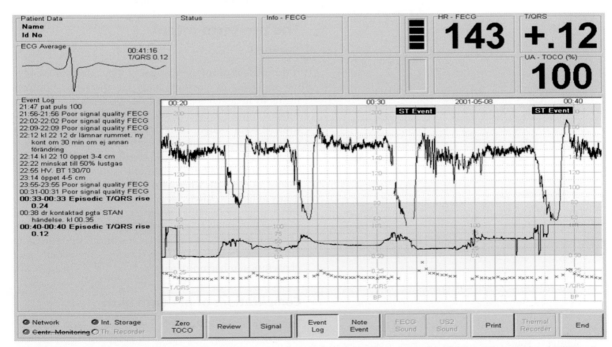

Fig.11.12 Screen of a fetal electrocardiogram (ECG) monitor that displays the fetal heart rate, fetal ECG and the calculated T/QRS ratio.

Spontaneous pre-term labour

Aetiology

A number of factors are known to be associated with spontaneous pre-term labour, although in many cases the cause is unknown.

Some of the major factors associated with pre-term labour are shown in Figure 11.13. There is an association with poor social conditions, nutritional status, antepartum haemorrhage, multiple pregnancy, uterine anomalies, cervical incompetence and PROM, which is often associated with infection. A previous history of pre-term delivery is the best single predictor. The relative risk is about 3, and the risk increases if there has been more than one pre-term delivery. Complications during a pregnancy may also precipitate pre-term labour; these includes over-distension of the uterus, such as multiple pregnancy and polyhydramnios. Other factors, such as haemorrhage in either the first or early second trimester, increase the risk of subsequent pre-term labour. Severe maternal illness, particularly febrile illness, may also promote the early onset of labour.

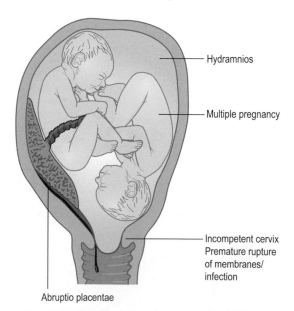

Fig. 11.13 Factors predisposing to premature labour.

Hydramnios

Multiple pregnancy

Incompetent cervix
Premature rupture
of membranes/
infection

Abruptio placentae

Box 11.1 Pre-term labour: social factors

- Poverty
- Maternal age (<20 and >35 years)
- Heavy stressful work
- Marital status
- Cigarette smoking
- Substance abuse

Social factors involve maternal age (under 20 or over 35 years), first pregnancy, ethnicity, marital status, cigarette smoking, substance abuse and heavy, stressful work (Box 11.1). Active social intervention appeared to reduce the incidence of pre-term labour in early studies but has not received unanimous support due to lack of good scientific evidence. Very recently, genetic markers have been identified in those who are likely to go into pre-term labour.

The role of genital tract infection

Genital tract infection may act either through promoting myometrial activity or by causing pre-labour rupture of the fetal membranes. Organisms that have been found to be associated with chorioamnionitis and the onset of pre-term labour include *Neisseria gonorrhoeae*, group B haemolytic streptococci, *Chlamydia trachomatis*, *Mycoplasma hominis*, *Ureaplasma urealyticum*, *Gardnerella vaginalis*, *Bacteroides* spp. and *Haemophilus* spp. Of these, group B streptococci are probably the most sinister.

The bacteria that have penetrated the mucus plug produce proteases, resulting in tissue destruction and PROM. Organisms may also release phospholipase A_2 and phospholipase C, which releases arachidonic acid from the amnion, causing the release of prostaglandins. Release of bacterial toxins may also initiate an inflammatory process in the decidua and membranes, resulting in the production of prostaglandins and cytokines, particularly interleukins (IL-1, IL-6) and tumour necrosis factor.

The pre-term infant

Survival

If the cause is of infective origin, it may affect the mother, but the effect is predominantly on the fetus. Improvements in neonatal services provide good chance of intact survival if the newborn is in good condition and is of reasonable birth weight. Each day of delay in birth after 24 weeks increases the chance of survival by 3–6%, and hence the need to conserve the pregnancy as long as possible. An infant born with a birth weight of less than 500 g has little chance of survival, whereas one born weighing 1500 g is nearly as likely to survive as a full-term infant. Between 500 and 1000 g, every 100-g increment produces a significant increase in survival (Fig. 11.14). The major causes of death in very-low-birth-weight infants are infection, respiratory distress syndrome (RDS), necrotizing enterocolitis and periventricular haemorrhage.

Complications of pre-term birth

Immediate complications are respiratory distress, jaundice, hypoglycaemia and hypothermia. Long-term complications include pulmonary dysplasia and neurodevelopmental delay.

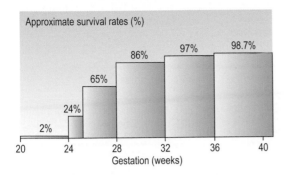

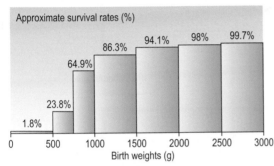

Fig. 11.14 Birth weight, gestational age and perinatal outcome.

The management of pre-term labour

The diagnosis of pre-term labour is based on the onset of regular painful uterine contractions associated with progressive cervical effacement and dilatation. Uterine contractions are common and a normal occurrence during pregnancy and do not always progress to established labour. Over 30% of hospital admissions for suspected pre-term labour may be discharged home undelivered. Ultrasound assessment of the length of the cervix of <2.5 cm after 24 weeks is a useful predictor of possible pre-term labour. The presence of the protein fetal fibronectin in the cervix can be used in the assessment of the risk of pre-term delivery. The test can be performed by taking a swab from the cervix, provided that the membranes are intact and the woman has not had intercourse or a vaginal examination within the previous 24 hours. A negative result makes delivery within the next 7 days unlikely (<3%), although a positive test result is of less value, as only 20% of such women will deliver in the same period. A combination of short cervix on ultrasound and positive fibronectin is more useful in predicting impending pre-term labour in a woman with pre-term contractions.

Prevention

Prevention has been approached from different directions, some of which appear to have been effective, while others have not been convincing. It has been difficult to prove efficacy with any interventional therapy for established pre-term labour because many labours stop spontaneously irrespective of treatment. Interventional studies have been based on the concept that heavy work and excessive physical activity should be kept to a minimum during pregnancy. Studies by Papiernik in Paris strongly supported social intervention programmes as the way to reduce the incidence of pre-term labour. Other studies have not supported these observations. However, it appears logical to suggest that those women who have a history of pre-term labour should be advised concerning lifestyle and diet and that they should avoid heavy or stressful work during pregnancy. The treatment of asymptomatic bacteriuria with antibiotics has been shown to reduce the likelihood of pre-term labour and, where β-haemolytic streptococci are detected in cervical swabs, antibiotic treatment appears to reduce the incidence of PROM. Recent randomized controlled trials investigated women with short cervical length on ultrasound and the role of 17-alpha-hydroxyprogesterone caproate. In women who have a short cervix of <2.5 cm beyond 24 weeks, the use of progesterone reduced the incidence of delivery. Large randomized trials which studied the role of prophylactic cervical cerclage for women with short cervix on ultrasound did not show any benefit. The Arabin cervical pessary, which changes the angulation of the cervix to the body of the uterus, and other pessaries have been advocated, but results from studies show different outcomes – some supporting its use whilst others do not.

Treatment

Once the woman is admitted to hospital in established pre-term labour, a decision must be made as to the approach to management. The long-term advantages of preventing pre-term labour are uncertain, although every day of delay in the early pre-term period increases the chance of survival and reduces morbidity and more dependence on intensive care. There is no controversy in postponing delivery long enough for the administration of corticosteroids to enable the release of fetal lung surfactant from type II pneumocytes with the aim of reducing the chance of hyaline membrane disease (HMD) and RDS (Fig. 11.15).

The decision on whether labour should be allowed to proceed or to inhibit uterine activity depends on the period of gestation, absence of infection, bleeding or fetal compromise, intact membranes and the cervix being less than 5 cm dilated. In cases where gestational age by ultrasound dating is less than 34 weeks, it is appropriate to inhibit uterine activity pharmacologically until corticosteroids can be administered to the mother to enhance fetal lung maturity. Magnesium sulphate 4 g IV (in some series followed by 1 g hourly for 24 hours as an infusion) has been shown to be neuroprotective, and its use is now recommended by professional organizations for use in pre-term labour less than 32 weeks.

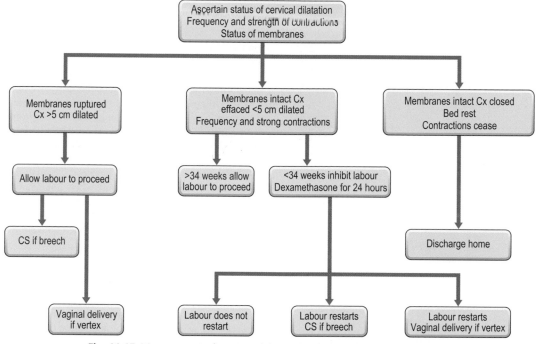

Fig. 11.15 Management of pre-term labour. *CS*, Caesarean section; *Cx*, cervix.

Tocolysis is contraindicated in the presence of bleeding, because of the risk of maternal haemodynamic compromise, and with infection, as delay may compromise the health of mother and fetus.

Box 11.2 **Drug treatment for pre-term labour**

- β-Adrenergic agonists
- Prostaglandin synthetase inhibitors
- Magnesium sulphate
- Slow calcium channel blockers
- Corticosteroids
- Oxytocin antagonists

Drug therapy to delay the delivery can be divided into groups operating on different principles (Box 11.2).

β-Adrenergic agonists

These drugs act on the β-2-adrenergic receptor sites on the membranes of the myometrial cells, with the activation of adenyl cyclase resulting in an increase in intracellular cAMP. Action is by inhibition of actin–myosin interaction, which inhibits uterine activity.

These drugs have potentially dangerous maternal side effects and hence must be used with caution.
The side effects include palpitations and tremor, ischaemic arrhythmias, fluid retention, pulmonary oedema and sometimes sudden death.

The most commonly used drugs are ritodrine, salbutamol and terbutaline. The drugs should not be used where there is a known history of cardiovascular disease or hypertension.

The drugs are administered diluted in 5% dextrose or dextrose/saline, and the infusion rate should be incrementally increased every 10–20 minutes until contractions are reduced to one every 15 minutes, or until the maternal heart rate has reached 140 beats/min. Careful monitoring of maternal pulse rate, BP, fluid input/output and plasma electrolytes is essential. Fluid overload due to IV fluids and drug action increasing antidiuretic hormone causing retention of fluids is the main cause of pulmonary oedema and heat failure, and this may be greater in multiple pregnancy.

β-Adrenergic drugs can cause hypokalaemia, hyperglycaemia (ketoacidosis in diabetics) and pulmonary oedema with prolonged use.

The dosage can be reduced slowly after the administration of corticosteroids to the mother. It is unlikely that any major benefit will accrue to the fetus if the gestational age exceeds 34 weeks. It is necessary to continue treatment until the mother is transferred to a tertiary care centre with neonatal intensive care facilities. Oral maintenance therapy remains unproven and is not recommended.

Prostaglandin synthetase inhibitors

Drugs such as Indocin (indomethacin) given at a dose of 1–3 mg/kg maternal body weight for 24 hours inhibit prostaglandin production and thus uterine activity. These drugs are very effective in preventing the progression of labour. However, they may result in in-utero closure of the ductus arteriosus and therefore adversely affect the fetal circulation. There may be occasions when they are the drug of choice and where the pre-term delivery of the infant constitutes a greater risk than the not-invariable early closure of the ductus. This drug also increases pulmonary and renal artery resistance and can cause oligohydramnios. Such consequences are best avoided by using the drug for 1–3 days at the minimum required dose. Usually it is given as 100-mg suppositories.

 Indomethacin also reduces liquor volume by its effect on fetal renal function and may be of additional benefit in cases of polyhydramnios.

Calcium antagonists

The effect of slow calcium channel blockers in inhibiting uterine activity is not in doubt. There has been some evidence in animal studies using very large doses of these compounds, particularly nifedipine, that they may cause rib fusions in the fetus if given during the period of organogenesis. However, if the drugs are administered in the late second and third trimesters, this is well past this period and there is no evidence that they pose a threat.

Nifedipine is administered with a starting oral dose of 20 mg followed by 10–20 mg every 4–6 hours thereafter. Severe side effects are rare.

Calcium antagonists, although not licensed for use in pregnancy in the UK, are recommended by the Royal College of Obstetricians and Gynaecologists as the drug of choice to inhibit the uterine activity because of its efficacy and low cost.

Corticosteroids

The use of corticosteroids in the prevention of respiratory distress is based on the action of these compounds in enhancing the release of surfactant from type II

pneumocytes, thus enabling rapid expansion of the alveoli at the time of delivery and the establishment of normal respiratory function. Controlled trials on the antenatal effects of corticosteroids in pre-term infants have shown that there are significant reductions in RDS, periventricular haemorrhage and necrotizing enterocolitis.

The dosage of betamethasone is two doses of 12 mg given intramuscularly 24 hours apart. Dexamethasone is given as four 6 mg doses intramuscularly 12 hours apart. Optimal benefit can be achieved if delivery is postponed for at least 24 hours and up to 7 days. Over 34 weeks' gestation, the administration of corticosteroids is not justified. The production of phosphatidylcholine can also be enhanced by the administration of thyrotropin-releasing hormone (TRH) to the mother.

 Failure to prescribe corticosteroids before delivery between 28 and 34 weeks may now be considered negligent.

Neuroprotection by magnesium sulphate

The use of magnesium sulphate as a tocolytic has largely been abandoned because of its low efficacy. However, large randomized studies have shown a neuroprotective effect in the neonate with its use prior to pre-term delivery. It stabilizes capillary membranes and reduces the incidence of intraventricular and periventricular haemorrhage. An IV dose of 4 g $MgSO_4$ is given followed by 1 g every hour for the next 24 hours. However, there is a trial that suggests that even a bolus dose of 4 g without subsequent continued dosing is effective and offers neuroprotection after 24 hours. Little information is available as to whether this regimen could be repeated if the delivery does not ensue and the mother restarts in pre-term labour. A pragmatic approach is to give another dose if the interval was greater than 1 week.

Method of delivery

On many occasions, it may not be either possible or desirable to inhibit labour. It is rare to inhibit labour when the gestation is over 34 weeks because the benefits of intervention do not outweigh those of allowing the labour to proceed. If the contractions are strong and frequent and the cervix is more than 5 cm dilated on admission, the likelihood of successfully stopping pre-term delivery is low. If the membranes have ruptured and there is no sign of infection, short-term inhibition of contractions to enable the administration of corticosteroids is worthwhile. If there is any antepartum bleeding, non-reassuring FHR or suspicion of intrauterine infection, it may be safer to allow progress of labour and for the fetus to be delivered, and at times the delivery may need to be expedited.

There is no proven evidence that the use of forceps or a wide episiotomy improves fetal outcome in the presence of a vertex presentation, although it is important that delivery be as gentle and controlled as possible. If the perineum is tight, it is not sensible to allow the soft, pre-term skull to be battered on the perineum for a long period. A sudden expulsive delivery may produce intracranial bleeding due to sudden decompression. Routine forceps delivery is not the norm, and a gentle controlled delivery is preferred.

In the presence of a breech presentation, delivery by caesarean section is the preferred option unless the gestation is greater than 34 weeks. Although there are no randomized studies, several large studies on the outcome comparing vaginal breech delivery and delivery by caesarean section overwhelmingly favour delivery by caesarean section because of lower perinatal mortality and long-term neurological deficits. The reason for this is that up to 34 weeks, the head is relatively larger than the trunk and the fetal trunk may be pushed through an incompletely dilated cervix and the head may get stuck. Forceful delivery causes sudden compression and decompression of the head and possible intracranial haemorrhage. Hence with caesarean section to deliver a pre-term breech, the incision type needs to be carefully planned, such as a lower segment midline incision extending upwards or use of a tocolytic to relax the uterus to prevent entrapment of the after-coming head.

Pre-labour rupture of the membranes

Pre-term labour may be associated with PROM, but spontaneous ROM may occur in isolation at term or pre-term without the onset of labour. Factors that are associated with pre-labour ROM are:

- The tensile strength of the fetal membranes, which may be weakened by infection.
- The support of the surrounding tissues, which is reflected in the dilatation of the cervix; the greater the dilatation of the cervix, the greater the likelihood that the membranes will rupture.
- The intra-amniotic fluid pressure.

Pathogenesis

Pre-labour ROM has no known major risk factor but is associated with first- and second-trimester haemorrhage and, less predictably, with smoking. However, the most common factor is infection. Various organisms have been described in this context; these include group B haemolytic streptococci, *C. trachomatis* and those organisms causing bacterial vaginosis.

Management

The mother will come with a history of sudden loss of amniotic fluid from her vagina. On admission to hospital, a speculum examination should be performed to confirm the presence of amniotic fluid, although sometimes it can be difficult to confirm the diagnosis. The use of nitrazine sticks, which shows colour change with pH, is of limited value. Tests using more specific markers based on the presence of α-fetoprotein and insulin-like growth factor (IGF) are more accurate but not widely used because of their cost.

The risks to the mother and baby are those of infection. Long-term drainage of amniotic fluid may result in fetal pulmonary hypoplasia. The difficulty is to decide when to deliver the fetus and how to effect delivery, as the uterus may not respond adequately to the action of oxytocic agents, especially in the very pre-term period.

> If the plan was not to stimulate labour immediately, avoid digital examination to reduce the risk of introducing infection.

Where there is doubt about PROM, it is better to continue observation to look for wetness of a sanitary pad worn to assist in the diagnosis. An ultrasound examination that shows the presence of normal quantities of amniotic fluid with a pocket of fluid between the presenting part and the cervix with no fluid escaping into the vagina is highly suggestive of intact membranes.

If there is clear evidence of amniotic fluid in the vagina, swabs should be taken for culture. Maternal infection may result in uterine tenderness, fetal and/or maternal tachycardia and pyrexia, as well as the presence of a purulent vaginal discharge. Monitoring for the presence of maternal sepsis is best performed by the measurement of blood white cell count and C-reactive protein (CRP). Increasing levels of CRP on subsequent estimations suggest the presence of infection.

> Corticosteroids may cause an increase in maternal white blood count and reduction in baseline variability in the CTG trace.

If there is a positive culture or evidence of maternal infection, the appropriate antibiotic should be administered. If there is evidence of infection, labour should be induced using an oxytocic infusion and delivery expedited in the interest of the fetus and the mother. If there is no evidence of infection, conservative management with erythromycin cover should be adopted. Tocolysis is generally ineffective in the presence of ruptured membranes if contractions are already well established, and one should consider whether the underlying triggering factor may be infection. If gestation is over 28 weeks, the infant probably has a better chance of survival if delivered. Most women with PROM will deliver spontaneously within 48 hours.

At term, women with PROM are induced with prostaglandins or Syntocinon on admission or after 24 hours of PROM. In the pre-term period, conservative management is adopted with the warning that there may be risks of infection, abruption, cord prolapse, pulmonary hypoplasia or stillbirth, but the need for conservatism is to advance to a mature gestation for better survival and outcome.

Induction of labour

Labour is induced when the risk to the mother or child of continuing the pregnancy exceeds the risks of inducing labour. It is the act of artificially initiating uterine activity with the aim of achieving vaginal delivery. The incidence of induction varies widely from country to country and centre to centre and can be from 5 to 25% depending on the high-risk population managed in the centre.

Indications

The major indications for induction of labour are:
- prolonged pregnancy (more than 42 weeks' gestation)
- pre-eclampsia
- placental insufficiency and intrauterine growth restriction
- antepartum haemorrhage: placental abruption and antepartum haemorrhage of uncertain origin
- Rhesus isoimmunization
- diabetes mellitus
- chronic renal disease

Prolonged pregnancy is defined as pregnancy exceeding 294 days from the first day of the last menstrual period in a woman with a 28-day cycle. The perinatal mortality rate doubles after 42 weeks and trebles after 43 weeks compared with 40 weeks' gestation. Although routine induction of labour has a minimal effect on the overall perinatal mortality rate, it is offered after 41+ weeks, as an adverse outcome is not an acceptable option for the individual mother. Conservative management of prolonged pregnancy is preferred by some, and it involves at least twice-weekly monitoring of the fetus with ultrasound assessment of liquor volume and non-stress test (NST) by antenatal CTG. Induction is undertaken if there is suspicion of fetoplacental compromise. However, many women request induction of labour based on the physical discomfort of the continuing pregnancy. The chance of successful vaginal delivery should be considered and explained to the mother based on parity and cervical score. Artificial separation of membranes just past 40 weeks reduces the number who may need induction after 41 weeks.

Cervical assessment

Clinical assessment of the cervix enables prediction of the likely outcome of induction of labour. The most commonly used method of assessment is the Bishop score or by modification of this score. This cervical score involves clinical examination of the cervix to formulate a numerical score based on the features of the position of the cervix in the pelvis, consistency, effacement, dilation and station of the head.

A Bishop score of more than 6 is strongly predictive of easy initiation of labour with successful clinical outcome of normal progress and vaginal delivery. A score of less than 5 is not that favourable and indicates the need for cervical ripening.

Methods of induction

The method of induction will be determined by whether membranes are still intact and the score on cervical assessment.

Forewater rupture of membranes

ROM should be performed under conditions of full asepsis in the delivery suite. Under ideal circumstances, the cervix should be soft, effaced and at least 2 cm dilated. The head should be presenting by the vertex and should be engaged in the pelvis. In practice, these conditions are often not fulfilled, and the degree to which they are adhered to depends on the urgency of the need to start labour. The mother is placed in the supine or lithotomy position and, after swabbing and draping the vulva, a finger is introduced through the cervix, and the fetal membranes are separated from the lower segment: a process known as *stripping the membranes*. The bulging membranes are then ruptured with Kocher's forceps, Gelder's forewater amniotomy forceps or an amniotomy hook (Fig. 11.16). The amniotic fluid is released slowly, and care is taken to exclude presentation or prolapse of the cord. The FHR should be monitored for 30 minutes before and following ROM.

Hindwater rupture of membranes

An alternative method of surgical induction involves ROM behind the presenting part. This is known as *hindwater rupture*. A sigmoid-shaped metal cannula known as the *Drewe–Smythe catheter* is introduced through the cervix and penetrates the membranes behind the presenting part (Fig. 11.17). The theoretical advantage of this technique is that it

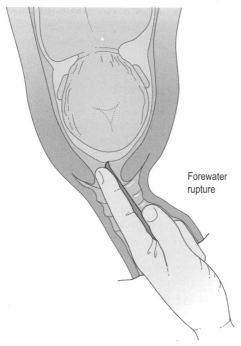

Fig. 11.16 Induction of labour by forewater rupture.

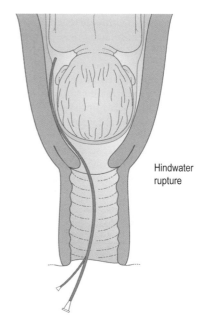

Fig. 11.17 Induction of labour by hindwater rupture.

reduces the risk of prolapsed cord. In reality, the risk is even lower with forewater rupture than with spontaneous ROM, and the technique of hindwater rupture is now rarely used.

Medical induction of labour following amniotomy

Various pharmacological agents can be used to stimulate uterine activity. It is common practice to combine surgical induction with a Syntocinon infusion. A suitable regimen would begin at 1 mU/min and increase by 3 mU/min every 30 minutes until three to four uterine contractions, each lasting >40 seconds, every 10 minutes become established.

The principal hazards of combined surgical and medical induction of labour are:

- **Hyper-stimulation:** Excessive or too frequent and prolonged uterine contractions reduce uterine blood flow and result in fetal asphyxia, i.e. contractions should not occur more frequently than every 2 minutes and should not last more than 1 minute. The Syntocinon infusion should be discontinued if excessive uterine activity occurs or if there are signs of a pathological FHR pattern of concern.
- **Prolapse of the cord:** This should be excluded by examination at the time of forewater ROM or, subsequently, if severe variable decelerations occur on the FHR trace.

- **Infection:** A prolonged induction–delivery interval increases the risk of infection in the amniotic sac, with consequent risks to both infant and mother. If the liquor becomes offensive and/or maternal pyrexia occurs, the labour should be terminated unless the delivery is imminent and the infant delivered.

Medical induction of labour and cervical ripening

This is the method of choice where the membranes are intact or where the cervix is unsuitable for surgical induction. The most commonly used forms of medical induction are:

- administration of prostaglandins by various routes
- mechanical dilation of the cervix

The National Institute for Health and Clinical Excellence recommends the use of prostaglandins PGE2 pessaries or gel every 6 hours or a long-term, slow-release, PGE2 polymer–based control release delivery system over 24 hours for all inductions of labour, including when the cervix is favourable.

Prostaglandins

The most widely used form is prostaglandin E_2 (PGE2). This is used to ripen the cervix and may be administered:

- **Orally:** Doses of 0.5 mg are increased to 2 mg/h until contractions are produced. However, this is not used in current practice due to the side effects of vomiting and diarrhoea.

- **By the vaginal route:** The most commonly used method is to insert prostaglandin pessaries or xylose gel into the posterior fornix. Nulliparous women with an unfavourable cervix (Bishop score of less than 4) are given an initial dose of 2 mg gel. Multiparous women and nulliparae with a Bishop score of more than 4 are given an initial dose of 1 mg. This is repeated if necessary after 6 hours and again the following day up to a maximum dose of 4 mg until labour is established or the membranes can be ruptured and the induction continued with oxytocin infusion. The pessaries come as 3-mg doses. If there is no response to the first pessary in 6 hours in the form of regular contractions or cervical changes, a second pessary is inserted. If the mother does not start labour or there is no cervical change, another pessary is inserted the next day.

Recent technological advances have allowed polymeric, non-biodegradable, controlled-release delivery systems to have 10 mg of PGE2 which can be released in small amounts uniformly over 24 hours (https://www.medicines.org.uk/emc/product/135/smpc). The chance of hyper-stimulation is low with such a system. Should it happen, it can be removed by pulling on the tape attached to the delivery system. Once removed, the hyper-stimulation settles, and if not, a short-acting beta mimetic drug such as terbutaline 0.25 mg subcutaneously can be used. Such long-acting inserts also have the advantage of avoiding repeated vaginal examination within 24 hours to insert repeated doses of PGE2 gel or pessaries (Fig. 11.18).

The WHO (2011) guidelines on induction of labour recommend oral misoprostol 25 µg every 2–4 hours. Misoprostol (prostaglandin E_1) is not licensed in many countries for use in obstetrics, and the 25- or 50-µg formulations are not available in all countries. Some take a 200-µg formulation and divide it into four or eight segments to get 50-µg or 25-µg doses. Some dissolve a 200-µg tablet in 20 mL, and small aliquots of dissolved solution are taken as appropriate. The use of prostaglandins is contraindicated in the presence of a previous uterine scar. Some use the prostaglandin E_2 pessaries or gel with caution but not prostaglandin E_1 (i.e. misoprostol), as there is increased incidence of uterine rupture that will compromise the fetus and the mother. The mother should be properly counselled before these drugs are used.

Mechanical cervical ripening

Commonly this involves the insertion of a balloon catheter through the cervix. The balloon is used to mechanically distend the cervical canal by inflating the balloon with 40 to 80 mL of sterile water or saline over a 12-hour period. Some may go into labour during this period. In a few, the balloon would be expelled with cervical dilatation, and in the others, the balloon could be removed after 12 hours, and if the cervix is favourable, an amniotomy could be performed. If they do not progress to established labour

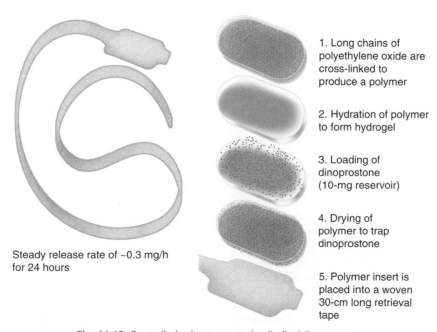

Steady release rate of ~0.3 mg/h for 24 hours

1. Long chains of polyethylene oxide are cross-linked to produce a polymer

2. Hydration of polymer to form hydrogel

3. Loading of dinoprostone (10-mg reservoir)

4. Drying of polymer to trap dinoprostone

5. Polymer insert is placed into a woven 30-cm long retrieval tape

Fig. 11.18 Controlled-release prostaglandin E_2 delivery system.

with uterine contractions in the next 4 hours, an oxytocin infusion could be commenced. Currently Foley catheters with a single balloon as well as a specially designed double balloon catheter are available for cervical ripening. Alternatively, synthetically manufactured osmotic dilators (e.g. Dilapan – http://www.dilapan.com/) can be used which absorbs the water content in the cervix and swells, thereby dilating the cervix.

Precipitate labour

Occasionally, at one end of the spectrum of normal labour, normal or slightly increased uterine activity may produce rapid cervical dilatation and an early delivery. A labour lasting less than 2 hours resulting in vaginal delivery is classified as precipitate. The hazards of such labours are that the child may be delivered in a rapid and uncontrolled manner and in an inconvenient environment such as into a toilet!

Fetal morbidity and mortality may be related to the lack of resuscitation facilities. Maternal morbidity may arise from severe perineal damage and from postpartum haemorrhage.

Precipitate labour tends to repeat itself with subsequent labours, and where there is such a history, the mother is best admitted to hospital near term to await the onset of labour or to have a planned induction.

Uterine hyper-stimulation

The commonest contemporary cause of uterine hyper-stimulation is the uncontrolled use of excessive amounts of oxytocic drugs. In extreme cases, this may result in uterine tetany with a continuous contraction. Leading up to this state, there will be frequent strong contractions and insufficient time between contractions to allow a return to normal baseline pressures. The condition can be rapidly corrected by turning off the oxytocin infusion. In fact, the condition should not arise if uterine activity is properly monitored by external or internal tocography. Contractions should not occur more frequently than five in 10 minutes. More than five contractions in 10 minutes is called *polysystole* and is likely to affect the placental perfusion and oxygenation of the fetus that can give rise to FHR changes.

The uterus becomes more and more sensitive to the same dose of oxytocin with advance in cervical dilatation. Hence, it is important to carefully monitor the contractions and reduce or stop the oxytocin infusion should the contraction frequency increase to more than five in 10 minutes.

Uterine hyper-stimulation can occur with the use of prostaglandins in various forms. This is due to rapid absorption of the drug from the vagina, as the rate of absorption is affected by the temperature and pH of the vagina and the

presence of infection/inflammation. This is best managed by removal of the PG pessary and the use of a bolus dose of a short-acting tocolytic such as 0.25 mg terbutaline as a subcutaneous dose or in 5 mL saline as a slow IV over 5 minutes.

Hyper-stimulation may also lead to uterine rupture, particularly where there is a uterine scar from a previous section or myomectomy. Such a rupture may sometimes occur even in the presence of normal uterine activity.

Delay in progress in labour

The view of what constitutes an abnormal labour has changed substantially over the last two decades. The definition of prolonged labour now relies more on the rate of progress than on absolute times. Nevertheless, it must be remembered that 90% of primigravid women deliver within 16 hours and 90% of multigravid women deliver within 12 hours. It is now rare to see a labour that lasts more than 24 hours. When labour becomes prolonged and progress is abnormally slow, the possibility of cephalopelvic disproportion must be considered, but in most cases slow progress is associated with inefficient uterine activity.

Efficiency of uterine activity

Efficiency of uterine activity is judged by the desired result of effacement and dilatation of the cervix and descent of the head. Few infrequent contractions may result in good progress in some women (efficient), whilst good frequent uterine contractions may not result in good cervical dilatation (inefficient). In the past, the terms *hypertonic* and *hypotonic* uterine activity were used, but they are hardly used in clinical practice during physiological labour because there are no specific criteria to define and they are difficult to diagnose. In pathological conditions such as abruptio placenta, the blood seeping into the myometrium may cause increased tone of the uterus (hypertonicity) and very frequent low-amplitude contractions (hypersystole/polysystole). On palpation, the uterus would be 'woody hard', tender and 'irritable'.

Despite the absence of an anatomical or physiological pacemaker in the uterus, contractions are usually coordinated and come at regular intervals increasing in frequency, duration and amplitude with progress of labour. In some women in labour, two or three contractions may come together followed by a small period of no activity, followed by another bout of two or three contractions. This is called *incoordinate uterine contractions*. Incoordinate contractions do not mean inefficient uterine activity if the desired

Case study

A 23-year-old primigravida was admitted to hospital in labour with regular and painful contractions. There was no evidence of antepartum haemorrhage. The cervix was found to be 2 cm dilated. Four hours later, the cervix was 4 cm dilated and the rate of progress was delayed. The cervicogram is shown in Figure 11.19. An epidural catheter was inserted and epidural analgesia commenced. The membranes were ruptured artificially, and clear amniotic fluid was released. Progress in labour continued to be slow – 3 hours later, the cervix was 5 cm dilated. A dilute oxytocin infusion was started. This resulted in rapid progress to full dilatation and vaginal delivery some 4 hours later.

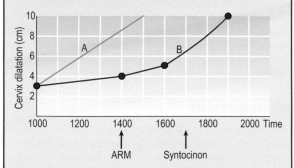

Fig. 11.19 Slow progress in the first stage of labour. The action time is line A, and line B is the actual cervical dilatation. *ARM*, Artificial rupture of membranes.

progress of cervical effacement, dilatation and descent of the head is achieved.

Management

Efficiency of uterine activity is usually recognized by the progress in labour. It is essential to evaluate the power (uterine contractions), passenger (fetus) and passage (maternal pelvis). Careful assessment of uterine activity, size and shape of the maternal pelvis and size of the fetus will guide the proper management.

The general principles of management of inefficient uterine activity involve:

- Reassurance to the mother and partner and explanation of the situation
- Adequate pain relief, principally with epidural analgesia
- Adequate fluid replacement by IV infusion of dextrose saline or Hartmann's solution
- Stimulation of uterine activity using an escalating dose infusion of oxytocin

Careful continuous monitoring of the mother and fetus with EFM should reassure maternal and fetal health.

Uterine activity may be stimulated by encouraging mobilization of the mother and, if the membranes are intact, by artificial ROM. If no progress is seen with the simple measures, an oxytocic infusion is commenced to augment labour and delivery. If progress continues to be slow, or there is evidence of fetal distress based on the CTG or there are signs of cephalopelvic disproportion as identified by poor progress of cervical dilation and descent of the head and increasing caput and moulding, delivery should be effected by caesarean section.

Continued uterine activity despite disproportion may lead to 'constriction ring'. The fetus is best delivered by caesarean section after relaxing the constriction ring using beta-sympathomimetic agents, or ether or halothane anaesthesia.

Cephalopelvic disproportion

This may arise because the fetus is large or where the pelvis, and especially the pelvic inlet, is small, or a combination of both factors. The head may not be engaged at the onset of labour but may engage with flexion and rotation of the head, moulding and progressive increase in pelvic dimensions. The pelvis can only be truly tested in the presence of strong uterine contractions over an adequate length of time in the absence of fetal compromise and signs of cephalopelvic disproportion.

Management

When the possibility of cephalopelvic disproportion is suspected, labour should be carefully monitored. Regular observations must be recorded of uterine activity; the rate of cervical dilatation; the descent of the presenting part; the position, station and caput and moulding; and the condition of both the mother and the fetus.

In primigravid women, the uterus may become exhausted late in the first stage and contractions may cease or become attenuated, and there may be no progress in cervical dilatation. If there is no change in cervical dilatation over a period of 4–6 hours, with no descent of head, increasing caput and moulding, the trial of labour should be abandoned. Similarly, if clinical signs of fetal distress or maternal exhaustion develop, the labour should be terminated by caesarean section.

> Multiparous women are at increased risk of uterine rupture if the labour becomes obstructed. Delay in progress in a multigravid patient should always be treated with caution, as it is likely to be associated with malposition or cephalopelvic disproportion and there is a greater risk of uterine rupture with the injudicious use of oxytocic agents.

Case study

A 38-year-old multigravid woman was admitted in labour at term. After good initial progress in labour, significant arrest occurred at 8 cm dilatation (Fig. 11.20). Vaginal examination confirmed the presence of an occipitoposterior position associated with marginal cephalopelvic disproportion. The cervix eventually became fully dilated, and the head was rotated and delivered with forceps.

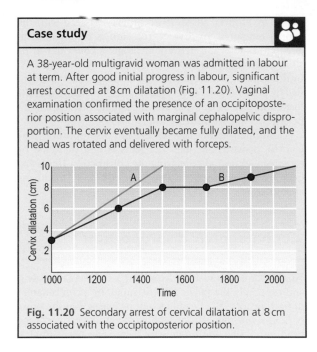

Fig. 11.20 Secondary arrest of cervical dilatation at 8 cm associated with the occipitoposterior position.

Cord presentation and cord prolapse

Cord presentation (Fig. 11.21) occurs when any part of the cord lies alongside or in front of the presenting part. The diagnosis is usually established by digital palpation of the pulsating cord, which may be felt through the intact membranes. When the membranes rupture, the cord prolapses and may appear at the vulva or be palpable in front of the presenting part.

Predisposing factors

Any condition that displaces the head or presenting part away from the cervix or where the presenting part is irregular and forms poor contact with the cervix will predispose to cord presentation or prolapse. Under these circumstances, if the membranes are ruptured artificially to induce labour, the cord may prolapse. In normal labour, the uterine contractions are likely to cause descent of the presenting part and fix it to the pelvic brim, and spontaneous ROM is much later in labour. The possibility of cord prolapse should be reduced by excluding cord presentation before artificial ROM. Slow release of amniotic fluid should be practised with high presenting part to allow the presenting part to slowly descend and snugly fit into the pelvis to avoid cord prolapse. With artificial ROM for induction of labour, the head may be higher with slightly increased incidence of cord prolapse. Hence, the procedure should be done in the labour room that is near an operating theatre (OT) so that the baby can be delivered rapidly should cord prolapse occur.

Management

The diagnosis of cord presentation is sometimes made prior to ROM and prolapse of the cord, but this is the exception rather than the rule. If the cord prolapses through a partially dilated cervix, delivery should be effected as soon as possible, as the presenting part will compress the cord or the cord arteries may go into spasm on exposure to cold air. Handling of the cord may cause the same effect. Cord spasm or compression leads to fetal asphyxia.

Prolapse of the cord is an obstetric emergency. Immediate assistance of a senior obstetrician, midwife, anaesthetist, paediatrician and OT staff should be summoned.

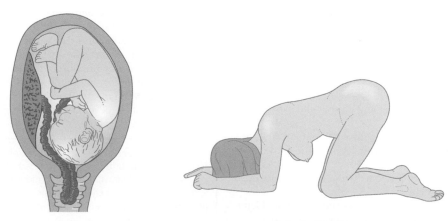

Knee–chest position

Fig. 11.21 Cord prolapse (left); pressure on the cord can be minimized by placing the mother in the knee–chest position.

Reduction of the loops of cord into the vagina and swab at the introitus may help to preserve the warmth and moisture content of the cord, thus reducing the chance of cord arterial spasm.

Unless spontaneous delivery is imminent, the woman should be placed in the knee–chest position, or the buttocks elevated by pillows or head tilt in a trolley to reduce pressure on the cord. Filling the urinary bladder may help to reduce pressure on the cord by the presenting part. It is difficult to replace the cord into the uterus, although there have been a few reports about this possibility.

Vaginal examination and digital displacement of the head to alleviate pressure of the head on the cord are a possibility, but it is difficult to transfer the woman to the theatre along the corridors with a hand in the vagina, although she would be covered. Each uterine contraction may further compress the cord at the pelvic brim against the presenting part, and a bolus dose of tocolytic (terbutaline 0.25 mg subcutaneously or slow IV in 5 mL saline over 5 minutes) may be of help to relieve this intermittent compression.

Delivery should be effected by caesarean section unless the cervix is fully dilated and delivery can be achieved rapidly by forceps or vacuum with the assistance of the maternal expulsive efforts.

Despite the acute asphyxial insult to the fetus, which is likely to be depressed at birth (hence the need for paediatrician to be on stand-by), the long-term prognosis in these infants is good. Provided there is no pre-existing impairment to gaseous transfer, the fetus can effectively withstand an acute asphyxial episode without suffering long-term damage.

Essential information

Normal labour

- Labour resulting in vaginal delivery
- <24 hours in a primigravida
- <16 hours in multigravida

Stages of labour

- First stage – onset of labour to full dilatation
- Second stage – full dilatation to delivery of the baby
- Third stage – delivery of the baby to delivery of the placenta and membranes

Onset of labour

- Regular painful contractions with cervical changes

Initiation of labour

- Complex interaction of fetal and maternal factors
- Principal components
  - Interaction of progesterone/oestradiol
  - Increased fetal cortisol
  - Local activity of prostaglandins
- Effects on myometrium of relaxin, activin A, follistatin, hCG and CRH
- A 'show'
- Rupture of fetal membranes

Uterine activity

- Increasing frequency, 'intensity' and duration of contractions
- Normal resting tonus increases slightly during labour
- Contractions cause shortening of myometrial cells
- Effacement and dilatation of the cervix
- Fundal dominance necessary for progression

The passages

- Softening of pelvic ligaments
- Increased distensibility of pelvic floor

The mechanism of normal labour

The fetal head adapts by:
- Descent throughout labour
- Flexion – to minimize diameter of presentation
- Internal rotation – as head reaches pelvic floor
- Extension – with delivery of head
- Restitution – head in line with shoulders
- External rotation – shoulders descend into pelvis
- Delivery of shoulders followed by rest of the body

The third stage

Following delivery:
- Placenta shears off uterine wall
- Uterus expels placenta and membranes into lower segment
- Oxytocic drugs given with delivery of the anterior shoulder
- Assisted delivery of placenta and membranes
- Check placenta and membranes
  Separation of the placenta is associated with:
- Lengthening of cord
- Elevation of uterine fundus and becoming hard and globular
- Trickling of fresh blood

Management of labour

- Observe cervical dilatation and descent of the head with the use of partogram
- Fluid balance and nutrition in labour

- Pain relief
  - Narcotic agents
  - Inhalation analgesia
  - Non-pharmacological methods
  - Regional analgesia

Fetal monitoring in labour

- Regular intermittent auscultation or fetal cardiotocography as appropriate
  - Interpretation (DrCBraVADO)
    - Dr: Define risks
    - C: Contractions
    - Bra: Baseline rate
    - V: Variability
    - A: Accelerations
    - D: Decelerations
    - O: Overall classification and Opinion
- The fetal electrocardiogram for changes in the ST waveform
- Fetal scalp blood sampling for acid–base balance

Pre-term labour

- Labour occurring prior to 37 weeks
- Occurs in 6–12% of pregnancies – varies from centre to centre
- Causes are:
  - Antepartum haemorrhage
  - Multiple pregnancy
  - Infection
  - Polyhydramnios
  - Socioeconomic
- Chances of survival same as at term by 34 weeks
- Prevention is by treatment of infection, use of progesterone pessaries and in selected cases cervical cerclage
- Management is by administration of corticosteroids and tocolysis that
  - Is not needed after 34 weeks
  - Contraindicated in cases of antepartum haemorrhage (APH), infection
  - Tocolytics may not be effective if cervix more than 5 cm
  - Delays delivery by 48 hours
  - Allows time to transfer or give steroids
  - May cause maternal pulmonary oedema

- Use of $MgSO_4$ – 4 g followed by 1 g IV per hour for 24 hours for neuroprotection for fetuses <32 weeks
- Is associated with an increased incidence of breech presentation
- Delivery by caesarean section considered in a pre-term breech presentation

Pre-labour rupture of membranes

- Rupture of membranes before onset of labour at term or pre-term period
- Causes are:
  - Infection
  - Multiple pregnancy
  - Polyhydramnios
  - Smoking
- Usually followed by labour within 48 hours
- If it occurs in the pre-term period, can be managed conservatively by monitoring for signs of infection before 36 weeks

Efficiency of uterine activity

- 90% of primigravidae deliver within 16 hours
- Diagnosis of efficient action is based on partogram
- Management
  - Reassurance and explanation of the situation
  - Pain relief
  - Fluid replacement
  - Mobilize if infrequent, weak contractions
  - Rupture membranes
  - Augment with oxytocin infusion
  - Operative delivery if lack of progress, cephalopelvic disproportion or fetal distress

Cord prolapse

- Predisposing factors
  - Multiple pregnancy
  - Malpresentation
  - Polyhydramnios
- Anticipation where presenting part is high
- Management
  - Reduction of cord into the vagina
  - Fill bladder with 500 mL saline/sterile water
  - Knee–chest position
  - Urgent delivery by caesarean section; if fully dilated and low station, by forceps or vacuum delivery

Chapter | 12 |

Management of delivery

Sabaratnam Arulkumaran

LEARNING OUTCOMES

After studying this chapter you should be able to:

Knowledge criteria

- Outline the mechanism of spontaneous vaginal delivery
- Describe the aetiology, diagnosis and management of the common malpresentations and malpositions in labour
- Define the different types of perineal trauma
- Describe indications, methods and complications of vaginal delivery and caesarean section
- List the risk factors and initial steps in management of shoulder dystocia
- Describe the complications in the third stage of labour, including postpartum haemorrhage, perineal trauma, haematoma and amniotic fluid embolism

Clinical competencies

- Conduct a normal vaginal delivery
- Carry out an episiotomy repair on a practice mannequin
- Explain the procedures of caesarean section and instrumental delivery

Professional skills and attitudes

- Consider the importance of choice of mode of delivery in partnership with the mother and respect the views of other health care workers
- Consider the emotional implications of birth for the woman, family and staff

Normal vaginal delivery

Normal vaginal delivery marks the end of the second stage of labour.

The second stage of labour is defined as the period from the time of complete cervical dilatation to the baby's birth. It is convenient to consider the second stage in two phases: the descent in the pelvis, i.e. the pelvic or 'passive' phase, and the perineal, or 'active', phase of the second stage. During the descent phase the mother does not normally experience the sensation of bearing down and, from a management point of view, this phase may be regarded as an extension of the first stage of the labour. In the perineal phase the urge to bear down is present, although this may be masked or diminished if epidural analgesia has been provided for the woman. Therefore, unless the head is visible with contractions, the dilatation of the cervix and the station of the presenting part should be confirmed by vaginal examination before encouraging the woman to bear down.

Provided no adverse clinical factors are present, a normal duration of the second stage is commonly regarded as lasting up to 2 hours in the nulliparous woman and 1 hour in the multipara. If the woman has received epidural analgesia, these times are extended by 1 hour for each group, respectively. Progress in the second stage is monitored by descent of the fetal head assessed by an abdominal and vaginal examination. The fetal head is engaged and it is favourable for mother to bear down when no more than one-fifth of the head is palpable abdominally and the bony part of the vertex has descended to the level of the ischial spines.

If the labour is normal, women may choose a variety of positions for delivery, but the supine position should be discouraged because of the risk of supine hypotensive syndrome. Many women adopt a semi-reclining position, which has the advantage of reducing the risk of supine hypotension and is a suitable position for assisted delivery or perineal repair should these procedures be required.

Normal vaginal delivery ABC

Women should be guided by their own urge to push. Pushing effort should allow for an unhurried, gentle delivery of the fetal head, and this can be achieved by combining short pushing spells with periods of panting, thus giving the vaginal and perineal tissues time to relax and stretch over the advancing head (Fig. 12.1). Several contractions may occur before the head crowns and is delivered. For the delivery of the head, either the 'hands-on' technique – supporting the perineum and flexing the baby's head – or the 'hands-poised' method – with the hands off the perineum but in readiness – can be used to facilitate spontaneous birth.

Episiotomy is not routinely required for spontaneous vaginal birth but may be indicated if the perineum begins to tear, if the perineal resistance prevents delivery of the head or if concern for the wellbeing of the fetus requires that the birth be expedited. Where an episiotomy is performed, the recommended technique is a mediolateral incision at the time of crowning, originating at the vaginal fourchette and directed usually to an angle of 60 degrees, which becomes a cut of 45 degrees when the head is delivered (Fig. 12.2).

With the next contraction, the head is gently pulled downwards along the longitudinal axis of the baby until the anterior shoulder is delivered under the sub-pubic arch, and then the baby is pulled anteriorly to deliver the posterior shoulder and the remainder of the trunk whilst protecting the perineum from tearing by the emerging posterior shoulders.

The infant will normally cry immediately after birth, but if breathing is delayed, the nasopharynx should be aspirated and, if needed, the baby's lungs inflated with oxygen using a face mask. If the onset of breathing is further delayed, intubation and ventilation may become necessary. The condition of the baby is assessed at 1 and 5 minutes using the Apgar scoring system (Table 12.1) and again at 10 minutes if the baby is depressed. If the baby is born in poor condition (Apgar score of less than 4 at 1 minute and less than 7 at 5 minutes), the cord should be double-clamped for paired cord blood gas analysis.

Management of the third stage

Active management of the third stage of labour is recommended, which includes the administration of oxytocin (10 I/U) intramuscularly to the mother, followed by late clamping (>2 minutes) and cutting of the cord. When the signs of placental separation are seen, i.e. the lengthening of the cord, trickle of blood and the uterus becoming globular and hard due to contraction and extruding the placenta into the lower segment, the placenta is delivered by controlled cord traction, a method commonly referred to as the *Brandt–Andrews technique* (Fig. 12.3).

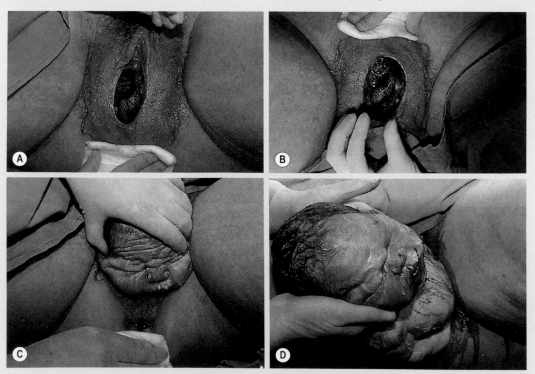

Fig. 12.1 Spontaneous vaginal delivery. (A) The second stage of labour, the scalp becomes visible with contractions and expulsive efforts by the mother. (B) Crowning of the head. (C) At delivery, the head is in the anteroposterior position. (D) Delivery of the head and shoulders.

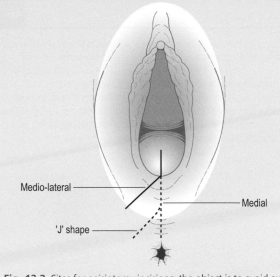

Table 12.1 Evaluation of Apgar score at 1 and 5 minutes			
	0	1	2
Colour	White	Blue	Pink
Tone	Flaccid	Rigid	Normal
Pulse	Impalpable	<100 beats/min	>100 beats/min
Respiration	Absent	Irregular	Regular
Response	Absent	Poor	Normal

Medio-lateral

Medial

'J' shape

Fig. 12.2 Sites for episiotomy incisions: the object is to avoid extension of the incision or tear into the anal sphincter or rectum.

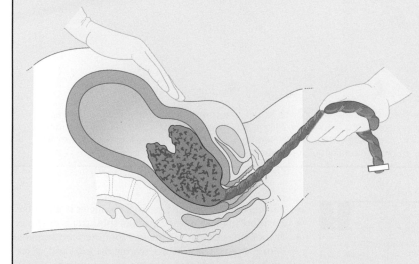

Fig. 12.3 Brandt–Andrews technique for assisted delivery of the placenta: the uterine fundus must be contracted with signs of placental separation (trickle of blood, lengthening of the cord) before this technique is attempted.

Repair of episiotomy or perineal injury

A careful examination of the mother's perineum should be made as soon as possible to identify the degree of perineal or genital tract trauma sustained during the birth. Perineal trauma caused either by episiotomy or tearing may be classified as first-, second-, third- or fourth-degree tears. A first-degree tear describes laceration to vaginal and perineal skin only. A second-degree tear involves the posterior vaginal wall and underlying perineal muscles but not the anal

sphincter. Third-degree injury to the perineum is damage that involves the anal sphincter complex, and a fourth-degree laceration is injury to the perineum that includes the ano/rectal mucosa.

In the case of a first-degree perineal tear, there is no need for suturing if the skin edges are already apposed, provided the wound is not bleeding. Episiotomies and second-degree lacerations should be sutured to minimize bleeding and to expedite healing. Third- and fourth-degree perineal lacerations should be repaired under epidural/spinal or general anaesthesia by an experienced surgeon in an operating theatre under good lighting conditions. This is discussed in more detail in the next section.

Episiotomy repair ABC

For episiotomy repair, the woman should be placed in the lithotomy position so that a good view of the extent of the wound can be obtained (Fig. 12.4). Repair should only be undertaken with effective analgesia in place using either local anaesthetic agent infiltration or epidural or spinal anaesthesia. Closure of the vaginal wound requires a clear view of the apex of the incision. It is recommended that an absorbable synthetic suture material be used for the repair, using a continuous technique for the vaginal wall and muscle layer and a continuous subcuticular technique for the skin.

On completion of the procedure, it is important to ensure that the vagina is not constricted and that it can admit two fingers easily. In addition, a rectal examination should be performed to confirm that none of the sutures have penetrated the rectal mucosa. If this occurs, the suture must be removed, as it may otherwise result in the formation of a rectovaginal fistula.

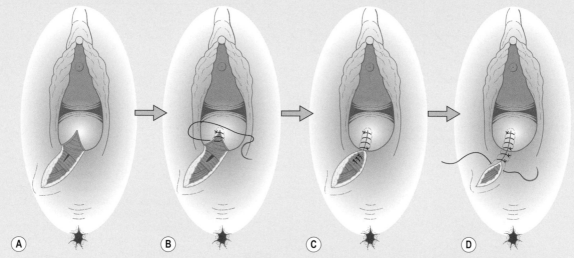

Fig. 12.4 Repair of the episiotomy: the posterior vaginal wall may be closed with continuous or interrupted sutures; apposition of the cut levator muscle ensures haemostasis before skin closure. (A) Episiotomy wound. (B) Continuous suture of posterior vaginal wall. (C) Interrupted sutures into the cut edge of the levator. (D) Interrupted suture into the perineal skin. Current evidence suggests subcuticular absorbable continuous suture for the skin.

> **!** Accurate repair of an episiotomy is important. Over-vigorous suturing of the wound or shortening of the vagina may result in dyspareunia and sexual disharmony with the partner. Failure to recognize and repair damage to the anal sphincter may result in varying degrees of incontinence of flatus and faeces.

Third- and fourth-degree injuries

Obstetric anal sphincter injuries are a complication of vaginal deliveries and lead to long-term **sequelae**: faecal and flatus incontinence (up to 25%), perineal discomfort, dyspareunia (up to 10%) and rarely rectovaginal fistulas. A third-degree tear is a partial or complete disruption of the external and internal sphincter; either or both of these may be involved. These tears are often sub-classified as:

- 3a: less than 50% of the external sphincter is disrupted
- 3b: more than 50% of the external sphincter is disrupted
- 3c: both the external and internal sphincters are disrupted

Fourth-degree tears involve tearing the anal and/or rectal epithelium in addition to sphincter disruption.

A number of risk factors have been identified, though their value in prediction or prevention of sphincter injury is limited (Box 12.1). It is important to examine a perineal injury carefully after delivery so as not to miss sphincter damage. This may increase the rate of sphincter damage, but it will help to reduce the rate of long-term morbidity.

Repair and management of third- and fourth-degree tears

An experienced obstetrician should be performing or supervising the repair. Good exposure, lighting and anaesthesia are prerequisites. The procedure should be covered with

Box 12.1 **Risk factors for anal sphincter damage**

- Large baby (>4 kg)
- First vaginal delivery
- Instrumental delivery (more with forceps than with ventouse)
- Occipitoposterior position
- Prolonged second stage
- Induced labour
- Epidural anaesthesia
- Shoulder dystocia
- Midline episiotomy

Data from Robson S, Higgs P (2011) Third- and fourth-degree injuries. RANZCOG 13(2); 20–22.

broad-spectrum antibiotics and an oral regimen carried on for at least 5 days following the repair. There are two recognized forms of repair that include the end-to-end method and overlapping of the sphincter ends. Documentation describing the extent of the tear, the method of repair, as well as the level of supervision is vital. Immediately after the repair, the women should be debriefed and referred for physiotherapy and stool softeners should be prescribed. At the 6-week postnatal appointment, women need to be specifically asked about control of faeces, flatus and bowel movements, as well as urgency and sexual dysfunction. An elective caesarean section for subsequent deliveries should be offered to all women who have sustained a sphincter injury if they remain symptomatic. Early referral to a colorectal surgeon is advised if physiotherapy has not relieved her symptoms.

Malpresentations

More than 95% of fetuses present with the vertex and are termed *normal*. Those presenting with other parts of the body (breech, face, brow, shoulder, cord) to the lower segment and cervix are known as *malpresentations*. There may be a reason for malpresentation, although in most instances there is no identifiable cause. They also present with specific problems in labour and during delivery. In modern obstetrics, the presentation needs to be diagnosed early in labour and appropriate management instituted to prevent maternal or fetal injury.

Breech presentation is discussed in Chapter 8.

Face presentation

In face presentation, the fetal head is hyperextended so that the part of the head between the chin and orbits, i.e. the eyes, nose and mouth, that can be felt with the examining finger is the presenting part. The incidence is about 1 in 500 deliveries. In most cases, the cause is unknown but is associated with high parity and fetal anomaly, particularly anencephaly. In modern obstetric practice where most pregnant women have an ultrasound scan for fetal abnormalities, it is rare to see such conditions as a cause of face presentation.

Diagnosis

Face presentation is rarely diagnosed antenatally, but rather is usually identified during labour by vaginal examination when the cervix is sufficiently dilated to allow palpation of the characteristic facial features. However, oedema may develop that may obscure these landmarks. If in doubt, ultrasound will confirm or exclude the diagnosis. The position of a face presentation is defined with the chin as the denominator and is therefore recorded as mentoanterior, mentotransverse and mentoposterior (Fig. 12.5).

Management

If the position is mentoanterior, progress can be followed normally with the expectation of spontaneous vaginal delivery. However, if progress is abnormally slow, it is preferable to proceed to caesarean section. In cases of persistent

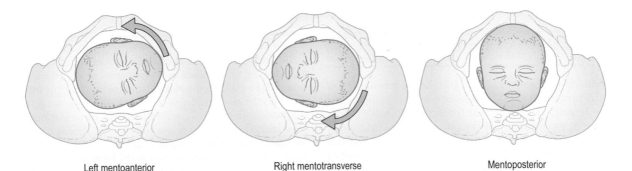

Left mentoanterior   Right mentotransverse   Mentoposterior

Fig. 12.5 Position of the face presentation. The denominator is the chin.

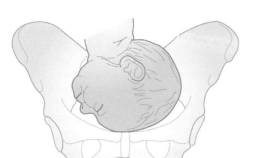

Brow presentation

Fig. 12.6 Brow presentation preventing delivery.

mentoposterior positions, vaginal delivery is not possible without manual or forceps rotation. Because the risk associated with these manoeuvres to the mother and infant is considerable, most obstetricians will perform a caesarean delivery.

Brow presentation

A brow presentation is described when the attitude of the fetal head is midway between a flexed vertex and face presentation (Fig. 12.6) and is the most unfavourable of all cephalic presentations. The condition is rare and occurs in 1 in 1500 births. If the head becomes impacted with a brow as the presenting diameter, the mentovertical diameter (13 cm), this is incompatible with vaginal delivery.

Diagnosis and management

The diagnosis is almost always made in labour when the anterior fontanelle, supraorbital ridges and root of the nose are palpable. In the normally grown term fetus, vaginal delivery is not possible as a brow because of the large presenting diameters. Therefore in the vast majority of cases with brow presentation, caesarean section is the method of choice for delivery.

Malposition of the fetal head

Position of the fetal head is defined as the relationship of the denominator to the fixed points of the maternal pelvis. The denominator of the head is the most definable prominence at the periphery of the presenting part. In 90% of cases, the vertex presents with the occiput in the anterior half of the pelvis in late labour, and hence is defined as the 'normal' or 'occipitoanterior' (OA) position. In about 10% of cases, there may be malposition of the head; i.e.

the occiput presents in the posterior half of the pelvis with the occiput facing the sacrum or one of the two sacroiliac joints – the occipitoposterior (OP) position – or the sagittal suture is directed along the transverse diameter of the pelvis – the occipitotransverse (OT) position. Malposition of the vertex is frequently associated with deflexion of the fetal head or varying degrees of asynclitism, i.e. one parietal bone, usually the anterior, being lower in the pelvis with the parietal eminences at different levels. Asynclitism is most pronounced in the OT position. Deflexion and asynclitism are associated with larger presenting diameters of the fetal head, thereby making normal delivery more difficult.

The occipitoposterior position

Some 10–20% of all cephalic presentations are OP positions at the onset of labour, either as a direct OP or, more commonly, as an oblique right or left OP position. During labour, the head usually undertakes the long rotation through the transverse to the OA position, but a few, about 5%, remain in the OP position. Where the OP position persists, progress of the labour may be arrested due to the deflexed attitude of the head that results in larger presenting diameters (11.5 cm × 9.5 cm) than are found with OA positions (9.5 cm × 9.5 cm). Prolonged and painful labour associated with backache is a characteristic feature of a posterior fetal position (Fig. 12.7).

Diagnosis and management

The diagnosis is usually made or confirmed on vaginal examination during labour when the cervix is sufficiently dilated to allow palpation of the sagittal suture with the posterior fontanelle situated posteriorly in the pelvis. In many cases, labour will progress normally, with the head rotating anteriorly and delivering spontaneously. Occasionally the head may rotate posteriorly and deliver in a persistent OP position.

> Because of the deflexed head and the relatively large presenting diameters, delivery in the posterior position may result in over-distension of the perineum, resulting in third- or fourth-degree tears.

Adequate pain relief and fluid replacement should be provided for the mother, and if progress of the labour is slower than average, the introduction of an oxytocin infusion should be considered, provided there are no other contraindications to its use and contractions were thought to be inadequate. If progress is judged to be slow or if there are other indications to expedite delivery, further management will depend on the station of the head, the dilatation of the cervix and the competence of the operator to perform rotational forceps or vacuum-assisted delivery.

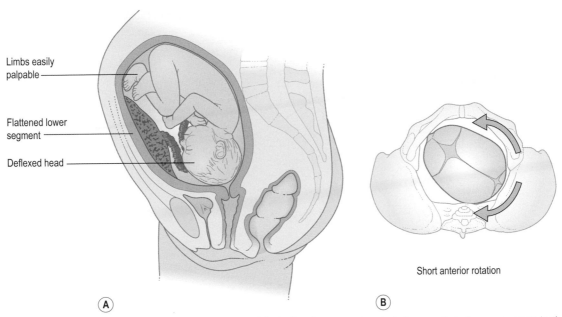

Limbs easily palpable

Flattened lower segment

Deflexed head

Short anterior rotation

(A)

(B)

Fig. 12.7 Clinical findings in the occipitoposterior position (A); the head may rotate anteriorly or posteriorly or may arrest in the occipitoposterior position (B).

If the cervix is not completely dilated or the head is not engaged, caesarean section will be the only option for delivery of the baby. On the other hand, if the head is engaged and the cervix is fully dilated, the choice of method will be between caesarean section and forceps or vacuum-assisted delivery, depending on the obstetric circumstances (station and position of the vertex and fetal condition) and the skill of the operator in performing rotational instrumental deliveries.

> ! When performing caesarean section for OP position, the head sometimes becomes impacted in the pelvis and may be difficult to dislodge. In such cases, it may be advisable to disimpact the head vaginally before extracting it abdominally. Occasionally a breech extraction is performed through the uterine incision.

Deep transverse arrest

The head normally descends into the pelvis in the OT or OP position and then the occiput rotates anteriorly to emerge under the pubic arch. Occasionally this anterior rotation of the occiput fails to occur or, in an OP position, fails to rotate beyond the transverse diameter of the pelvis. Labour will then become arrested due to the large presenting diameters resulting from asynclitism of the head that characterizes a fetal OT position. This clinical situation is referred to as *deep transverse arrest*.

Diagnosis and management

The diagnosis of deep transverse arrest is made during labour by vaginal examination when the second stage is prolonged and the cervix is fully dilated. As with OP arrest, the choice of method of delivery will be between caesarean section and instrumental delivery. However, provided the head is engaged in the pelvis and the station is at or below the spines, it can usually be rotated to the anterior position, either manually or by rotational forceps or vacuum extraction (auto-rotation with descent) and delivered vaginally.

There is no longer any place for 'heroic' procedures using excessive force to rotate and extract the head. Such procedures may result in fetal intracranial injury and laceration of major cerebral vessels. If the fetal head does not rotate and descend easily, the procedure should be abandoned and delivery completed by caesarean section.

Instrumental delivery

Two main types of instruments are employed for assisted vaginal delivery: the obstetric forceps (Fig. 12.8) and the obstetric vacuum extractor (ventouse; Fig. 12.10). The forceps were introduced into obstetric practice some three centuries ago, whereas the vacuum extractor as a practical alternative to the forceps only became popular over the past half-century.

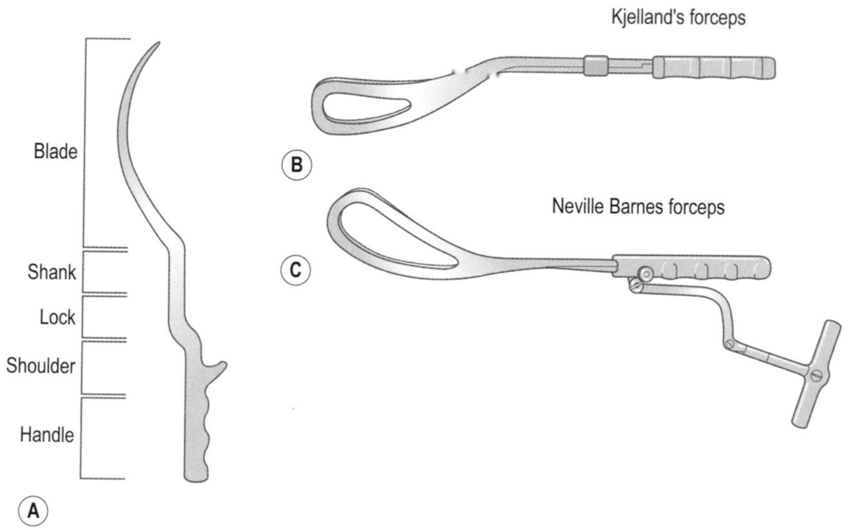

Fig. 12.8 Forceps parts (A) and commonly used forceps (B, C); the absence of the pelvic curve in Kjelland's forceps enables rotation of the fetal head.

Indications for instrumental delivery

With few exceptions, both instruments are used for similar indications, but the technique with the forceps differs completely from that of vacuum extraction.

The common indications for forceps or vacuum-assisted delivery are:
• delay in the second stage of labour
• non-reassuring fetal status ('fetal distress')
• maternal exhaustion and medical disorders

Clinical factors that may influence the need for assisted vaginal delivery include the resistance of the pelvic floor and perineum, inefficient uterine contractions, poor maternal expulsive effort, malposition of the fetal head, cephalopelvic disproportion and epidural analgesia.

Prerequisites for instrumental delivery

The mother should be placed in a modified lithotomy position, and the thighs, vulva and perineum should be washed and draped. The following prerequisites should be confirmed before proceeding:
• full cervical dilatation
• vertex presentation
• head engaged, not palpable abdominally and station at or below the spines
• known position and attitude of the head
• empty bladder
• adequate analgesia

Method of instrumental delivery

It is customary to classify instrumental deliveries into three categories according to the station of the fetal head, i.e. outlet, low and midpelvic deliveries, and into two types according to position of the fetal head, i.e. non-rotational and rotational deliveries.

Non-rotational instrumental delivery

Forceps
Examples of the types of forceps used when no anterior rotation of the head is required are the Neville Barnes and Simpson's forceps (see Fig. 12.8). Both of these forceps have cephalic and pelvic curves. The two blades of the forceps are designated according to the side of the pelvis to which they are applied. Thus the left blade is applied to the left side of the pelvis (Fig. 12.9A). There is a fixed lock between the blades (Fig. 12.9B). The two sides of the forceps should lock at the shank without difficulty. The sagittal suture should be perpendicular to the shank, the occiput 3–4 cm above the shank and only one finger space between the heel of the blade and the head on either side. Intermittent traction is applied coinciding with the uterine contractions and maternal bearing-down efforts in the direction of the pelvic canal (Fig. 12.9C) until the occiput is on view, and then the head is delivered by anterior extension (Fig. 12.9D).

Vacuum delivery
All vacuum extractors consist of a cup that is attached to the baby's head, a vacuum source that provides the

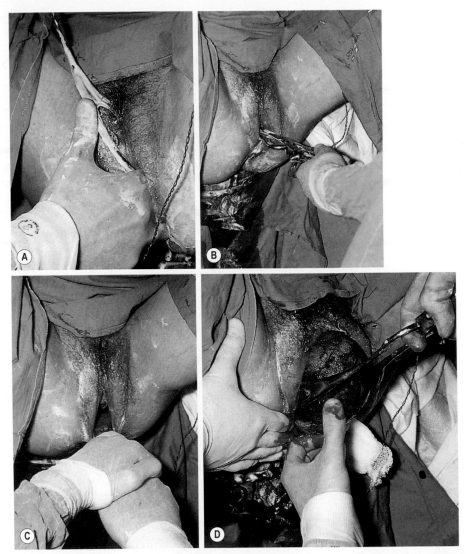

Fig. 12.9 Forceps. (A) Left blade for left side of pelvis. (B) Fixed lock between blades. (C) Application of intermittent traction in direction of pelvic canal. (D) Delivery of head by anterior extension.

means of attachment of the cup and a traction system or handle that allows the operator to assist the birth (see Fig. 12.10). As with forceps, there are two main design types of vacuum devices: the so-called *anterior* cups for use in non-rotational OA extractions and the *posterior* cups for use in rotational OP and OT deliveries. The cup is applied to the baby's head at a specific point on the vertex (the flexion point) (Fig. 12.11A), and traction is directed along the axis of the pelvis (Fig. 12.11B) until the head descends to the perineum (Fig. 12.11C). With

crowning, traction is directed upwards and the head is delivered (Fig. 12.11D).

Rotational instrumental delivery

If the position of the fetal head is OP or OT, forceps and vacuum extractors specifically designed for use in these positions must be used to achieve anterior rotation of the head.

For example, Kjelland's forceps (see Fig. 12.8) has a sliding lock and minimal pelvic curve so that rotation of

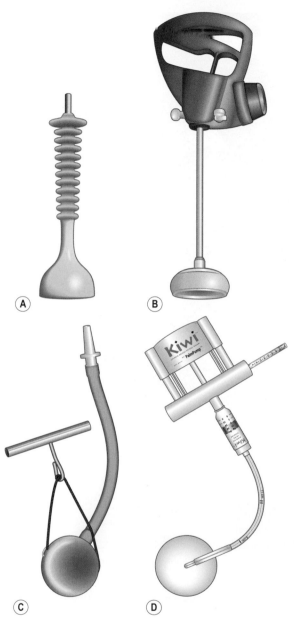

Fig. 12.10 Vacuum-assisted delivery devices. (A, B) Anterior cups for use in non-rotational (occipitoanterior) vacuum deliveries. (C, D) Posterior cups for use in rotational (occipitoposterior and occipitotransverse) vacuum deliveries.

the fetal head with the forceps can be achieved without causing damage to the vagina by the blades. For rotational vacuum-assisted delivery, a 'posterior' cup (see Fig. 12.10) will allow the operator to manoeuvre the cup towards and over the flexion point, thereby facilitating

flexion and *auto-rotation* of the head to the OA position at delivery.

Trial of instrumental delivery

Where some difficulty with a forceps or vacuum delivery is anticipated, e.g. if there is a suspicion of borderline dispro-portion, the procedure should be attempted in the operating room as a 'trial' of instrumental delivery, with preparation made to proceed to caesarean section. If some descent is not evident with each traction, the procedure should be abandoned in favour of caesarean section. In this way, significant trauma to the infant and mother should be avoided.

Caesarean section

Caesarean delivery is the method by which a baby is born through an incision in the abdominal wall and uterus. There are two main types of caesarean section, namely, the more common and preferred lower uterine segment operation (Fig. 12.12) and the much less common 'classical' caesarean section that involves incising the upper segment of the uterus.

Indications for caesarean section

Although caesarean section rates show considerable variation from place to place, there has been a consistent increase in this method of delivery over recent years to such an extent that in many developed countries, rates of 25–30% or even higher are not unusual. Common indications for caesarean section are:

- non-reassuring fetal status ('fetal distress')
- abnormal progress in the first or second stages of labour (dystocia)
- intrauterine growth restriction due to poor placental function
- malpresentations: breech, transverse lie, brow
- placenta praevia and/or severe antepartum haemorrhage, e.g. abruptio placentae
- previous caesarean section, especially if more than one
- severe pre-eclampsia and other maternal medical disorders
- cord presentation and prolapse
- miscellaneous uncommon indications

Depending on the urgency of the clinical indication, caesarean sections have been classified into four categories based on time limits within which the operation should be performed. The most urgent, *category 1*, describes indications where there is immediate threat to the life of the woman or fetus; *category 2*, where maternal or fetal compromise is present but is not immediately life threatening; *category 3*, where there is no maternal or fetal compromise but early delivery is required; and *category 4* refers to elective planned caesarean section.

Women who have had one previous uncomplicated, lower segment caesarean section for a non-recurrent indication may attempt a vaginal delivery in a subsequent labour provided no other adverse clinical factors are present. The major concern is risk of dehiscence of the uterine scar, but this is low with a previous lower uterine segment incision. The figures quoted are 5/1000 with spontaneous labour, 8/1000 with the use of oxytocin infusion and 25/1000 with the use of prostaglandins. The risk is higher and may occur before the onset of labour where a classical (upper segment) caesarean section has been performed. Signs of impending or actual scar dehiscence include suprapubic pain and tenderness, fetal distress, maternal tachycardia, vaginal bleeding and collapse. Thus, women attempting a vaginal birth after caesarean section should deliver in a hospital where there are facilities for close monitoring of maternal and fetal wellbeing; ready accessibility to an operating theatre; an experienced obstetric, anaesthetic and paediatric team; and blood transfusion services.

Complications

Although the risks of caesarean delivery for a woman have decreased significantly, as with all major surgical operations, immediate and late complications are associated with this method of delivery. The main immediate complication is perioperative haemorrhage, which may occasionally result in shock. Rarely injury to the bladder or ureters may occur during the procedure. Late complications of caesarean section include infection of the wound or uterine cavity, secondary postpartum bleeding and, less commonly, deep vein thrombosis and pulmonary embolus.

Shoulder dystocia

Shoulder dystocia is a serious condition that occurs when the fetal head has delivered but the shoulders fail to deliver spontaneously or with the normal amount of downward traction. The head recoils against the mother's perineum to form the so-called *turtle sign*. If delivery is delayed, the baby may become asphyxiated and, unless care is exercised when assisting the birth, may suffer brachial plexus palsy or limb fractures from over-vigorous manipulations. Shoulder dystocia is associated with the birth of macrosomic infants (>4500 g), especially if the mother has diabetes. Other predisposing factors are prolonged second stage of labour and assisted vaginal delivery.

Unfortunately, shoulder dystocia is unpredictable; only a minority of macrosomic infants will experience shoulder dystocia, and the majority of cases will occur in normal labours with infants weighing less than 4000 g. For this reason, all birth attendants should be skilled in the recognition and the specific steps in the management of this potentially serious emergency.

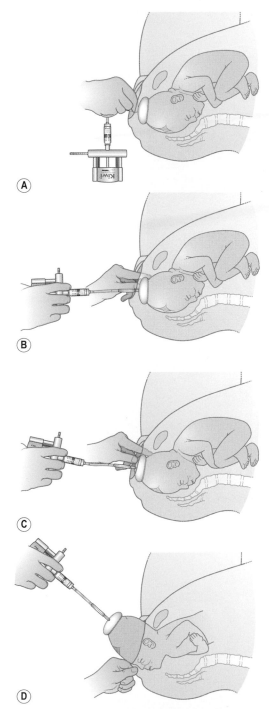

Fig. 12.11 Vacuum-assisted delivery. (A) Application of the cup over the flexion point to achieve a flexing median application. (B) Traction downwards with a finger on the cup and anther on the skull to detect and avoid any cup displacement. (C) Change of direction of pull from downwards to horizontal with descent of head. (D) Traction upwards with the protection of the perineum.

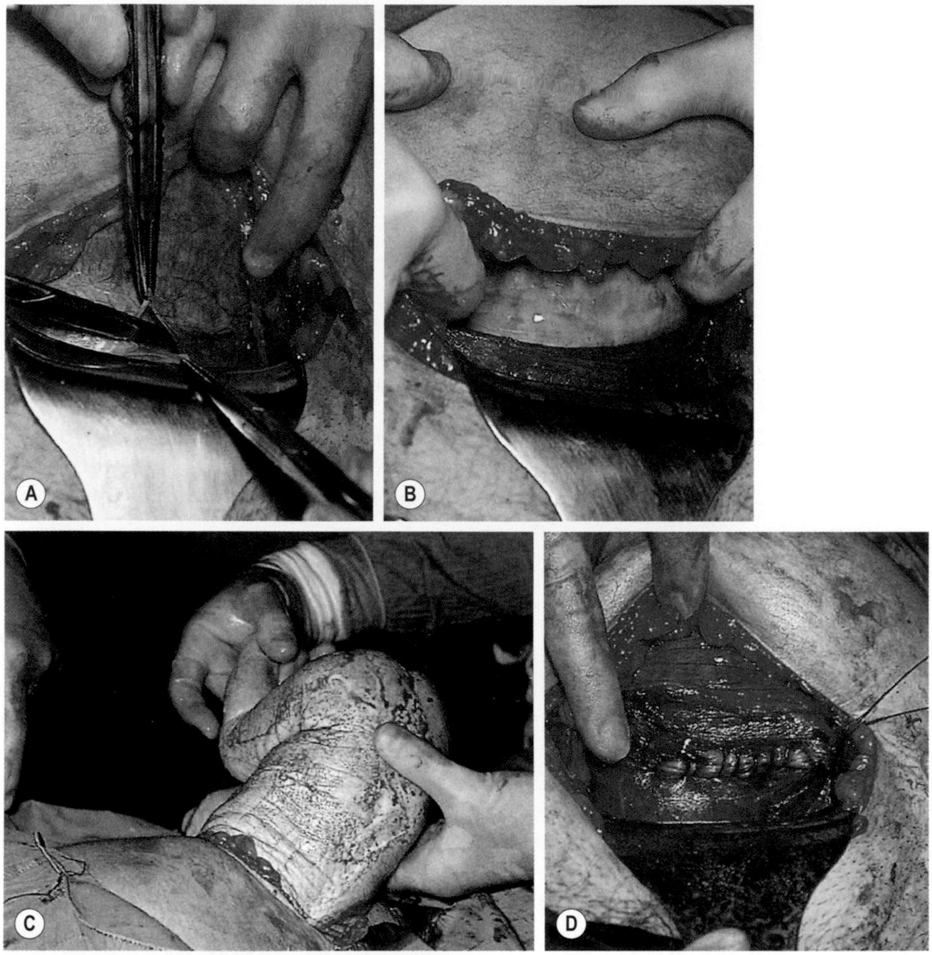

Fig. 12.12 Caesarean section. (A) Bladder is reflected from the lower segment. (B) Incision made in lower segment. (C) Presenting part delivered. (D) Wound closure.

Normally, delivery of the anterior shoulder is achieved with gentle downward traction (Fig. 12.13) and then followed by upward traction to deliver the posterior shoulder (Fig. 12.14). If this is not successful, the recommended first-line treatment for shoulder dystocia is McRobert's manoeuvre (Box 12.2). The woman is placed in the recumbent position with the hips slightly abducted and acutely flexed with the knees bent up towards the chest. At the same time, an assistant applies directed suprapubic pressure to help dislodge the anterior shoulder and for it to be in the oblique diameter of the pelvic inlet.

McRobert's manoeuvre and directed suprapubic pressure are successful in the majority of cases of shoulder dystocia. Other more complex internal manoeuvres are described, such as rotation of the fetal shoulders to one or another oblique pelvic diameter by inserting the whole hand into the pelvis, or manual delivery of the posterior

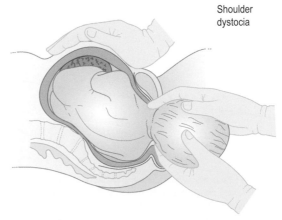

Shoulder dystocia

Fig 12.13 Disimpaction of the anterior shoulder.

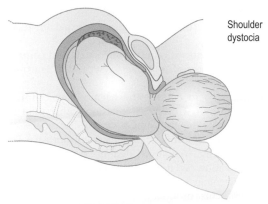

Fig 12.14 Impacted shoulders. It is sometimes necessary to rotate the fetus to disimpact the posterior shoulder.

Box 12.2 Difficulty delivering shoulders: actions to be taken

- Summon help, including senior obstetrician, paediatrician and anaesthetist
- Place mother in recumbent position with the hips and knees fully flexed and slightly abducted (McRobert's manoeuvre)
- Apply suprapubic pressure on the anterior shoulder to displace it downwards and laterally
- Make or extend an episiotomy
- Insert a hand into the vagina and rotate the fetal shoulders to the oblique pelvic diameter
- Deliver the posterior arm by flexing it at the elbow and sweeping the arm across the chest

---

arm to reduce a larger bi-acromial diameter to a slightly smaller acromio-axillary diameter. These steps may be facilitated by a generous mediolateral episiotomy.

Abnormalities of the third stage of labour

The third stage of labour lasts from the delivery of the infant to delivery of the placenta. This is normally accomplished within 10–15 minutes and should be complete within 30 minutes.

Postpartum haemorrhage

Primary postpartum haemorrhage is defined as bleeding from the genital tract in excess of 500 mL in the first 24 hours after delivery (Fig. 12.15).

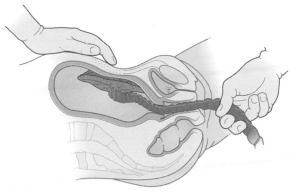

Fig. 12.15 Primary postpartum haemorrhage may occur in the presence of a retained placenta.

Secondary postpartum haemorrhage refers to abnormal vaginal bleeding occurring at any subsequent time in the puerperium up to 6 weeks after delivery.

Primary postpartum haemorrhage

Predisposing causes
Haemorrhage may occur from any part of the genital tract for reasons listed next but arises most commonly from the placental site. Low implantation of the placenta appears to be associated with inadequate constriction of the uterine blood vessels at the placental implantation site.

Causes of primary haemorrhage are due to one of four 'Ts' – tone, tissue, trauma or thrombin (referring to clotting problems).

Uterine atony accounts for 75–90% of all causes of postpartum haemorrhage. Predisposing factors include:
- uterine over-distension, e.g. multiple pregnancy, polyhydramnios
- prolonged labour, instrumental delivery
- antepartum haemorrhage: placenta praevia and abruption
- multiparity
- multiple fibroids, uterine abnormalities
- general anaesthesia
- genital tract trauma
- episiotomy
- lacerations to perineum, vagina and cervix
- uterine rupture and caesarean scar dehiscence
- haematomas of the vulva, vagina and broad ligament
- tissue: retained placenta or placental tissue
- thrombin: acquired in pregnancy, e.g. HELLP syndrome, sepsis or disseminated intravascular coagulation (DIC)

Management
Postpartum bleeding may be sudden and profound and may rapidly lead to cardiovascular collapse. Treatment is directed towards controlling the bleeding and replacing the blood and fluid loss (Fig. 12.16).

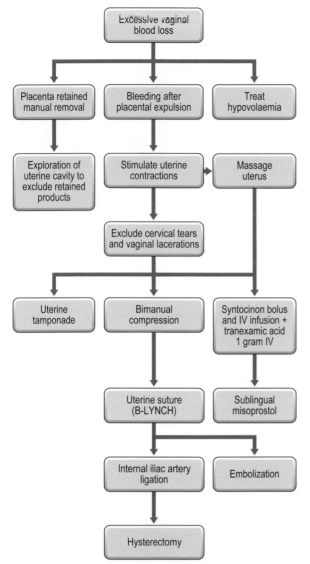

Fig. 12.16 Flow chart showing management of postpartum haemorrhage.

Controlling the haemorrhage

A brief visual inspection will suffice to estimate the amount of blood loss and whether the placenta has been expelled.

If the placenta is retained:

- Massage the uterus to ensure it is well contracted.
- Attempt delivery of the placenta by controlled cord traction.
- If this fails, proceed to manual removal of the placenta under spinal, epidural or general anaesthesia when the mother is adequately resuscitated.

If the placenta has been expelled:

- Massage and compress the uterus to expel any retained clots.
- Inject IV oxytocin 5 units immediately and commence an IV infusion of 40 units in 500 mL of Hartmann's solution.
- If this fails to control the haemorrhage, administer ergometrine 0.2 mg by IV injection (other than those women with hypertension or cardiac disease).
- If bleeding continues, administer misoprostol 800 µg sublingually (recommended by the World Health Organization (WHO) and the International Federation of Gynecology and Obstetrics (FIGO)).
- Intramuscular or intramyometrial injection of 15-methyl prostaglandin $F_{2\alpha}$ 0.25 mg can be given and repeated every 15 minutes for up to a maximum of eight doses.
- Tranexamic acid (anti-fibrinolytic agent) 1 g should be given by slow IV and, if bleeding continues, the dose should be repeated in 30 minutes. If bleeding restarts within 24 hours the tranexamic acid 1 g could be repeated. Administration of tranexamic acid within 3 hours of postpartum haemorrhage reduces maternal mortality due to bleeding by 30%.
- Two size 14-gauge (orange – 240 mL/min) or 16-gauge (grey – 180 mL/min) IV cannulas should be used to adequately infuse fluids or transfuse blood.
- Collect blood sample to check for Hb%, coagulation disorders and for cross-matching.
- Check that the placenta and membranes are complete. If they are not, manual exploration and evacuation of the uterus are indicated.
- At the same time, the vagina and cervix should be examined with a speculum under good illumination and any laceration should be sutured.
- Replacement of blood loss and resuscitation: It is essential to replace blood loss throughout attempts to control uterine bleeding. Hypovolaemia should be actively treated with IV crystalloid, colloid, blood and blood products. One or two packed cell volumes to one pack of plasma is shown to reduce morbidity and improve survival.

If these measures fail, a number of surgical techniques can be implemented, including:

- bimanual compression of the uterus –should be maintained for 8–10 minutes to allow clotting within the intramyometrial blood vessels
- uterine tamponade with balloon catheters
- uterine compression sutures (B-Lynch or modified compression suture)
- internal iliac and uterine artery ligation
- major vessel embolization where invasive radiological facilities and expertise are available
- total or subtotal hysterectomy

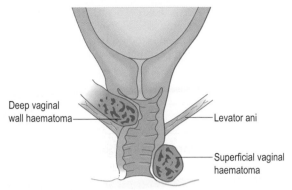

Fig. 12.17 The sites of vaginal wall haematomas.

Secondary postpartum haemorrhage

Causes and predisposing factors
Causes of secondary postpartum haemorrhage includes:
- retained placental tissue
- intrauterine infection
- rare causes, e.g. trophoblastic disease or abnormal vasculature like intrauterine arteriovenous malformation

Management
Treatment will depend on whether the bleeding is mild or heavy and whether it is associated with signs of possible sepsis. If the bleeding is slight, the uterus is not tender and there are no other signs of infection, observation with a course of antibiotics is justified. However, if the bleeding is heavy and particularly if there are signs of infection, IV broad-spectrum antibiotics (to cover aerobes and anaerobes) and uterine exploration under anaesthesia are indicated.

Vaginal wall haematomas

Profuse haemorrhage may sometimes occur from vaginal and perineal lacerations, and bleeding from these sites should be controlled as soon as possible. Venous bleeding may be controlled by compression alone, but arterial bleeding will require vessel ligation. Vaginal wall haematomas may occur in one of two sites (Fig. 12.17):
- **Superficial:** The bleeding occurs below the insertion of the levator ani, and the haematoma will be seen to distend the perineum, causing the mother considerable pain. The haematoma must be drained and any visible bleeding vessels ligated, although they are rarely identified. For this reason, a drain should be inserted before the wound is re-sutured.
- **Deep:** The bleeding occurs deep to the insertion of the levator ani muscle and is not visible externally. It is more common after instrumental delivery than after spontaneous birth and presents with symptoms of continuous pelvic pain, retention of urine and unexplained anaemia. It can usually be diagnosed by vaginal examination as a bulge into the upper part of the vaginal wall. Alternatively, ultrasound examination will confirm the diagnosis. If the pulse and blood pressure (BP) are stable and within the normal range and there are no signs of increase in the size of the haematoma, i.e. self-limiting, then the management can be conservative. If there is increasing pain with rise in pulse rate and drop in BP or there is increase in size of the haematoma, the haematoma should be evacuated by incision and a large drain inserted into the cavity. The vagina should be firmly packed and an indwelling catheter inserted into the bladder. Antibiotic therapy should be administered and, if necessary, a blood transfusion is instituted.

Uterine inversion

This is a rare complication usually occurring during attempted delivery of the placenta, where the uterine fundus inverts and protrudes through the cervix. The condition is more likely to occur when the placenta is fundal and adherent. The symptoms are severe lower abdominal pain and maternal shock with haemorrhage. The management is to leave the placenta attached to the uterus, initiate fluid resuscitation and attempt to push the fundus back through the cervix manually or using hydrostatic pressure. If this cannot be accomplished immediately, it will be necessary to perform replacement under general anaesthesia in theatre with the use of uterine relaxants. If these measures fail, laparotomy and a surgical procedure may be needed to correct the inversion.

Perineal wound breakdown

Breakdown of episiotomy or perineal wound repairs may occur due to infection or haematoma in the wound. Small areas of breakdown can be treated by regular cleaning and antibiotics and left to granulate until healed. More extensive wound breakdowns should be treated by antibiotics and cleansing and debridement of sloughing tissues. When signs of active infection have subsided, a secondary repair can then be performed. With third- and fourth-degree-tear wound breakdown, bowel preparation should precede the secondary repair, which is best undertaken in the operation room by an experienced operator.

Amniotic fluid embolism

Amniotic fluid embolism (AFE) is a potentially catastrophic and often fatal complication that usually occurs suddenly during labour and delivery. The clinical diagnosis is based on the sudden development of acute respiratory distress and cardiovascular collapse in a patient in labour or who has recently delivered. Amniotic fluid enters the maternal circulation and triggers a syndrome like that seen with anaphylactic shock. If the woman survives the initial event, she has high chances of developing severe DIC. Therefore, effective resuscitation and treatment require a multidisciplinary team with expertise in the fields of obstetrics, intensive care, anaesthesia and haematology. Although AFE is a rare condition, that occurs in about 1/80,000 pregnancies, it has a disproportionately high maternal mortality rate.

Essential information

Management of the second stage

- Delivery of the head
  - Controlled descent
  - Minimize perineal damage
- Delayed clamping of the cord
- Evaluation of Apgar score

Management of the third stage

- Recognition of placental separation
- Assisted delivery of the placenta with cord traction
- Routine use of oxytocic agents with crowning of the head or delivery of the anterior shoulder

Rare presentations

- Face presentation: 1/500
- Brow presentation: 1/1500
- Unstable lie associated with:
  - High parity
  - Polyhydramnios
  - Uterine anomalies
  - Low-lying placenta

Occipitoposterior position

- 10–20% cephalic presentations
- Associated with backache and prolonged labour
- Treatment:
  - Adequate analgesia
  - Syntocinon
  - Caesarean section
  - Rotational forceps or posterior cup vacuum extraction

Management of postpartum haemorrhage

- Massage and compress the uterus to expel any retained clots
- Inject IV oxytocin 5 units immediately and commence an IV infusion of oxytocin
- Ergometrine 0.2 mg by IV injection once hypertension and cardiac disease are excluded
- Intramuscular or intramyometrial injection of 15-methyl prostaglandin $F_{2\alpha}$ 0.25 mg
- Tranexamic acid 1 g slow IV over 10 minutes and repeat in 30 minutes if bleeding continues or recurs within 24 hours; the earlier, the better – less beneficial after 3 hours of onset of postpartum haemorrhage
- Collect blood sample to check for Hb%, coagulation disorders and for cross-matching
- Manual exploration and evacuation of the uterus if indicated
- Look for lower genital tract trauma and, if present, treat promptly and appropriately
- Replacement of blood loss and resuscitation

Repair of perineal damage

- Four degrees of perineal damage
- Third- and fourth-degree tears should be repaired by experienced staff with good analgesia and usually in theatre
- Following repair, check:
  - No retained swabs
  - No rectal suture
  - Vagina not abnormally constricted

Chapter | 13 |

Postpartum and early neonatal care

Shankari Arulkumaran

LEARNING OUTCOMES

After studying this chapter you should be able to:

Knowledge criteria

- Describe the normal maternal changes in the puerperium
- Describe the aetiology, diagnosis and management of the common abnormalities/emergencies in the postpartum period, including maternal collapse, thromboembolism, puerperal infections, anaemia and problems with lactation
- Discuss the sequelae of obstetric complications (e.g. pre-term delivery)
- Describe the principles of resuscitation of the newborn
- Describe the normal changes in the neonatal period

Clinical competencies

- Carry out a routine postnatal clinical review
- Provide contraceptive advice to a woman in the postnatal period
- Carry out a newborn baby examination

Professional skills and attitudes

- Consider the importance of breast-feeding on childhood health

The normal postpartum period

Puerperium is the Latin word for childbirth, so we use it with license to mean the postpartum period from the birth of the baby through to involution of the uterus at 6 weeks. Delivery of the baby and the placenta is necessary for lactation or a return to fertility.

Physiological changes

Genital tract

The uterus weighs 1 kg after birth but less than 100 g by 6 weeks. Uterine muscle fibres undergo autolysis and atrophy, and within 10 days the uterus is no longer palpable abdominally (Fig. 13.1). By the end of the puerperium, the uterus has largely returned to the non-pregnant size. The endometrium regenerates within 6 weeks, and menstruation occurs within this time if lactation has ceased. If lactation continues, the return of menstruation may be deferred for 6 months or more.

Discharge from the uterus is known as *lochia*. At first this consists of blood, either fresh or altered (lochia rubra), and lasts 2–14 days. It then changes to a serous discharge (lochia serosa) and finally becomes a slight white discharge (lochia alba). These changes may continue for up to 4–8 weeks after delivery. Abnormal persistence of lochia rubra may indicate the presence of retained placental tissue or fetal membranes.

Cardiovascular system

Cardiac output and plasma volume return to normal within approximately 1 week. There is a fluid loss of 2 L during the first week and a further loss of 1.5 L over the next 5 weeks. This loss is associated with an apparent increase in haematocrit and haemoglobin (Hb) concentration. There is an increase of serum sodium and plasma bicarbonate as well as plasma osmolality. An increase in clotting factors during the first 10 days after delivery is associated with a higher risk of deep vein thrombosis (DVT) and pulmonary embolism. There is also a rise in platelet count and greater platelet adhesiveness. Fibrinogen levels decrease during labour but increase in the puerperium.

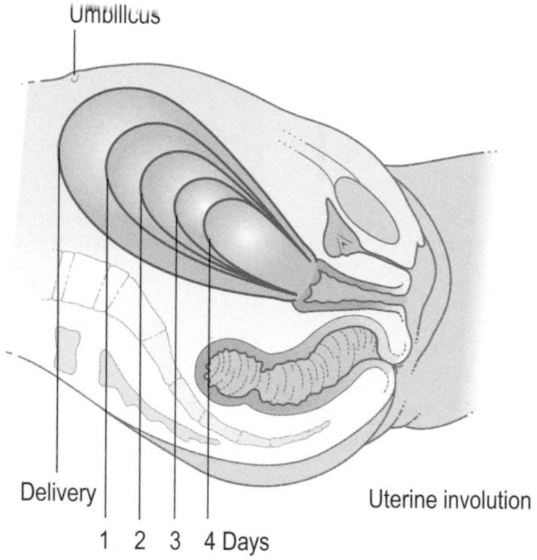

Umbilicus

Delivery   Uterine involution

1   2   3   4 Days

Fig. 13.1 Uterine involution in the puerperium results in a rapid reduction in size.

Endocrine changes

There are rapid changes in all facets of the endocrine system. There is a rapid fall in the serum levels of oestrogens and progesterone, and they reach non-pregnant levels by the seventh postnatal day. This is associated with an increase in serum prolactin levels in those women who breast-feed. By the tenth postnatal day, human chorionic gonadotrophin (hCG) is no longer detectable.

The importance of breast-feeding

Colostrum

Colostrum is the first milk and is present in the breast from 12 to 16 weeks of pregnancy. Colostrum is produced for up to 5 days following birth before evolving into transitional milk, from 6 to 13 days, and finally into mature milk from 14 days onwards. It is thick and yellow in colour due to β-carotene and has a mean energy value of 67 kcal/dL, compared to 72 kcal/dL in mature milk. The volume of colostrum per feed varies from 2 to 20 mL in keeping with the size of the newborn's stomach.

Linked with the importance of the baby having colostrum as its first food is the importance of the baby being skin to skin with its mother after birth. This has the benefit of the baby being colonized by its mother's bacteria. Colonizing starts during the birth process for vaginally born infants, while those born via caesarean section are more likely to colonize bacteria from the air. Early breast-feeding also promotes tolerance to antigens, thus reducing the number of food allergies in breast-fed babies. The development of healthy intestinal flora also reduces the incidence

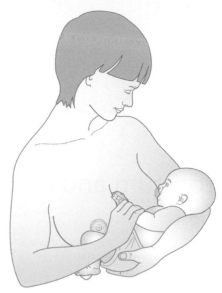

Fig. 13.2 The mother should be comfortable and the child placed well on to the breast to ensure adequate suckling.

of allergic disease, inflammatory gut disease and rotavirus diarrhoea in infants.

While breast-feeding is desirable and women should be encouraged, the overall wishes of the woman should not be ignored. There are social and often emotional reasons why a woman may choose not to breast-feed. In some cases, it is not possible or even advisable, such as inverted nipples, previous breast surgery, breast implants, cracked or painful nipples or the mother may have a condition (e.g. HIV) or may be on medical treatment (e.g. chemotherapeutic agents) that serve as a contraindication to breast-feeding.

Breast-feeding

The breasts and nipples should be washed regularly. The breasts should be comfortably supported and aqueous-based emollient creams may be used to soften the nipple and thus avoid cracking during suckling. Suckling is initially limited to 2–3 minutes on each side, but subsequently this period may be increased. Once the mother is comfortably seated, the whole nipple is placed in the infant's mouth, taking care to maintain a clear airway (Fig. 13.2). Correct attachment of the baby to the breast is essential to the success of breast-feeding. The common problems such as sore nipples, breast engorgement and mastitis usually occur because the baby is poorly attached to the breast or is not fed often enough. Most breast-feeding is given on demand, and the milk flow will meet the demand stimulated by suckling. Once the baby is attached correctly to the nipple, the sucking pattern changes from short sucks to long deep sucks with pauses. It may, on occasions, be necessary to express milk and store it, either because of breast discomfort or cracked nipples or because the baby is sick. Milk can be expressed manually or by using hand or electric pumps. Breast milk can be safely stored in a refrigerator at 2–4°C for 3–5 days or frozen and stored for up to 3 months in the freezer.

In women who choose not to breast-feed, have suffered a stillbirth or intrauterine death or where there is a contraindication to breast-feeding, suppression of lactation may be achieved by conservative methods or by drug therapy. Firm support of the breasts, restriction of fluid intake, avoidance of expression of milk and analgesia may be sufficient to suppress lactation. The administration of oestrogens will effectively suppress lactation but carries some risk of thromboembolic disease. The preferred drug therapy is currently the dopamine receptor agonist cabergoline. This can be given as a single dose and will inhibit prolactin release and hence suppress lactation. Bromocriptine is also effective, but the dosage necessary to produce this effect tends to create considerable side effects.

Complications of the postpartum period

Puerperal infections

Puerperal sepsis has been reported as far back as the 5th century BC. Sepsis is a leading cause of maternal morbidity and mortality according to the *Mothers and Babies: Reducing Risk through Audits and Confidential Enquiries across the UK* (MBRRACE-UK) report in 2016. Despite the UK direct death rate from sepsis falling from 0.67 to 0.29 per 100,000 maternities between 2009 and 2014, it remains the second commonest cause of total (combined direct and indirect) deaths in the UK. However, in London, it was the leading cause of direct maternal deaths in 2016. Once a diagnosis of sepsis is suspected, a sepsis care bundle should be instituted. Prospective analyses have indicated that immediate of these care pathways reduces mortality from sepsis. The UK Sepsis Trust produced one such care bundle in 2013, the 'Sepsis Six Care Bundle', and recommend that this be completed within an hour of diagnosis of sepsis, as shown in Table 13.1.

Common causes of sepsis include urinary tract infections (UTIs), wound infections (perineum or caesarean section scar) and mastitis (Box 13.1 and Fig. 13.3).

Endometritis

In the puerperium, the placental surface in the womb is vulnerable to infection. It is exposed to the vagina, which harbours aerobic and anaerobic bacteria. Peripartum events, such as prolonged rupture of membranes, chorioamnionitis,

Table 13.1 Sepsis Six Care Bundle

Inform consultant obstetrician and consultant anaesthetist
1. Take an arterial blood gas and give high-flow oxygen if required Aim to keep SpO_2 >94%
2. Take blood cultures And consider other cultures, e.g. urine, vaginal swabs
3. Start IV antibiotics According to local protocol
4. Start IV fluid resuscitation if hypotensive or lactate ≥4, give 30 ml/kg of crystalloid immediately
5. Take blood for haemoglobin and lactate levels If lactate is over 4 mmol/L, obtain critical care/intensive treatment unit advice
6. Measure hourly urine output. Insert a urinary catheter if needed

Adapted from The UK Sepsis Trust. ED/AMU Maternal Sepsis Tool. Available at: https://sepsistrust.org/professional-resources/clinical/ (accessed 7 November 2018).

Box 13.1 Complications of the puerperium

- Genital tract infections
- Urinary infection
- Wound infection
- Mastitis
- Thromboembolism
- Incontinence/urinary retention
- Anal sphincter dysfunction
- Breakdown of episiotomy wound
- Postnatal depression

repeated vaginal examinations, poor personal hygiene, bladder catheterization, invasive fetal monitoring, instrumental deliveries, caesarean sections, perineal trauma and manual removal of the placenta, lead to introduction of pathogens into the uterus and thus contribute to puerperal infections.

The patient with endometritis usually presents with fever, lower abdominal pain, secondary postpartum haemorrhage (PPH) and foul-smelling vaginal discharge. The organisms involved are group A β-haemolytic streptococci, aerobic Gram-negative rods and anaerobes. On examination, the patient often has a fever, is tachycardic and is tender on palpation of the lower abdomen. There may be foul-smelling vaginal discharge, bleeding and cervical excitation. The white cell count and C-reactive protein may be raised. Vaginal or blood cultures may identify the organism responsible. Broad-spectrum antibiotics are the first-line treatment, and resolution should start to occur within the

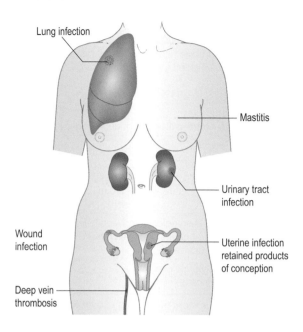

Lung infection

Mastitis

Urinary tract
infection

Wound
infection

Uterine infection
retained products
of conception

Deep vein
thrombosis

Fig. 13.3 The pathogenesis of puerperal pyrexia.

first 48 hours. The complications of endometritis are parametritis, peritonitis, septic pelvic thrombophlebitis, pelvic abscesses and, rarely, toxic shock syndrome.

Urinary tract infections

UTIs are the most common cause of puerperal infections. The predisposing factors include a history of previous UTIs, polycystic kidneys, congenital abnormalities of the renal tract, neuropathic bladder and urinary tract calculi, but most are idiopathic. Patients present with voiding difficulties (e.g. urgency and frequency), dysuria, fever and pain in the renal angle. Urine analysis may be positive for protein and leucocytes, though nitrites are more sensitive. Urine should be sent for culture before commencing antibiotic treatment. The commonest organisms are *Escherichia coli*, *Enterococcus*, *Klebsiella*, *Proteus* and *Staphylococcus epidermidis*.

Mastitis and breast abscess

Presenting symptoms include breast pain, fever and erythema. The commonest organisms are *S. aureus*; *S. epidermidis*; or group A, B and F streptococci. Oral antibiotics are usually sufficient for mastitis, but intravenous treatment is required for an abscess. In the case of an abscess, fluctuance will be elicited and surgical drainage may be warranted.

Caesarean wound infections and perineal infections

Puerperal infection is more common in caesarean sections than vaginal deliveries. Intraoperative antibiotics have helped reduce the incidence. The commonest organisms involved are *S. aureus*, methicillin-resistant *S. aureus* (MRSA), skin flora and those involved with endometritis. Complications include wound dehiscence and necrotizing fasciitis. Infection may also occur in episiotomy wounds or perineal tears, although these infections are relatively uncommon because the vascularity of the perineum provides a higher resistance to infection. The perineum becomes tender and reddened and may be seen to exude purulent discharge. Where wound breakdown occurs, the wound should be kept clean and allowed to heal by secondary intention. Resuturing should not be performed unless the wound is clean and there is no residual inflammation around the wound margins.

Other infections

Once more common sites of infection have been excluded, one must consider other sites of infection or sepsis. These include pneumonia; meningitis; bacterial endocarditis; or even influenza, malaria and H1N1. The incidence of chest infection is greater in caesarean sections than vaginal births due to reduced mobility and reduced air entry secondary to pain or if the patient has had a general anaesthetic. Between 2006 and 2010 in the UK, almost half of the deaths from sepsis were from influenza and another 10% were secondary to pneumonia. The period 2006–2010 covered the H1N1 influenza pandemic, which caused 17,000 deaths worldwide. H1N1 is a strain of influenza A that was discovered in Mexico in early 2009 and spread globally, causing outbreaks up until August 2010. During this period, it became apparent that pregnant women and those in the puerperium were particularly vulnerable, with a four times greater admission rate to hospital and seven times greater admission rate to an intensive treatment unit (ITU) than the general population. It has subsequently been recognized that there was a delay in starting appropriate treatment for these women, as it was frequently delayed until the influenza swab results were available.

Thromboembolism
Thrombophlebitis

This is the commonest form of thromboembolic disease and tends to arise within the first 3–4 days after delivery. Localized inflammation, tenderness and thickening occur in the superficial leg veins. Although the condition is painful and may spread along the leg veins, it rarely leads to serious embolic disease and does not require anticoagulant treatment. Anti-inflammatory drugs and local applications of glycerine and ichthyol should be used.

Phlebothrombosis (see also Chapter 9)

DVT is a much more serious complication that tends to arise 7–10 days after delivery and is particularly likely to occur after operative delivery or prolonged immobilization. Clotting occurring in deep veins may be silent and presents only when the clot breaks loose and lodges in the lung as a pulmonary embolus (PE), with consequent chest pain, dyspnoea and haemoptysis. Clinical signs include local rhonchi and pleural rub on auscultation and a pulmonary perfusion. A ventilation scan or chest computed tomography (CT) scan should help to confirm or refute the diagnosis. Massive PE results in sudden death unless treated by prompt surgical management. Successful treatments with antithrombolytic agents and fragmenting the clots with percutaneous arterial catheters have been reported.

Postnatal anticoagulation

National guidelines in the UK recommend that in non-pregnant patients, anticoagulant therapy should be continued for 6 weeks for calf vein thrombosis and 3 months for proximal DVT or PE when venous thromboembolism (VTE) has occurred in relation to a temporary risk factor and 6 months for a first episode of idiopathic VTE. The presence of continuing risk factors and the safety of low-molecular-weight heparin (LMWH) have led authorities to propose that anticoagulant therapy be continued for the duration of the pregnancy and until at least 6 weeks postpartum, and to allow a total duration of treatment of at least 3 months. Both heparin and warfarin are satisfactory for use postpartum.

Neither heparin nor warfarin is contraindicated in breast-feeding. If the woman chooses to continue with LMWH postnatally, then either the doses that were employed antenatally can be continued or the manufacturers' recommended doses for the non-pregnant patient can be employed. If the woman chooses to commence warfarin postpartum, this should be avoided until at least the third postnatal day. Daily testing of the international normalized ratio (INR) is recommended during the transfer from LMWH to warfarin to avoid over-anticoagulation. Warfarin administration should be delayed in women with risk of PPH.

Postnatal clinic review for women who develop VTE during pregnancy or the puerperium should ideally be at an obstetric medicine clinic or a joint obstetric haematology clinic. At the postnatal review, the continuing risk of thrombosis should be assessed, including a review of personal and family history of VTE and any thrombophilia screen results. Advice should be given on the need for thromboprophylaxis in any future pregnancy and at other times of increased risk. Hormonal contraception should be discussed.

Primary and secondary postpartum haemorrhage

Please see Chapter 12.

Anaemia

If the Hb is less than 7–8 g/dL in the postnatal period, where there is no continuing or threat of bleeding, the decision to transfuse should be made on an informed individual basis. In fit, healthy, asymptomatic patients, there is little evidence of the benefit of blood transfusion. If severe bleeding was encountered and if bleeding disorders were suspected, appropriate investigations should be made. These investigations should be repeated on a non-urgent basis at least 3–6 months after delivery when pregnancy-related coagulation changes have settled.

Oral iron should be the preferred first-line treatment for iron deficiency. Parenteral iron is indicated when oral iron is not tolerated or absorbed or patient compliance is in doubt. Parenteral therapy offers a shorter duration of treatment and a quicker response than oral therapy. It is, however, more invasive and expensive to administer. Iron sucrose is given in multiple doses, whereas iron dextran may be given as a single total-dose infusion. Recombinant human erythropoietin (rHuEPO) is mostly used in the anaemia of end-stage renal disease.

Maternal collapse

Maternal collapse is defined as an acute event involving the cardiorespiratory systems and/or brain, resulting in a reduced or absent conscious level (and potentially death) at any stage in pregnancy and up to 6 weeks after delivery. An obstetric early-warning score chart should be used routinely for all women to allow early recognition of the woman who is becoming critically ill. In some cases, maternal collapse occurs with no prior warning, although there may be existing risk factors that make this more likely. Antenatal care for women with significant medical conditions at risk of maternal collapse should include multidisciplinary team input with a pregnancy and delivery management plan in place.

There are many causes of collapse, and these may be pregnancy related or result from conditions not related to pregnancy and possibly existing before pregnancy. The common reversible causes of collapse in any woman can be remembered using the 4 Ts and the 4 Hs employed by the

Table 13.2 Reversible causes of collapse in pregnancy/postpartum

Reversible cause		Cause in pregnancy
4 Hs	Hypovolaemia	Bleeding, relative hypovolaemia of dense spinal block, septic or neurogenic shock
	Hypoxia	Peripartum cardiomyopathy, myocardial infarction, aortic dissection, large-vessel aneurysms
	Hypo/hyperkalaemia (and other electrolyte imbalances)	No more likely
	Hypothermia	No more likely
4 Ts	Thromboembolism	Amniotic fluid embolus, pulmonary embolus, air embolus, myocardial infarction
	Toxicity	Local anaesthetic, magnesium, other
	Tension pneumothorax	Following trauma/suicide attempt
	Tamponade (cardiac)	Following trauma/suicide attempt
Eclampsia and pre-eclampsia		Includes intracranial haemorrhage

Reproduced from: Royal College of Obstetricians Green Top Guideline 56 Maternal Collapse in Pregnancy and the Puerperium, London, RCOG, January 2011, with the permission of the Royal College of Obstetricians and Gynaecologists.

Resuscitation Council (UK) (Table 13.2). In the pregnant woman, eclampsia and intracranial haemorrhage should be added to this list.

Haemorrhage is the most common cause of maternal collapse. In most cases of massive haemorrhage leading to collapse, the cause is obvious, but concealed haemorrhage should not be forgotten, including following caesarean section. Other rare causes of concealed haemorrhage include splenic artery rupture and hepatic rupture.

In the UK, thromboembolism is the most common cause of direct maternal death and may present as maternal collapse. Appropriate use of thromboprophylaxis has improved maternal morbidity and mortality, but improvements in clinical risk assessment and prophylaxis are still required.

Amniotic fluid embolism (AFE) presents as collapse during labour or delivery or within 30 minutes of delivery in the form of acute hypotension, respiratory distress and acute hypoxia. Seizures and cardiac arrest may occur. There are different phases to disease progression; initially, pulmonary hypertension may develop secondary to vascular occlusion either by debris or by vasoconstriction. This often resolves, and left ventricular dysfunction or failure develops. Coagulopathy often occurs, resulting in massive PPH. The underlying pathophysiological process has been compared to anaphylaxis or severe sepsis. Clinically, an AFE can be suspected,

but a definitive diagnosis can only be made on postmortem.

Cardiac disease is currently the leading cause of indirect maternal death in the UK. The majority of deaths secondary to cardiac causes occur in women with no previous history. The main cardiac causes of death are myocardial infarction, aortic dissection and cardiomyopathy. Primary cardiac arrest in pregnancy is rare, and most cardiac events have preceding signs and symptoms. Aortic root dissection can present with central chest or interscapular pain and a wide pulse pressure, mainly secondary to systolic hypertension. A new cardiac murmur must prompt referral to a cardiologist and appropriate imaging. The incidence of congenital and rheumatic heart disease in pregnancy is increasing secondary to improved management of congenital heart disease and increased immigration. Other cardiac causes include dissection of the coronary artery, acute left ventricular failure, infective endocarditis and pulmonary oedema.

Bacteraemia, which can be present in the absence of pyrexia or a raised white cell count, can progress rapidly to severe sepsis and septic shock leading to collapse. The most common organisms implicated in obstetrics are the streptococcal groups A, B and D; *Pneumococcus;* and *E. coli.*

Drug toxicity/overdose should be considered in all cases of collapse, and illicit drug overdose should be remembered as a potential cause of collapse outside of hospital. In terms of therapeutic drug toxicity, the common sources in obstetric practice are magnesium sulphate in the presence of renal impairment and local anaesthetic agents injected intravenously by accident. Effects initially include a feeling of inebriation and light-headedness followed by sedation, circumoral paraesthesia and twitching; convulsions can occur in severe toxicity. On intravenous injection, convulsions and cardiovascular collapse may occur very rapidly. Local anaesthetic toxicity resulting from systemic absorption of the local anaesthetic may occur sometime after the initial injection. Signs of severe toxicity include sudden loss of consciousness, with or without tonic–clonic convulsions, and cardiovascular collapse.

Eclampsia as the cause of maternal collapse is usually obvious in the inpatient setting, as often the diagnosis of pre-eclampsia has already been made and the seizure witnessed. Intracranial haemorrhage is a significant complication of uncontrolled, particularly systolic, hypertension but can also result from ruptured aneurysms and arteriovenous malformations. The initial presentation may be maternal collapse, but often severe headache precedes this.

Anaphylaxis causes a significant intravascular volume redistribution, which can lead to decreased cardiac output. Acute ventricular failure and myocardial ischaemia may occur. Upper airway occlusion secondary to angioedema, bronchospasm and mucous plugging of smaller airways all contribute to significant hypoxia and difficulties with ventilation. Common triggers are a variety of drugs, latex, animal allergens and foods.

Other causes of maternal collapse include hypoglycaemia and other metabolic/electrolyte disturbances, other causes of hypoxia such as airway obstruction secondary to aspiration/foreign body, air embolism, tension pneumothorax and cardiac tamponade secondary to trauma and, rarely, hypothermia.

The management of maternal collapse in the UK follows the Resuscitation Council (UK) guidelines using the standard A, B, C approach: airways, breathing and circulation. The airway should be protected as soon as possible by intubation with a cuffed endotracheal tube, and supplemental oxygen should be administered. Bag and mask ventilation should be undertaken until intubation can be achieved. In the absence of breathing despite a clear airway, chest compressions should be commenced immediately. Two wide-bore cannulae should be inserted as soon as possible to enable an aggressive approach to volume replacement. Abdominal ultrasound by a skilled operator can assist in the diagnosis of concealed haemorrhage. The same defibrillation energy levels should be used as in the non-pregnant patient. There should normally be no alteration in algorithm drugs or doses. Common reversible causes of maternal cardiopulmonary arrest should be considered throughout the resuscitation process. If cardiac output is not restored after 3 minutes of cardiopulmonary resuscitation (CPR) in a woman who is still pregnant, the fetus should be delivered by caesarean section, as this will improve the effectiveness in maternal resuscitation efforts and may save the baby. Resuscitation efforts should be continued until a decision is taken by the consultant obstetrician and consultant anaesthetist in consensus with the cardiac arrest team. Senior staff with appropriate experience should be involved at an early stage. Accurate documentation in all cases of maternal collapse, whether or not resuscitation is successful, is essential. Debriefing is recommended for the woman, her family and the staff involved in the event. All cases of maternal collapse should generate a clinical incident form, and the care should be reviewed through the clinical governance process. All cases of maternal death should be reported to MBRRACE-UK (Mothers and Babies: Reducing Risk through Audits and Confidential Enquiries across the UK).

Contraception in the postnatal period

A conversation regarding contraception is best before the woman leaves hospital, but further follow-up is essential. Discussion should ideally cover all options, including lactational amenorrhoea, condoms, diaphragm, progestogen-only pills, progestogen implants or injection (Depo-Provera) and an intrauterine contraceptive device (IUCD) such as a copper coil or levonorgestrel-releasing device (Mirena). This consultation should include the indications and contraindications, as well as the risks and benefits of each.

Condoms are a good first option. They are low cost, unlikely to have side effects and, with partner compliance, have a 95% success rate in preventing pregnancy whilst offering protection from sexual health infections. The copper IUCD is popular, as it has a lifespan of 10 years. Those women who have a history of menorrhagia may benefit from a Mirena. These can be inserted immediately after delivery of the placenta or within 48 hours, or after the uterus has involuted at 6 weeks.

The combined oral contraceptive pill cannot be used in fully breast-feeding women because the oestrogen will suppress lactation. The progesterone-only pill and injectable/implantable progestogenic contraceptives can be safely given to the fully breast-feeding woman. These are normally started 6 weeks postpartum because of the potential for side effects or irregular bleeding, but where the risk of unplanned pregnancy is high can be commenced immediately after delivery.

Neonatal problems

Passage through the birth canal is a hypoxic experience for the fetus, since significant respiratory exchange at the placenta is prevented for the 50- to 75-second duration of the average contraction. Though most babies tolerate this well, the few who do not may require help to establish normal breathing at delivery. Newborn life support is intended to provide this help and comprises the following elements: drying and covering the newborn baby to conserve heat, assessing the need for any intervention, opening the airway, aerating the lung, rescue breathing, chest compression and, rarely, the administration of drugs.

If subjected to sufficient hypoxia in utero, the fetus will attempt to breathe. If the hypoxic insult is continued, the fetus will eventually lose consciousness. Shortly after this, the neural centres controlling these breathing efforts will cease to function because of lack of oxygen. The fetus then enters a period known as *primary apnoea*. Up to this point, the heart rate remains unchanged but soon decreases to about half the normal rate as the myocardium reverts to anaerobic metabolism: a less fuel-efficient mechanism. The circulation to non-vital organs is reduced in an attempt to preserve perfusion of vital organs. The release of lactic acid, a by-product of anaerobic metabolism, causes deterioration of the biochemical environment.

If the insult continues, shuddering (whole-body gasps) is initiated by primitive spinal centres. If for some reason these gasps fail to aerate the lungs, they fade away and the neonate enters a period known as *secondary* or *terminal apnoea*. Until now, the circulation has been maintained, but as terminal apnoea progresses, cardiac function is impaired. The heart eventually fails, and without effective intervention, the baby dies.

Thus, in the face of asphyxia, the baby can maintain an effective circulation throughout the period of primary apnoea, through the gasping phase, and even for a while after the onset of terminal apnoea. The most urgent requirement for any asphyxiated baby at birth is that the lungs be aerated effectively. Provided the baby's circulation is sufficient, oxygenated blood will then be conveyed from the aerated lungs to the heart. The heart rate will increase, and the brain will be perfused with oxygenated blood. Following this, the neural centres responsible for normal breathing will, in many instances, function once again and the baby will recover. Merely aerating the lungs is sufficient in the vast majority of cases. Although lung aeration is still vital, in a few cases cardiac function will have deteriorated to such an extent that the circulation is inadequate and cannot convey oxygenated blood from the aerated lungs to the heart. In this case, a brief period of chest compression may be needed. In a very few cases, lung aeration and chest compression will not be sufficient, and drugs may be required to restore the circulation. The outlook in the latter group of infants is poor.

Most babies born at term need no resuscitation, and they can usually stabilize themselves during the transition from placental to pulmonary respiration very effectively. Provided attention is paid to preventing heat loss and a little patience is exhibited before cutting the umbilical cord, intervention is rarely necessary. However, some babies will have suffered stresses or insults during labour, and resuscitation is then required. Significantly, pre-term babies, particularly those born below 30 weeks' gestation, are a different matter. Most babies in this group are healthy at the time of delivery and yet all can be expected to benefit from help in making the transition. Intervention in this situation is usually limited to maintaining a baby's health during this transition and is called *stabilization*.

Examination of the newborn	ABC

The purpose of the examination is to ascertain parental concerns, identify risks (e.g. perinatal/family history), reassure parents where possible and offer advice on health promotion (e.g. prevention of sudden infant death syndrome (SIDS), immunizations). The ideal time for this is between 24 and 72 hours, though it may be undertaken after 6 hours of age and no later than 7 days of age.

Babies should be examined undressed. Look at their general appearance and alertness as well as facial features and colour. Listen to their heart and feel the anterior fontanelle and sutures. Examine their ears/eyes, nose/mouth (including palatal sweep), neck (including clavicles), arms and hands, legs and feet, as well as genitalia and anus. Palpate the abdomen and feel for femoral pulses. Turn the baby to the prone position and examine their back and spine. Place the baby supine and examine their hips. Measure the head circumference and clearly document.

Conducting a routine postnatal clinical review

The postnatal period marks a significant transition point in a woman's life. The period of postnatal care extends from the hospital stay to the community and home and is provided by multiple caregivers. The objectives of care of mother and baby in the postnatal period include provision of rest and recovery following birth, supporting maternal attachment and assisting in the development of maternal self-esteem. The family unit should be supported, and risks need to be identified and managed appropriately. If the mother wishes to breast-feed, this should be initiated and encouraged. Steps should be taken to prevent, identify and manage postnatal depression.

Most of a woman's care in the community is conducted by the community midwives and general practitioners. If a woman is returning for a clinical review in the hospital, it is either for debriefing following a complication during her pregnancy, labour, delivery or postnatal period or for the medical management of medical conditions such as diabetes or hypertension. The opportunity should be utilized to discuss family planning and contraception, as well as cervical screening. Letters regarding the woman's pregnancy and postnatal needs should be sent out in a timely fashion, as they are helpful to general practitioners and in many cases are the only link between the services. An ideal model of maternity care should seek to maximize the health of women across their reproductive life rather than focus on a single pregnancy.

Essential information

Physiological changes

- Uterine involution
- Lochial loss
- Endometrial regeneration
- Reduction of cardiac output
- Fluid loss 2 L first week

Endocrine changes

- Oestrogen/progesterone falls, prolactin rises
- hCG undetectable 10 days

Lactation and breast-feeding

- Colostrum
- Milk flow 2–3 days
- Suckling process, lactation suppression

Psychological changes

- Puerperal depression (see Chapter 14)

Puerperal pyrexia

- Genital tract infection
- Urinary tract infection
- Breast infection
- Wound infection

Chapter | 14 |

Mental health and childbirth

Jo Black

LEARNING OUTCOMES

After studying this chapter you should be able to:

Knowledge relating to mental disorders

- Demonstrate an awareness of the range of possible mental health disorders in the perinatal period
- Understand the importance of identification of mental health history and working in a proactive and preventative way with women at risk of illness
- Identify of symptoms of mental illness in the perinatal period
- Understand and manage risk in the perinatal period
- Understand the risk of misattribution in the perinatal period
- Describe the principles of prescribing in the perinatal period
- Discuss capacity issues in perinatal mental illness

Clinical competencies

- Take an adequate mental health history
- Make a clinical management plan for someone with a mental health diagnosis
- Assess and manage physical health for those with a mental health diagnosis
- Assess, communicate and manage risk in the perinatal period

Professional skills and attitudes

- Develop of active listening skills
- Develop professional curiosity about the mental wellbeing of all expectant and new mothers
- Understand the barriers women with mental health disorders may have and can experience in health care
- Show leadership in respectful and inclusive use of language, attitude and decision-making when offering care to those at risk of or experiencing poor mental health

Understanding the importance of good maternal mental health is expected core knowledge of every obstetrician. Knowledge of adult mental health, infant mental health, psychopharmacology, embryology, psychology, endocrinology, medicolegal frameworks and pregnancy- and postnatal-specific mental health issues is necessary.

This chapter is designed to be a practical introductory guide to achieve a better understanding of common mental health problems which women can experience during and after pregnancy. The role of the obstetrician is prevention, detection, early intervention, assessing risk and providing safe, evidence-based care.

Mental health disorders can be debilitating and can affect both mother and child. Untreated they are a common cause of morbidity and are one of the leading causes of maternal deaths. One hundred sixty-one women died from mental health–related causes between 2009 and 2013. This represents a rate of 3.7 deaths from mental health–related causes during or up to 1 year after the end of pregnancy per 100,000 maternities in the UK and Ireland for 2009–2013 (95% CI 3.2–4.4) (MBRACCE-UK).

Poor maternal mental health increases the risk to the infant of poorer health during infancy and childhood, the possibility of speech and language delay or lower educational attainment (Avon Longitudinal Study of Parents and Infants).

It is important to recognize that measures which improve the mental health of mothers can directly improve the life chances of the next generation.

Midwives and obstetricians are uniquely placed to support women to stay mentally well throughout their pregnancies and to identify emerging mental health issues quickly and ensure access to appropriate treatment. To do this effectively, it is crucial to take a holistic view of the needs of women in your care, respecting strengths, preferences, attitudes and cultural heritage of women. Women with mental health histories will bring a range of views, opinions and wishes to decisions with regard to their pregnancy, birth and postnatal period. Women, including women with mental health issues, need to have access to accurate, understandable and comprehensive information in order to help them consider their options and make informed decisions.

No one expects an obstetrician or midwife to be a mental health expert. You are not expected to know about every diagnosis, every therapy or every treatment in mental health. You are not expected to diagnose a disorder or initiate treatment. However, an obstetrician needs to be able to take an adequate history and assess current mental health and to ensure women have access to high-quality information, further assessment and treatment if required. Health care systems vary. Within the system in which you work, it is necessary to have measures in place for women to be able to access accurate information, advice and treatment. Primary care, reliable online resources, the voluntary sector, midwives, health visitors, counselling and therapy services all have a part to play. For those women with the most complex or serious mental health issues, access to a specialist mental health service (preferably a perinatal mental health service) is recommended.

The role of the obstetrician as relates to mental illness and childbirth

In antenatal clinic or at a postnatal review, there are three specific questions to consider in relation to mental illness

- Does the expectant mother have a **history** of mental illness?

- Does the expectant mother have any **current symptoms** of a mental illness or disorder?
- Does the expectant mother use any **treatment** for a mental illness or disorder?

Taking a basic mental health history

As in any branch of medicine, your role is to take an adequate history and perform the necessary examination. Taking a basic mental health history is an expected competency of an obstetrician (Box 14.1).

To have a productive conversation with a woman about her mental health, you should consider whether you are at ease talking about mental health. Always use respectful language and open questioning and take notice of verbal and non-verbal cues in the conversation; actively listen; and allow adequate time.

In 2017, the Royal College of Obstetricians and Gynaecologists invited women to share their experiences. The themes were collated in their *Women's Voices Publication 2017*. They concluded:

'The current system relies too heavily on women coming forward and disclosing their own conditions. The lack of understanding of various perinatal mental health conditions means that, without women coming forward and disclosing, symptoms are being completely missed and are damaging women's confidence in the system. A number of women reported how it was all too easy to evade healthcare professionals' questions and hide symptoms. Many women are reluctant to talk about how they are feeling and about their history

---

Box 14.1 **A basic mental health history**

Suggested questions
1. Have you had any issues with your mental health in the past?
2. How many episodes have you had?
3. (For multiparous women) What was your mental health like during/after your previous pregnancies?
4. Can you tell me a bit more about what that was like for you when things were at their worst?
5. Were you given a diagnosis? What was it?
6. What treatment did you receive?
7. Did the treatment you received work?
8. What else helped with your mental health?
9. Did you ever need hospital care? Did you accept hospital care or was admission under the Mental Health Act?
10. Have you ever felt life was not worth living?

11. Have you ever thought about or tried to end your life? Can you say a bit more about that?
12. Do you use medication or are you engaged in treatment or receive ongoing support for your mental health? Can you describe these?
13. If not using medication (and you have used it previously), when did you stop and why?
14. Does anyone else in your family have a diagnosis of significant mental illness?
15. Are you worried about mental health in this pregnancy or after childbirth?
16. How are things currently with your mental health?
17. Is there anything I haven't asked you about in relation to your mental health that you think I should have or that you think it's important for me to know?

of mental health, and simple tick box "yes" and "no" questions do not encourage a dialogue that allows a woman to open up. This means that only those who are confident and able to speak up are doing so, leaving many vulnerable women to fall through the gaps.

A number of women highlighted incidents of failings by healthcare professionals, ranging from bad experiences of not being listened to after repeatedly asking for help to being told that they were being referred but with no support then ever materialising. Women felt frustrated that their concerns had not been taken seriously and many only had access to support once they had found a healthcare professional who was willing to listen.

A lot of respondents commented that they did not feel that they had had enough time with healthcare professionals to discuss their mental health, or that appointments had been rushed. Many of these commented that they felt had been due to an overstretched service, not because the healthcare professional did not care. Where conversations about mental health were being had, they were often not held in a personal or an open way, or felt like simple "tick box" exercises.'

Maternal Mental Health-Women's Voices RCOG 2017

If you do enable a woman to disclose a mental health history or concern, it is important you and she have a shared understanding about what will happen with the information she has given. Making a plan undoubtedly involves including all those who work with her in the perinatal period.

Always ask for a woman's consent to liaise with other health care professionals with whom she may be involved. Why?

'In at least 16 of the 57 women with a prior history of mental health problems, who died by suicide, there was evidence that significant aspects of the woman's past psychiatric history were not communicated between primary care and maternity services. In several instances, maternity services had not been informed of a woman's past psychiatric history and in some circumstances the GP was unaware that the women had booked for maternity care.'

Saving Lives, Improving Mothers' Care 2015

> Frequently, women report that because they were articulate, well groomed, in employment and/or in a committed relationship, health care professionals made assumptions that mental health issues would not be present, so did not ask, and an opportunity to intervene was lost.
>
> Similarly other women from a range of socioeconomic and cultural backgrounds report they felt assumptions were made about their mental health, their resilience and their support network without any evidence to support these views.
>
> It is important to be aware of unconscious bias with regard to mental health.
>
> Unconscious bias happens by our brains making quick judgements and assessments of people and situations. Our biases are influenced by our background, cultural environment and personal experiences. We may not even be aware of these views or aware of their full impact or implication.

Making a mental health plan

Women with established mental health diagnoses need a **mental health plan** for their pregnancy, delivery and postnatal period which takes into account their mental health and the treatment (including medication) that they use for their mental health disorder.

Case study 1

Sarah is 24 years old and a PhD student in astrophysics. She has a diagnosis of bipolar affective disorder and used lithium since her last acute episode 2 years ago to good effect.

She stopped her lithium abruptly on discovering her pregnancy. The pregnancy was not planned.

She and her partner are happy to be expecting a baby. Sarah's family lives overseas, and her partner's family is local. They do not know anything about her past mental health.

Case study 2

Thelma is 29 years old and works in retail. She is in the first trimester of her first pregnancy. Thelma's body mass index (BMI) is in the low/normal range and has fallen in the last 4 weeks. She has a history of anorexia nervosa and has had two hospital inpatient spells for treatment. Both admissions were involuntary under the Mental Health Act, and nasogastric (NG) feeding was administered on both occasions. She has been well for over a year, and this pregnancy was planned. She is horrified by her enlarging breasts and is dreading her body changing further. She admits to some temptation to restrict calories.

Case study 3

Angela is 34 years old and works as a local general practitioner. She knows several obstetricians in the department socially. Angela has had episodes of depression throughout her teenage years and early twenties. She discloses at 28 weeks she is low in mood, regrets being pregnant and feels resentful of the baby, as she blames it for her sore back and hips and her ongoing nausea. She is not sleeping well and sometimes thinks it is too hard to go on. She does not want you to share this information with anyone or to include it in her clinical record.

Case study 4

Selma is 30 years old, is 28 weeks' pregnant and is attending her first antenatal contact. She has a diagnosis of schizophrenia and sees a community psychiatric nurse monthly. She lived in supported accommodation and has had frequent hospital admissions for her mental health. She says she is not currently taking any medication. She seems distracted and guarded in her responses. She asks some questions and makes some remarks which strike you as odd. 'How do you know it's a human baby?' and 'The baby is chosen and will protect me from the pain.'

Making a mental health plan for pregnancy, birth and the postnatal period

What is a mental health plan?

A mental health plan enables a mother with a mental health concern or history to have planned, joined-up care

when she is pregnant. It considers her and her unborn baby's needs in pregnancy, during delivery and during the postnatal period. It takes into account her protective factors, her support network, her cultural and religious beliefs and her choices.

It recognizes any risks or potential challenges related to her mental health and creates with her a plan of what can minimize these, or in the event of a significant mental health episode, what the plan of treatment will be.

Creating a mental health plan

- A robust mental health plan should be completed before the thirty-second week of pregnancy.
- Adequate time is needed to complete a thorough plan.
- All health care professionals involved with the mother and family should be invited to contribute.
- The plan should include the needs of the mother, the infant and the rest of the family.
- The plan should identify any current mental health symptoms and any treatment/therapy which is recommended.
- The plan should describe any medication used in pregnancy and any monitoring recommended for the mother and baby postdelivery because of this.
- The plan needs to address actions and responsibilities should a mental health crisis occur.
- A copy of the plan should be included in all copies of the mother's notes.
- The plan must identify factors to ensure priority is given to the relationship between the mother and baby.
- The plan will detail how the baby will be fed and identify early any questions or concerns with breast-feeding if the mother uses medication.

Specific mental health diagnoses in pregnancy and the postnatal period

Bipolar affective disorder

Bipolar affective disorder is a major affective disorder marked by severe mood swings (manic or major depressive episode) and a tendency to remission and recurrence (ICD 10).

Bipolar affective disorder has a lifetime prevalence of approximately 1% of the adult population.

At booking, a woman with bipolar affective disorder may be completely well if in remission, and it is tempting to assume she does not have a major mental illness. Nonetheless, the risk of a postnatal episode is real, and it is crucial you and she can discuss this openly.

Bipolar affective disorder is a highly significant risk factor and predictor for postpartum psychosis (see later). If you work in a health care system where a perinatal psychiatry service is available, it is imperative that a referral to this service is prioritized for all women with a diagnosis of bipolar affective disorder.

Women with this condition may use mood stabilizers to stay well and at booking of pregnancy are highly likely to want to consider the risks and benefits of medication options. Ideally this should be done in collaboration with a consultant perinatal psychiatrist and a specialist pharmacist. A sudden discontinuation of any psychotropic medication is not advisable (NICE CG192).

Postpartum (puerperal) psychosis

Postpartum psychosis is the most florid and often the most serious of the postpartum conditions, occurring in 2/1000 deliveries in women of all ages, backgrounds and cultures and countries in the world. Risk factors include a family history of bipolar illness; a maternal family history of postpartum psychosis; and previous episodes of bipolar illness, schizo-affective disorder or postpartum psychosis.

Approximately 50% of women with a previous bipolar illness or postpartum psychosis will become ill. This risk justifies assessment and monitoring during pregnancy, and with the woman's consent, prophylactic intervention following delivery.

The illness is characterized thus:
- Sudden onset in the early days following delivery, deteriorating on a daily basis.
- Half will present within the first postpartum week, the majority within 2 weeks and almost all within 3 months of delivery.
- Psychosis, delusions, fear and perplexity, confusion and agitation and sometimes hallucinations are apparent.
- Agitation and severe disturbance may also manifest.

In the early days of the illness, the picture changes frequently and is often called *an acute undifferentiated psychosis*. Later it is more clearly a bipolar illness. A third will be manic and the rest usually mixed with some symptoms of mania but a predominantly depressive content.

Management

Urgent admission to an inpatient mother and baby unit is usually necessary. These women should not be admitted to a general adult psychiatric unit. Specialized medical and nursing care is required. The admission of the baby with the mother is not only humane but will facilitate the mother's treatment and ensure a good relationship with her infant.

These illnesses respond rapidly to treatment. Antipsychotics, antidepressants and mood stabilizers may be used and, on occasion, electroconvulsive therapy (ECT). The prognosis for a full recovery is good.

Postpartum psychosis can be a life-threatening condition with an elevated risk of suicide and accidental harm from disturbed behaviour. There is risk to physical health from not eating and drinking and not accessing medical care, and the woman may be temporarily unable to care for the baby.

Treatment needs to be continued for some time after recovery because the risk of relapse in the early weeks is high, particularly if she has been manic and may relapse into a depressive state.

The risk of recurrence following all future pregnancies is at least 1 in 2. She should therefore be referred early in her next pregnancy and a management plan put into place.

Antenatal and postnatal depression

- Taking a history (see previous section) is crucial. A woman with a mild, self-limiting depression will need a different conversation and management plan from a woman with severe, debilitating and hard-to-treat symptoms.
- Women who use antidepressants to stay well may have been advised to discontinue medication without full consideration of the risks and benefits. Staying well is preferable to having to deal with relapse.
- Psychological therapies are effective and can be used for depression and anxiety in pregnancy if women are symptomatic and wish to avoid medication.
- Take care not to misattribute physical symptoms to 'mental health' if you note a past mental health history.
  - Women with anxiety and depression can have fatigue, headaches, palpitations, nausea or dizziness as a manifestation of their mental health problem or as a symptom of a physical illness. Being thorough in history taking and examination is key. Misattribution of symptoms to 'mental health' has contributed to maternal death (CEMACE), so it is essential to remain curious, open minded and thorough.
- A significant antenatal or postnatal depression is a serious and treatable complication of pregnancy. Depressive symptoms can be similar to depression at any other time. It is common for health care professionals to miss the severity of a perinatal depression and attribute the symptoms to exhaustion of motherhood. Women sometimes can and do successfully mask symptoms.

The following are 'red flag' signs for severe maternal illness and require urgent senior psychiatric assessment:
- recent significant change in mental state or emergence of new symptoms
- new thoughts or acts of violent self-harm
- new and persistent expressions of incompetency as a mother or estrangement from the infant

Admission to a mother and baby unit should always be considered where a woman has any of the following:
- rapidly changing mental state
- suicidal ideation (particularly of a violent nature)
- pervasive guilt or hopelessness
- significant estrangement from the infant
- beliefs of inadequacy as a mother
- evidence of psychosis

Eating disorders

Women who are relatively well but have a history of anorexia nervosa or bulimia nervosa may well have specific issues in pregnancy and postnatally.
- Morning sickness may well be more challenging for women with bulimia nervosa.
- Bodily changes in pregnancy may be very uncomfortable to tolerate.
- Even 'well' women may still have significant restriction pre-pregnancy, and trying to 'eat well' in pregnancy is often highly uncomfortable.
- Others noticing or even touching a woman's changing body can be deeply distressing.
- Her postpartum body can be shocking and distressing to the mother, and even if pregnancy was uneventful, a significant postpartum episode is a possibility.

Women with active eating disorders present both psychological and physical issues in pregnancy which, without active management, present significant risk.
- Active bulimia nervosa can contribute to grossly abnormal blood biochemistry, specifically clinically significant hypokalaemia.
- Hypercoagulability is a concern for those with restriction, binge-purging, general malaise and reduced mobility.
- Some associations with anorexia and low birth weight or prematurity have been found, but these findings have not been reproduced in all studies.
- The relationship between mother and her unborn is often affected. Mothers who have ambivalent or regretful emotions about being pregnant are more likely to have difficulty establishing a warm relationship with their baby.
- It is highly likely that postnatally, the eating disorder behaviours will escalate further.
- It is probable that mothers with active eating disorders may be concealing the extent of their illness.

- Maternal weight and BMI have limited use as a measure of severity of eating disorder in pregnancy, but a static or falling BMI is significant.

Borderline personality disorder/ emotionally unstable personality disorder

This is a diagnosis which can cause concern or confusion.

Someone who has an established diagnosis of borderline personality disorder/emotionally unstable personality disorder (EUPD) is likely to have experienced an emotionally invalidating early life. They have often experienced neglect or abuse, including possibly sexual abuse. As a result, they struggle with a range of emotional scars which can manifest in a variety of ways.

Women with EUPD may struggle to form and maintain relationships, particularly in times of uncertainty or disagreement. They are highly attuned to threat and often respond when threat is perceived. They often experience rapidly changing and hard-to-predict extremes of emotion. At times they can experience strong senses of hopelessness, rage or desperation. Some difficult behaviours can be used to cope with these overwhelming emotions. These can be directed towards themselves (self-harm, including overdoses, cutting, binging/purging, substance or alcohol misuse) or others (interpersonal conflict, aggression, dependency, relationship issues).

Staff can feel really challenged to provide respectful and consistent care for those with personality disorder. It is never acceptable to use demeaning, flippant, derogatory or patronizing language to or about anyone with a mental health problem. This could include using terms such as 'she's a PD/manipulative/irrational/a pain/ungrateful/a nightmare' to other colleagues. You have a responsibility to lead by example and recognize all the challenges presented as a result of earlier trauma.

It is worth considering for a moment that if she is a survivor of abuse, particularly childhood sexual abuse, vaginal examinations, being immobile, experiencing pain beyond her control, being touched and feeling powerless could all be very traumatic and retriggering for her.

She may well be avoiding previous coping strategies such as overdosing, binge drinking or cutting in her pregnancy for the wellbeing of her child but, in avoiding these, her emotional pain may feel even more acute.

She is likely to be struggling to imagine how she can parent and keep her baby safe in the face of such a hostile world. If she did not experience kind and adequate parenting, she may be terrified that she lacks the skills to parent. Or she may be so fearful that others will see her as inadequate that they will remove her baby at birth.

In light of all this, one can begin to see how this pregnancy and imminent birth could cause a mother with personality disorder to feel extremely anxious, vigilant and defensive, and so may be seen within the health care system as 'challenging' or 'difficult'.

This mother needs kind, truthful, respectful, proactive care. She needs to understand you and your team are professional and human and practise evidence-based medicine. She needs to know that, as with any other woman, in the presence of capacity, she can accept or decline investigations, examinations and interventions. Any concerns about her mental health or about her baby's welfare need to be discussed with her openly and honestly.

Obsessive-compulsive disorder

Obsessive-compulsive disorder (OCD) is characterized by the presence of either obsessions or compulsions, but commonly both. The symptoms can cause significant functional impairment and/or distress. An obsession is defined as an unwanted intrusive thought, image or urge that repeatedly enters the person's mind. Compulsions are repetitive behaviours or mental acts that the person feels driven to perform. A compulsion can either be overt and observable by others, such as checking that a door is locked, or a covert mental act that cannot be observed, such as repeating a certain phrase in one's mind.

It is thought that 1–2% of the population have OCD, although some studies have estimated 2–3%.

Perinatal OCD can be particularly problematic. A mother experiencing a recurrent intrusive thought or image relating to her baby can be so horrified by its content that asking for help is exceptionally difficult, so she suffers in silence. Some rituals can be incredibly time consuming, and either the obsessional thought or the compulsion can dramatically interfere with the mother's comfort in carrying out day-to-day baby care tasks.

Psychological therapy and pharmacotherapy are effective in the treatment of OCD and are a priority as a mother's and baby's ability to be comfortable together and to enjoy one another are very important for the healthy development of the infant. Treatment as soon as possible minimizes the impact the mother's mental health has on the infant, which is critical.

Post-traumatic stress disorder

Post-traumatic stress disorder (PTSD) is frequently missed in pregnancy or misdiagnosed as a generalized anxiety disorder, panic attacks or depression.

Symptoms of PTSD include flashbacks, nightmares, hypervigilance and physical symptoms of significant anxiety

PTSD can contribute to significant mental health problems in the perinatal period.

High-risk groups include asylum seekers, refugees, services personnel and those who have been exposed to recent trauma, such as those involved in the Grenfell disaster or Manchester bombings. It is always advisable to be mindful of the communities who use your service and any specific groups you need to be aware of.

PTSD is also experienced by those not from these high risk populations, so broader awareness is necessary for a history of trauma, including previous birth trauma.

Psychological therapy is effective and should be prioritized in the pregnant and postnatal population.

For antenatal women with marked PTSD, a careful birth plan can also be helpful to ensure her intrapartum care is designed specifically to reduce triggers or stimuli which could be distressing. Women who have experienced previous birth trauma can have some very specific challenges in subsequent pregnancies. Re-entering the delivery suite, the same lighting, noises and smells can be very challenging and need to be thought about carefully in advance. Women who have raised complaints or concerns about previous episodes of care may fear less favourable treatment and may need reassurance from senior staff that this will not be the case.

Principles of prescribing psychotropic medication in pregnancy

Including medication-specific advice in a textbook is problematic. The evidence base continues to grow and evolve, and using this resource years after publication could result in the reader using data which are no longer valid or that have been superseded by more up-to-date research and prescribing guidance.

Prescribing psychotropic medication in pregnancy follows the principles outlined in Box 14.2.

Box 14.2 Prescribing psychotropic medication in pregnancy

1. Use the lowest effective dose of the minimum number of medications.
2. If possible, use what has been used successfully in the past.
3. Do not abruptly stop medication on discovery of pregnancy.
4. Women need to be able to have a timely risks/benefits conversation with a prescriber or pharmacist.
5. Breast-feeding should be discussed when thinking about medication with any pregnant woman.
6. Medication may need to be increased during pregnancy given the increasing maternal circulating volume.
7. Consider the monitoring needed for both mother and infant during the antenatal, perinatal and postnatal phases if psychotropic medication has been used.

As a clinician and a prescriber, it is important to access up-to-date information to ensure your knowledge and advice is current. The UK Teratology Information Service (UKTIS) and the British Association of Psychopharmacology Perinatal Guideline 2017 are helpful resources.

Special mention of sodium valproate

Medicines containing valproate taken in pregnancy can cause malformations in 11% of babies and developmental disorders in 30–40% of children after birth.

Valproate treatment must not be used in girls and women, including in young girls below the age of puberty, unless alternative treatments are not suitable and unless the conditions of the pregnancy prevention programme are met. Valproate must not be used in pregnant women. See also the MHRA toolkit to ensure female patients are better informed about the risks of taking valproate during pregnancy (NICE CG192 2014).

Capacity and mental health

Women have the right to make decisions about their care and treatment if they have the capacity to do so. Capacity assessment is a core skill every clinical practitioner must have, and she or he must keep the medical records accurately to give assurance that capacity was considered and an assessment was done.

Women with mental illness must be assumed to have capacity, even when mentally ill. A thorough capacity assessment for a specific decision is essential. Women detained under the Mental Health Act with ongoing symptoms of psychosis must still be assumed to have capacity to make decisions about their medical treatment.

If it is established that a mental illness has affected capacity (see the following example), you should consult the legal team for your hospital to consider the need for an application to a court to proceed.

Case study

Mary is 44 years old and has a diagnosis of paranoid schizophrenia. She believes she is not pregnant and her abdominal swelling is because she has cancer after being experimented on by the Secret Services. She is 35 weeks' pregnant and has high blood pressure, but she thinks the antihypertensive treatment is poison, so no one is sure if she is taking it or not. She admits to frequent headaches which have started recently, and you note ankle swelling.

Because Mary does not believe she is pregnant, she will not engage in a conversation about the baby's movements.

You believe she is at risk of worsening pre-eclampsia and would like to admit her for assessment and treatment. She refuses.

Consider what you think needs to happen next.

What additional information do you need to know?

Who else needs to be involved?

Summary

Maternal mental health is as important as maternal physical health. Early detection and prevention of possible poor mental health are always preferable to treatment. To advise and support a woman at risk to stay well in pregnancy takes time, expertise, patience, curiosity and kindness. Treatment of mental health problems are effective, and we should all be ambitious for the full recovery of the women with whom we work.

Perinatal mental health problems affect women from every walk of life, every socioeconomic background and every ethnicity. They are common, and at the severe end of the spectrum are a leading cause of maternal death. Treatments are effective, and recovery is absolutely achievable. Ideally for those with serious mental health problems, treatment should be coordinated by perinatal mental health teams, if suitable in the community, but where risk is identified in the acute episode, an admission to a mother and baby unit should be sought.

Essential information

- Deaths related to mental illness remain a leading cause of maternal deaths.
- A significant past history is the most reliable predictor of serious mental illness in the perinatal period.
- Obstetricians and midwives are uniquely positioned to enable women to share their histories, without fear of judgement, shock, overreaction or rejection.
- Obtaining a history of mental illness is as important as obtaining a history of heart disease, diabetes or epilepsy in the perinatal period.
- Mental illness is treatable in the perinatal period. Instillation of hope for those experiencing poor mental health is part of good clinical care.

Essential gynaecology

Chapter | 15 |

Basic clinical skills in gynaecology

Ian Symonds

LEARNING OUTCOMES

After studying this chapter you should be able to:

Knowledge criteria

- Recognize the logical sequence of eliciting a history and physical signs in gynaecology
- Describe the pathophysiological basis of symptoms and physical signs in obstetrics and gynaecology (O&G)
- List the relevant investigations used in the management of common conditions in O&G

Clinical competencies

- Elicit a history from a gynaecology patient
- Perform an abdominal examination in women in the non-pregnant state and in early pregnancy (under 20 weeks) and recognize normal findings and common abnormalities
- Perform a vaginal examination (bimanual, bivalve speculum) and recognize normal findings and common abnormalities
- Recognize the acutely unwell patient in gynaecology (pain, bleeding, hypovolaemia, peritonitis)

- Perform, interpret and explain the following relevant investigations: genital swabs (high vaginal swab, endocervical swab) and cervical screening test
- Summarize and integrate the history, examination and investigation results; formulate a management plan in a clear and logical way; and make a clear record in the case notes

Professional skills and attitudes

- Conduct an intimate examination in keeping with professional guidelines (e.g. Royal College of Obstetricians and Gynaecologists [RCOG], General Medical Council [GMC])
- Have a chaperone present when undertaking intimate examination
- Demonstrate an awareness of the importance of empathy
- Acknowledge and respect cultural diversity
- Demonstrate an awareness of the interaction of social factors with the patient's illness
- Maintain patient confidentiality
- Provide explanations to patients in language they can understand

---

The term *gynaecology* describes the study of diseases of the female genital tract and reproductive system. There is a continuum between gynaecology and obstetrics so that the division is somewhat arbitrary. Complications of early pregnancy (less than 20 weeks) such as miscarriage and ectopic pregnancy are generally considered under the title of gynaecology.

History

When taking a history start by introducing yourself and explaining who you are. Details of the patient's name, age

and occupation should always be recorded at the beginning of a consultation unless this information has already been provided (e.g. in a referral letter). The age of the patient will influence the likely diagnosis for a number of presenting problems. The history should be comprehensive but not intrusive in a manner that is not relevant to the patient's problem. For example, whilst it is essential to obtain a detailed sexual history from a young woman presenting with a genital tract infection, some women may find the discussion of sexual history uncomfortable. It is important to approach the clinical history with respect, regardless of age, religion or social situation, and tailor this approach to each individual patient.

Up to 30% of patients presenting to gynaecological services have psychiatric morbidity, and there is a significant association between adverse life events, depression and gynaecological symptoms. Remember, the presenting symptom may not always be related to the main anxiety of the patient and that some time and patience may be required to uncover the various problems that bring the patient to seek medical advice.

The presenting problem(s)

The patient should be asked to describe the nature of her problem, and a simple statement of the presenting symptoms should be made in the case notes. A great deal can be learnt by using the actual words employed by the patient. It is important to ascertain the time scale of the problem and, where appropriate, the circumstances surrounding the onset of symptoms and their relationship to the menstrual cycle. It is also important to discover the degree of disability experienced for any given symptom.

More detailed questions will depend on the nature of the presenting problem(s). Disorders of menstruation are the commonest reason for gynaecological referral, and a full menstrual history should be taken from all women of reproductive age (see later). Another common presenting symptom is abdominal pain, and the history must include details of the time of onset and precipitants, i.e. intercourse, associated symptoms, the distribution and radiation of the pain and the relationship to the menstrual cycle

If vaginal discharge is the presenting symptom, the colour, odour and relationship to the periods should be noted, as well as any over-the-counter medications used to treat this. It may also be associated with vulval pruritus or skin changes, i.e. rash/lesions, particularly in the presence of specific infections. The presence of an abdominal mass may be noted by the patient or may be detected during the course of a routine examination. Symptoms may also result from pressure of the mass on adjacent pelvic organs, such as the bladder and bowel.

Vaginal and uterine prolapse is associated with symptoms of a mass protruding through the vaginal introitus or difficulties with micturition and defecation. Common urinary symptoms include frequency of micturition, pain or dysuria, incontinence and the passage of blood in the urine, or haematuria.

Where appropriate a sexual history should include reference to the coital frequency, the occurrence of pain during intercourse – *dyspareunia* – and functional details relating to libido, sexual satisfaction and sexual problems (see Chapter 19).

Menstrual history

The first question that should be asked in relation to the menstrual history is the date of the last menstrual period (LMP). In relation to the menstrual cycle, you should ascertain her normal cycle length, duration of bleeding, regularity/irregularity of cycle and whether any hormonal contraception is being used. It is also very common for women to now track their menstrual cycle with phone applications, especially if attempting to conceive.

The time of onset of the first period, the **menarche,** commonly occurs at 12 years of age and can be considered to be abnormally delayed over 16 years or abnormally early at 8 years. The absence of menstruation in a girl with otherwise normal development by the age of 16 is known as **primary amenorrhoea**. The term should be distinguished from the **pubarche**, which is the onset of the first signs of sexual maturation. Characteristically, the development of breasts and nipple enlargement predate the onset of menstruation by approximately 2 years (see Chapter 16).

Failure to check the date of the last period may lead to serious errors in subsequent management.

The length of the menstrual cycle is the time between the first day of one period (i.e. first day of bleeding) and the first day of the following period. Whilst there is usually an interval of 28 days, the cycle length may vary between 21 and 42 days in normal women and may only be significant where there is a change in menstrual pattern. It is important to be sure that the patient does not describe the time between the last day of one period and the first day of the next period, as this may give a false impression of the frequency of menstruation.

Absence of menstruation for more than 6 months in a woman who is not pregnant and has previously had periods is known as **secondary amenorrhoea**. **Oligomenorrhea** is the occurrence of five or fewer menstrual periods over 12 months.

The amount and duration of the bleeding may change with age but may also provide a useful indication of a disease process. Normal menstruation lasts from 4 to 7 days, and normal blood loss varies between 30 and 40 mL (6–8 teaspoons). A change in pattern is often more noticeable and significant than the actual time and volume of loss. In practical terms, excessive menstrual loss is best assessed on the history of the number of pads or tampons used during a period and the presence or absence of clots and symptoms of anaemia.

Abnormal uterine bleeding (AUB) is any bleeding disturbance that occurs between menstrual periods or is excessive, prolonged or irregular. **Intermenstrual bleeding**

is any bleeding that occurs between clearly defined, cyclical, regular menses. **Postcoital bleeding** is non-menstrual bleeding that occurs during or after sexual intercourse. AUB always requires investigation, as it may be the first symptom of an underlying potential medical condition.

The term **heavy menstrual bleeding (HMB)** is now used to describe any excessive or prolonged menstrual bleeding which is greater than 5–6 tablespoons of blood (>80 mL), irrespective of whether the cycle is regular (**menorrhagia**) or irregular (**metrorrhagia**).

The cessation of periods at the end of menstrual life is known as *menopause,* and bleeding which occurs more than 12 months after this is described as **postmenopausal bleeding.** A history of irregular vaginal bleeding or blood loss that occurs after coitus or between periods should be noted.

Previous gynaecological history

A detailed history of any previous gynaecological problems and treatments must be recorded. It is also important, where possible, to obtain any records of previous gynaecological surgery. Patients are often uncertain of the precise nature of their operations. The amount of detail needed about previous pregnancies will depend on the presenting problem. In most cases the number of previous pregnancies and their outcome (miscarriage, ectopic or delivery after 20 weeks, caesarean section delivery) is all that is required. If previous births have occurred, it is important to know the mode of delivery, i.e. normal vaginal delivery, caesarean section or assisted instrumental delivery via forceps or vacuum. Furthermore any injury to the perineum either via tear or episiotomy should be noted.

For all women of reproductive age who are sexually active, it is essential to ask about contraception and any screening for sexually transmitted infections. This is important not only to determine the possibility of pregnancy but also because the method of contraception used may itself be relevant to the presenting complaint (e.g. irregular bleeding may occur on the contraceptive pill or when an intrauterine device is present). For women over the age of 25, ask about the date and result of the last cervical screening test. Recent changes to cervical screening in Australia mean that women now begin testing at the age of 25 and every 5 years instead of the previous 2-year interval. The new cervical screening test combines human papilloma virus (HPV) genotype testing and liquid-based cytology (LBC) where appropriate.

Previous medical and surgical history

A comprehensive medical and surgical history is vital to any medical history, and gynaecology is no different. This should take particular account of any history of chronic lung disease, disorders of the cardiovascular system and previous surgeries and anaesthetics, as these are highly relevant where any surgical procedure is likely to be necessary. A record of all current medications (including non-prescription and over-the-counter treatments) and any known drug allergies should be made. If she is planning a pregnancy in the near future, check if she is taking folic acid supplements.

Psychosocial history

A psychosocial history is important with all medical presentations but is particularly relevant where the presenting difficulties relate to abortion or sterilization. For example, a 15-year-old female requesting a termination of pregnancy may be put under substantial pressure by her parents to have an abortion and yet may not really be happy about following this course of action. Ask about smoking, alcohol and other recreational drug use. It is important to ask about mental health history, including anxiety, depression and if they are currently being treated or seen by a mental health professional. Domestic violence is a significant issue for society and is particularly important in women's health care and should be kept in mind when seeing women in clinic. In Australia, screening in pregnancy for domestic violence and sexual abuse is now a Medicare requirement. Up to 40% of women presenting for a well-woman check will give a history of domestic violence, although the figure is lower in gynaecology clinics.

Examination

A general examination should always be performed at the first consultation, including assessment of pulse, blood pressure and temperature. Careful note should be taken of any signs of anaemia. The distribution of facial and body hair is often important, as hirsutism may be a presenting symptom of various endocrine disorders. Body weight and height should also be recorded to calculate a body mass index (BMI).

The intimate nature of gynaecological examination makes it especially important to ensure that every effort is made to ensure privacy and that the examination is not interrupted by phone calls, pagers or messages about other patients. The examination should ideally take place in a separate area to the consultation. The patient should be allowed to undress in privacy and, if necessary, empty her bladder first (unless the presenting problem is incontinence, in which case an empty bladder may mask signs of stress incontinence). Always offer a blanket for the patient to cover herself after undressing for the examination. After undressing there should be no undue delay

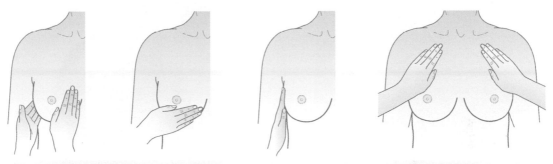

Fig. 15.1 Systematic examination of the four quadrants of the breasts.

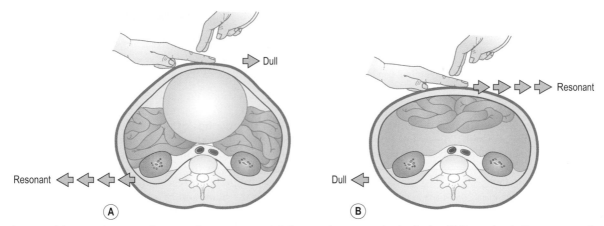

Fig. 15.2 (A) Percussion over a large ovarian cyst – central dullness and resonance in the flanks. (B) Percussion in the presence of ascites – dullness in the flanks and central resonance.

prior to examination. Before starting the examination and whilst the woman is fully dressed, explain what will be involved in the vaginal examination, and verbal consent should be obtained and documented. The woman should be informed that she can ask for the examination to be stopped at any stage and that she is in control. A chaperone should generally be present, irrespective of the gender of the gynaecologist.

Breast examination

The breast examination should be performed if there are symptoms or at the first consultation in women over the age of 45. The presence of the secretion of milk at times not associated with pregnancy, known as *galactorrhoea*, may indicate abnormal endocrine status or medication with dopamine antagonists such as psychotropic medication. Systematic palpation with the flat of the hand should be undertaken to exclude the presence of any nodules in the breast or axillae (Fig. 15.1).

Examination of the abdomen

Inspection of the abdomen may reveal the presence of a mass. The distribution of body hair should be noted, and the presence of scars, striae and hernias. Palpation of the abdomen should take account of any guarding and rebound tenderness. It is important to ask the patient to outline the site and radiation of any pain in the abdomen, and palpation for enlargement of the liver, spleen and kidneys should be carried out. If there is a mass, try to determine if it is fixed or mobile, smooth or regular, and if it arises from the pelvis (you shouldn't be able to palpate the lower edge above the pubic bone). Check the hernial orifices and feel for any enlarged lymph nodes in the groin. Percussion of the abdomen may be used to outline the limits of a tumour, to detect the presence of a full bladder or to recognize the presence of tympanitic loops of bowel. Free fluid in the peritoneal cavity will be recognized by the presence of dullness to percussion in the flanks and resonance over the central abdomen (Fig. 15.2).

235

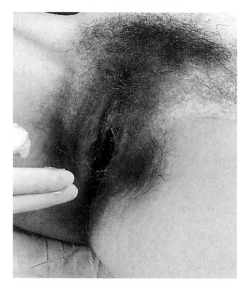

Fig. 15.3 Inspection of the external genitalia.

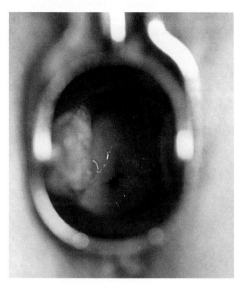

Fig. 15.4 View of normal cervix on speculum examination.

Auscultation of bowel sounds is indicated in patients with postoperative abdominal distension or acute abdominal pain where obstruction or an ileus is suspected.

> ✓ Remember to look in particular in the umbilicus for scars from previous laparoscopies and in the suprapubic region where transverse incisions from caesarean sections and most gynaecological operations are found.

Pelvic examination

The pelvic examination should not be considered an automatic or inevitable part of every gynaecological consultation. You should consider what information will be gained by the examination, whether this is a screening or diagnostic procedure and whether it is necessary at this time.

The patient should be examined resting supine with the knees drawn up and separated or in stirrups in the lithotomy position, especially for older women with weak hip flexors or painful joints secondary to arthritis (Fig. 15.3). Gloves should be worn on both hands during vaginal and speculum examinations.

Parting the lips of the labia minora with the left hand, look at the external urethral meatus and inspect the vulva for any discharge, redness, ulceration and old scars. Speculum examination should be performed before digital examination to avoid any contamination with lubricant. A bivalve/duckbill or Cusco's speculum is most commonly used and enables a clear view of the cervix to be obtained, with a variety of sizes available.

Holding the lips of the labia minora open with the left hand, insert the speculum into the introitus with the widest dimension of the instrument in the transverse position, as the vagina is widest in this direction. When the speculum reaches the top of the vagina, gently open the blades and visualize the cervix (Fig. 15.4). Make a note of the presence of any discharge or bleeding from the cervix and of any polyps or areas of ulceration. Remember that the appearance of the cervix is changed after childbirth, with the external os more irregular with a horizontal slit. The commonest finding is of a so-called **erosion** or **ectropion.** This is an area of cervical epithelium around the cervical os that appears a darker red colour than the smooth pink of the rest of the cervix. It is not an erosion at all but normal columnar epithelium extending from the endocervical canal onto the ectocervix. If the clinical history suggests possible infection, take swabs from the posterior vaginal fornices and cervical os and place in transport medium to look for *Candida* and *Trichomonas* and a separate swab without culture medium from the endocervix for polymerase chain reaction nucleic acid amplification testing (PCR NAAT) for *Chlamydia/Gonorrhoea*. PCR testing for *Chlamydia* and *Neisseria* can also be performed on the same sample used for cervical screening if this is collected using the cytobrush for liquid-based cytology.

Where vaginal wall prolapse is suspected, a Sims' speculum might be required, as it often provides a clearer view of the vaginal walls. Where the Sims' speculum is used, it is preferable to examine the patient in the semi-prone or Sims' position (Fig. 15.5).

Performing a cervical screening test (Fig. 15.6)

This should be done in accordance with local guidelines and at least 3 months after pregnancy and not during normal menstruation due to contamination by blood. Explain the purpose of the test and warn the patient that she may notice some spotting afterwards.

Record the date, patient's name and hospital number or date of birth on a suitable slide. After consent and appropriate positioning, insert the speculum gently, as noted earlier, and wipe away any discharge or blood. Note the appearance of the cervix. A 360-degree sweep should be taken with the central bristles of the cervical brush pressed firmly into the cervical os and the outer bristles against the ectocervix. Rotate the brush in a clockwise direction five times.

In liquid-based screening tests (LBT – which has in most jurisdictions replaced cervical cytology) the sampling device is transferred into the preservative solution and agitated vigorously (avoiding spillage) to separate the cells from the device. In the laboratory, the solution is passed through a filter, which traps the large squamous cells but allows smaller red cells, debris and bacteria to pass through. The squamous cells are analyzed for HPV DNA replication, and in some circumstances cells might also be transferred to a glass slide to perform conventional cytology ('Pap smear'). If so, the specimen is spread immediately onto a clear glass slide in a thin, even layer. The slide is fixed with 95% alcohol alone or in combination with 3% glacial acetic acid. Fixation requires 30 minutes in solution. The rate of unsatisfactory smears is lower in LBT, and LBT accuracy appears unaffected by the presence of blood. In Australia, the replacement of conventional cytology by LBT and high-risk HPV typing is anticipated to reduce the incidence of invasive cervical cancer by 15%. LBT also allows for PCR-based testing for *Chlamydia* and gonorrhoea.

Finally, complete the cervical screening test request form. Required details are usually specified in bespoke forms produced for centralized screening registration units; otherwise, ensure that clinical indications for the test and any relevant history, e.g. previous test results, date of LMP, is recorded.

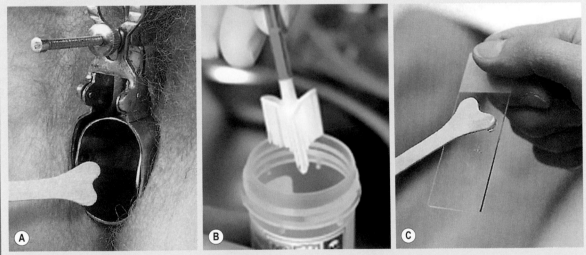

Fig. 15.6 (A) A cervical smear is taken using an Ayres spatula. (B) A sample being taken for liquid-based cytology using the broom-like device. (C) The material obtained is plated onto a glass slide and fixed.

Taking vaginal swabs

The indications are for symptoms of vaginal discharge, irregular bleeding and pelvic inflammatory disease. Swabs may also be taken to screen for sexually transmitted infection in asymptomatic women.

A high vaginal swab is taken as part of a speculum examination by dipping the tip of a culture swab moistened in culture media in the posterior vaginal fornix and then placing the swab immediately back into a suitable culture medium. This is used mainly to identify organisms such as *Candida* or *Trichomonas* and in the assessment of bacterial vaginosis.

Endocervical swabs need preparation of the endocervical area by first using a cotton swab to clean the area, which can then be discarded. Following this, the tip of the swab is placed into the external cervical os and rotated two or three times. Using standard culture media as for the high vaginal swab, this can be used to test for fungal infections such as *Candida* species or bacterial infections such as *Escherischia coli, Ureaplasma urealyticum* or *Mycoplasma pneumoniae*.

Bimanual examination

The bimanual examination is an important part of the gynae-cological series of examinations but is not necessarily routine or indicated for every patient. It is performed by introducing the middle finger of the examining hand into the vaginal introitus and applying pressure towards the rectum (Fig. 15.7). As the introitus opens, the index finger is introduced as well. The cervix is palpated and has the consistency of the cartilage of the tip of the nose. Assessment of the cervix for elicitation of pain through its movement/rubbing is called *cervical excitation* and suggests possible pelvic pathology, particularly inflammation secondary to infection or surrounding blood.

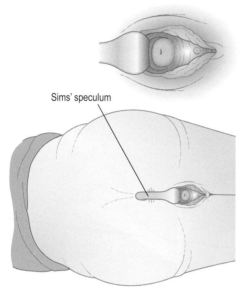

Sims' speculum

Fig. 15.5 Examination in the lateral semi-prone position with a Sims' speculum enables inspection of the vaginal walls.

It must be remembered that the abdominal hand is used to compress the pelvic organs onto the examining vaginal hand. The size, shape, consistency and position of the uterus must be noted. The uterus is commonly pre-axial or anteverted but will be postaxial or retroverted in some 10% of women. Provided the retroverted uterus is mobile, the position is rarely significant. It is important to feel in the pouch of Douglas for the presence of thickening or nodules and then to palpate laterally in both fornices for the presence of any ovarian or tubal masses. An attempt should be made to differentiate between adnexal and uterine masses, although this is often not possible. For example, a pedunculated fibroid may mimic an ovarian tumour, whereas a solid ovarian tumour, if adherent to the uterus, may be impossible to distinguish from a uterine fibroid. The ovaries may be palpable in the normal pelvis if the patient is thin, but the Fallopian tubes are only palpable if they are significantly enlarged.

In a child or in a woman with an intact hymen, speculum and pelvic examination is usually not performed unless as part of an examination under anaesthesia. It should always be remembered that a rough or painful examination rarely produces any useful information and might result in future refusal to be examined, as well as in certain situations, such as tubal ectopic pregnancy, being dangerous. Throughout the examination, remain alert to verbal and non-verbal indications of distress from the patient. Any request that the examination be discontinued should be respected. For these reasons and those noted earlier, it is prudent to always have a chaperone present during any pelvic or gynaecological examination (Box 15.1).

Special circumstances

Except in an emergency situation, pelvic examination should not be carried out for non–English-speaking patients without an interpreter. You should be aware of, and sensitive

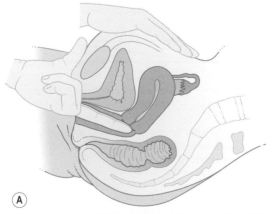

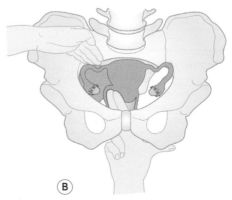

(A)

(B)

Fig. 15.7 (A) Bimanual examination of the pelvis. (B) Examination of the lateral fornix.

BOX 15.1 GMC Guidelines: intimate examination and chaperones

Intimate examinations

Intimate examinations can be embarrassing or distressing for patients and whenever you examine a patient you should be sensitive to what they may think of as intimate. This is likely to include examinations of breasts, genitalia and rectum, but could also include any examination where it is necessary to touch or even be close to the patient.

In this guidance, we highlight some of the issues involved in carrying out intimate examinations. This must not deter you from carrying out intimate examinations when necessary. You must follow this guidance and make detailed and accurate records at the time of the examination, or as soon as possible afterwards.

Before conducting an intimate examination, you should:

a. explain to the patient why an examination is necessary and give the patient an opportunity to ask questions
b. explain what the examination will involve, in a way the patient can understand, so that the patient has a clear idea of what to expect, including any pain or discomfort
c. get the patient's permission before the examination and record that the patient has given it
d. offer the patient a chaperone (see paragraphs 8–13 below)
e. if dealing with a child or young person[†]
   • you must assess their capacity to consent to the examination[‡]
   • if they lack the capacity to consent, you should seek their parent's consent[**]
f. give the patient privacy to undress and dress, and keep them covered as much as possible to maintain their dignity; do not help the patient to remove clothing unless they have asked you to, or you have checked with them that they want you to help.

During the examination, you must follow the guidance in consent: patients and doctors making decisions together. In particular you should:

a. explain what you are going to do before you do it and, if this differs from what you have told the patient before, explain why and seek the patient's permission
b. stop the examination if the patient asks you to
c. keep discussion relevant and don't make unnecessary personal comments.

Intimate examinations of anaesthetised patients

Before you carry out an intimate examination on an anaesthetised patient, or supervise a student who intends to carry

one out, you must make sure that the patient has given consent in advance, usually in writing.

Chaperones

When you carry out an intimate examination, you should offer the patient the option of having an impartial observer (a chaperone) present wherever possible. This applies whether or not you are the same gender as the patient.

A chaperone should usually be a health professional and you must be satisfied that the chaperone will:

a. be sensitive and respect the patient's dignity and confidentiality
b. reassure the patient if they show signs of distress or discomfort
c. be familiar with the procedures involved in a routine intimate examination
d. stay for the whole examination and be able to see what the doctor is doing, if practical
e. be prepared to raise concerns if they are concerned about the doctor's behaviour or actions.

A relative or friend of the patient is not an impartial observer and so would not usually be a suitable chaperone, but you should comply with a reasonable request to have such a person present as well as a chaperone.

If either you or the patient does not want the examination to go ahead without a chaperone present, or if either of you is uncomfortable with the choice of chaperone, you may offer to delay the examination to a later date when a suitable chaperone will be available, as long as the delay would not adversely affect the patient's health.

If you don't want to go ahead without a chaperone present but the patient has said no to having one, you must explain clearly why you want a chaperone present. Ultimately the patient's clinical needs must take precedence. You may wish to consider referring the patient to a colleague who would be willing to examine them without a chaperone, as long as a delay would not adversely affect the patient's health.

You should record any discussion about chaperones and the outcome in the patient's medical record. If a chaperone is present, you should record that fact and make a note of their identity. If the patient does not want a chaperone, you should record that the offer was made and declined.

[†]You must also follow our guidance on *Protecting Children and Young People: The Responsibilities of All Doctors*. General Medical Council (2012), London, GMC.
[‡]When assessing a young person's capacity to consent, you should bear in mind that:
   at 16 a young person can be presumed to have the capacity to consent
   a young person under 16 may have the capacity to consent, depending on their maturity and ability to understand what is involved.
General Medical Council (2007) *0–18 Years: Guidance for all Doctors*. London, GMC, paragraphs 24–26.
[**]General Medical Council (2007) *0–18 Years: Guidance for All Doctors*, London, GMC, paragraphs 27–28.
General Medical Council March 2013 Available at:
https://www.gmc-uk.org/ethical-guidance/ethical-guidance-for-doctors/intimate-examinations-and-chaperones [accessed 7 May 2019]

to, factors that may make the examination more difficult for the woman with particular cultural or religious expectations. Furthermore some women have undergone female genital mutilation or female circumcision, which can limit the opening of the vaginal introitus, making speculum and bimanual examinations difficult and painful.

Women who experience difficulty with vaginal examination should be given every opportunity to facilitate disclosure of any underlying previous childhood sexual abuse, sexual abuse such as rape or current sexual and/or marital difficulties. However, it must not be assumed that all women who experience difficulty with pelvic examination have a background history of sexual abuse, domestic violence or sexual difficulties.

The basic principles of respect, privacy, explanation and consent that apply to the conduct of gynaecological examinations in general apply equally to the conduct of such examinations in women who have temporary or permanent learning disabilities or mental illness.

When examining anaesthetized patients, all staff should treat the woman with the same degree of sensitivity and respect as if she were awake.

Exceptional gentleness should be displayed in the examination of victims of alleged sexual assault. The woman should be given a choice about the gender of the doctor and be allowed to control the pace of, and her position for, the examination. In the event of post-alleged sexual assault examination, a discussion with the nearby rape and sexual assault centre is crucial to avoid the disruption and contamination of forensic evidence. Furthermore, it may be that early samples can be collected, such as first urinary voids, underwear worn and oral rinses, to help preserve forensic evidence until an appropriately trained health professional can attend. In some areas, there are on-call forensic doctors trained in this type of examination.

Rectal examination

Rectal examination may be indicated if there are symptoms such as change of bowel habit or rectal bleeding, which may suggest bowel disease or severe endometriosis with associated rectal disease. It is occasionally used as a means of assessing a pelvic mass and, in conjunction with a vaginal examination, can provide additional information about disease in the rectovaginal septum.

Presenting your findings

Start by introducing the patient by name and age, and give the main reason for presentation and in turn admission.

If there are several problems, deal with each in turn. If the history consists of a long narrative of events, try to summarize these rather than recap each event. Present the remainder of the history in a logical structured way, not skipping back and forward between items. At the end of your history give a summary in no more than one or two sentences.

Case study: Example of a typical history

This is Ms Smith, a 29-year-old gravida 2 para 2 accountant who has been referred by her general practitioner to the clinic because of bleeding and a positive pregnancy test. Ms Smith has had three episodes of small painless vaginal bleeding over the last 3 days. Her LMP was 7 weeks ago, and prior to this she had a regular 28-day menstrual cycle. She has no previous gynaecological history of note, and her only cervical screening test was 4 years ago and was negative. This is a planned pregnancy, and before conceiving she was using the combined oral contraceptive pill until 3 months ago. She has had two previous pregnancies with uncomplicated normal vaginal deliveries at term. She underwent an appendectomy at the age of 14 and had no problems with the general anaesthetic at the time. She is currently taking folic acid and has no known allergies. She lives with her partner and two children. She does not smoke or drink.

In summary, Ms Smith is a 29-year-old woman with a history of painless vaginal bleeding at 7 weeks in her third pregnancy.

Unless you are asked only to discuss one particular part of the examination, always start by commenting on the patient's general condition, including pulse and blood pressure. For abdominal examinations, list the findings on inspection first followed by those on palpation and percussion (if there is abdominal distension or a mass). If there is a mass arising from the pelvis, describe it terms of a pregnant uterus (e.g. a mass reaching the umbilicus would be a 20-week-size pelvic mass). If there are areas of tenderness, specify whether they are associated with signs of peritonism (guarding and rebound). On pelvic examination, describe the findings on inspection of the vulva and then of the cervix (if a speculum examination was carried out). Describe the size, position and mobility of the uterus and any tenderness. Finally, say whether there were any palpable masses or tenderness in the adnexae.

Case study: Example of presentation of clinical findings

On general examination, Ms Smith looked well. She was not clinically anaemic, and her BMI was 31. Her blood pressure was 110/70, and her pulse 88 and regular. Examination of the chest and heart was unremarkable. On abdominal examination, there was a scar in the right lower quadrant consistent with a previous open appendectomy. On palpation, the abdomen was soft and non-tender with no palpable masses and no organomegaly. On pelvic examination, the external genitalia were normal, apart from an old scar on the perineum consistent with a previous tear or episiotomy. On speculum examination, the cervix was closed and there was a small amount of free blood in the vagina. She had a an 8-week-size, mobile, anteverted uterus, and there were no palpable adnexal masses.

Essential information

History

Presenting complaint

- Onset and duration of main complaint
- Associated symptoms, relationship to menstrual cycle
- Previous treatment and response
- Specific closed questions

Previous gynaecological history

- Previous investigations or treatment
- Contraceptive history
- Sexual history
- Cervical smear
- Menstrual history

Previous pregnancies

- How many (gravidity)
- Outcome (parity)
- Surgical deliveries, including forceps/vacuum delivery and any perineal trauma

Past surgical and medical history

- Previous abdominal surgery
- Major cardiovascular/respiratory disease
- Endocrine disease
- Thromboembolic disease
- Breast disease
- Drug history and allergies

Psychosocial and family history details

- Home and living circumstances
- Support
- Mental health history
- Smoking
- Family history

Examination

General examination

- General condition, weight, height
- Pulse, blood pressure
- Anaemia
- Goitre
- Breast examination (if indicated)
- Secondary sex characteristics, body hair

Abdominal examination

- Inspection – distension, scars
- Palpation – masses, organomegaly, tenderness, peritonism, nodes, hernial orifices
- Percussion –- ascites

Pelvic examination

- Explanation, comfort, privacy, chaperone
- Inspection of external genitalia
- Speculum examination, cervical screening, swabs
- Bimanual examination
- Rectal examination if indicated

Chapter | 16 |

Gynaecological disorders

Ian S. Fraser

LEARNING OUTCOMES

After studying this chapter you should be able to:

Knowledge criteria

- Describe the causes, significance and management of disorders of menstruation, including intermenstrual, postcoital and postmenopausal bleeding, menstrual irregularity, heavy menstrual bleeding, dysmenorrhoea and secondary amenorrhoea.
- Describe the PALM COEIN concept of assessment and classification of causes of abnormal uterine bleeding.
- Describe the problems of puberty, including precocious puberty and delayed puberty. Recognize that endometriosis is a condition that often starts in adolescence.
- Describe problems of the perimenopause, including abnormal bleeding, vasomotor and other symptoms, osteoporosis and hormone-replacement therapy.
- Describe benign conditions of the lower genital tract, including vulval pruritus, vaginal discharge and pelvic pain.
- Describe the causes, significance and management of Bartholin's abscess/cyst, abdominal pain of uncertain origin and acute unscheduled vaginal bleeding.

Clinical competencies

- Assess and plan the initial investigation of a patient presenting with abnormal uterine bleeding, pelvic pain, vaginal discharge and amenorrhoea.
- Interpret the results of the common investigations in benign gynaecological disorders.
- Counsel a patient about indications, contraindications, principles and complications of the common surgical procedures in gynaecology.

Introduction

Benign gynaecological conditions affect women's lives in ways that often remain hidden from society and from health systems. Many aspects of benign conditions such as heavy menstrual bleeding (HMB) and debilitating pelvic pain are often tolerated by women and sometimes dismissed as normal by health care professionals. Many of these conditions do have significant implications for women's health and wellbeing, family and social relationships, the working lives of women and their ability to conceive. The recognition of benign gynaecological conditions requires education of women about what symptoms can be considered part of normal reproductive life and what symptoms may require investigation and treatment. Full appreciation of benign gynaecological conditions also requires that health care professionals develop a deeper understanding of managing reproductive health issues and of identifying potential pathological conditions.

Benign conditions of the upper genital tract

The uterus

The formation of the uterus results from the fusion of the two Müllerian ducts; this fusion gives rise to the upper two-thirds of the vagina, the cervix and the body of the uterus. Congenital anomalies arise from the failure of fusion, or the absence or partial development of one or both ducts. Thus, the anomalies may range from a minor indentation of the uterine fundus to a full separation of each uterine horn and cervix (Fig. 16.1). These conditions are also commonly associated with vaginal septa.

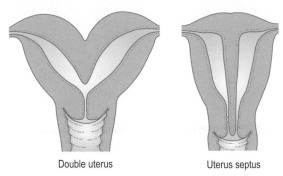

Double uterus   Uterus septus

Fig. 16.1 Common congenital abnormalities of the uterus include uterus bicornis unicollis (double uterus, one cervix, *left*) and the subseptate uterus (uterus septus, *right*).

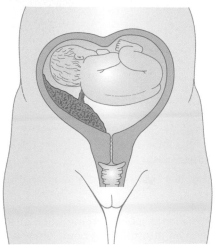

Fig. 16.3 Malpresentation and a subseptate uterus.

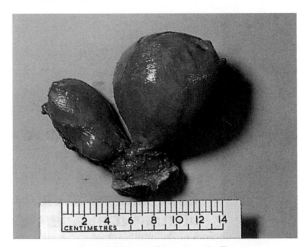

Fig. 16.2 Uterus bicornis unicollis.

Symptoms and signs

The majority of uterine anomalies are asymptomatic and are usually diagnosed in relation to complications of pregnancy. However, the presence of a vaginal septum may result in dyspareunia and postcoital bleeding (PCB).

The presence of a double uterus may also be established at routine vaginal examination, when a double cervix may be seen. The separation of the uterine horns is sometimes palpable on bimanual vaginal examination, but in most cases the uterus feels normal and there is a single cervix. When only one horn is present, the uterus may be palpable as lying obliquely in the pelvis. The abnormality of two uterine horns and one cervix is known as *uterus bicornis unicollis* (Fig. 16.2).

Partial atresia of one horn of the uterus or a septate vagina resulting in obstruction to menstrual outflow from one horn of the uterus may result in a unilateral haematocolpos and haematometra with retrograde spill of menstrual fluid. In this case, the patient may present with symptoms of dysmenorrhoea and will have a palpable mass arising from the pelvis.

The complications of pregnancy in women with these uterine anomalies include:

- Recurrent miscarriage: the role of congenital abnormalities in early pregnancy loss is unclear. For example, the incidence of uterine septa is the same in women with normal reproductive histories. However, there is an association with cervical incompetence, which may lead to mid-trimester miscarriage. This problem is usually associated with the subseptate uterus and is not common in unicornuate uterus or uterus bicornis bicollis.
- Pre-mature labour.
- Malpresentation of the fetus (Fig. 16.3).
- Retained placenta.

Diagnosis and management

As many cases are asymptomatic, the diagnosis may arise only as a coincidental finding and requires no treatment or intervention. Where the diagnosis is suggested by the history, further investigation should include hysterography and hysteroscopy.

Surgical treatment

The role of surgical reconstruction of a double uterus in women with infertility is difficult to assess, as there are no controlled studies demonstrating the benefits in pregnancy outcome. Consideration should be confined to women who have a history of recurrent miscarriage and where the abnormality is one of uterus bicornis unicollis or there is a uterine septum.

243

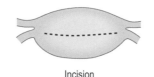
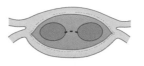
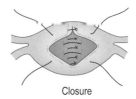

Septate uterus

Incision   Septum divided   Closure

Fig. 16.4 Metroplasty *(right)* for the reunification of a bicornate uterus or the division of a uterine septum *(left)*.

The operation of plastic reconstruction of the uterus with unification of two uterine horns or excision of the uterine septum is known as **metroplasty** (Fig. 16.4). An incision is made across the fundus of the uterus between the uterotubal junctions, taking care not to involve the intramural portion of the tube. The cavities are then reunited by suturing the surfaces together in the anteroposterior plane. If there is a septum, it is simply divided by diathermy, and the cavity is then closed by suturing the transverse incision in the anteroposterior plane. Surgery of this type is associated with postoperative infertility in some cases and with a risk of uterine rupture in subsequent pregnancy.

An alternative surgical management is to divide the septum by diathermy through a hysteroscope inserted through the cervix.

Endometrial polyps

Endometrial polyps (EPs) are localized outgrowths from the surface of the endometrium. They appear at any age from the early reproductive years through to the postmenopausal period. EPs are usually benign lesions but have been implicated in subfertility, as removal of these lesions may improve rates of pregnancy and/or reduce pregnancy loss. There are differences in morphology, function and symptoms between different polyps, and attempts are now being made to develop a detailed subclassification system, as a component of the FIGO PALM-COEIN system (see later), which will allow clarification and improved understanding of the different types of polyps.

Symptoms

EPs are usually asymptomatic lesions, but they may contribute to abnormal uterine bleeding (AUB) manifesting as either intermenstrual bleeding (IMB), HMB or postmenopausal bleeding. Occasionally, protrusion of the polyp through the cervix may result in PCB. Attempts by the uterus to expel the polyp may cause colicky, dysmenorrhoeic pain.

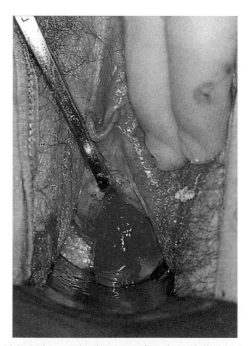

Fig. 16.5 Endometrial polyp protruding through the cervical os.

Signs

EPs are usually detected during the investigation for AUB and infertility. If the polyp protrudes through the cervix, it may be difficult to distinguish from an endocervical polyp (Fig. 16.5). EPs can be visualized on transvaginal ultrasound. They are most easily detected in the secretory phase of the menstrual cycle when the non-progestational type of glands in the polyp stand out in contrast to the normal surrounding secretory endometrium. If their presence is suspected either clinically or on transvaginal ultrasound, further clarification can be undertaken by performing a transvaginal sonohysterography (Fig. 16.6) and/or office or inpatient hysteroscopy, with or without directed excisional biopsy.

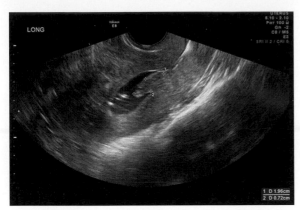

Fig. 16.6 Sonohysterogram demonstrating the endometrial polyp *(outlined by the markers)* extending into the fluid-filled cavity.

Pathology

EPs are localized overgrowths of the surface endometrium. Grossly, they are smooth, cylindrical structures, tan to yellow in colour after removal. Microscopically, they consist of a fine fibrous tissue core covered by columnar epithelium glands. The endometrium encasing the polyps varies from normal endometrium to endometrium that is unresponsive to cyclical hormonal influences. Occasionally the endometrial surface develops simple or complex hyperplasia and, rarely, malignant change occurs.

Treatment

Small (1 cm or less) asymptomatic polyps may resolve spontaneously, and in these cases watchful waiting can be the treatment of choice. However, in women suffering from bleeding symptoms or infertility, surgical excision with removal of the polyp base is required. Traditionally, EPs were removed by dilatation and curettage (D&C) under general anaesthesia, but because blind curettage may miss EPs in 50–85% of cases, removal is best performed under hysteroscopic guidance or by performing curettage followed by reintroducing the hysteroscope to ensure that all the lesions have been removed. Using modern equipment, this can often be done without anaesthesia or with injection of local anaesthetic into the cervix.

Benign tumours of the myometrium
Uterine leiomyomas ('fibroids')

Uterine fibroids (or, more accurately, leiomyomas) are the most common benign tumour of the female genital tract and are clinically apparent in around 25% of women. They are smooth muscle tumours that vary enormously in size from microscopic growths to large masses that may weigh as much

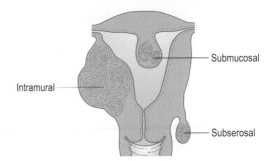

Fig. 16.7 Uterine fibroids produce symptoms that are determined by their site.

as 30–40 kg. Fibroids may be single or multiple and may occur in the cervix or in the body of the uterus. There are three main types of fibroids according to their anatomical location. The most common of these lie within the myometrium (intramural fibroids). Those located on the serosal or outer surface that extend outwards and deform the normal contour of the uterus are subserosal fibroids. These may also be pedunculated and only connected by a small stalk to the serosal surface (Fig. 16.7). Fibroids that develop near the inner surface of the endometrium distend the endometrium and extend into the endometrial cavity, either causing a distortion of the cavity or filling the cavity if they are pedunculated are submucous fibroids. Cervical fibroids are similar to other sites in the uterus. They are commonly pedunculated but may be sessile and grow to a size that will fill the vagina and distort the pelvic organs.

The size and site of the tumour have a considerable effect on the symptoms. Subserosal fibroids can put pressure on adjacent organs and cause bowel and bladder symptoms. Submucosal fibroids can lead to HMB and infertility. This HMB can be exceedingly heavy with submucous lesions. Cervical fibroids have symptoms similar to other cervical polyps, and in addition, during attempted extrusion, acute local pain can occur, as well as when there is degeneration of a fibroid or torsion of a pedunculated fibroid. Nowadays there is a strong recommendation to use the FIGO PALM-COEIN classification system (see later) to describe the location of individual fibroids and link these characteristics with symptoms.

The aetiology of fibroids is not well understood, although there is a significant genetic contribution. They are more common in women who are of Afro-Caribbean ethnicity, are overweight, are nulliparous, have polycystic ovary syndrome (PCOS), have diabetes, have hypertension and have a family history of fibroids. Pregnancy causes enlargement, and menopause is associated with some shrinkage.

Histopathology

Myomas consist of whorled masses of unstriated muscle cells, varying amounts of fibrous tissue and accompanying connective tissue. The main blood supply of a fibroid is localized within the pseudo-capsule around the outside of the main muscle mass, and it is these thin-walled venules which contribute to HMB.

Pathological changes

Fibroids can undergo a range of pathological changes, including hyaline degeneration, cystic degeneration, calcification, infection and abscess formation and necrobiosis. The latter, known as *red degeneration*, can occur in pregnancy or after treatment with embolization. Rarely, with an incidence of between 0.13% and 1%, sarcomatous change can occur.

Symptoms and signs

Some 50% of women with fibroids are asymptomatic, and the condition may only be discovered during routine pelvic examination: either at the time of cervical cytology or in the management of a pregnancy. Where symptoms do occur, they are often related to the site of the fibroids. The common presenting symptoms are as follows:

- *Abnormal uterine bleeding:* Submucous and intramural fibroids commonly cause HMB. Submucous fibroids may cause irregular vaginal bleeding, particularly if associated with overlying endometritis or if the surface of the fibroid becomes necrotic or ulcerated. Although a rare occurrence, submucous fibroids may prolapse through the cervix, resulting in profuse bleeding.
- *Pain:* Pelvic pain is a fairly common symptom that may occur in association with HMB. Acute pain is usually associated with torsion of the pedicle of a pedunculated fibroid, prolapse of a submucous fibroid through the cervix or the 'red degeneration' associated with pregnancy where haemorrhage occurs within the leiomyoma, causing an acute onset of pain.
- *Pressure symptoms:* A large mass of fibroids may become apparent because of palpable enlargement of the abdomen or because of pressure on the bladder or rectum. Women may describe reduced bladder capacity with urinary frequency and nocturia. A posterior-wall fibroid exerting pressure on the rectosigmoid can cause constipation or tenesmus.
- *Complications of pregnancy:* Recurrent miscarriage is more common in women with submucous fibroids. Fibroids tend to enlarge in pregnancy and are more likely to undergo red degeneration. A large fibroid in the pelvis may obstruct labour or make caesarean section more difficult. There is an increased chance of postpartum haemorrhage, and the presence of fibroids increases the risk of threatened pre-term labour and perinatal morbidity.

- *Infertility:* Obvious fibroids are found in 3% of women with infertility, but ultrasound scanning demonstrates a substantially higher number. The proportion increases greatly with age (up to 50% by the age of menopause). Up to 30% of women with uterine fibroids will have difficulty conceiving. Submucous and intramural fibroids are more likely to impair infertility than subserous ones. The mechanism may be mediated by mechanical, hormonal and local molecular regulatory factor effects.

The diagnosis can usually be confirmed by transvaginal ultrasound scans of the pelvis. However, a solid ovarian tumour may occasionally be mistaken for a subserous fibroid, and a fibroid undergoing cystic degeneration may mimic an ovarian cyst.

Management

Most fibroids are asymptomatic and do not require treatment. In symptomatic women the choice of approach may be dictated by factors such as the patient's desire for future fertility, the importance of uterine preservation, symptom severity and tumour characteristics.

Medical treatment

The oral contraceptive pill, progestogens and non-steroidal anti-inflammatory drugs (NSAIDs) have no effect on the size of fibroids but may be of value in controlling menstrual loss. A reduction of up to 45% in size can be achieved using gonadotrophin-releasing hormone (GnRH) analogues. However, the long-term use of these drugs is limited by their effect on bone density, and the fibroids return to their original size when treatment is stopped. The progesterone receptor modulator mifepristone has been found to be effective in reducing blood loss and fibroid size over a 6-month period, but there is still a lack of long-term data to support its use. Other selective progesterone receptor modulators, such as ulipristal, may also have a role, but their utility awaits the outcome of clinical trials, formal marketing and the clarification of potential side effects and rare hepatotoxicity.

Uterine artery embolization

Uterine artery embolization (UAE) involves the catheterization of the uterine arteries via the femoral artery and the injection of polyvinyl particles to reduce the blood supply to the uterus and to the fibroids. The fibroid shrinks because of ischaemia. The advantages of this technique are that it avoids the risks of major surgery and allows the preservation of fertility, although there is evidence that fertility can be impaired and that in those women who do conceive, there may be an increased chance of an adverse pregnancy outcome. Impairment of fertility may be associated with a small risk of ovarian damage from the embolization. The side effects of UAE include pain from uterine ischaemia and risk of sepsis in the degenerating fibroid. At present its use is recommended only in selected cases.

Surgical treatment

Where the preservation of reproductive function is not important, the surgical treatment of choice is hysterectomy. Indeed, fibroids account for about a third of all hysterectomies in the UK. In younger women or where the preservation of reproductive function is important, the removal of fibroids by surgical excision or myomectomy is indicated. This procedure involves incision of the pseudocapsule of the fibroid, enucleation of the bulk of the tumour and closure of the cavity by interrupted absorbable sutures. Myomectomy is associated with similar morbidity to hysterectomy. There may be haematoma formation in the cavity of the excised fibroid if care is not taken with surgical haemostasis. It is also impossible to be certain that all fibroids are removed without causing excessive uterine damage; there is always a possibility that residual seedling fibroids may regrow.

 Recurrence of fibroids occurs within 5 years in up to 60% of cases after myomectomy.

Endoscopic resection of many submucous fibroids can be performed using the hysteroresectoscope, and resection of subserous and intramural myomas can often be accomplished using laparoscopic techniques. In skilled hands, these procedures tend to be associated with lower morbidity and recurrence rate compared to open procedures. If the fibroid is more than 3 cm in diameter, pre- or perioperative measures such as the use of GnRH analogues can used to reduce the size of the fibroid prior to surgery.

Treatments in development

Clinical trials have shown that magnetic resonance imaging (MRI)–guided, focused ultrasound (that is only available in a few centres), which utilizes directed energy to heat and destroy the fibroid, is a potentially less invasive treatment option. The method requires treatment of one fibroid at a time and cannot be used for the management of pedunculated fibroids. Pregnancy is not recommended after the procedure, and long-term data are lacking.

Adenomyosis

Adenomyosis is a condition characterized by the invasion of endometrial glands and stroma into myometrium with surrounding smooth muscle hyperplasia. It probably affects around 5–10% of women and until recently the diagnosis was most commonly made only after histological assessment of tissue removed at hysterectomy. Diagnosis

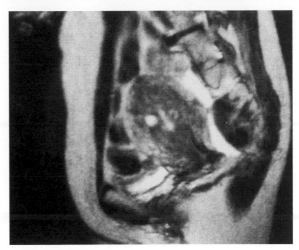

Fig. 16.8 Sagittal view using magnetic resonance imaging of a uterus enlarged by adenomyosis.

is now being made increasingly frequently with modern ultrasound equipment, increasing skills of the operators in recognizing the features or using MRI.

Symptoms and signs

This condition, unlike endometriosis, typically occurs in parous women and is usually diagnosed in the fourth decade. It is associated with HMB and dysmenorrhoea of increasing severity. On clinical examination, the uterus is symmetrically enlarged and tender. The condition regresses after menopause.

Pathology

The macroscopic appearances of the uterus are those of diffuse enlargement. Adenomyosis and myomas often co-exist, although the uterus is rarely enlarged to the size seen in the presence of myomas. The posterior wall of the uterus is usually thicker than the anterior wall. The cut surface of the uterus presents a characteristic, whorl-like, trabeculated appearance, but occasionally circumscribed nodules with dark haemorrhagic spots can be seen in the myometrium.

Both transvaginal ultrasound and MRI show high levels of accuracy for the non-invasive diagnosis of moderate to severe adenomyosis, but MRI is the most sensitive technique (Fig. 16.8). The microscopic diagnosis is based on the presence of a poorly circumscribed area of endometrial glands and stroma invading the smooth muscle layers of the myometrium. The International Federation of Gynecology and Obstetrics (FIGO) and others are developing improved classifications of different degrees and characteristics for improved management.

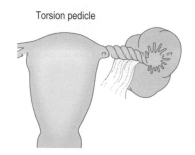
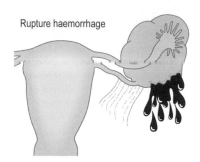

Fig. 16.9 Common complications of ovarian tumours that precipitate a request for medical advice.

Treatment

Adenomyosis can be managed conservatively with medical treatment, with UAE or surgically. Both medical and surgical approaches to treatment are controversial. Medical therapy, as for endometriosis, is effective in some cases, and symptomatic relief of dysmenorrhoea and heavy bleeding can best be obtained with insertion of a levonorgestrel-releasing intrauterine system. Prostaglandin synthetase inhibitors may sometimes help. UAE is often an effective alternative. Hysterectomy is the surgical procedure of choice, although less invasive techniques whereby the area of adenomyosis is specifically excised can sometimes be undertaken in specialized units with experienced endoscopic surgeons. Other new techniques that may gain credence include high-intensity focused ultrasound to thermally ablate the adenomyotic foci.

Lesions of the ovary

Ovarian enlargement is commonly asymptomatic, and the silent nature of malignant ovarian tumours is the major reason for the advanced stage of presentation of this cancer. Ovarian tumours may be cystic or solid, functional, benign or malignant. There are common factors in the presentation and complications of ovarian tumours, and it is often difficult to establish the nature of a tumour without direct pathological examination. The diagnosis and management of ovarian neoplasms are discussed in more detail in Chapter 20.

Symptoms

Tumours of the ovary that are less than 10 cm in diameter rarely produce symptoms. The common presenting symptoms include:

- Abdominal enlargement: in the presence of malignant change, this may also be associated with ascites.
- Symptoms from pressure on surrounding structures such as the bladder and rectum.

- Symptoms relating to complications of the tumour (Fig. 16.9); these include:
  - **Torsion:** acute torsion of the ovarian pedicle results in necrosis of the tumour; there is acute pain and vomiting followed by remission of the pain when the tumour has become necrotic.
  - **Rupture:** the contents of the cyst spill into the peritoneal cavity and result in generalized abdominal pain.
  - **Haemorrhage** into the tumour is an unusual complication but may result in abdominal pain and shock if the blood loss is severe.
  - **Hormone-secreting tumours** may present with disturbances in the menstrual cycle. In androgen-secreting tumours, the patient may present with signs of virilization. Although a greater proportion of the sex-cord stromal type of tumour (see later) are hormonally active, the commonest type of secreting tumour found in clinical practice is the epithelial type.

Signs

On examination, the abdomen may be visibly enlarged. Percussion over the swelling will demonstrate central dullness and resonance in the flanks. These signs may be obscured by gross ascites. Small tumours can be detected on pelvic examination and will be found by palpation in one or both fornices. However, as the tumour enlarges, it assumes a more central position and, in the case of dermoid cysts, is often anterior to the uterus. Most ovarian tumours are not tender to palpation; if they are painful, the presence of infection or torsion should be suspected. Benign ovarian tumours are palpable separately from the uterine body and are usually freely mobile.

Endometriosis

Endometriosis is a disease characterized by the presence of extrauterine endometrial-like tissue consisting of glands

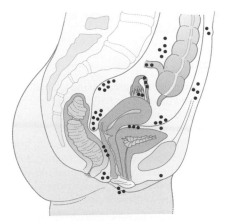

Fig. 16.10 Common sites of endometriotic deposits.

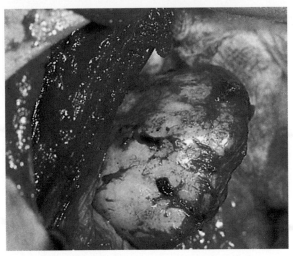

Fig. 16.11 Endometriotic patches on the surface of the ovary.

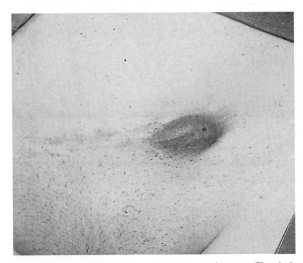

Fig. 16.12 Endometriosis in a caesarean section scar. The dark tender mass at the left of the wound becomes tender and enlarged during menstruation.

and stroma, often infiltrated by an inflammatory response. This is clearly an inflammatory condition. It affects between 5% and 15% of reproductive-age women. In women presenting with pelvic pain or infertility, or in adolescents with severe dysmenorrhoea or chronic pelvic pain, the prevalence is significantly higher. Women suffering from endometriosis very often present with a complex of debilitating symptoms, including pelvic pain, dyspareunia, dysuria, dyschezia and dysmenorrhoea. Although benign, endometriosis causes a substantial burden to the woman's health, partly because of an average delay of 8–10 years between the onset of the symptoms and diagnosis. If undiagnosed, the condition can progress in severity and result in many years of untreated or ineffectively treated pelvic pain.

Pathophysiology

Aberrant endometriotic deposits occur in many different sites (Fig. 16.10). Endometriosis commonly occurs in the ovaries (Fig. 16.11), the uterosacral ligaments and the rectovaginal septum. It may also occur in the pelvic peritoneum covering the uterus, tubes, rectum, sigmoid colon and bladder. Remote ectopic deposits of endometriotic tissue may occasionally be found in the umbilicus, laparotomy scars (Fig. 16.12), hernial scars, the appendix, vagina, vulva, cervix, lymph nodes and, on rare occasions, the pleural cavity.

Nowadays, endometriosis is usually recognized to present in one or more of three phenotypes, peritoneal surface lesions (superficial or deep), ovarian surface or deep cystic endometriomas, or as deep pelvic lesions, especially in the rectovaginal septum.

Ovarian endometriosis occurs in the form of small superficial deposits on the surface of the ovary or as larger cysts known as *endometriomas* (Fig. 16.13), which may grow up to 10 cm in size. These cysts have a thick, whitish capsular layer and contain altered blood, which has a chocolate-like appearance. For this reason, they are known as *chocolate*

cysts. Endometriomas are often densely adherent both to the ovarian tissue and to other surrounding structures.

These cysts may leak or occasionally rupture, and in 8% of cases, patients with endometriosis present with symptoms of acute peritoneal irritation.

The microscopic features of the lesions may be of endometrium (Fig. 16.14) that cannot be distinguished from the normal tissue lining the uterine cavity, but there is wide variation, and in many long-standing cases, desquamation and repeated menstrual bleeding may result in the loss of all characteristic features of endometrium. Underneath the lining of the cyst, there is often a broad zone containing

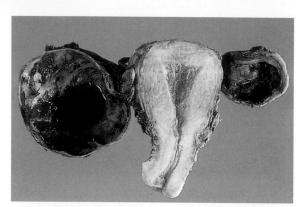

Fig. 16.13 Bilateral endometriomas removed at hysterectomy.

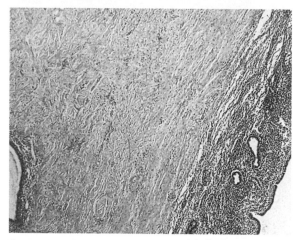

Fig. 16.14 High-powered magnification showing active epithelial lining of the cavity of an endometriotic deposit in scar tissue.

phagocytic cells with haemosiderin. There is also a broad zone of hyalinized fibrous tissue. One of the characteristics of endometriotic lesions is the intense fibrotic reaction that surrounds them, and this may also contain muscle fibres. The intensity of this reaction often leads to great difficulty in dissection at the time of any operative procedure. The pathogenesis of endometriosis remains obscure, although a genetic component is frequently recognized. There is a great deal of ongoing research geared to improve the accuracy of diagnosis and assessment of this disease.

Sampson (1921) originally suggested that the condition was associated with retrograde spill of endometrial cells during menstruation and that some of these cells would implant under appropriate conditions in the peritoneal cavity and on the ovaries. This hypothesis does not account for endometriotic deposits outside the peritoneal cavity. An alternative theory suggests that endometrial lesions may arise from metaplastic changes in epithelium surfaces throughout the body.

Diagnosis

The initial assessment involves taking a detailed history of the duration and nature of pelvic pain with attention to the relationship to the menstrual cycle, the presence of bowel and bladder symptoms, the presence of dyspareunia and the impact of posture and movement on pain. Initial investigations may include urinalysis, screening for sexually transmitted infections and a transvaginal ultrasound scan. The ultrasound, if performed in expert hands, has a high degree of sensitivity and specificity for diagnosing ovarian endometriotic cysts and deep infiltrating bowel endometriosis but is of little use in identifying the commoner types of peritoneal disease. As there is no consistently reliable non-invasive test, diagnostic laparoscopy by an experienced gynaecological endoscopist remains the best way of confirming or excluding most types of endometriosis.

Management

Endometriosis is a chronic disease that often requires life-long management. Medical treatment involves suppression of ovulation (and ovarian oestrogen secretion) and creating a steady hormone environment. Commonly used medication includes oral progestogens, progestogen subdermal implants and/or the levonorgestrel intrauterine system. Combined oral contraceptive pills are widely used, but it does not make logical sense to use an oestrogen-containing preparation in a woman with an oestrogen-sensitive disease. However, modern pills have a high progestogen balance and may work well. These medications are all generally well tolerated and are initially preferable to alternatives such as danazol, GnRH agonists and aromatase inhibitors. Medical therapy needs to be integrated with use of surgical therapies.

Surgical management of endometriosis usually involves complete excision of visible lesions. This is preferable to attempted diathermy ablation of the lesions and reduces pain and improves quality of life in 67–80% of operated patients. To prevent recurrences, preventive medical therapy after surgery should always be considered, unless pregnancy is immediately desired. Deep infiltrating pelvic endometriosis that involves the sigmoid colon or rectum requires a multidisciplinary approach with a colorectal surgeon. Laparoscopic resection of the rectovaginal endometritic nodule by a 'shaving technique' with reconstruction by expert laparoscopic gynaecologists is increasingly practised instead of bowel resection and anastomosis.

There is usually amelioration of endometriosis symptoms during pregnancy, and there may sometimes be long-term improvement in pain after pregnancy. However, many women with endometriosis will experience recurrence of symptoms as soon as pregnancy and breast-feeding have been completed.

Abnormal uterine bleeding

AUB is any bleeding disturbance that occurs during or between menstrual periods, or that is excessive, frequent or prolonged. This is the overarching term to describe any significant disturbance of menstruation or the menstrual cycle. FIGO has recently designed a classification system and precise terminologies for underlying causes of AUB – The FIGO AUB Systems. These recommend that causes can be grouped under categories using the acronym PALM COEIN (Table 16.1). The most common menstrual abnormalities are intermenstrual (often associated with PCB) and heavy or irregular menstrual bleeding.

The FIGO classification is a very useful and flexible system, which can easily be used both for initial training in understanding underlying causes and for application to more complex specialized or research classifications.

Intermenstrual bleeding

IMB generally occurs between clearly defined, cyclical, regular menses.

The bleeding may occur at the same time in each cycle or may be random. This symptom is typically associated with surface lesions of the genital tract, and these women may also experience PCB. Undiagnosed pregnancy-related bleeding, including ectopic pregnancy and hydatidiform molar disease, may result in irregular bleeding mimicking IMB. In 1–2% of women, IMB may be physiological, with spotting occurring around the time of ovulation.

> ! IMB is commonly associated with the use of hormonal contraception (when it is known as *unscheduled* or *breakthrough bleeding*), particularly the combined oral contraceptive pill, intrauterine systems and use of progestogen-only methods, including the pills and implants.

In women with new onset of IMB, sexually transmitted infection of the cervix or vagina should be considered as a possible cause, especially *Chlamydia*. Less common causes are vaginitis (non-sexually transmitted), cervical ectropion, endometrial or cervical polyps, endometritis, adenomyosis, submucous myomas and sometimes cervical or endometrial cancers.

After a careful examination of the lower genital tract, the investigation of IMB should always exclude pregnancy

Table 16.1 FIGO recommendations on classification of causes underlying symptoms of abnormal uterine bleeding

	Examples
Structural lesions ('PALM')	
Polyps (endometrial, endocervical) **A**denomyosis **L**eiomyoma (uterine fibroids) **M**alignancy and hyperplasia	
Non-structural causes ('COEIN')	
Coagulopathies	Von Willebrand disease Platelet dysfunctions Rare clotting factor deficiencies Thrombocytopenia (low platelets)
Ovulatory dysfunction	Anovulatory or disturbed ovulatory cycles (disturbance of oestrogen positive feedback or other ovarian mechanisms) Polycystic ovary syndrome Thyroid disease
Endometrial primary causes	Errors of endometrial molecular pathways affecting local vascular function
Iatrogenic	A category including all causes from therapeutic or human interference. This includes AUB side effects of medicinal therapies, drugs or use of devices, e.g. IUCDs.
Not yet classified	Rare or novel causes which do not immediately or obviously fit into any of the other categories at this time. These may change with new research. Two examples of such conditions are uterine arteriovenous malformations, which can cause very heavy menstrual bleeding, or the novel diagnosis of 'isthmocoele' (the lower segment 'niche' frequently found following caesarean section).

AUB, Abnormal uterine bleeding; *FIGO*, The International Federation of Gynecology and Obstetrics; *IUCD*, intrauterine contraceptive device. Reproduced from Munro MG, Critchley HO, Fraser IS, et al. (2011) The FIGO classification system (PALM-COEIN) of causes of abnormal uterine bleeding in non-gravid women of reproductive age. Int J Gynecol Obstet 113:3–13.

and infection as a cause. Ensure that cervical screening is up to date, and if all these are negative, pelvic ultrasound or hysteroscopy may reveal an intrauterine cause.

Postcoital bleeding

PCB is non-menstrual bleeding that occurs during or after sexual intercourse. The symptom is reported by around 6% of women per year. Causes of PCB include surface lesions of the genital tract, typically infection; cervical or EPs; cervical, endometrial or (rarely) vaginal cancer; and trauma. PCB occurs in 1–39% of women with cervical cancer, and if there is a history of recurrent PCB, with or without IMB, colposcopy examination of the cervix is recommended even if the Pap smear is normal.

Postmenopausal bleeding

Vaginal bleeding that occurs more than 1 year after the last natural menstrual period is known as *postmenopausal bleeding*. Although it is not the commonest cause of this symptom, the possibility of carcinoma of the body of the uterus should be considered, and an assessment of the endometrium is advised for all women, whether with diagnostic hysteroscopy and endometrial biopsy or with a high-quality transvaginal ultrasound measurement of the endometrial thickness and appearance. When the endometrium is measured at less than 3 mm, significant endometrial pathology is very unlikely.

Other causes of postmenopausal bleeding include other benign and malignant tumours of the genital tract, stimulation of the endometrium by exogenous (or endogenous) oestrogen (e.g. hormone replacement therapy [HRT] and oestrogens from ovarian tumours), infection and postmenopausal atrophic vaginitis.

Heavy menstrual bleeding

HMB, defined in research studies as more than 80 mL per month of loss, affects approximately 10% of women. The recommended 'clinical' definition of HMB (for use in the clinic) is 'excessive menstrual loss leading to interference with the physical, emotional, social and material quality of life of a woman, and which occurs alone or in combination with other symptoms'. HMB should be recognized as having a major impact on a woman's quality of life. Although HMB is usually caused by benign conditions, it commonly leads to iron deficiency or iron-deficiency anaemia, which can be part of the serious impact on a woman's social, family and working life (through the burden of managing the practical difficulties of excessive blood loss and having to curb normal activities). HMB can commonly arise from an imbalance in the clotting and other regulatory molecular factors at a local endometrial level, without the presence of obvious structural pathology. However, it also can be associated with a number of benign gynaecological conditions, including leiomyomata, EPs, adenomyosis, endometrial hyperplasia and sometimes endometrial cancer. The causes of HMB include most of the overall causes of AUB.

Causes

Structural lesions (PALM component of the FIGO classification of causes)

Leiomyomata (discussed later) are the commonest structural lesions to cause heavy regular bleeding, although most women with fibroids do not experience abnormal loss. Endometrial carcinoma is rare under the age of 40 years and is more likely initially to cause irregular bleeding. Adenomyosis is usually associated with a uniformly enlarged tender uterus, HMB and dysmenorrhoea. EPs are a common cause of HMB but usually also cause IMB. Endometrial hyperplasia is a common structural lesion causing HMB and may be associated with irregular, anovulatory cycles. It may be a premalignant condition. It may overlap with the disturbed ovulation discussed in the next section.

Non-structural conditions (COEIN component of the FIGO classification)

Disturbed ovulation or anovulation can result in very irregular, especially infrequent, cycles with prolonged, heavy and irregular bleeding of such severity that it may occasionally be life threatening. In this situation, unopposed oestrogen often leads to the endometrium becoming greatly thickened and hyperplastic. This unstable endometrium eventually breaks down in a patchy and erratic fashion. Most ovulatory disorders occur in the menopause transition and in adolescence or can be traced to endocrinopathies, e.g. PCOS and hypothyroidism.

When there is regular heavy bleeding with no underlying structural lesion, HMB is usually the result of a primary endometrial disorder where the mechanisms regulating local endometrial 'haemostasis' are disturbed. There may be excessive local production of fibrinolytic factors (especially tissue plasminogen activator), deficiencies in local production of vasoconstrictors and increased local production of substances that promote vasodilation. The commonest iatrogenic cause of heavy bleeding is the presence of a copper-bearing intrauterine contraceptive device (IUCD).

History and examination

An accurate history is essential to establish the pattern of bleeding and the duration of symptoms. Clinical estimation of the degree of blood loss is very subjective, although the presence of clots, the need to change sanitary protection at night and 'flooding' (the soiling of bedclothes or underwear during menstruation) are more likely to indicate significant bleeding. A recent change in the pattern of menstruation and associated pain are more likely to be associated with the development of structural pelvic pathology. Pain is typically associated with adenomyosis and chronic pelvic inflammatory disease (PID). Women are more likely to complain of HMB if the bleeding is accompanied by pain. Endometriosis sometimes causes HMB (as well as pain). Structural surface lesions of the uterus and cervix more typically cause IMB and PCB. Endometrial malignancy is rare under the age of 40 years, but women with a history of diabetes, hypertension, PCOS and obesity are at increased risk of endometrial hyperplasia and carcinoma.

Women with heavy periods should have a general examination for signs of anaemia and thyroid disease and a pelvic examination, including cervical screening test, if indicated. The finding of a pelvic mass on pelvic examination is most likely to indicate the presence of uterine leiomyomata (fibroids) but may indicate a uterine malignancy, adenomyosis or ovarian tumour.

Investigations

A full blood count with platelets (and sometimes serum ferritin and serum transferrin receptor saturation to assess iron status) is the only investigation needed before starting treatment, provided that clinical examination is normal. It should be remembered that iron deficiency is the commonest deficiency disease worldwide. Patients should be referred for further investigation if:

- There is a history of repeated or persistent irregular or IMB or of risk factors for endometrial carcinoma.
- The cervical screening test is abnormal.
- Pelvic examination is abnormal.
- There is significant pelvic pain unresponsive to simple analgesia.
- They do not respond to first-line treatment after 6 months.

Additional investigation is mainly to confirm or exclude the presence of pelvic pathology and in particular of endometrial malignancy. The main methods of investigation are ultrasound, endometrial biopsy, hysteroscopy and transvaginal ultrasound (with or without saline sonohysterography). Investigations for systemic causes of abnormal menstruation, such as a partial coagulation screen for the disorders of haemostasis – a coagulopathy – (of which mild von Willebrand disease is the commonest of these causes associated with HMB), are only indicated if a screening history for coagulopathies is suggestive or in young women. Thyroid disease is a rare cause of HMB, and investigation is only indicated if there are other features on examination or a previous history. Endometrial biopsy can be performed as an outpatient procedure either alone or in conjunction with hysteroscopy.

Hysteroscopy allows visualization of the uterine cavity using a 3-mm endoscope introduced through the cervix. It can be performed under general anaesthetic or as an outpatient investigation using local anaesthesia. Hysteroscopy with endometrial biopsy has largely replaced the traditional and unreliable blind D&C. Transvaginal ultrasound is of value in distinguishing the structural lesions of the genital tract. In premenopausal women, ultrasound-measured endometrial thickness will vary at different times of the menstrual cycle, but it is usually possible to visualize structural lesions such as polyps in the endometrial cavity.

Management

Medical treatment

In the absence of malignancy, the treatment chosen will depend on whether contraception is required, whether irregularity of the cycle is a problem and the presence of contraindications to certain treatments. Where a copper IUD is in place, mefenamic or tranexamic acid can be used, or the device may be replaced by a levonorgestrel intrauterine system (Mirena).

Non-hormonal treatments

NSAIDs, such as mefenamic acid or ibuprofen, inhibit prostaglandin synthetase enzymes. They reduce blood loss by around 30%, and their analgesic properties may be an advantage if there is associated dysmenorrhoea. The principal side effect is mild gastrointestinal irritation. Tranexamic acid is an anti-fibrinolytic agent that reduces blood loss by about 50%. It is safe and available over the counter without prescription in many countries. It does not cause venous thrombosis, but it is wise to avoid its use in patients with a previous history of thromboembolic disease. Both groups of drugs have the advantage of only needing to be taken during menstruation.

Hormonal treatments

Use of the combined oral contraceptive pill or the levonorgestrel intrauterine system is associated with around 30% and 90% reduction in average monthly blood loss, respectively (Fig. 16.15). The levonorgestrel-releasing intrauterine system is widely recommended as the first choice for medical therapy of HMB in those women who do not have contraindications to its use. Synthetic oral progestogens, such as norethisterone or medroxyprogesterone acetate, can be given for 21 days out of 28 over prolonged periods to effectively control irregular, heavy bleeding but do tend to be associated with a higher incidence of nuisance-value side effects. They can also be used in higher doses in an acute situation to control severe HMB (oral norethisterone 5 mg, or medroxyprogesterone acetate 10 mg, three times daily for 21 days). Danazol is a synthetic, mild impeded androgen derivative that acts

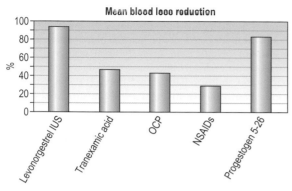

Fig. 16.15 Mean percentage reduction in measured blood loss with different therapies in women with heavy menstrual bleeding due to non-structural causes. *IUS*, Intrauterine system; *OCP*, Oral Contraceptive Pill ; *NSAIDs*, non-steroidal anti-inflammatory drugs.

on the hypothalamic–pituitary axis and endometrium and is uncommonly used nowadays. Given at high doses, it will normally cause amenorrhoea but is associated with significant side effects in 10% of patients. The efficacy of various medical therapies in reducing HMB is documented in Figure 16.15.

Surgical treatment

Endometrial resection or ablation

The endometrium can be removed or destroyed using an operating hysteroscope or with a number of modern third-generation intrauterine heating or cooling devices that ablate the endometrium. The first- and second-generation techniques involve using laser or diathermy resection with a wire loop or coagulation with a rollerball or a combination of the two (Fig. 16.16). The endometrium can be thinned prior to treatment with danazol or GnRH analogues for 4–8 weeks before surgery, allowing for more effective ablation. The uterine cavity is distended with an irrigation fluid such as glycine or normal saline. There is a rare risk of intraoperative uterine perforation and possibly damage to other organs requiring laparotomy and repair. The other potential complication is fluid overload from excessive absorption of the irrigation fluid. Hysteroscopic procedures have now been largely replaced by newer semi-automatic techniques that do not require the same hysteroscopic skills. Balloon ablation involves inserting a fluid-filled balloon into the endometrial cavity, which is then very precisely heated so that it destroys the entire endometrium. A range of other devices are available, which are all based on the principle of excessively heating or cooling the endometrium using different energy sources so that it is very precisely destroyed without damaging adjacent structures. Around 30–70% of patients will become amenorrhoeic, with a further 20–30% achieving major reduction in HMB. A minority of patients will eventually need further surgery and hysterectomy.

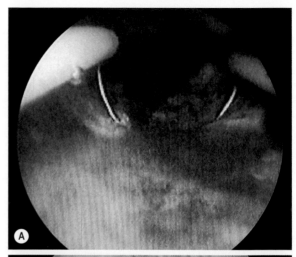
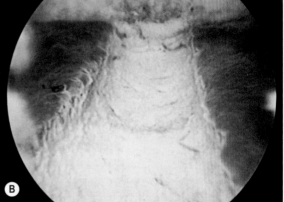

Fig. 16.16 Endometrial resection. View of the uterine cavity (A) before and (B) after excision using a resectoscope.

Hysterectomy

This remains the definitive treatment and is more likely to be appropriate for those women with pelvic pathology, such as adenomyosis and fibroids, than medical treatment or endoscopic surgery. Hysterectomy is associated with a mortality of around 1 in 2000, although the mortality for women with benign gynaecological diseases should be less. Significant complications occur in 25–40% of patients and tend to be more common in patients undergoing abdominal hysterectomy. Intraoperative bleeding is the major concern, and intraoperative precautions should always be taken to minimize postoperative venous thromboembolism. The commonest postoperative complications are infections (urinary, respiratory or at the operation sites), but any postoperative complication may occasionally occur in individual cases. Hysterectomy can be undertaken abdominally, vaginally or laparoscopically.

Abdominal hysterectomy is carried out through a transverse lower abdominal or midline incision. The round ligaments, Fallopian tubes and ovarian vessels are cut and ligated on each side, either medial or distal to the ovaries, depending on whether these are to be conserved (see later). The uterovesical peritoneum is opened, and the bladder is reflected off the lower part of the uterus and cervix so as to displace the ureters away from the uterine vessels, which are then cut and ligated. Finally, the transverse cervical ligaments are cut and the vagina opened around the cervix, allowing removal of the uterus. If there has been no history of cervical disease, the cervix can be conserved by removing the uterine corpus just below the internal os after the uterine vessels have been ligated (*subtotal hysterectomy*). This may be indicated if other pelvic disease makes dissection of the cervix difficult in order to reduce the risk of ureteric damage or because of patient preference. Radical abdominal hysterectomy involves removing the uterus, cervix, upper vagina and supporting tissues and is performed when there is known uterine or cervical cancer.

In *vaginal hysterectomy* (with approach through the vaginal introitus), the vaginal skin is opened around the cervix and the bladder and reflected up into the pelvis. The peritoneum over the uterovesical and rectovaginal space is opened, and the cervical ligaments are clamped, cut and ligated. The uterine and ovarian vessels are clamped and ligated, the uterus is removed and the peritoneum and vaginal skin are closed. Removal of the ovaries is possible but is less commonly carried out by this route. The absence of an abdominal wound substantially reduces postoperative morbidity, making this the method of choice for most cases of hysterectomy. It is contraindicated where malignancy is suspected. Other relative contraindications include a uterine size of over 14 weeks, the presence of endometriosis and in women who require concurrent removal of the diseased ovaries.

Laparoscopic hysterectomy involves dividing and occluding or fixing the attachments of the uterus under direct visualization through the laparoscope and then removing the uterus either vaginally or through the abdominal ports after reducing it to strips (morcellation). Laparoscopic hysterectomy by a skilled endoscopist is the best approach to hysterectomy when a vaginal hysterectomy cannot be performed because of the presence of diseases such as endometriosis, adhesions or when the ovaries need be removed.

Conservation of the ovaries, if normal, is usually recommended for women under the age of 50 years undergoing hysterectomy for HMB to avoid the onset of a surgically induced early menopause. For women near menopause, this advantage has to be offset against the small possible risk of later ovarian malignancy, and the option of oophorectomy should be discussed. Family history of ovarian cancer is usually considered in this decision.

Secondary amenorrhoea and oligomenorrhoea

Secondary amenorrhoea is defined as the cessation of menses for 6 or more months in a woman who has previously menstruated. Oligomenorrhoea is the occurrence of five or fewer menstrual periods over 12 months. In practice, the distinction between the two can be somewhat arbitrary, as they share many of the same causes.

Aetiology
Physiological

Physiological causes, including pregnancy and lactation, account for most cases of amenorrhoea in the reproductive years. Breast-feeding causes a rise in prolactin, which inhibits GnRH release and prevents normal ovarian stimulation. The duration of amenorrhoea depends on the extent, frequency and length of time of breast-feeding.

Pathological

Pathological causes can be divided into disorders of the hypothalamus, anterior pituitary, ovary and genital tract (Fig. 16.17).

Hypothalamic disorders

Functional hypothalamic amenorrhoea (FHA) is defined as a non-organic and reversible disorder in which the impairment of GnRH pulsatile secretion plays a key role. There are three types of FHA: weight loss–related amenorrhoea, stress-related amenorrhoea and exercise-related amenorrhoea. FHA is characterized by low or normal levels of follicle-stimulating hormone (FSH) and luteinizing hormone (LH), normal prolactin levels, normal imaging of the pituitary fossa and hypo-oestrogenism.

There is a critical relationship between body weight and menstruation. A loss of body weight of 10–15% of normal weight for height is likely to cause oligomenorrhoea or amenorrhoea. This may result from vigorous dieting, or it may be a manifestation of *anorexia nervosa*, a psychiatric condition characterized by disturbed body image and an intense fear of weight gain even in those already underweight. Those affected strive to reduce their body mass through intense exercising and limiting their food intake or inducing vomiting after meals. Secondary amenorrhoea of 3 months' duration forms part of the basic criteria for diagnosis of the condition in women.

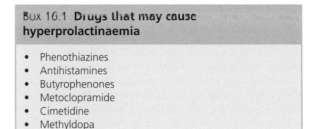

Fig. 16.17 Causes of secondary amenorrhoea. *FSH*, Follicle-stimulating hormone; *GnRH*, gonadotrophin-releasing hormone; *LH*, luteinizing hormone; *PIF*, prolactin-inhibiting factor; *PRL*, prolactin.

Women who participate in sports that require strenuous training, such as long-distance running or gymnastics, or ballet dancing, may develop secondary amenorrhoea (exercise-related amenorrhoea). Several factors combine to contribute to this FHA, including low body fat, psychological and physical stress and high energy expenditure.

Emotional stress from change in work, family, housing or relationship situations can also result in FHA. Individuals who cope less well with stress seem to release higher cortisol levels and are more prone to FHA.

> ✔ Although the combined oral contraceptive pill causes suppression of the hypothalamic–pituitary–ovarian axis, there is no evidence that this persists when the pill is discontinued.

Pituitary disorders

The pituitary causes of secondary amenorrhoea are most commonly the result of high prolactin levels. Around 40% of cases are associated with a prolactin-secreting tumour of the anterior pituitary (microadenoma or macroadenoma), and secretion of breast milk (*galactorrhoea*) occurs in about one-third of patients. All patients with secondary amenorrhoea should have a prolactin estimation and, if the levels are abnormally raised, imaging of the pituitary fossa with computed tomography (CT) or MRI. Pituitary microadenomas are common, but macroadenomas are rare and usually present to an endocrinologist because of associated endocrine effects. Growth of a macroadenoma may cause bitemporal hemianopia as a result of compression of the optic chiasma, but this and other cranial nerve compressions are unusual findings.

The release of prolactin from the anterior pituitary is inhibited by the neurotransmitter dopamine. Drugs with anti-dopaminergic effects (Box 16.1) will result in iatrogenically elevated prolactin levels and amenorrhoea.

Rarely (in high-resource countries), pituitary amenorrhoea may result from postpartum necrosis of the anterior pituitary from severe obstetric haemorrhage and hypotension (Sheehan's syndrome).

Ovarian disorders

Ovarian failure

Premature ovarian failure (POF) is usually defined as the cessation of ovarian function before the age of 40 and is characterized by amenorrhoea and raised gonadotrophin levels. It affects 1% of women and is most often non-reversible. Genetic factors play an important role, and 20–30% of women with POF have an affected relative. A range of genetic syndromes lead to POF, of which Turner's syndrome is the most obvious. Autoimmune oophoritis is found in around 4% of women who present with spontaneous POF. This condition is most often associated with autoantibodies to multiple endocrine and other organs but has also been seen in women with systemic lupus erythematosus and myasthenia gravis.

Surgical removal of the ovaries or destruction by radiation or infection inevitably results in secondary amenorrhoea. All these conditions are characterized by high levels of gonadotrophins and hypo-oestrogenism (*hypergonadotropic hypogonadism*). Rare ovarian neoplasms, particularly those associated with excessive, abnormal production of oestrogen or testosterone, may cause amenorrhoea but constitute only a very small percentage of known causes.

Polycystic ovary syndrome

PCOS affects 5–10% of reproductive-age women and is associated with 75% of all anovulatory disorders causing infertility and with 90% of women with oligomenorrhoea (Box 16.2). PCOS is found in women with symptoms of androgen excess: in 90% of women with hirsutism and 80% of women with acne. Approximately 50% of women with the condition are overweight or obese. PCOS was first described by American gynaecologists Irving Stein and Michael Leventhal in 1935, who noticed the association between polycystic ovaries, amenorrhoea and hirsutism. The ovaries in PCOS appear enlarged and contain multiple (more than 10–12), small (less than 10 mm) fluid-filled structures just under the ovarian capsule. These are small, normal antral and atretic follicles and are not true 'cysts'. They are present in much greater numbers than are present in the normal ovary, but they have the same functions as normal (Fig. 16.18). The polycystic ovary also has a greatly increased ovarian stroma, which may have abnormal endocrine properties.

The presence of polycystic ovaries on ultrasound is very common, and around 25% of women in the population may have such appearances. Only a small proportion of these women will have the polycystic ovary *syndrome* (which comprises polycystic ovary appearances on ultrasound, associated with at least one of the androgenic or ovulation symptoms).

Biochemical investigations (Fig. 16.19) indicate abnormally raised LH levels and absence of the LH surge. Oestrogen and FSH levels are normal and, as a result, there is an increase in the LH:FSH ratio. There may be increased ovarian secretion of testosterone, androstenedione and dehydroepiandrosterone. Prolactin levels are increased in 15% of cases.

Pathogenesis. The exact aetiology of PCOS is unknown, but there is a strong genetic component. The primary disorder may be abnormalities in androgen biosynthesis and insulin resistance. As a result of insulin resistance and hyperlipidaemia, women with PCOS are prone to developing non–insulin-dependent diabetes and are at greater risk of metabolic syndrome. Many women with PCOS have

---

Box 16.2 Features of polycystic ovarian syndrome

Oligomenorrhoea/amenorrhoea Hirsutism/acne Obesity Infertility	} Abnormal androgen production
Ultrasound – ovaries Polycystic ovaries; the presence of 12 or more follicles in either ovary measuring 2–9 mm in diameter and/or increased ovarian volume (>10 mL)	{ Size >8 cm 8 ovarian cysts <8 mm in diameter Echogenic ovarian stroma

---

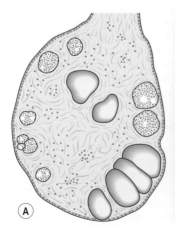 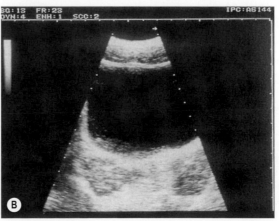

Fig. 16.18 Polycystic ovaries. (A) The capsule of the ovary is thickened and there are numerous small cysts in the ovarian cortex. (B) Ultrasound showing mottled appearance of both ovaries characteristic of multiple small cysts.

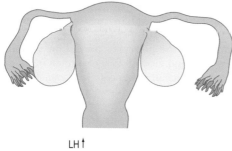

LH ↑
LH surge absent
Δ^4-androstenedione ↑
Dehydroepiandrosterone ↑
Normal oestradiol levels
Normal FSH levels

Fig. 16.19 Biochemical features of Stein–Leventhal syndrome. *FSH*, Follicle-stimulating hormone; *LH*, luteinizing hormone.

substantial obesity. Inappropriate exposure of antral follicles to excessive concentrations of androgens results in inhibition of FSH release and may result in the 'polycystic' changes in the ovaries. The primary source of androgens may be both the ovary and/or the adrenals. The excretion of dehydroepiandrosterone sulphate – an exclusively adrenal steroid – is elevated in up to 50% of all women with PCOS. The principal androgens raised in PCOS and produced by the ovary include testosterone and androstenedione. Their production is significantly increased by insulin and insulin-like growth factors. They will not be suppressed by adrenal steroids but can be suppressed by GnRH agonists. About 10% of women with PCOS have type 2 diabetes, and 30% have impaired glucose tolerance.

Diagnosis. Diagnosis (and criteria for the definition) is controversial. An international consensus meeting in Rotterdam proposed the following definition of PCOS, which has been widely adopted.

Any two of the following three are sufficient to confirm the diagnosis:

1. Oligoovulation or anovulation
2. Hyperandrogenism (biochemical or clinical)
3. Polycystic ovaries on ultrasound examination

Uterine causes

Surgical removal of the uterus will result in secondary amenorrhoea. Other conditions that scar the endometrium and cause intrauterine adhesions and loss of menses include infection from tuberculosis and Asherman's syndrome. The latter occurs mostly following dilatation and sharp curettage procedures for postpartum haemorrhage with retained, adherent placental fragments; where there has been damage to the full depth of endometrium by the sharp curettage; and where there is concurrent low-grade endometrial infection.

Cryptomenorrhoea (literally 'hidden menstruation')

Cervical stenosis from surgical procedures or infection can cause blockage of menses through obstruction of outflow.

Investigations in women with amenorrhoea or oligomenorrhoea

The possibility of pregnancy should always be considered and, if necessary, excluded by pregnancy test. The history should include details of recent emotional stress, changes in weight, menopausal symptoms and current medication. In the majority of cases, nothing abnormal is found on clinical examination, although a body mass index (BMI) of less than $19\,kg/m^2$ is likely to be associated with weight-related amenorrhoea. In the absence of clinical evidence of thyroid or adrenal diseases, it is unusual to find biochemical evidence. The differential diagnosis is established by the measurement of FSH and LH, prolactin, oestradiol and thyroid function tests (TFTs). A pelvic ultrasound can provide additional evidence of PCOS, ovarian tumours and abnormalities of the lower genital tract. Nowadays, it is not usual to do routine imaging of the pituitary fossa, unless there is an elevated prolactin or some unusual features in the history suggesting other intracranial pathology. If such imaging is needed, MRI is now usually recommended.

Pregnancy should be excluded in all women who are sexually active and who present with delayed or absent menses, even of long-standing menses.

The progesterone challenge test, in which medroxyprogesterone acetate 10 mg daily for 5 days is administered, should produce withdrawal bleeding 2–7 days after completing the course and is sometimes used as a diagnostic tool. This is really an in vivo bioassay of oestrogen presence. A positive test indicates a functional uterus with an intact endometrium and a patent outflow tract where circulating levels of oestrogen are adequate. Modern measurement of serum oestradiol levels is now usually sufficient to provide this evidence.

Management

The treatment depends on the cause. Outside the 'physiological' group, the majority of cases are hypothalamic or PCOS in origin. Most of these will eventually resolve spontaneously, and where weight loss is the main underlying factor, the emphasis should be on restoring normal body mass. However, oestradiol levels are low, and in some cases it is useful to administer cyclical oestrogen–progestogen therapy. Hyperprolactinaemia will usually respond to stopping any dopamine-inhibiting drugs or to treatment with dopamine agonists such as cabergoline, bromocriptine or quinagolide. Treatment for PCOS depends on which of the presenting symptoms predominate. Lifestyle changes, including weight loss and exercise, are the cornerstone, and a loss of as little as 5% in weight can improve the menstrual pattern, endocrine profile and fertility.

Hirsutism can be treated by the local use of depilatory aids and electrolysis, but the presence of hirsutism, acne and alopecia may also respond to antiandrogens such as cyproterone acetate combined with an oestrogen such as ethinylestradiol given on a cyclical basis. If the problem is primarily one of subfertility, then clomiphene citrate or carefully monitored human menopausal gonadotrophin can be used to stimulate ovulation. Approximately 15–40% of women with PCOS have clomiphene resistance, which may result from its antioestrogenic effects on the endometrium and cervical mucus. Second-line treatment has previously involved laparoscopic ovarian drilling, whereby the ovarian surface is punctured multiple times, but early evidence suggests the use of aromatase inhibitors may be more effective than surgical intervention. Medical management with the oral hypoglycaemic, insulin-sensitizing agent metformin also appears to be effective in some cases. The long-term sequelae of PCOS need to be considered. Prolonged unopposed oestrogen action may result in the development of endometrial hyperplasia, which may rarely undergo malignant change. Hyperplasia will often regress following the administration of a progestational agent, such as norethisterone or medroxyprogesterone acetate. PCOS is associated with metabolic disturbances, and regular testing for the development of late-onset (type 2) diabetes and lipid abnormalities should occur.

Dysmenorrhoea

Dysmenorrhoea, or painful menstruation, is the commonest of all gynaecological symptoms. It is usually characterized as colicky pain that starts with the onset of bleeding and is maximal in the first 1–5 days of the period.

Primary dysmenorrhoea occurs in the absence of any significant pelvic pathology and is caused by excessive myometrial contractions producing uterine ischaemia in response to local release of prostaglandins (especially $PGF_{2\alpha}$) from the endometrium. It often begins with the onset of ovulatory cycles between 6 months and 2 years after the menarche, and it may occur more frequently or be more severe in young women whose periods start at an early age. There is often a family history of painful periods, and the mother's own experience can impact on the daughter's perception of her condition. The pain may be severe in some women, and the intense cramping can be associated with nausea, vomiting, diarrhoea and dizziness, which can be incapacitating and cause a major disruption to social activities. The pain usually only occurs in ovulatory cycles and is lower abdominal and pelvic in nature but sometimes radiates down the anterior aspect of the thighs. Commonly the pain disappears or improves after the birth of the first child. Pelvic examination reveals no abnormality.

Secondary or *acquired dysmenorrhoea* occurs in association with some form of pelvic pathology and usually, but not always, has its onset sometime after menarche. The pain typically precedes the start of the period by several days and may last throughout the period. It tends to be of a heavy, dragging nature (often called *congestive*) and may radiate to the back, loins and legs. Secondary dysmenorrhoea may occur as a result of endometriosis, fibroids, adenomyosis, pelvic infections, adhesions and developmental anomalies. Endometriosis pain often begins with severe dysmenorrhoea in adolescence, and this potential diagnosis should not be overlooked. A high degree of suspicion of the presence of endometriosis should be entertained if the features of 'dysmenorrhoea' in adolescence are unusual or do not respond to initial therapies. There is commonly a major delay (of more than 10–12 years) in making a diagnosis of endometriosis in those women in whom the symptom onset is in adolescence because of lack of medical awareness of this association.

Investigations

A careful history is important with attention to the timing of the onset and characteristics of pain and associated symptoms, such as dyspareunia and dysuria. Pelvic examination is to be avoided in those women with primary dysmenorrhoea who have never been sexually active. The decision to perform a vaginal examination should be individually assessed, taking into account sexual activity and the need for a Pap smear. In women with primary dysmenorrhoea, there is usually no pelvic tenderness or any abnormality on vaginal examination.

In secondary dysmenorrhoea, a pelvic examination is essential to assess uterine and adnexal tenderness, masses and uterine mobility, as well as the posterior fornix and cervical movement pain. Swabs should be taken for pelvic infection and a pelvic ultrasound organized. Although transvaginal ultrasound is a good investigation for fibroids, it is less reliable for adenomyosis and will not commonly detect endometriosis, unless an endometrioma or deep lesion is present. Laparoscopy is required for women with persistent or progressive pain symptoms that are unresponsive to medical therapies.

Management

An explanation of the causes of menstrual pain is helpful and, where appropriate, reassurance that there is no underlying pathology. Clinicians should adopt a holistic approach with attention to diet and lifestyle factors, as well as to medical therapies. There is good evidence that smoking increases dysmenorrhoea and some evidence that exercise can be beneficial. Using a heat pack on the lower abdomen anecdotally provides relief, and several dietary supplements have been investigated, with vitamin B_1 indicated to be a helpful treatment.

Pharmacological

NSAIDs are the most commonly used drugs for the treatment of dysmenorrhoea due to their inhibition of prostaglandin synthesis. These drugs include aspirin, mefenamic acid, naproxen or ibuprofen. Adolescents and young adults with symptoms that do not respond to treatment with NSAIDs within three menstrual periods should be offered a combined oral contraceptive pill for the next three menstrual cycles (the NSAID therapy can be continued).

The combined oral contraceptive pill, in addition to suppressing ovulation, reduces uterine prostaglandin release. It can be used in a continuous manner to reduce symptom frequency. Progestogen-only methods such as depo-medroxyprogesterone acetate injections, subdermal implants and the levonorgestrel intrauterine system can also be used. Adolescents and young adults who do not respond to these treatments should be evaluated for an underlying structural or infective cause.

In cases of secondary dysmenorrhoea, the treatment is dependent on the nature of the associated pathology. Intensive medical therapies may assist, but may also need to be combined with surgery. If the condition is not amenable to medical therapy, occasionally the symptoms may only be relieved by hysterectomy and excision of the associated pathology (such as adenomyosis or endometriosis).

Premenstrual syndrome

Premenstrual syndrome (PMS) is defined as recurrent moderate psychological and physical symptoms that occur during the luteal phase of the menstrual cycle and resolve with the onset of bleeding. It affects around 20% of reproductive-age women. In the more severe form, premenstrual dysphoric disorder (PMDD), women experience somatic, psychological and behavioural symptoms severe enough to disrupt social, family or occupational life.

Symptoms and signs

The symptoms associated with PMS and PMDD are listed in Table 16.2.

Table 16.2 The most commonly expressed physical and psychological symptoms in women suffering from PMS or PMDD

Physical	Psychological
Abdominal bloating	Anger, irritability
Body pains	Anxiety
Breast tenderness or fullness	Changes in appetite (increased appetite, food cravings)
Abdominal pain and cramps	Changes in libido
Tiredness	Decreased concentration
Headaches	Depressed mood
Nausea	Feelings of loss of control
Peripheral oedema	Mood swings
Weight gain	Poor sleep
	Withdrawal from social and work activities

PMDD, Premenstrual dysphoric disorder; PMS, premenstrual syndrome.

Pathogenesis

The aetiology of PMS and PMDD is not known, but women appear to be more 'physiologically' sensitive to changes in circulating levels of oestrogen and progesterone, and may have altered central neurotransmitter function, particularly for serotonin.

Management

Clinical history is the key to diagnosis, and the correct diagnosis is best established by asking women to prospectively collect a detailed menstrual diary of their symptoms ideally over two cycles. This will clarify whether there are non-luteal symptoms that may suggest other medical or psychological disorders. The goal of treatment is relief of symptoms and involves both non-pharmacological and pharmacological options.

Non-pharmacological options frequently recommended are increasing exercise and reducing caffeine and refined carbohydrate intake, but there is little evidence to support these. A number of dietary supplements have been studied, and women with high intakes of calcium and vitamin D are less likely to have PMS symptoms. Vitamin B_6 and evening primrose oil are frequently self-prescribed for PMS. Vitamin B_6 (pyridoxine) is a co-factor in neurotransmitter synthesis. Although there is no evidence of any actual deficit of these substances in PMS, the largest controlled study showed an 82% response rate to vitamin B_6 compared to 70% on placebo. Peripheral neuropathy has been reported at high doses, but a dose of 100 mg is probably safe.

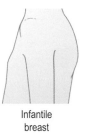
Infantile
breast

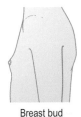
Breast bud

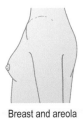
Breast and areola
enlarged

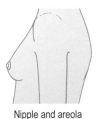
Nipple and areola
enlarged

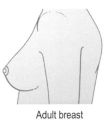
Adult breast

Fig. 16.20 Development of the female breast during thelarche.

Evening primrose oil contains the unsaturated fatty acid precursors of prostaglandins. There is some evidence of improvement in selected symptoms, but the recommended dose of eight capsules a day is difficult to sustain. Anti-prostaglandin painkillers, such as ibuprofen, may be useful for breast pain and headaches. Diuretics such as spironolactone may be of benefit in the small group of women who experience true water retention but should only be used for symptoms of bloating where there is measurable weight gain. The dry extract of the *Agnus castus* fruit (20 mg daily) may also be effective in reducing symptoms of irritability, mood change, headache and breast fullness. Cognitive behaviour therapy, although useful for other affective disorders, has no evidence to support its use in PMD or PMDD.

Pharmacological

The first-line medications for severe PMS and PMDD are the selective serotonin reuptake inhibitors (SSRIs) or the serotonin–norepinephrine reuptake inhibitors (SNRIs). These medications, such as sertraline, citalopram and fluoxetine, taken either daily or during the luteal phase of the cycle, have been found to significantly reduce the physical and psychological symptoms of PMS compared to placebo. The positive impact on PMS is often seen within a few weeks of taking the medication, but improvement in mood, if there is associated depression, may take up to a month to improve.

The combined oral contraceptive pill has been commonly used to treat PMS, but there are no data to support its effectiveness, with the exception of some studies of pills containing progestogens with antidiuretic properties. Several studies suggest that pills containing drospirenone, a spironolactone derivative, in a 24-day pack are better than placebo in reducing the symptoms of PMS. Further, taking the pills in a continuous manner (hormone tablets every day without a break) is beneficial compared with taking a conventional 28-day pill with 7-day break.

GnRH agonists suppress ovarian function and relieve symptoms during treatment. However, these recur when treatment is stopped. They are unsuitable for long-term use because of their cost and adverse side effects, including menopausal symptoms and osteoporosis.

Disorders of puberty

Puberty and menarche

Puberty represents a period of significant growth and profound hormonal changes that will lead to the development of an adult body and in the majority of cases the ability to reproduce. It needs also to be noted that these changes are usually occurring contemporaneously with educational, social and physical challenges. Precocious or delayed puberty may present the young girl or woman and her family with added psychosocial difficulties. The clinician needs to be sensitive to these issues, with the goal of any therapeutic intervention being to alleviate distress while maximizing potentials for growth, development and future fertility.

Normal pubertal development occurs in an ordered sequence and involves acquisition of secondary sex characteristics associated with a rapid increase in growth that culminates in reproductive capability. The process is initiated by increased amounts of GnRH secreted in a pulsatile manner from the hypothalamus, but the exact trigger of this event is not known. The release of pulsatile GnRH leads to release of the pituitary hormones, i.e. LH and FSH. The former stimulates androstenedione production in the ovary, and the latter stimulates oestradiol synthesis. The pulses are initially nocturnal, becoming eventually diurnal. At the same time there is an increase in amplitude of growth hormone from the pituitary. Both androgens and oestrogens may regulate this amplification. Sex steroids have also been shown to stimulate skeletal growth directly.

Puberty in females is characterized by accelerated linear growth, development of breasts, thelarche, axillary and pubic hair, adrenarche and eventual onset of menses, i.e. menarche (Figs 16.20 and 16.21). Generally, there is a forward progression through these stages. However, several variations can occur such as premature thelarche or adrenarche. Puberty is complete once oestrogen rises to the level where positive

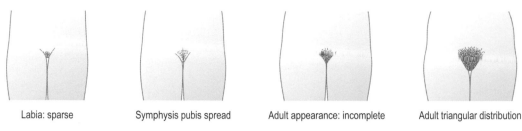

| Labia: sparse | Symphysis pubis spread | Adult appearance: incomplete | Adult triangular distribution |

Fig. 16.21 Pubic hair distribution leading up to full sexual maturation during adrenarche.

feedback occurs on the hypothalamus and ovulatory cycles establish. The entire process is seen to vary in length considerably being between 18 months and 6 years.

The timing of puberty was documented in longitudinal studies of North American girls performed by Tanner and Davies in the 1980s. Their studies found that breast budding occurred at the average age of 10.7 years with a standard deviation (SD) of 1 year and menarche at 12.7 (SD 1.3) years. The onset of breast development more than 2.5 SD from the mean or occurring in girls under the age of 8 is defined as precocious.

The age at onset of puberty is seen to be influenced by race, family history and nutrition. It was felt for some time that a critical weight, as postulated in the 1970s by Frisch and Revelle, of approximately 45 kg was necessary to stimulate pubertal development. This suggested that fat tissue itself was responsible. However, this view has not been upheld by subsequent studies, and the relationship between height, weight and pubertal development is significantly more complex. Although more recent studies have suggested that the average age of onset of puberty is declining, possibly triggered by increasing rates of obesity, the definition of precious puberty has not changed.

Thelarche

Breast tissue development begins with a subareolar breast bud and occurs under the influence of initially unopposed oestradiol. Puberty begins with breast development in approximately 80% of girls, with the others experiencing adrenarche first.

Adrenarche

The normal onset of adrenal androgen production occurs approximately 1–2 years before pubarche, the onset of puberty. Adrenarche is independent of gonadarche, the maturation of the gonads and the secretion of sex steroids, but occurs prior.

Menarche

Reproductive maturity occurs with the onset of menstruation. In the UK, the average age is 12–13 years. Menarche usually occurs after the peak in growth velocity. The menstrual cycle is often irregular in the first 6–18 months as ovulation can initially be infrequent.

Growth spurt

The acceleration in the rate of growth accompanies or precedes pubertal development. The onset of the growth spurt occurs between 9.5 and 14.5 years and is dependent on growth hormone as well as gonadal steroids. The first development is lengthening of legs followed by increase in shoulder breadth and trunk length. The pelvis enlarges and changes shape. Most girls reach maximum growth velocity approximately 2 years after thelarche and 1 year prior to menarche. Maximal height is reached between 17 and 18 years with fusion of the femoral epiphyses.

Precocious puberty

In girls, precocious puberty is defined as the development of the physical signs of puberty before the age of 8 years. It usually progresses from premature thelarche to menarche because breast tissue responds faster to oestrogen than does the endometrium. It is useful to categorize possible causes as central, i.e. dependent on GnRH secretion, and peripheral, i.e. GnRH independent. The majority of cases do not have a pathological basis. In girls older than 4 years old, specific causes are less likely to be found, with the majority being idiopathic (80%). Below this age, central nervous system (CNS) causes predominate.

Central (GnRH dependent) in order of frequency:

- idiopathic
- CNS tumours
- hydrocephaly
- CNS injury secondary to trauma or infection, recent or past
- CNS irradiation
- neurofibromatosis

Patients with central precocious puberty have unregulated GnRH release. FSH and LH levels fluctuate, so multiple samples may be required, remembering a propensity to nocturnal secretion. A GnRH stimulation test will show a pubertal, threefold response in LH levels. FSH also rises but to a lesser degree. In central precocious puberty the progression follows the usual pattern, albeit earlier.

Peripheral or GnRH independent causes:

- hormonal secreting tumour of the adrenal gland or ovaries
- gonadotrophin-producing tumours
- congenital adrenal hyperplasia (non-classical)
- McCune–Albright syndrome
- hypothyroidism
- exogenous oestrogens
- follicular cysts of the ovary

Evaluation

The first step in evaluating a girl with precocious puberty is to obtain a complete family history, including the age of onset of puberty in parents and siblings. The heights of both parents should be recorded and the projected height of the child calculated (Fig. 16.22). The history of pubertal development needs to be documented along with other symptoms such as headache or visual disturbance. A history of illness, trauma, surgery and medications is also pertinent. Physical examination should include documentation of the Tanner stage and examination for other signs to indicate a peripheral cause, such as skin lesions or ovarian masses. Signs of virilization must be looked for, including acne, hirsutism and clitoromegaly.

Investigations

This is the most important step in determining which category of precocious puberty is responsible and narrowing the differential diagnosis. Plasma FSH, LH and oestradiol are essential, as is a TFT. X-ray of the hand to determine bone age is important. Bone age is advanced in the constitutional and cerebral forms and may need to be repeated at an interval of 6 months to confirm maturation. Ultrasound of the abdomen and pelvis should be conducted, looking for adrenal or ovarian tumours and to establish normal anatomy. The ovary may show a multicystic appearance in normal puberty and in cerebral and idiopathic forms. Follicular cysts need to be distinguished from predominantly solid oestrogen-secreting granulosa or theca cell tumours. Radiological skeletal survey of the long bones may indicate osteolytic lesions of McCune–Albright syndrome. If results are consistent with a central cause, cranial CT or MRI should be arranged, looking for abnormalities of the sella turcica, suprasellar calcification and other lesions.

Management

The key aims of treatment are to arrest and even reverse the physical signs of puberty and to avert the rapid development in bone age, which can result in initial growth advancement compared to peers but ultimately premature epiphyseal fusion and smaller-than-normal stature. The main treatment for central progressive precocious puberty is the GnRH agonist, which desensitizes the pituitary and leads to a reduction in LH and FSH output. This may be

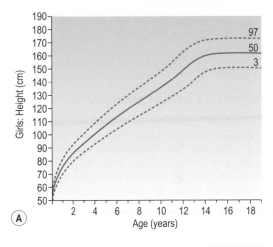

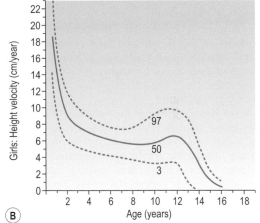

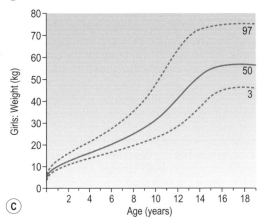

Fig. 16.22 (A) Centile change for height in the female. (B) Height velocity indicates the slowing down of the rate of growth with a secondary acceleration around the time of puberty. (C) Changes in weight show a wider scatter than with height.

administered as monthly or trimonthly injections or as intranasal preparations. Once an appropriate chronological age is reached, the agent is withdrawn, allowing pubertal development to advance.

Variations on normal puberty

Premature adrenarche

This refers to the secretion of adrenal androgens before the age of 8 years. This frequently is idiopathic and non-progressive. It presents usually with complaints of axillary hair and/or pubic hair plus the emergence of body odour, sometimes with acne and hirsutism. It is very important to exclude enzyme deficiencies, e.g. chronic adrenal hyperplasia or androgen-secreting tumours, while recognizing that the majority of cases will be self-limiting.

Premature thelarche

Defined as breast budding prior to age 8 years, this condition needs to be differentiated from precocious puberty, as approximately 10% will progress. It is more common in infants and tends to resolve spontaneously in this group.

Precocious menarche

This is the least common of the variants and is defined as cyclic vaginal bleeding without secondary sexual characteristics. It may be caused by a transitory rise in oestrogen as the result of follicular activity or a heightened endometrial sensitivity. A careful history is necessary to establish cyclicity, as other causes of prepubertal vaginal bleeding, including infection, foreign body and neoplasm, need exclusion.

Delayed puberty

Delayed puberty is defined by the absence of breast development in girls beyond 13 years. The diagnosis is also made in the absence of menarche by age 16 or within 5 years after the onset of puberty. Mostly delayed puberty is constitutional, arising from inadequate GnRH from the hypothalamus. It may also be secondary to chronic illness such as anorexia nervosa, asthma, chronic renal disease and inflammatory bowel disease. Anatomical considerations such as outflow obstruction in haematocolpos need exclusion. The hypogonadism that characterizes this state may occur with both elevated and lowered levels of gonadotrophins. As with precocious puberty, it is essential to establish the status of the gonadotrophins to determine causation (Table 16.3).

Investigations

Physical examination, noting height, weight, BMI, Tanner staging and vital signs, may draw attention to possible aetiologies such as low BMI and cold peripheries, with postural drop being suggestive of a possible eating disorder.

Table 16.3 Causes of delay in some aspects of puberty

Delayed puberty types (% frequency)	Causes
Constitutional eugonadism (25%)	
Anatomical	Imperforate hymen Transverse vaginal septum Müllerian agenesis: Mayer–Rokitansky–Küster–Hauser syndrome and variant
Chronic anovulation	PCOS
Hypergonadotrophic hypergonadism (45%)	
Normal chromosomes	Gonadal dysgenesis XY Androgen insensitivity Swyer's syndrome Premature ovarian failure de novo or iatrogenic/environmental Resistant ovary syndrome
Abnormal chromosome array	Turner's syndrome XO Mixed gonadal dysgenesis
Hypogonadotrophic hypogonadism (30%)	Constitutional Congenital or acquired CNS tumours Infection Trauma
Psychosocial	Drug ingestion, opiates and marijuana inhalants Eating disorders Exercise Stress
Illness including endocrine	Kallman's syndrome Isolated GnRH deficiency
Pituitary destruction	Pituitary destruction
Delayed puberty with virilization	C-21 hydroxylase deficiency Neoplasm Partial androgen insensitivity

GnRH, Gonadotrophin-releasing hormone; *PCOS*, polycystic ovary syndrome.

However, once again laboratory tests hold the key to the category of causal agent. FSH, LH, oestradiol, prolactin and TFTs will illustrate gonotrophin function and ovarian response together with the major endocrine disorders that may be responsible. Pelvic ultrasound will define genital tract architecture, bearing in mind that the prepubertal uterus may be very difficult to see on an abdominal pelvic ultrasound. If the gonadotrophins are elevated, first check the patient's karyotype to determine whether Turner's syndrome, androgen sensitivity or Swyer's syndrome is present. If the karyotype is normal, explore for autoimmune disease. It is important to ensure that karyotyping explores at least 40 cells to exclude the possibility of a Y-cell line in mosaicism. If the gonadotrophins are low or normal, investigate for eating disorders, rigorous training and congenital or acquired cerebral lesions. Eugonadism requires a thorough exclusion of anatomical abnormalities, which may require MRI to adequately assess genital tract agenesis or dysgenesis.

Management

Delayed puberty can be treated initially with unopposed oestrogens beginning at 0.3 mg daily and slowly increasing to facilitate adequate breast development. Once adequate growth is achieved, progesterone should be added for endometrial protection and cyclicity.

The goal is to treat any underlying cause to maximize growth and fertility potentials. Fertility counselling and help with accepting a diagnosis can be extremely difficult and require sensitivity. Peer support has been shown to be valuable for young women facing infertility and struggling with difference. A multidisciplinary approach, including genetics, endocrine, psychology and gynaecology, is suggested.

Menopause

Menopause is the last natural menstrual period defined as the permanent cessation of menstruation resulting from the loss of ovarian follicular activity, and it marks the end of a woman's reproductive function. The definition is made retrospectively once a woman has had no periods for 12 consecutive months. For most women, menopause occurs naturally between the ages of 45 and 55 years, with an average age of around 51 years. 'Premature menopause' may occur before the age of 40 due to either the cessation of natural ovarian function or after surgical removal of the ovaries or following chemotherapy or radiotherapy.

Menopause transition

The menopausal transition, or 'perimenopause', is defined by the World Health Organization (WHO) as 'that period of time immediately before menopause when the endocrinological, biological and clinical features of approaching menopause commence'. The menstrual cycle shortens in women over the age of 40 years, and the change in the cycle length is related to shortening of the follicular phase. FSH levels are higher at all stages of the cycle than levels seen in younger women, whilst oestradiol levels may be lower with erratic elevations. In the early part of the menopause

transition, associated with rising FSH and LH levels, menstrual cycle irregularity often occurs with a predominance of short, normal-length or long cycles. These cycles may be associated with delayed follicle development, or intermittent 'luteal out-of-phase' (LOOP) cycles, and are often accompanied by erratically heavy periods.

In the later stages where there are further elevations in FSH and LH, cycle irregularity occurs with a predominance of elongated menstrual cycles. Although AUB is common in perimenopause, persistent irregular bleeding should never be considered normal because it may be associated with uterine neoplasms.

Hormone changes after menopause

There is a marked reduction in ovarian production of oestrogen and, in particular, of oestradiol. Some oestrogen production occurs in the adrenal gland, but the major source of oestradiol arises from peripheral conversion of both oestrone and testosterone in fat tissue. Thus, women with a high BMI have higher circulating oestrogen levels than slender women. There is considerable variation in the circulating levels of oestradiol in menopause, and this may account for the variation in severity of menopausal symptoms. The absence of any significant oestrogen production results in excessive release of FSH and LH, with the major increases occurring in FSH. The levels of gonadotrophins continue to show pulsatile release similar to the pattern seen in the premenopausal phase. Androgens produced in the ovary and adrenal glands are mainly androstenedione and testosterone, and these levels fall in menopausal women. There is also a reduction in adrenal androgen secretion, including that of dehydroepiandrosterone (DHEA) and DHEA sulphate. Oestrogen production by the ovary is reduced, but the production of testosterone persists.

Symptoms and signs of menopause

Numerous symptoms are described in relation to menopause, but the two that are the most significant are hot flushes (often associated with insomnia) and vaginal dryness. These symptoms are experienced by 70% of women and result from reduced oestrogen levels. A range of other symptoms, both physical and psychological, are associated with menopause, including palpitations, headaches, bone and joint pain, asthenia, tiredness and breast tenderness. Most women will have little or only mild symptoms. Around 20% of women seek help for management of their symptoms.

Physical symptoms

Vascular disturbances. The commonest symptom, occurring in around 75% of women, is the development of hot flushes.

These episodes usually last for 4–5 minutes and consist of flushes and perspiration affecting the face, neck and chest. Hot flushes are typically experienced maximally in the first year after menopause and last up to 5 years. Although the exact pathophysiology remains elusive, the flushes coincide with pulsatile release of LH, an acute rise in the skin temperature of several degrees centigrade, a transient increase in heart rate and fluctuations in the electrocardiographic baseline. The administration of oestrogens relieves these symptoms, but the mechanism is unknown. Night sweats and insomnia also occur.

Urogenital tract. The urogenital tissues of the uterus, vagina and bladder contain oestrogen and progesterone receptors. Loss of oestrogen results in epithelial thinning, reduced vascularity, decreased muscle bulk and increased fat deposition. Up to half of women experience urogenital symptoms after menopause, including uterovaginal prolapse, dry vagina and urinary symptoms.

The vaginal walls lose their rugosity and become smooth and atrophic. In severe cases, this may also be associated with chronic infection and atrophic vaginitis. The complaint of vaginal and vulval dryness can manifest as discomfort or pain during intercourse, as well as bleeding or spotting after sex. The cervix diminishes in size, and there is a reduction in cervical mucus production. The uterus also shrinks in size, and the endometrium becomes atrophic. The bladder epithelium may also become atrophic with the development of frequency, dysuria and urge incontinence. It is important to recognize these symptoms because they can be relieved by oestrogen replacement therapy.

Other physical symptoms. The skin over the body becomes thinner and drier, and body and facial hair become coarser. The reduction in ovarian oestrogen production results in involution and regression of target organs, including breasts that become less dense and reduce in size (Fig. 16.23).

Psychological and emotional symptoms

Many women experience psychological symptoms around the time of menopause such as anxiety, depression, loss of memory, irritability, poor concentration, tiredness and loss of confidence. The emotional disturbances of menopause may be associated with feelings of inadequacy and uncertainty about the woman's role if they have been the primary caregiver of children who are leaving home. Although there is no evidence that these symptoms are directly related to oestrogen deficiency, hormone therapy (HT)/HRT may improve mild depressive symptoms; however, moderate to severe depression should be treated with antidepressant and other therapies.

Other symptoms

Oestradiol can affect the heart's electrophysiological parameters, and women commonly experience palpitations,

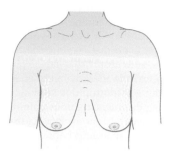

Involution of breast structure

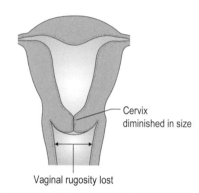

Cervix diminished in size

Vaginal rugosity lost

Fig. 16.23 Characteristic changes in the breasts and genitalia following menopause.

especially in the perimenopausal period, that impact on quality of life. Although often benign, this symptom can also be brought on by a variety of cardiac disorders, such as cardiomyopathy, valvular heart disease and coronary artery disease, although primary cardiac arrhythmias is the most common cause.

Headaches. Menses, pregnancy and menopause affect the frequency and treatment of headaches in women.

In the Women's Health Study, current use of HT was associated with higher reported rates of migraines than in non-users.

Bone and joint pain. Many women complain of bone and joint pain around the time of menopause, and osteoarthritis may manifest at this stage of life. For all women, exercise is an important way of managing these symptoms, and, in some women, HRT is beneficial.

Consequences of menopause

Bone changes

Osteoporosis is a condition characterized by loss of trabecular bone. Oestrogen plays an important role in maintaining bone strength and, with a drop in oestrogen levels after menopause, bone loss occurs at a rate of about 2.5% per year for the first 4 years. Fractures become a major source of morbidity in the menopausal female, with at least half of all women over the age of 60 years reporting to have at least one fracture due to osteoporosis.

Bone loss is most severe in women who have an artificial menopause. Hip fractures increase in incidence from 0.3/1000 at age 45 years to 20/1000 at age 85 years, and there is also a 10-fold increase in Colles' fractures.

The diagnosis of osteoporosis is commonly made using a specialized X-ray technique called dual-energy X-ray absorption (DXA or DEXA). DXA test results are presented as a T-score and a Z-score. The T-score compares the bone density of the woman being scanned with that of a young woman (when peak bone mass is at its best). The Z-score compares the bone density of the woman being scanned with that of a woman of the same age as you. T-scores, not Z-scores, are used in premenopausal women:

- T-score greater than –1 indicates **normal bone density.**
- T-score between –1 and –2.5 indicates **low bone density,** sometimes called *osteopoenia.* This means there is some loss of bone mineral density but not severe enough to be called osteoporosis.
- T-score of –2.5 or less indicates **osteoporosis.** When a person has a minimal impact fracture, regardless of the T-scores, osteoporosis is also diagnosed.

Cardiovascular complications

The prevalence and incidence of cardiovascular events and death from cardiovascular events are higher in women who experience early menopause compared to those having late menopause. The changes in serum lipoproteins that occur after menopause include a rise in cholesterol levels and an increase in all lipoprotein fractions, with a decrease in the ratio of the high- to low-density fractions. This can explain some, but not all, of the increased cardiovascular morbidity, and it is now evident that ovarian hormone deprivation has a widespread impact on the cardiovascular system, with a direct harmful effect on vessel wall physiology.

Treatment of menopause

Many women pass through menopause without any symptoms, and there is considerable variation in serum oestradiol levels between individuals after menopause. Oestrogen therapy is the most effective treatment for symptomatic relief but may be associated with significant adverse effects in a small minority of women. The decision to use HRT is made on an individual basis taking into account each woman's history, risk factors and personal preferences (Table 16.4). This should be done in a way that can be understood so that each woman can make an informed choice.

Hormone replacement therapy

Oestrogen therapy may be given on its own or as a combined or sequential therapy with a progestogen. The type of

Table 16.4 Relative risks and benefits seen in women taking combined oestrogen and progestogen hormone replacement therapy

	Relative risk vs. placebo group at 5 years
Heart attacks	1.29
Stroke	1.41
Breast cancer	1.26
Venous thrombosis	2.11
Fractured neck of femur	0.66
Colorectal cancer	0.63

Adapted from Rossouw JE, Anderson GL, Prentice RL, et al. (2002) Risks and benefits of estrogen plus progestin in healthy postmenopausal women: principal results from the Women's Health Initiative randomized controlled trial. JAMA 2002; 288:321–333.

therapy recommended will depend on whether the uterus has been removed and whether the therapy planned is to be short or long term. There should be regular reappraisal of the risk and benefits on any woman taking long-term HRT.

Oral therapy. Micronized oestradiol or conjugated equine oestrogen (Premarin) is given continuously with concomitant administration of a progestogen in women with an intact uterus to prevent the development of endometrial hyperplasia or malignancy. Progestogens are commonly given for 10–14 days every 4 weeks to produce a monthly withdrawal bleed, but there is no loss of protective effect when this is reduced to 12-weekly intervals. Those women who have previously stopped their periods and wish to avoid further bleeds can be offered combination therapy that includes continuous progestogen administration with an oestrogen.

Parenteral therapy. Oestrogen can also be administered by injection or by subcutaneous implants. This can be achieved with crystalline oestradiol 100 mg in a pellet inserted in the subcutaneous tissue of the anterior abdominal wall. This is often combined with testosterone 50 mg, which has the advantage of a mild anabolic effect and of enhancing libido. The pellets usually last for 6–12 months and are useful in women who have experienced surgical menopause. Tachyphylaxis with progressively shorter intervals between implants and the return of symptoms even in the presence of normal or high oestradiol levels can occasionally be a problem. If the implants are given to a woman with an intact uterus, it is important to give a progestogen, such as norethisterone acetate 5 mg, for the first 14 days of each month. This will provoke withdrawal bleeding as long as active oestrogen absorption occurs.

Topical therapy. Oestradiol can be given percutaneously by self-adhesive patches or gel. Patches are applied to any area of clear, dry skin other than the face or breast and changed twice a week. The gel is rubbed into the skin once a day. A progestogen can be given either orally or transdermally. This route has the advantage of bypassing the 'first pass' liver metabolism and gives more stable serum hormone levels than with implants. The major complication is one of skin irritation.

Contraindications. HRT is contraindicated in the presence of endometrial and breast carcinoma, thromboembolic disease (including family history), acute liver disease and ischaemic heart disease. Other conditions such as fibrocystic disease of the breast, uterine fibroids, familial hyperlipidaemia, diabetes and gallbladder disease provide a relative contraindication, but relief of symptoms may sometimes be more important than other considerations.

Risks. The potential complications of HRT include an increased incidence of carcinoma of the endometrium, breast and possibly ovary. The risk of these cancers is very small but may increase the longer that HRT is taken. Previous observational studies had suggested a protective effect against heart disease and stroke, but this is complex and uncertain. The risk of venous thrombosis is increased, but the overall incidence is very low. Some women develop hypertension on oestrogen therapy, and periodic checks on blood pressure are therefore important. Caution should be taken when there is a history of gallbladder disease. The development of irregular uterine bleeding after more than 6 months on HRT is an indication for endometrial biopsy.

> HRT should no longer be prescribed for the specific indication of prevention of coronary heart disease.

Benefits. The principal benefits of HRT use are in the relief of menopausal symptoms and the prevention of osteoporosis. HRT use is associated with a reduction in the risk of fracture of the neck of the femur and in the incidence of colorectal cancer.

Alternatives to oestrogen-containing HRT

As the principal indication for long-term use of HRT is the prevention of osteoporosis, patients need to be aware of the possible increased risk of some conditions with long-term use and the alternative treatment options available to prevent osteoporosis.

Tibolone is a synthetic weak androgen with oestrogenic properties. It does not cause endometrial proliferation, so there is no withdrawal bleed, but it is only advisable for women more than a year after menopause. It is effective at reducing vasomotor symptoms and osteoporosis. Selective oestrogen receptor modulators (SERMs) act on oestrogen receptors in bone without affecting the breast or endometrium. Those currently available are effective at doing this but do not relieve vasomotor symptoms and are associated

with the same increased risk of thrombosis as conventional oestrogen therapy.

Clonidine is an antihypertensive agent that has some effect on vasomotor symptoms but no effect on other symptoms or long-term health. The serotonergic antidepressants, the SSRIs and SNRIs, seem to be effective in hot flushes, and relief, if any, is rapid. The use of these medications in the long term, particularly in women who have had breast cancer as there may be an interaction with tamoxifen, remains in doubt. Gabapentin, an anticonvulsant drug, is more effective than placebo in reducing the severity and frequency of hot flushes and is likely to be safe in women on tamoxifen.

Herbal therapies such as black cohosh are widely used but in randomized controlled trials fare no better than placebo in relieving menopausal symptoms. Phyto-oestrogens are non-steroidal plant compounds that, because of their structural similarity with oestradiol, have mild oestrogenic effects. There is still a lack of well-controlled clinical trials for the use of these compounds as alternatives to HRT. They probably have a weak positive impact on cardiovascular disease and may be protective against breast cancer. They are not potent enough to impact on bone loss.

Benign conditions of the lower genital tract

Vulval pruritus

Pruritus, or itch, is the most commonly described symptom of those complaining of discomfort in the vulval area. The itch, so often accompanied by scratching with its attendant trauma to the epithelium, may often be chronic. Women may experience sexual difficulties as a consequence and often report problems in discussing their symptoms or seeking help. Diagnosis and management may be difficult for the clinician, as symptoms and signs tend to cluster, biopsy results can be equivocal and irritant or allergic reactions may develop to various medications and remedies tried.

Fortunately the majority of causes of vulval pruritus are benign (Table 16.5). However, care must be taken not to overlook or misdiagnose the rarer malignant causes. The vulva is skin and therefore may express conditions seen elsewhere on the body, e.g. psoriasis and dermatitis. Because of the nature of this area, the appearance of skin conditions may vary greatly. The vulva, in such proximity to the vagina, may also express features of bacterial or viral vaginitis or cervicitis with hypersensitivity reaction to productive discharge, as seen in candidiasis. It is therefore extremely important when assessing a patient with pruritus of the vulva to take a very wide-ranging history to include

Table 16.5 Benign causes of vulval pruritus

Condition	Presentation	Management
Dermatitis	Itchy, erythematous rash (endogenous) Atopic/seborrhoeic Allergic or irritant induced (exogenous)	Mild to moderate corticosteroid reducing as symptoms abate (regardless of the cause)
Lichen simplex chronicus	Chronic irritation results in thickening and hypertrophy of skin, erythema, excoriations Mucosa not involved	Isolate and remove provoking and exacerbating factors High-potency steroid locally Reducing after symptom control
Candidiasis	Itch discomfort, white discharge dyspareunia, dysuria Hypersensitivity reaction on vulva Requires positive culture to confirm diagnosis	Mild: pessaries of clotrimazole Moderate: prolonged treatment ± oral drugs Severe/recurrent: 2–3 months oral fluconazole. Maintenance of oral 150 mg weekly or clotrimazole pessary 500 mg
Lichen sclerosis (LS)	Whitened parchment-like plaques Classic hourglass appearance involving perianal skin Loss of labial/clitoral architecture, introital narrowing May have tearing or subepithelial haemorrhage/petechiae Mucosa not involved	High-potency corticosteroids Nightly until clinical improvement (1–2 months) then reduce Maintenance 1–2 per week Increase treatment to original intensity for 2 weeks if symptoms recur
Lichen planus (LP)	Chronic LS difficult to differentiate from LP Introits of vagina involved Adhesions and erosions may occur not responsive to surgical division Oral/gingival involvement possible	High-potency corticosteroids Except in mild cases that are very resistant to treatment
Psoriasis	Itchy, scaly, red plaques not as well demarcated as elsewhere on the skin; examine hair/scalp, nails also	As for psoriasis in general; high-potency corticosteroid plus tar products Local tacrolimus

personal and family history of skin conditions; autoimmune disease; and exposures to possible irritants such as soaps, perfumes, sanitary products, etc. and to examine the rest of their skin. Particular attention should be paid to the scalp, elbows, anterior cubital fossae and knees. Inspection of the genitalia does not generally require colposcopic examination, but it is important to obtain bacterial and viral cultures both from vulval lesions and vaginal or cervical mucosa when indicated.

In adult women, the threshold to perform punch biopsy should be low. Itchy, scaly lesions with increased vascularity or poor treatment response should be biopsied to exclude malignancy. Further, as several dermatological conditions have similar presentations, biopsy may be necessary to confirm the diagnosis and ascertain treatment plans.

A cornerstone of treatment for all cases involving pruritus of the vulva is to ensure irritant or allergic stimuli are removed, that the area is kept dry and well ventilated to promote healing and that barrier preparations to prevent repeated insult are prescribed. Soap, perfumed hygiene products, talcum and flavoured lubricants should all be avoided. Washing with water alone or oil-based, hypoallergenic products; cotton underwear; loose clothing; and frequent moisturization with sorbolene or similar form an essential core of management.

Vulval neoplasia

Skin cancers will occur on the vulva and present with itchiness and need to be differentiated from benign dermatoses. Suspicion should be increased in any persistently eroded or scaly and hypervascular lesions with a very low threshold for biopsy (see Chapter 20).

Vaginal discharge

Vaginal discharge describes any fluid loss through the vagina. While most discharge is normal and can reflect physiological

Table 16.6 Vaginal discharge: Causes and treatment

Features of discharge and associated symptoms	Possible causes	Treatment
Thick, white, non-itchy	Physiological	
Thick, white, cottage cheese, vulval itching, vulval soreness and irritation, pain or discomfort	*Candida albicans*	Topical or oral anti-yeast medication
Yellow-green, itchy, frothy, foul-smelling ('fishy' smell) vaginal discharge	*Trichomonas*	Metronidazole and treatment of sexual partners
Thin, grey or green, fishy odour	Bacterial vaginosis	Metronidazole
Thick, white discharge, dysuria and pelvic pain, friable cervix	Gonorrhoea	Variable but cephalosporins

changes throughout the menstrual cycle, some discharge can occur because of infection or trauma. White discharge usually occurs in response to hormonal changes at the beginning and the end of the cycle, whilst mid-cycle, with high oestrogen levels, the discharge is clear. The common causes and management of vaginal discharge are summarized in Table 16.6. Further details on the common infections of the genital tract and their treatment can be found in Chapter 19.

Cervical polyps

Benign polyps arise from the endocervix and are pedunculated, with a covering of endocervical epithelium and a central fibrous tissue core. The polyps present as bright red, vascular growths that may be identified on routine examination. The presenting symptoms may include irregular vaginal blood loss or PCB.

Less frequently, the polyps arise from the squamous epithelium, when the appearance will resemble the surface of the vaginal epithelium.

Small polyps can be avulsed in the outpatient clinic by grasping them with polyp forceps and rotating through 360 degrees. Larger polyps may need ligation of the pedicle and excision of the polyp under general anaesthesia.

Benign tumours of the vulva and vagina

Benign cysts of the vulva include sebaceous, epithelial inclusion and wolffian duct cysts (Fig. 16.24), which arise from the labia minora and the periurethral region, and Bartholin's cysts (see later). A rare cyst may arise from a peritoneal extension along the round ligament, forming a hydrocele in the labium major. Benign solid tumours include fibromas, lipomas and hidradenomas. True squamous papillomas appear as warty growths and rarely become malignant. All these lesions are treated by simple biopsy excision.

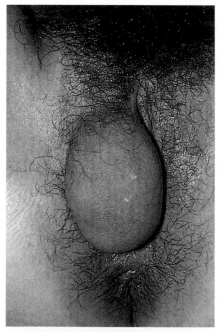

Fig. 16.24 Benign vulval cyst arising from remnant of the wolffian duct.

Vaginal cysts
Congenital

Cysts arise in the vagina from embryological remnants; the commonest varieties are those arising from Gartner's duct (wolffian duct remnants). These are not rare and occur in the anterolateral wall of the vagina. They are usually asymptomatic and are found on routine examination.

Histologically, the cysts are lined by cuboidal epithelium, but sometimes a flattened layer of stratified squamous epithelium is seen.

The cysts are treated by simple surgical excision and rarely give rise to any difficulties.

Vaginal inclusion cysts

Inclusion cysts arise from inclusion of small particles or islands of vaginal epithelium under the surface. The cysts commonly arise in episiotomy scars and contain yellowish thick fluid. They are treated by simple surgical excision.

Endometriosis

Endometriotic lesions may appear anywhere in the vagina but occur most commonly in the posterior fornix. The lesions may appear as dark brown spots or reddened ulcerated lesions. The diagnosis is established by excision biopsy. If the lesions are multiple, then medical therapy should be instituted as for lesions in other sites.

Solid benign tumours

These lesions are rare but may represent any of the tissues that are found in the vagina. Thus, polypoid tumours may include fibromyomas, myomas, fibromas, papillomas and adenomyomas. These tumours are treated by simple surgical excision.

Neoplastic lesions of the vaginal epithelium

Neoplastic lesions of the vaginal epithelium are covered in Chapter 20.

Emergency gynaecology

Pelvic infection

PID comprises a spectrum of inflammatory disorders of the upper female genital tract mainly caused by ascending infection from the cervix or vagina. Acute PID is covered in detail in Chapter 19.

Bartholin's abscess/cyst

The Bartholin's glands lie in the posterior vaginal wall at the introitus and secrete mucus-like fluid via a short duct into the vagina. They are normally the size of a pea, but when the duct becomes blocked, a cyst can form. These cysts may present acutely as an oval-shaped lump in the posterior labia, sometimes growing to the size of a golf ball or larger. They are unusually unilateral and cause discomfort with walking, sitting and sexual intercourse. When the gland is infected, most commonly with skin or genitourinary bacteria, e.g. *Staphylococcus* or *Escherichia coli*, an abscess can

develop. These arise more acutely than the Bartholin's cysts and are particularly painful.

Small asymptomatic cysts may not require treatment, and abscesses can sometimes resolve with antibiotics. However, treatment of large cysts and abscesses requires surgery. The procedure, called *marsupialization*, involves making a pouch-like opening to the gland by incising into the cyst wall and then suturing it to the overlying skin to ensure the new opening continues to drain the fluid from the glands (see Chapter 19, Fig. 19.13).

Vulval and vaginal trauma

Injuries to the vulva and vagina may result in severe haemorrhage and haematoma formation. Vulval bruising may be particularly severe because of the rich venous plexus in the labia and commonly results from falling astride. Lacerations of the vagina are often associated with coitus. Vulval haematomas often subside with conservative management but sometimes need drainage. It is important to suture vaginal lacerations and be certain that the injury does not penetrate into the peritoneal cavity.

Acute abdominal pain of uncertain origin

In a woman of reproductive age presenting with acute abdominal pain, it is first important to take a good history about the nature of the pain and the presence of associated symptoms. A thorough examination will identify the site of maximal tenderness, rebound tenderness and guarding. It is vital to always exclude pregnancy and particularly ectopic pregnancy. Gynaecological disorders in women with a negative pregnancy test and acute pelvic pain include PID, functional ovarian cysts, ovarian or peritoneal endometriosis and adnexal torsion. The most common gastrointestinal causes that can present with acute pelvic pain include appendicitis, acute sigmoid diverticulitis and Crohn's disease.

It is important in the assessment of a woman with acute pelvic pain to exclude those diagnoses that require urgent intervention: PID, ovarian torsion and appendicitis. The investigation and diagnosis of PID were discussed earlier. Ovarian torsion usually occurs in the presence of an enlarged ovary (see Chapter 20). Women with torsion present with sudden onset of sharp unilateral pelvic pain that is often accompanied by nausea and vomiting. The sonographic findings in ovarian torsion are variable. The ovary is enlarged and can be seen in an abnormal location above or behind the uterus. The absence of blood flow is an important sign, and a lack of venous waveform on Doppler ultrasound has a high positive predictive value. However, the presence of arterial and venous flow does not exclude torsion, and any cases where it is suspected clinically require laparoscopy to visualize the adnexae. If the torsion is reversed early in the process, the ovary may be saved.

Acute appendicitis

The classic history of anorexia and periumbilical pain followed by nausea, right lower quadrant (RLQ) pain and vomiting occurs in only 50% of cases. Nausea is present in 61–92% of patients; anorexia is present in 74–78% of patients.

Acute and excessively heavy unscheduled vaginal bleeding

The entity of acute HMB has recently been defined by FIGO as heavy uterine bleeding not associated with pregnancy that is of sufficient volume to require urgent or emergent medical intervention. Women presenting with acute bleeding most often have ovulatory dysfunction but may also have an underlying coagulopathy. The management of acute AUB/HMB can require D&C but can be usually managed non-surgically with the administration of gonadal hormones, and/or intrauterine tamponade. Previously, parenteral conjugated oestrogens were used, and more recently oral progestogens and sometimes double doses of the combined oral contraceptive pill have been shown to be successful. The safer option is high doses of progestogens, sometimes in combination with the anti-fibrinolytic agent, tranexamic acid. Intravenous tranexamic acid is widely used with benefit for 'acute' HMB, but there are no clinical trials to confirm the degree of this benefit.

A regimen of norethisterone 5 mg tds can be used to settle the bleeding. Follow-up is required to establish the cause of the bleeding. For really severe cases, the insertion of a small inflated Foley catheter balloon into the uterine cavity can be useful to achieve endometrial tamponade.

Essential information

Puberty

- Normal sequence is thelarche, adrenarche, growth spurt, menarche
- Menarche normally between 11 and 15 years
- Early cycles anovulatory
- Most cases of precocious puberty are constitutional
- Primary amenorrhoea not always synonymous with delayed puberty

Secondary amenorrhoea

- Absence of menstruation for more than 6 months
- Physiological causes – pregnancy, breast-feeding
- Pathological causes – hypothalamic dysfunction, hyperprolactinaemia, polycystic ovarian syndrome
- Ask about – weight, stress, chronic illness, medication, contraception
- Investigations – pregnancy test, FSH, LH, prolactin, ultrasound

Heavy menstrual bleeding

- Prolonged and/or heavy bleeding
- Commonest diagnoses are disturbance of endometrial molecular function and submucous uterine fibroids
- Only routine investigations needed are full blood count and serum ferritin
- Mainstay of treatment is medical

Premenstrual syndrome

- Cyclical changes occurring in the luteal phase of the cycle and ceasing at the onset of menstruation
- Commonest symptoms – mood changes, breast tenderness, bloating and gastrointestinal symptoms
- Treatment options are pyridoxine, evening primrose oil, suppression of ovulation
- High placebo response rate

Menopause

- Part of climacteric
- Onset 50–51 years
- Hypergonadotrophic, hypogonadic
- Associated with vasomotor instability, atrophic changes in genital tract and breast, cardiovascular changes and osteoporosis
- HRT effective in symptom relief and osteoporosis

Congenital abnormalities of the uterus

- Due to failure of müllerian ducts to fuse or develop
- Usually asymptomatic unless menstrual flow obstructed
- May cause recurrent miscarriage, malpresentation or retained placenta

Benign uterine tumours

- Commonest are EPs and fibroids
- 25% of women over 30 years old have fibroids
- Symptoms depend on size and site and include menstrual disorders, pressure symptoms and complications of pregnancy
- May undergo secondary change, including necrosis or malignant change (0.13–1%)

Endometriosis and adenomyosis

- 'Ectopic' endometrium
- Commonest sites are ovaries, uterosacral ligaments and pelvic peritoneum
- May arise from metaplastic change or implantation
- Presents as subfertility and/or crescendic dysmenorrhoea

Chapter | 17 |

Infertility

Eloïse Fraison and William Ledger

LEARNING OUTCOMES

At the end of this chapter you should be able to:

Knowledge criteria

- Describe the common causes of male and female infertility
- Describe the indications for and interpretation of investigations used in the assessment of the infertile couple
- Discuss the principles of, indications for and complications of the common methods of treatment of infertility

Clinical competencies

- Take a history from a couple presenting with infertility
- Plan appropriate initial investigation of an infertile couple

Professional skills and attitudes

- Reflect on the impact of infertility on a couple
- Reflect on the social and ethical issues relevant to the management of infertility

Estimates of the prevalence of infertility in different parts of the world give remarkably similar results, with a 12-month prevalence rate ranging from 3.5 to 16.7% in more developed nations and from 6.9 to 9.3% in less developed nations, with an estimated overall median prevalence of 9%. In the UK, for instance, one in seven couples consult due to problems in conceiving. Only half of all infertile couples seek medical help, with the proportion being similar in developed and less developed nations. Based on these estimates and on the current world population, 72.4 million women are currently infertile, and of these, 40.5 million are currently seeking infertility medical care. Although firm evidence is hard to find, it seems that the prevalence of infertility in the Western world is increasing due to a number of factors, including the increase in number of young people with sexually transmitted diseases, increase in obesity and increasing numbers of women deferring plans for childbearing until later in life.

Primary infertility is defined as infertility without a previous pregnancy or live birth, and *secondary infertility* as failure to conceive after one or more pregnancies, whether successful or ending in miscarriage, ectopic pregnancy or voluntary termination. Improved methods for investigation of infertility frequently reveal a problem in both partners, leading to the concept of relative *subfertility*. A highly fertile female partner will often compensate for a male with poor sperm quality and conceive without difficulty, and vice versa.

At the age of 25 years old, the conception rate per cycle is approximately 25%; at 35 years old, it is 12%; and at 40 years old, it is only 6% per cycle. For a couple of reproductive age, if conception does not occur after 12 months of regular sexual intercourse, the couple should be considered potentially infertile, as 80% of couples normally conceive within 1 year. It is therefore reasonable to proceed with investigations at this time. However, this definition should be tempered by common sense. For example, a woman who has lost both Fallopian tubes because of ectopic pregnancies or a man who is known to have had testicular torsion in his youth should not be denied early investigation and treatment.

Both partners should be seen and investigated together, as infertility may result from male or female factors and is often associated with a combination of both. Indeed, in 30% the cause is due to male factor, 30% to female factor, 20% to both female and male factor and 20% cases of infertility are 'unexplained'.

Long-term follow-up studies of couples with unexplained infertility have shown that 30–40% will conceive over a 7-year period after investigation. Many 'unexplained' cases involve women over age 35 years who may later be shown to have a poor response to ovarian stimulation and oocyte abnormalities

Table 17.1 Female age and live birth rate per embryo transfer (fresh and frozen) in the UK (2015).

	Under 35	35–37	38–39	40–42	43–44	Over 44
Fresh	30	22	16	9	4	1
Frozen	25	23	18	14	9	6

Data sourced from www.HFEA.gov.uk.

Table 17.2 Causes of infertility

Diagnosis*	Primary infertile group (n = 167) N (%)	Secondary infertile group (n = 151) N (%)	P-value
Ovulation problems	54 (32.3)	35 (23.2)	0.069
Sperm quality problems	49 (29.3)	36 (23.8)	0.268
Blocked Fallopian tubes	20 (12)	21 (13.9)	0.607
Unexplained infertility	49 (29.3)	45 (29.8)	0.928
Endometriosis	19 (10.7)	15 (10)	0.677
Others	23 (13.8)	32 (21.2)	0.081

*Women have reported more than one diagnosis.
Data derived from a Scottish general practice–based survey (Bhattacharya S, et al. (2010) The epidemiology of infertility in the North East of Scotland. Hum Reprod 24:3096-3107). Self-reported cause of infertility amongst women who reported a diagnosis (northeast Scotland). The data reflect unsuccessful attempted conception for 12 months or longer and/or had sought medical help with conception.

if in vitro fertilization (IVF) is performed. Age, particularly female age, undoubtedly affects fertility. IVF success rates, defined by a live birth rate, fall sharply after age 38 (Table 17.1). The effect of age on the male is less pronounced, but older men exhibit more sperm abnormalities and DNA fragmentation.

The relative incidence of causative factors will vary according to country and whether the problem is primary or secondary. Furthermore, in many couples there are multiple reasons for the infertility. Table 17.2 shows the pattern of causative factors of primary infertility in a Western population.

History and examination

As mentioned, the initial consultation should involve both partners. Many clinics use a pro forma questionnaire to elicit basic information, allowing better use to be made of the time available in the consultation. Basic investigations, including baseline blood tests for both partners, and semen analysis can be organized through the general practice with results available at the initial meeting.

The history should include the following:

- Age, occupation and educational background of both partners

- Number of years that conception has been attempted and the previous history of contraception
- Previous conceptions of either partner in this or previous relationships
- Details of any complications associated with previous pregnancies, deliveries and postpartum
- Full gynaecological history, including regularity, frequency and nature of menses; cervical smears; intermenstrual bleeding; and vaginal discharge
- Coital history, including frequency of intercourse, dyspareunia, postcoital bleeding and erectile or ejaculatory dysfunction
- History of sexually transmitted diseases and their treatment
- A general medical history to include concurrent or previous serious illness or surgery, particularly in relation to appendicitis in the female or herniorrhaphy in the male; a history of undescended testes or of orchidopexy

Examination of both partners should be considered, although examination of the male is unlikely to reveal anything of significance in the presence of a normal semen analysis; that of the woman may well be equally unremarkable if there is a normal high-quality pelvic ultrasound. Azoospermic men should be examined for congenital bilateral absence of the vas deferens (CBAVD), which is associated with cystic fibrosis mutations.

Case study

Mrs and Mr Y were referred to the gynaecology clinic after trying to conceive for 5 years now without success. Mrs Y was 32 years old; her mother died of breast cancer at 38 years of age. She had no other personal or familial past history. Her menses were regular and painless, with regular ovulation. Her last cervical smear was 1 year previously and normal. Her body mass index (BMI) was 23 and clinical examination normal.

Mr Y was 33 years old. He had no personal medical history. He had one brother older than him, with no children.

The results of initial investigations for the couple showed that Mrs Y had an anti-müllerian hormone (AMH) of 30 pmol/mL, a follicle-stimulating hormone (FSH) of 5 IU/L, luteinizing hormone (LH) of 3 IU/L and E2 of 130 pMol/L. She was ovulating normally with a day-21 progesterone of 53 nMol/L. Her ultrasound was normal with evidence of tubal patency. She also saw a geneticist and did not have a detectable *BRCA* mutation. Mr Y was found to be azoospermia and with an acid seminal pH.

Mr Y was referred to an andrologist. He had a clinical examination and scrotal ultrasound. Clinical examination suggested CBAVD, which was confirmed by ultrasound. The patient was referred to a geneticist and was found to have a heterozygous mutation of the *CFTR*. His wife was also tested for the mutation and was negative.

In many cases of CBAVD it is possible to retrieve sperm from the epididymis or testis by surgical extraction. This can be used in an IVF cycle for intracytoplasmic sperm injection (ICSI). Use of donor sperm may be necessary in cases in which this is not possible.

Female infertility

General factors such as age, serious systemic illness, inadequate nutrition, excessive exercise and emotional stress may all contribute to female infertility. The majority of cases of female infertility follow from disorders of tubal or uterine anatomy or function, or ovarian dysfunction leading to anovulation. Less frequently observed disorders include cervical mucus 'hostility', endometriosis and dyspareunia.

Disorders of ovulation

Disorders of ovulation are divided into four categories, defined by the World Health Organization (WHO):
- Type I – Hypogonadal hypogonadism resulting from failure of pulsatile gonadotrophin secretion from the pituitary. This relatively rare condition can be congenital (as in Kallman's syndrome) or acquired, for example,

Case study

Mrs and Mr X presented with a 2-year history of trying to conceive without success. They were having regular intercourse.

Mrs X was 26 years old and had no personal or familial past history. She had irregular menses and struggled with facial acne for which she took Roaccutane before her desire to become pregnant. Her BMI was 28. On clinical examination, she was found to have abnormal hirsutes on her breast and abdomen. Her blood pressure was normal.

Mr X was 30 years old and had no personal or familial past history.

Mr X had a normal semen analysis. A pelvic ultrasound showed that Mrs X had an anteverted uterus, normal tubal patency and polycystic ovaries. Her blood test on day 3 showed an AMH of 35 pmol/L, FSH 7 IU/L, LH 9 IU/L, E2 at 110 pmol/L and testosterone at 3.2 nMol/L.

Progesterone on day 21 was 3.0 nMol/L. Her prolactin, thyroid-stimulating hormone (TSH) and fasting glucose lipid profiles were normal. Her cervical smear was normal, and she was rubella immune.

As the patient is under 30 years old, the first consideration should be a lifestyle modification program to help her improve physical fitness and lose weight. This should continue for at least 6 months. Five percent weight loss can restore normal ovulation in 50% of women with PCOS. She can be advised to track her ovulation with a Clearblue stick.

If she has not conceived after 6 months, consider use of clomiphene citrate or letrozole, which can restore ovulation in approximately 70% of women with anovular PCOS, with a pregnancy rate of approximately 60% after six cycles.

Third-line treatment may be either laparoscopic ovarian diathermy (LOD) or low-dose FSH ovarian stimulation, although there is a significant risk of multiple pregnancy with the latter approach.

The ultimate approach to treatment if there is no success with ovulation induction would be an IVF with a low-dose FSH stimulation in an antagonist-controlled cycle, with an agonist trigger and 'freeze all' embryos to avoid risk of ovarian hyperstimulation syndrome (OHSS).

after surgery or radiotherapy for a pituitary tumour. Serum concentrations of LH and FSH and oestradiol are abnormally low/undetectable, and menses will be absent or very infrequent.
- Type II – Normogonadotropic anovulation, most commonly caused by polycystic ovary syndrome (PCOS; see Chapter 16). Serum concentrations of FSH will be normal and LH normal or raised. Serum AMH will be elevated, and there may also be elevation of serum testosterone or free androgen index.

- Type III – Hypergonadotropic hypogonadism, frequently described as *premature ovarian failure*, describes cessation of ovulation due to depletion of the ovarian follicle pool before age 40 years. Serum gonadotrophin concentrations will be greatly raised and AMH low/undetectable, with postmenopausal (low) concentrations of oestradiol.
- Type IV – Hyperprolactinaemia, with elevated serum prolactin and low/normal serum FSH and LH. Frequently due to a pituitary microadenoma, although it is important to rule out a space-occupying macroadenoma using pituitary magnetic resonance imaging (MRI) or computed tomography (CT).

Anovulation is usually associated with amenorrhoea or oligomenorrhoea. Alterations in the menstrual cycle are commonly associated with periods of stress and with excessive weight gain or obesity, worsening the impact of PCOS on ovulation, or, at the other extreme, with anorexia nervosa or excessive exercise leading to hypogonadal (type I) anovulation.

Tubal factors

The Fallopian tube must first collect the ovum from its site of ovulation from the ruptured Graafian follicle and then transport the ovum to the ampullary segment, where fertilization occurs. The fertilized ovum must then be transported to the uterine cavity to arrive at the correct point in the menstrual cycle at which the endometrium becomes receptive to implantation (the 'implantation window'). Tubal factors account for about 10–30% of cases of infertility: this figure varies considerably according to the population involved. Occasionally, congenital anomalies occur, but the commonest cause of tubal damage is infection. Infection may cause occlusion of the fimbrial end of the tube, with the collection of fluid (hydrosalpinx) or pus (pyosalpinx) within the tubal lumen (Fig. 17.1).

The commonest cause of acute salpingitis in the UK is infection with *Chlamydia trachomatis*, but it may also result from infection with other organisms such as *Neisseria gonorrhoeae*, *Escherichia coli*, anaerobic and haemolytic streptococci, staphylococci and *Clostridium welchii*. The incidence of tubal damage is approximately 8% after the first episode of pelvic infection, 16% after two and 40% after three episodes. Tubal or uterine tuberculosis has begun to be seen more frequently in the UK in the immigrant population or their relatives.

Disorders such as appendicitis associated with peritonitis or inflammatory conditions, including Crohn's disease or ulcerative colitis, can result in peritubal and peri-ovarian adhesions, leaving the internal structure of the Fallopian tube relatively unaffected.

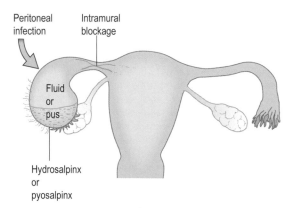

Fig. 17.1 The pathogenesis of tubal occlusion and subfertility; intramural tubal obstruction results from intrauterine infection.

> ! Even in the presence of a patent tube, damage to the internal structure with depletion of cilia and impairment of tubal peristalsis may result in loss of tubal function.

Uterine factors

Implantation is less likely to occur if there is distortion of the uterine cavity due to submucous fibroids or congenital abnormalities such as an intrauterine septum. These disorders are often amenable to surgical correction. Subserous or entirely intramural fibroids do not appear to affect implantation. The effect of adenomyosis on implantation is unclear, although the disorder has been linked to recurrent implantation failure and miscarriage. Intrauterine adhesions or synechiae following over-vigorous curettage or infection (Asherman's syndrome) result in inadequate endometrial development, absent or light periods and recurrent implantation failure.

Endometriosis

Endometriosis is an enigmatic condition with numerous theories related to aetiology and poorly defined links to infertility. Severe disease with large ovarian cysts and extensive adhesions distorting tubal anatomy and potentially interfering with approximation of the fimbriae to the mature follicle are likely to lead to subfertility due to impairment of ovulation and entrapment of the oocyte by the Fallopian tube. However, milder forms of the disorder have also been linked to problems of subfertility, and surgical treatment of grade I and II endometriosis led to a significant improvement in spontaneous pregnancy and live birth rates in a large randomized trial.

Case study

A 30-year-old woman, Mrs Z, presented complaining of painful and heavy periods. She had stopped using the contraceptive pill 3 months earlier in order to conceive. She had no relevant general medical history, and her husband was equally healthy. She had one sister who had her first child at 22 years old and her second at 24. Her mother was healthy, having reached menopause at age 52.

Mrs Z described surgery 1 year previously at which she was diagnosed with stage 4 endometriosis with bilateral endometriomata, which were completely excised. She was prescribed the combined oral contraceptive pill from the time of surgery. Her cycles were regular. She changed her sanitary protection every hour on the first day of her period. She had moderate dyspareunia but no symptoms relating to bowel or bladder function. Her preoperative AMH was 15 pMol/L.

Pelvic ultrasound showed normal ovaries, but the antral follicle count (AFC) was 3, and her right tube was not patent to contrast. Her AMH was 2 pmol/L, FSH 10 IU/L, LH 5 IU/L and E2 130 pMol/L. There was no evidence of recurrence of her endometriosis. The uterus was bulky with suspicion of early diffuse adenomyosis. Semen analysis was normal.

The investigations indicated that she has a decreased ovarian reserve, and her right tube had probably been damaged, both probably due to consequences of endometriosis and ovarian surgery. She was advised to commence IVF treatment with a long agonist protocol involving at least 6 weeks of pituitary downregulation with a gonadotropin-releasing hormone (GnRH) agonist.

Cervical factors

At the time of ovulation, endocervical cells secrete copious, clear, watery mucus, with high water content and elongated glycoprotein molecules containing channels that facilitate passage of spermatozoa into the uterine cavity. Sperm penetration occurs within 2–3 minutes of deposition. Between 100,000 and 200,000 sperm colonize the cervical mucus and remain at this level for approximately 24 hours after coitus. Approximately 200 sperm eventually reach the Fallopian tube. After ovulation, mucus produced by the cervix under the influence of progesterone is hostile to sperm penetration. Cervical infection or antisperm antibodies in cervical mucus or seminal plasma can inhibit sperm penetration and result in subfertility.

Male infertility

Male infertility can be divided into three categories: obstructive azoospermia, non-obstructive azoospermia and mixed (association of obstructive and non-obstructive azoospermia).

Obstructive azoospermia

Obstructive azoospermia may result from infection, trauma or side effects of surgery such as herniorrhaphy, leading to an obstruction of the genital tract. It can also be due to CBAVD or a stenosis of the ejaculatory duct.

If a CBAVD is found, the patient should have a genetic consultation and mutations in genes causing the patient to be a carrier for cystic fibrosis should be sought, since this has obvious implications for the potential offspring.

Non-obstructive azoospermia

Non-obstructive azoospermia can be due to primary testicular disorders or be secondary to central hypogonadal hypogonadism.

Testicular causes include androgen insensitivity, chromosomal abnormalities such as Klinefelter's syndrome, past history of cryptorchidism, treatment with gonadotoxic chemotherapy or a number of other medications, bilateral anorchia, testicular tumour or varicocele. Hypogonadal hypogonadism in the male can result from congenital abnormalities including Kallman's syndrome, genetic abnormalities such as Prader–Willi syndrome or haemocromatosis or may follow surgery or radiotherapy to a pituitary tumour. Hypogonadal hypogonadism may also result from hyperprolactinaemia as a result of micro or macro adenoma or use of medications, including those commonly used to treat male alopecia or in bodybuilding.

Investigation of infertility

Investigation of the female partner

All women presenting with infertility should have their rubella immunity checked and, if seronegative, be offered vaccination before undertaking further treatment for their infertility. They should also be advised to take folic acid supplementation from the outset of investigation and treatment of their fertility problem to reduce chances of spina bifida in their child.

Detection of ovulation

The assessment of ovulation depends on the menstrual history. In the presence of a regular menstrual cycle, ovulatory status can be investigated by changes in basal body temperature (BBT), cervical mucus or hormone levels; by endometrial biopsy; or by ultrasound. However, measurement of BBT is difficult for many women to achieve and requires daily charting, increasing stress with a daily reminder of failure to conceive. Hence measurement of BBT is no longer recommended. Similarly, many women find assessment of cervical mucus changes difficult and challenging, and this method is also not recommended. Ovulation can be inferred by detection of the LH surge in blood or urine, with a peak that occurs approximately 24 hours before ovulation. Modern commercially available LH surge detection kits can provide reassurance and allow timing of intercourse. Formation of the corpus luteum can be demonstrated by measurement of serum progesterone in the luteal phase of the cycle. A mid-luteal concentration above 25 nmol/L is usually accepted as evidence of ovulation, although values vary from laboratory to laboratory.

> There is no need to measure thyroid function or prolactin levels in women with regular menstrual cycles unless they have symptoms of galactorrhoea or thyroid disease.

Ultrasonography

Transvaginal ultrasound examination of the ovaries can be used to track follicle growth. Follicular diameter increases from 11.5 mm 5 days before ovulation to 20 mm on the day before ovulation and decreases to approximately half this size on the day after ovulation, with opacification of the follicular remnant as the corpus luteum forms. This is a helpful, although time-consuming, way of monitoring the time of ovulation. Ultrasound may also be of value in the diagnosis of PCOS or ovarian endometrioma.

Investigation of anovulation

If there is evidence of anovulation, further investigation should include measurement of:
- Serum FSH, LH and oestradiol on day 2 or 3 of a natural or induced menstruation, along with measurement of AMH
- Serum prolactin and thyroid function
- MRI or CT of the sella turcica if prolactin levels are raised

Assessment of ovarian reserve

Advancing female age is one of the strongest prognostic factors that determines the success or otherwise of IVF treatment. Ovarian reserve testing using measurement of AMH in serum and/or AFC with transvaginal ultrasound allows an individual estimate of 'ovarian reserve' to be made. An age-related low AMH or low AFC predicts poor oocyte yield at IVF and a lower-than-average chance of pregnancy, whereas higher-than-average values predict a better ovarian response to gonadotrophin stimulation. However, although these markers are helpful in identifying predicted oocyte *quantity* after stimulation, they do not identify oocyte *quality* with the same precision. Quality (potential for fertilization and implantation leading to healthy live birth) seems to be more closely related to female age, such that a young 'poor responder' to stimulation has a good chance of pregnancy, whereas an older 'good responder' may obtain a larger-than-usual number of oocytes but there is still a reduced chance of pregnancy.

Investigation of tubal patency

It is essential to establish tubal patency before beginning ovulation induction or intrauterine insemination. Tubal patency need not be established if the couple are to proceed directly to IVF if, for example, there is a severe male factor. However, uterine anatomy should then be checked with high-resolution transvaginal ultrasound or hysterosalpingography (HSG).

Hysterosalpingography

A radio-opaque contrast medium is injected into the uterine cavity and Fallopian tubes. General anaesthesia is unnecessary. The contrast medium outlines the uterine cavity and will demonstrate any filling defects. It will also show whether there is evidence of tubal obstruction and the site of the obstruction (Fig. 17.2). HSG should be performed within the first 10 days of the menstrual cycle to avoid inadvertent irradiation of a newly fertilized embryo. Women should be screened for *C. trachomatis* infection or given appropriate antibiotic prophylaxis before HSG in order to reduce the risk of reactivation of infection leading to pelvic abscess formation.

Hysterosonocontrast sonography

Hysterosonocontrast sonography (HyCoSy) using transvaginal ultrasound to observe filling of the uterine cavity and Fallopian tubes has recently been introduced as an alternative to HSG. HyCoSy avoids exposure to ionizing radiation and allows real-time observation of uterine and tubal anatomy. High-quality ultrasound equipment and a degree of technical expertise are necessary to obtain good images.

Laparoscopy and dye insufflation

Laparoscopy enables direct visualization of the pelvic organs and allows assessment of pelvic pathologies such as endometriosis or adhesions. Methylene blue is injected through the cervix in order to test tubal patency. Laparoscopy can be combined with hysteroscopy to assess the uterine cavity. A 'see-and-treat' policy allows for rapid surgical treatment of minor degrees of endometriosis or adhesions, although surgery that may result in damage to pelvic structures is better left to another occasion to allow full discussion of the implications of surgery to take place with the patient and her partner. Laparoscopy almost invariably requires general anaesthesia, and there are small but significant risks of damage to pelvic structures, including bowel,

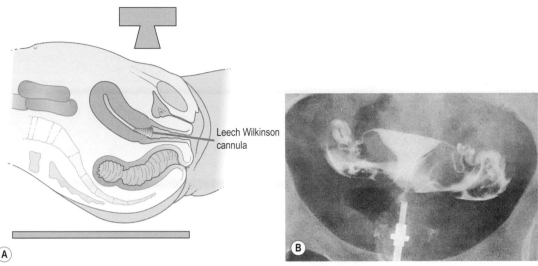

Fig. 17.2 (A) Hysterosalpingography enables assessment of the site of tubal obstruction and the presence of pathology in the uterine cavity. (B) The triangular outline of the uterine cavity can be seen and the spill of dye on both sides from the fimbrial ends of the Fallopian tubes. The dye spreads over the adjacent bowel.

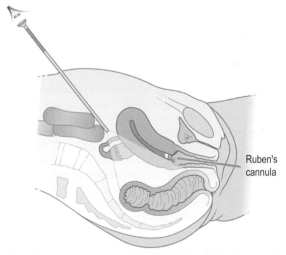

Fig. 17.3 Dye laparoscopy for evaluation of tubal patency.

bladder and ureter at laparoscopy, so less invasive methods are preferred as first-line investigations unless there is a specific indication, such as a history of pelvic inflammatory disease or appendicitis with peritonitis (Fig. 17.3).

Investigation of cervical factor infertility

'Cervical factor' infertility tests, such as postcoital tests, are not recommended in the routine investigation of the infertile couple because of the lack of established normal criteria and poor correlation between findings and fertility. Modern treatments for infertility, such as intrauterine insemination (IUI) or IVF, will bypass cervical mucus and circumvent any possible cervical causes for infertility.

Investigation of the male partner

The most useful investigation of the male partner is by semen analysis. Semen should be collected by masturbation into a sterile container after 3 days abstinence and examined within 2 hours of collection. The sample is best collected in a private facility adjacent to the andrology laboratory to avoid cooling during transportation and allow accurate identification of the male partner.

The lower reference limits and 95% confidence intervals for sperm parameters (WHO 2010) are given in Table 17.3. The major features of the semen analysis are:

- Volume: 80% of fertile males ejaculate between 1 mL and 4 mL of semen. Low volumes may indicate androgen deficiency, and high volumes abnormal accessory gland function.
- Sperm concentration: The absence of all sperm (azoospermia) indicates sterility, although sperm may well be recoverable by percutaneous epididymal aspiration (PESA) or testicular aspiration (TESA) or testicular biopsy. The lower limit of normal is between 15 million and 20 million sperm/mL, but the findings should not be accepted on a single sample, as there is significant fluctuation from day to day. Abnormally high values, in excess of 200 million sperm/mL, may be associated with subfertility.

Table 17.3 Lower reference limits (5th centiles and their 95% confidence intervals) for semen characteristics

Parameter	Lower reference limit
Semen volume (mL)	1.5 (1.4–1.7)
Total sperm number (10^6 per ejaculate)	39 (33–46)
Sperm concentration (10^6/mL)	15 (12–16)
Total motility (PR + NP, %)	40 (38–42)
Progressive motility (PR, %)	32 (31–34)
Vitality (live spermatozoa, %)	58 (55–63)
Sperm morphology (normal forms, %)	4 (3.0–4.0)
Other consensus threshold values	
pH	≥ 7.2
Peroxidase-positive leukocytes (10^6/mL)	<1.0
MAR test (motile spermatozoa with bound particles, %)	<50
Immunobead test (motile spermatozoa with bound beads, %)	<50
Seminal fructose (μmol/ejaculate)	≥ 13
Seminal neutral glucosidase (mU/ejaculate)	≥ 20

Data from Cooper TG, Noonan E, von Eckardstein S, et al. (2010) World Health Organization reference values for human semen characteristics. Hum Reprod Update 16:231–245.

- A normal analysis should show good motility in 60% of sperm within 1 hour of collection. The characteristic of forward progression is equally important. The WHO grades sperm motility according to the following criteria:
  - Grade 1 – rapid and linear progressive motility
  - Grade 2 – slow or sluggish linear or non-linear motility
  - Grade 3 – non-progressive motility
  - Grade 4 – immotile
- Sperm morphology shows great variability even in normal fertile males and is less predictive of subfertility than count or motility. It is important to look for leukocytes, as they may indicate the presence of infection. If pus cells are present, the semen should be cultured for bacteriological growth.

Spermatogenesis and sperm function may be affected by a wide range of toxins and therapeutic agents. Various toxins and drugs may act on the seminiferous tubules and the epididymis

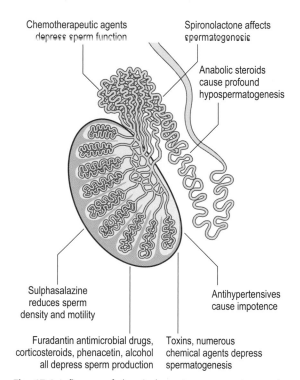

Fig. 17.4 Influence of chemical agents on spermatogenesis.

to inhibit spermatogenesis. Chemotherapeutic agents, particularly alkylating agents, depress sperm function, and sulfasalazine frequently used to treat Crohn's disease, reduces sperm motility and density. Patients who are prescribed chemotherapy or pelvic radiotherapy should be offered sperm cryopreservation before treatment to allow them to start a family later in life once their disease has been successfully treated (Fig. 17.4).

Additionally, antihypertensive agents can cause erectile dysfunction, and anabolic steroids used for bodybuilding may produce profound hypospermatogenesis.

Analysis of sperm DNA

Standard tests of sperm concentration, motility and morphology are poorly predictive of the ability of a couple to conceive. The integrity of sperm chromosomal DNA is essential for normal fertilization and transmission of paternal genetic information, and tests of sperm DNA integrity generally correlate with routine semen variables, including impaired sperm concentration or motility. Sperm DNA is protected from damage while the sperm is transported through the male and female reproductive tracts, and damage to sperm DNA may lead to impaired fertility.

The most frequently used measure of sperm DNA damage is the sperm chromatin structure assay (SCSA) that measures the stability of sperm chromatin in acid media with acridine orange. The dye gives rise to green fluorescence when bound to intact DNA and red when bound to fragmented DNA; the proportion of sperm with fragmented DNA is determined by flow cytometry and expressed as the DNA fragmentation index (DFI). Other commonly used tests include the deoxynucleotidyl transferase-mediated dUTP nick end labelling (TUNEL) assay in which fluorescence-activated cells are sorted by flow cytometry, the single cell electrophoresis assay (Comet) that measures single-strand and double-strand DNA breaks using electrophoresis and the Halo (SCD) test that identifies sperm with fragmented DNA because they fail to produce the characteristic halo when mixed with aqueous agarose following acid/salt treatment. Each assay has its strengths and weaknesses, and results imputing normality or abnormality do not always concur between assays.

In clinical studies, sperm DNA integrity is impaired among infertile compared with fertile men and with poor semen quality. Time-to-pregnancy studies with apparently normally fertile couples at the time of stopping contraception showed that results of the SCSA test were significantly associated with the probability of pregnancy. However, IVF and ICSI studies have been less conclusive in relating sperm DNA integrity results to fertilization or pregnancy rates. At present, assessment of sperm DNA damage should remain as a research tool, and routine use as a diagnostic test should await further evidence of ability to discriminate between those couples who will or will not conceive.

Endocrine assessment of the male

High serum concentrations of FSH and low AMH indicate testicular damage, whereas normal levels may indicate obstructive disease. Low or undetectable serum concentrations of FSH and LH are found in males with hypopituitarism, which may be treated with FSH/LH replacement therapy. The presence of high FSH, low AMH and azoospermia obviates the need for further investigation, as these findings indicate spermatogenic failure. However, testicular biopsy may reveal intratesticular foci of spermatogenesis, allowing retrieval of sperm for use in ICSI, even if FSH is raised and AMH suppressed.

Hyperprolactinaemia may occur in the male in association with a pituitary adenoma and may cause impotence or oligospermia.

Cytogenetic studies

Chromosome analysis in males with azoospermia may indicate the presence of a karyotype of XXY or XYY and, occasionally, autosomal translocation in the presence of oligospermia. Oligospermic men (fewer than 5 million motile sperm) should be screened for cystic fibrosis gene mutations. Carriers for such mutations may be healthy but could conceive a child with cystic fibrosis after IVF if their partner is also a carrier for the mutation.

Testicular/epididymal biopsy

Testicular biopsy may demonstrate the presence of spermatogenesis even if there are elevated concentrations of gonadotrophins. Sperm may be aspirated and cryopreserved for later use in ICSI. Men with obstruction of the vas deferens, e.g. postvasectomy, may undergo PESA with a high chance of obtaining sperm that are suitable for ICSI.

Retrograde ejaculation

Retrograde ejaculation is a rare cause of infertility. It should be suspected following a transurethral resection of the prostate. The diagnosis is made by detecting spermatozoa in the urine following orgasm. Sperm can be retrieved from an alkalinized postorgasm urine sample for use in ICSI.

Immunological tests for male infertility

Immunity to sperm may occur in the male: autoimmunity to sperm antigens can be related to infertility. Antigen–antibody reactions may lead to autoimmune infertility by neutralizing sperm capacitation or by blocking sperm receptors on the oocyte zona pellucida. Sperm antibodies in seminal plasma appear in the IgG and IgA class (IgG and IgA are different kinds of immunoglobins) and can be detected using the mixed agglutination reaction (MAR). Sperm-bound antibodies appear to have a significant negative effect on fertility when there is more than 50% binding.

Treatment of female subfertility

If the history, examination and systematic investigation in both partners are normal and the duration of infertility is less than 18 months, the couple should be reassured and advised regarding coital frequency and simple lifestyle changes that may improve chances of conception. Both partners should be advised to stop smoking and limit their intake of alcohol. Women or men with a BMI of more than 30 should be encouraged to join a supervised programme of weight loss.

However, if the woman is over 30 years of age, this 'wait and see' policy is unwise, since delay will have a significant adverse impact on her lifetime chance of conception using IVF. The couple should be referred rapidly to a specialist infertility clinic that has access to the full range of assisted reproductive technologies (ARTs), including IVF and ICSI, IUI and donor sperm and oocyte treatments.

Anovulation

In the presence of WHO group II anovulation with stigmata of PCOS, normal FSH and prolactin levels, the drug of choice remains clomiphene citrate. Clomiphene will produce ovulation in 80% of subjects, leading to pregnancy in about one-half of those who ovulate. Clomiphene is administered from day 2 to 6 of the cycle with an initial dosage of 50 mg/day, increased to 100 and 150 mg/day where necessary. Ovulation can be monitored by measurement of day-21 progesterone levels, although restoration of a regular menstrual cycle is frequently followed by pregnancy as ovulation resumes. Rates of twin pregnancy of 6–10% have been reported, with higher-order pregnancies being reported in approximately 1:1000 patients. Ultrasound monitoring of follicle growth is recommended, with abstention from intercourse if there are more than two mature follicles to reduce the incidence of multiple pregnancy. More recently, the aromatase inhibitor letrozole has been used as an oral alternative to clomiphene and is now recommended as the first-line therapy, with an increase in the percentage of women who ovulate and possibly better pregnancy rates. However, letrozole remains unlicensed for treatment of infertility.

Second-line management of anovulation may involve LOD, which induces ovulation in over 70% of PCOS patients. LOD has the advantage of inducing natural mono-ovulation with a risk of multiple pregnancy no higher than background and, when successful, allowing a drug-free and more natural conception. Alternatively, ovulation may be induced with daily injection of recombinant or urinary-derived FSH, although this may be costly, and monitoring with ultrasound and blood tests is required due to the possibility of over-response and risk of multiple pregnancy. Careful management using a low-dose, step-up regimen can produce acceptable pregnancy rates with a low multiple pregnancy rate.

Anovulation associated with hyperprolactinaemia in the absence of macroadenoma can be treated with a dopamine receptor agonist such as cabergoline. Cabergoline is preferred to bromocriptine due to its ease of administration and reduced incidence of side effects.

Tubal pathology

Tubal microsurgery has been almost completely supplanted by IVF in the management of tubal infertility. Laparoscopic surgery may still be necessary to perform salpingectomy or tubal clipping prior to IVF in the presence of hydrosalpynx to reduce chances of contamination of the endometrial cavity with 'toxic' hydrosalpyngeal secretions, or for preliminary ovarian cystectomy or myomectomy.

Salpingolysis to release peritubal adhesions still has a place if the fimbrial ends of the tubes are well preserved. However, it is important not to lose too much time if the woman is over 30 years of age. At times the blocked tubal end can be opened, i.e. salpingostomy (Fig. 17.5). There is an increased risk of ectopic pregnancy after all forms of tubal surgery.

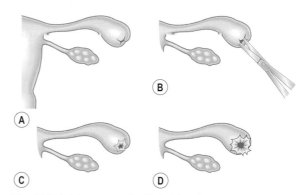

Fig. 17.5 Salpingostomy for fimbrial occlusions and hydrosalpynx. (A) Intact hydrosalpynx. (B, C) Opening of the fimbriae. (D) Suturing the opened hydrosalpinx.

Intrauterine insemination

Placement of a sample of sperm into the uterine cavity using a soft, flexible catheter has been performed for many years. The technique has been enhanced by preparation of the semen sample by washing and isolation of motile sperm and by stimulation of ovulation using low-dose gonadotrophins. IUI can be seen as a specific treatment for coital dysfunction and for abnormalities of cervical mucus but is also used frequently to treat unexplained infertility and mild male factor infertility. IUI requires healthy, patent Fallopian tubes. Live birth rates in high-quality centres are between 15% and 20% per cycle, although IUI remains a cost-effective alternative to IVF because of the lower doses of gonadotrophins, reduced level of monitoring and simplified laboratory requirements.

In vitro fertilization and embryo transfer

IVF and its many variants have revolutionized the management of infertility since the birth of Louise Brown in 1978. Forty years on, more than 7 million children have been born following IVF, and generally reassuring data on safety of IVF, ICSI and embryo cryopreservation have been compiled by the European Society for Human Reproduction and Embryology and the American Society for Reproductive Medicine. Essentially, IVF involves stimulation of multiple ovarian follicle development using recombinant or urinary-derived gonadotrophins, with concurrent use of a GnRH agonist or antagonist to prevent a premature LH surge and ovulation before oocytes are harvested. Oocytes are collected using transvaginal ultrasound-guided needle follicle aspiration, with the oocytes being isolated from the follicular fluid and cultured in the presence of a washed sample of the partner's sperm. Fertilized oocytes (embryos) can be cultured for up to 5 days, at which point they reach the blastocyst stage of division and it becomes possible to

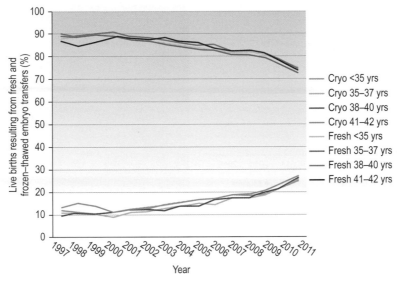

Fig. 17.6 The contribution of fresh and frozen-thawed embryo transfers to the number of total live birth rate. Data derived from a U.S. study showing the increasing contribution of frozen embryo transfer in total live birth rate after assisted reproductive technology per age. *Cryo*, Cryopreserved. Reprinted by permission from the American Society for Reproductive Medicine (Fertility and Sterility 2014;102(1):19–26).

make a detailed assessment of their morphological quality. The 'best' one or two blastocysts are then transferred to the uterine cavity using a simple catheter, with remaining blastocysts being cryopreserved for use later if conception does not follow the fresh embryo transfer (Fig. 17.6).

There are many variations on this theme – embryos can be transferred on day 2 or 3 of development rather than as blastocysts, or all embryos may be cryopreserved without a fresh transfer if there is risk of OHSS. Embryos can also be biopsied for preimplantation genetic diagnosis (PGD) or screening (PGS) of chromosomal or genetic disorders with transfer only of those screened as normal. ICSI is widely used in cases of moderate to severe male factor infertility to inject a single spermatozoon directly into the cytoplasm of the oocyte, giving similar fertilization and pregnancy rates to IVF. Female age remains the main determinant of outcome, and an increasing number of women are resorting to treatment with donated oocytes from younger women as a means of achieving pregnancy at a time of life when their own ovarian reserve is too low to allow them the opportunity of healthy pregnancy and live birth. Whilst treatment with donor oocytes has a high chance of a healthy live birth, the child does not have the DNA of his or her birth mother, and the shortage of altruistic donors has led to development of an international market in oocytes from paid donors. Payment to oocyte or sperm donors remains illegal in the UK, although at time of writing a Human Fertilisation and Embryology Authority (HFEA) consultation is underway to assess societal attitudes to this ethical dilemma.

In the UK, ART is regulated by the HFEA that oversees all aspects of IVF treatment. The HFEA has proven a useful interface between the public and government, on one hand, and IVF clinics, on the other, allowing for ethical debate and imposition of 'best practice' in areas of clinical and laboratory safety. HFEA also collates treatment results from all clinics in the UK, providing a snapshot of what can be achieved by ART. Fertilization rates after IVF are between 60% and 80%, depending largely on the age of the woman, and most patients who undertake IVF will have an embryo transfer. However, implantation rates remain relatively low, leading to a live birth in 30–40% of cycles in most centres.

The most frequent cause of obstetric and paediatric problems in offspring from IVF is the result of multiple pregnancy leading to premature birth. Transfer of two, three or more embryos in a single IVF cycle was commonplace in the early days of ART, but many countries, led by those in Scandinavia, have adopted a policy of single embryo transfer (SET) in the majority of IVF cycles. Multiple pregnancy rates remain at approximately 15% in the UK but are falling steadily (Fig. 17.7). Improved success rates from transfer of frozen embryos after cryopreservation using vitrification have made SET a more attractive option to couples, since their chances of a live birth after sequential transfer of one fresh then one frozen embryo are equivalent to those seen after transfer of two fresh embryos but without the risk of multiple pregnancy. The higher percentage of multiple pregnancies seen in the older patient groups reflects the lower overall chances of pregnancy, leading

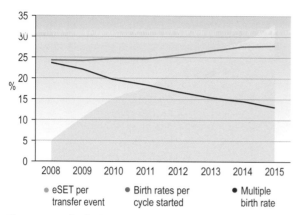

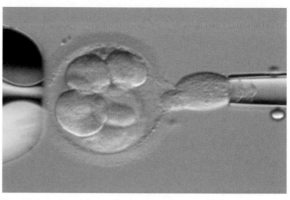

Fig. 17.8 Embryo biopsy day 3, cleavage-stage blastomere biopsy.

Fig. 17.7 UK live birth rate (per cycle started) and multiple birth rate (per live birth), fresh and frozen: 2008–2015. *eSET*, Elective single embryo transfers. (Data sourced from www.HFEA.gov.uk.)

patients and practitioners to resort to desperate measures in order to try and achieve a pregnancy.

Preimplantation genetic diagnosis or preimplantation genetic screening

The first preimplantation genetic testing was performed in the 1990s. Early studies used fluorescent in situ hybridization (FISH), but as this only probed a limited number of chromosomes, results were often disappointing. New technologies, first comparative genomic hybridization (CGH) and, more recently, next-generation sequencing (NGS), are now used. Biopsy of the embryo is now usually done, collecting cells from the trophectoderm to avoid damage to the inner cell mass (Figs 17.8 and 17.9).

PGD is used to detect specific single gene abnormalities that have been shown to exist in one or both parents, such as autosomal-recessive diseases in which both parents are carriers (e.g. cystic fibrosis), autosomal-dominant diseases (e.g. Huntington's disease), X-linked diseases (e.g. haemophilia A) or balanced chromosomal translocations or inversions. The diagnosis may be known by the potential parents due to the presence of an affected family member or found during a recurrent miscarriage screen. The aim is to avoid the birth of an affected child, preferably replacing a homozygous normal embryo. The purpose of PGS is to screen for aneuploidy in embryos, although both parents have no identified genetic abnormality. PGS has been used in cases of recurrent pregnancy loss, advanced maternal age, repeated unsuccessful IVF cycles or severe male factor infertility. The aim is to use PGS to select the best embryo for transfer. The use of PGS for aneuploidy screening in all cases of IVF has been advocated, but the contribution to improve success rates when used indiscriminately remains to be proven.

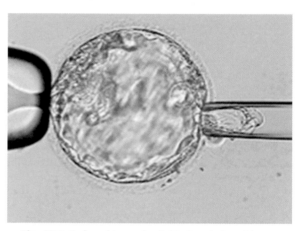

Fig. 17.9 Embryo biopsy day 5, blastocyst-stage biopsy.

Ovarian hyperstimulation syndrome

OHSS is the consequence of over-dosing with gonadotrophins, leading to excessive follicle development and high circulating concentrations of oestrogens and vascular endothelial growth factor (VEGF). OHSS is potentially lethal and is almost completely avoidable if a conservative approach to ovarian stimulation is used. In its severe form, the condition results in marked ovarian enlargement with fluid shift from the intravascular compartment into the third space, leading to ascites, pleural effusion, sodium retention and oliguria. Patients may become hypovolaemic and hypotensive and may develop renal failure, as well as thromboembolic phenomena and adult respiratory distress syndrome. The pathophysiology of this condition appears to be associated with an increase in capillary vascular permeability.

Treatment

If the haematocrit is below 45% and the signs and symptoms are mild, the patient can be managed at home, but where there is significant ascites as judged by ultrasound examination, she should be hospitalized. Baseline electrolyte values and liver and kidney function should be assessed. Volume expansion can be performed using human albumin, sometimes with crystalloid, and if there is severe ascites or pleural effusion, fluid should be drained to reduce the fluid load. Drugs such as indomethacin and angiotensin-converting enzyme inhibitors may be useful in reducing the severity of the episode. Eventually, the cysts will undergo resorption, and the ovaries will return to their normal size. Further attempts at ovarian stimulation should take into account the dosage regimens used during the episode of OHSS.

Avoidance of OHSS

More recently, new strategies have been developed that allow almost total avoidance of risk of OHSS (Devroey et al. 2011).

The process involves 'segmentation' of the IVF cycle, separating the stimulation phase from embryo transfer, luteal support and pregnancy, along with use of a GnRH agonist 'trigger'. The ovarian stimulation phase is regulated with a GnRH antagonist. Once the criteria for final oocyte maturation are reached (usually if at least three follicles exceed 17 mm in diameter), a single dose of a GnRH agonist is administered. This elicits an endogenous LH surge as in the natural cycle. The LH surge induces final oocyte maturation and luteinization. However, the duration of the effect is considerably less than seen with the traditional hCG 'trigger', lasting less than 36 hours compared with 4–5 days. Oocytes are collected using a transvaginal ultrasound-guided approach as usual, fertilized and cultured to blastocyst. All high-quality blastocysts are then frozen, avoiding fresh embryo transfer. The risk of OHSS is therefore avoided due both to the short half-life of the natural LH trigger and avoidance of exposure to human chorionic gonadotropin (hCG) following pregnancy. A blastocyst is then transferred later in a natural or medicated cycle.

Treatment of male infertility

Specific treatment is possible in only a small proportion of infertile males. Testicular size is important, and with the finding of small testes, azoospermia, high FSH and low AMH levels, it is unlikely that any therapy will help.

Where FSH levels are normal and testicular size is normal, ductal obstruction should be suspected and testicular biopsy performed. If normal spermatogenesis is demonstrated, it is necessary to proceed to vasography and exploration of the scrotum. Surgical anastomosis may re-establish fertility. Gonadotrophins are effective in the rare cases of men with hypogonadotropic hypogonadism, and dopamine agonists are used in men with hyperprolactinaemia. Unproven but widely practised treatments for male infertility include ligation of a varicocele and antioxidants and supplements to reduce sperm DNA fragmentation.

The most successful treatment for male infertility is ICSI. ICSI involves the direct injection of a single immobilized sperm into the cytoplasm of the oocyte. This technique produces pregnancy rates similar to those of in vitro fertilization. Anxieties remain concerning the slightly higher rate of abnormality in children conceived after ICSI. Abnormalities are mainly observed in the development of the genital tract (hypospadias, testicular maldescent), although cases of imprinting disorders such as Angelman and Beckwith–Widemann syndromes may also be seen more commonly after ICSI.

Donor insemination

If sperm cannot be obtained for ICSI or if the man is a carrier of a genetic disorder that the couple wish to avoid transmitting to their child, donor insemination should be discussed with the couple.

The implications of the procedure from both a legal and a personal point of view should be discussed in depth, with independent counselling for both partners. Anonymity for sperm donors was removed in the UK in 2004, and the resultant shortage of donor sperm has led many couples to seek treatment overseas or to import sperm from Denmark, the United States and elsewhere. Children conceived using donor oocyte or sperm collected after 2004 are legally allowed to meet their genetic parent under supervised conditions when they reach the age of 18. They can also check whether a potential partner was conceived using the same donor by referring to the HFEA database, although the name of the donor will not be released if the treatment preceded the change in the law regarding anonymity.

Waiting lists for treatment in the UK are lengthy, although this does at least give adequate time for reflection.

Essential information

Infertility

- Incidence about 9% in Western Europe
- Couple potentially infertile if no conception after 12 months
- Fertility declines progressively from the age of 25 years
- Causes (primary/secondary):
  - Disorders of ovulation: 3%2/23%
  - Tubal: 12%/14%
  - Endometriosis: 10%
  - Male: 29%/24%
  - Unexplained: 30%
- PCOS most common cause of anovulation
- Pituitary tumours can cause secondary amenorrhoea
- Infection (often chlamydial) commonest cause of tubal damage
- Infections associated with intrauterine devices (IUDs), abortion and the puerperium commonly cause cornual blockage
- Poor cervical penetration by sperm may be caused by infection, antisperm antibodies or abnormal mucus

Investigation of infertility

- Luteal-phase progesterone is the most useful method of detecting ovulation
- Hormone levels in anovulation
- HSG/laparoscopy/ultrasound to investigate tubal patency
- Semen analysis:
  - Total sperm count >50 million per ejaculate
  - 60% motile
  - Morphology
- Hormone levels in infertile males
- Chromosome analysis in males with azoospermia – abnormal karyotype

Treatment of infertility

- Anovulation:
  - Clomiphene or tamoxifen
  - If unsuccessful, human menopausal gonadotropin (hMG) (beware OHSS)
- Hypogonadotropic hypogonadism – GnRH
- Tubal pathology:
  - Surgery
  - IVF
- Treatment of male infertility only possible in a small proportion of cases

Chapter | 18 |

Early pregnancy care

Ian Symonds

LEARNING OUTCOMES

After studying this chapter you should be able to:

Knowledge criteria

- List the causes of bleeding and/or pain in early pregnancy.
- Describe the epidemiology, aetiology and clinical features of:
  - Miscarriage
  - Ectopic pregnancy
  - Molar pregnancy
- Discuss the use of ultrasound and endocrine assessments in early pregnancy problems
- Describe the management of the common problems and complications of early pregnancy, including the conservative, medical and surgical management of:
  - Miscarriage (including cervical shock)
  - Recurrent miscarriage
  - Ectopic pregnancy
  - Molar pregnancy
  - Hyperemesis gravidarum

Clinical competencies

- Take a relevant gynaecological history in a woman complaining of vaginal bleeding and/or abdominal pain in early pregnancy
- Perform a urinary pregnancy test and interpret the result
- Perform a circulatory assessment and abdominal examination of a woman with an early pregnancy problem, and identify those requiring immediate intervention
- Initiate appropriate resuscitation of a woman presenting in early pregnancy with cardiovascular collapse
- Be able to communicate effectively and sensitively with patients and relatives

Professional skills and attitudes

- Consider the need for a supportive environment that addresses religious and cultural issues around early pregnancy loss

Bleeding in early pregnancy

Vaginal bleeding occurs in up to 25% of pregnancies prior to 20 weeks. It is a major cause of anxiety for all women, especially those who have experienced previous pregnancy loss, and may be the presenting symptom of life-threatening conditions such as ectopic pregnancy. Bleeding should always be considered abnormal in pregnancy and investigated appropriately.

A small amount of bleeding may occur as the blastocyst implants in the endometrium 5–7 days after fertilization (implantation bleed). If this occurs at the time of expected menstruation, it may be confused with a period and so affect calculations of gestational age based the last menstrual period.

The common causes for bleeding in early pregnancy are miscarriage, ectopic pregnancy and benign lesions in the lower genital tract. Less commonly it may be the presenting symptom of hydatidiform mole or cervical malignancy.

Miscarriage

The recommended medical term for pregnancy loss under 24 weeks is *miscarriage*. In some countries, such as the United States, this term is used to describe pregnancy loss before fetal viability or a fetal weight of less than 500 g. In some states in Australia, the term is used for any pregnancy loss under 20 weeks. Most miscarriages occur in the second or third month and occur in 10–20% of clinical pregnancies. It has been suggested that a much higher proportion of pregnancies miscarry at an early stage if the diagnosis is based on the presence of a significant plasma level of beta-subunit human chorionic gonadotrophin (hCG).

The aetiology of miscarriage

In many cases no definite cause can be found for miscarriage. It is important to identify this group, as the prognosis for future pregnancy is generally better than average.

Epidemiological factors

Maternal age and the number of previous miscarriages are independent risk factors for further miscarriage. The risk of miscarriage increases from 11% in women aged 20–24 to more than 50% in women conceiving over the age of 45. This is in part related to the increased risk of chromosome abnormalities (see later) in the conceptus and in part a decline in the number and quality of the woman's remaining oocytes. The risk of miscarriage is also higher in couples where the man is over the age of 40.

Genetic abnormalities

Chromosomal abnormalities are a common cause of early miscarriage and may result in failure of development of the embryo, with formation of a gestation sac without the development of an embryo or with later expulsion of an abnormal fetus. In any form of miscarriage up to 57% of products of conception will have an abnormal karyotype. The most common chromosomal defects are autosomal trisomies, which account for half the abnormalities, while polyploidy and monosomy X account for a further 20% each. Although chromosome abnormalities are common in sporadic miscarriage, parental chromosomal abnormalities are present in only 2–5% of partners presenting with recurrent pregnancy loss. These are most commonly balance reciprocal or Robertsonian translocations or mosaicisms.

Endocrine factors

Progesterone production is predominately dependent on the corpus luteum for the first 8 weeks of pregnancy, and this function is then assumed by the placenta. Progesterone is essential for the maintenance of a pregnancy, and early failure of the corpus luteum may lead to miscarriage. However, it is difficult to be certain when falling plasma progesterone levels represent a primary cause of miscarriage and when they are the index of a failing pregnancy. The prevalence of polycystic ovarian syndrome (PCOS) is significantly higher in women with recurrent miscarriage than in the general population. Women with poorly controlled diabetes and untreated thyroid disease are at higher risk of miscarriage and fetal malformation.

Maternal illness and infection

Any severe maternal febrile illnesses associated with infections, such as influenza, pyelitis and malaria, predispose to miscarriage. Specific infections such as syphilis, *Listeria monocytogenes*, mycoplasma and *Toxoplasma gondii* may also be associated with sporadic miscarriage, but there is no evidence that these organisms cause recurrent miscarriage, particularly in the second trimester. The presence of bacterial vaginosis has been reported as a risk factor for pre-term delivery and second-trimester, but not first-trimester, miscarriage. Other severe illnesses involving the cardiovascular, hepatic and renal systems may also result in miscarriage.

Maternal lifestyle and drug history

Antidepressant use and periconceptual non-steroidal anti-inflammatory drugs have been associated with miscarriage. Smoking, alcohol (more than 5 units a week), caffeine (more than 3 cups per day), cocaine and cannabis have been associated with an increase in the risk of miscarriage, although current evidence is insufficient to confirm a causal link. There is some evidence that obesity may also be associated with pregnancy loss.

Abnormalities of the uterus

The exact contribution that congenital abnormalities of the uterine cavity, such as a bicornuate uterus or subseptate uterus, make to miscarriage remains controversial. The reported incidence of uterine anomalies in women with recurrent miscarriage varies from less than 2% to up to 38%. The impact of the abnormality depends on the nature of the anomaly, and the prevalence appears to be higher in women with second-trimester miscarriage. The fetal survival rate is best where the uterus is septate and worst where the uterus is unicornuate. It must also be remembered that over 20% of all women with congenital uterine anomalies also have renal tract anomalies. Following damage to the endometrium and inner uterine walls, the surfaces may become adherent, thus partly obliterating the uterine cavity (Asherman's syndrome). The presence of these synechiae may lead to recurrent miscarriage.

Cervical incompetence

Cervical incompetence typically results in second-trimester miscarriage or early pre-term delivery. The miscarriage tends to be rapid, painless and bloodless. The diagnosis is established by the passage of a Hegar 8 dilator without difficulty in the non-pregnant woman or by ultrasound examination or by a premenstrual hysterogram. Cervical incompetence may be congenital and associated with other congenital uterine malformations but most commonly results from physical damage caused by mechanical dilatation or surgery of the cervix or by damage inflicted during childbirth.

Autoimmune factors

Antiphospholipid antibodies – lupus anticoagulant (LA) and anticardiolipin antibodies (aCL) – are present in

15% of women with recurrent miscarriage but only 2% of women with normal reproductive histories. Without treatment, the live birth rate in women with primary antiphospholipid syndrome may be as low as 10%. Pregnancy loss is thought to be due to thrombosis of the uteroplacental vasculature and impaired trophoblast function. In addition to miscarriage there is an increased risk of intrauterine growth restriction, pre-eclampsia and venous thrombosis.

Thrombophilic defects

Defects in the natural inhibitors of coagulation – antithrombin III, protein C and protein S – are more common in women with recurrent miscarriage. The majority of cases of activated protein C deficiency are secondary to a mutation in the factor V (Leiden) gene.

Alloimmune factors

Research into the possibility of an immunological basis of recurrent miscarriage has generally explored the possibility of a failure to mount the normal protective immune response or if the expression of relatively non-immunogenic antigens by the cytotrophoblast may result in rejection of the fetal allograft. There is evidence that unexplained spontaneous miscarriage is associated with couples who share an abnormal number of human leukocyte antigen (HLA) antigens of the A, B, C and DR loci. Treatment with paternal lymphocytes and immunoglobulins has been shown not to be effective and is potentially dangerous.

Clinical types of miscarriage

Threatened miscarriage

The first sign of an impending miscarriage is the development of vaginal bleeding in early pregnancy (Fig. 18.1). The uterus is found to be enlarged, and the cervical os is closed. Lower abdominal pain is either minimal or absent. Most women presenting with a threatened miscarriage will continue with the pregnancy irrespective of the method of management.

Inevitable/incomplete miscarriage

The patient develops abdominal pain usually associated with increasing vaginal bleeding. The cervix opens, and eventually products of conception are passed into the vagina. However, if some of the products of conception are retained, the miscarriage remains incomplete (Fig. 18.2).

> ! Distension of the cervical canal by products of conception can cause hypotension and bradycardia (cervical shock).

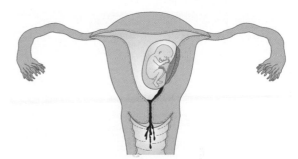

Fig. 18.1 Threatened miscarriage: blood loss in early pregnancy.

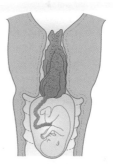

Fig. 18.2 Incomplete miscarriage: progression to expulsion of part of the conceptus is accompanied by pain and bleeding.

Case study: Incomplete miscarriage

A 32-year-old Asian woman presented with a history of 12 weeks amenorrhoea and vaginal bleeding followed by severe lower abdominal pain. On admission to hospital, she was sweating, pale and hypotensive. Her pulse rate was 68 beats/minute. She complained of generalized lower abdominal pain. Initially, a ruptured tubal pregnancy was suspected because of the pain and shock, until vaginal examination revealed copious products of conception protruding from an open cervical os. Removal of these products largely relieved the pain and allowed the uterus to contract, thus reducing the blood loss. Subsequent evacuation of retained products of conception was performed after appropriate resuscitation and preparation.

Complete miscarriage

An incomplete miscarriage may proceed to completion spontaneously, when the pain will cease and vaginal bleeding will subside with involution of the uterus. Spontaneous completion of a miscarriage is more likely in miscarriages over 16 weeks' gestation than in those between 8 and 16 weeks' gestation, when retention of placental fragments is common.

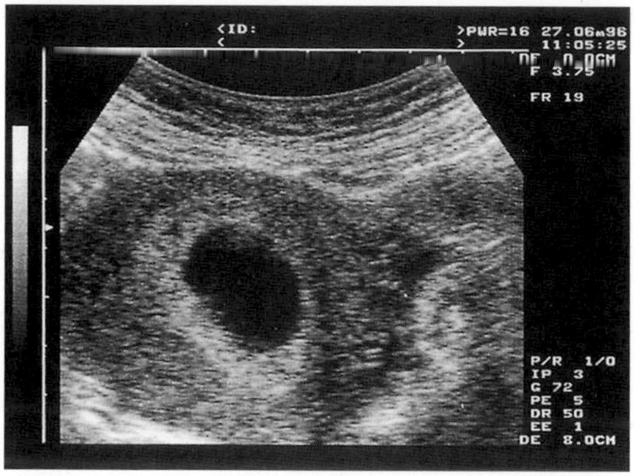

Fig. 18.3 The empty gestation sac of anembryonic pregnancy seen on ultrasound scan.

Miscarriage with infection (sepsis)

During the process of miscarriage – or after therapeutic termination of a pregnancy – infection may be introduced into the uterine cavity. The clinical findings of septic miscarriage are similar to those of incomplete miscarriage with the addition of uterine and adnexal tenderness. The vaginal loss may become purulent and the patient pyrexial. In cases of severe overwhelming sepsis, endotoxic shock may develop with profound and sometimes fatal hypotension. Other manifestations include renal failure, disseminated intravascular coagulopathy and multiple petechial haemorrhages. Organisms which commonly invade the uterine cavity are *Escherichia coli*, *Streptococcus faecalis*, *Staphylococcus albus* and *aureus*, *Klebsiella* and *Clostridium welchii* and *perfringens*.

Missed miscarriage (empty gestation sac, embryonic loss, early and late fetal loss)

In empty gestation sac (anembryonic pregnancy or blighted ovum), a gestational sac of ≥25 mm is seen on ultrasound (Fig. 18.3), but there is no evidence of an embryonic pole or yolk sac or change in size of the sac on rescan 7 days later. Embryonic loss is diagnosed where there is an embryo ≥7 mm in size without cardiac activity or where there is no change in the size of the embryo after 7 days on scan. Early fetal demise occurs when a pregnancy is identified within the uterus on ultrasound consistent with 8–12 weeks size but no fetal heartbeat is seen. These may be associated with some bleeding and abdominal pain or be asymptomatic and diagnosed on ultrasound scan. The pattern of clinical loss may indicate the underlying aetiology; for example, antiphospholipid syndrome tends to present with recurrent fetal loss.

Spontaneous second-trimester loss

Pregnancy loss occurs between 12 and 24 weeks associated with spontaneous rupture of membranes or cervical dilation despite the presence of fetal heart activity

Recurrent miscarriage

Recurrent miscarriage is defined as three or more successive pregnancy losses prior to viability. The problem affects 1% of all women, approximately three times the number that would be expected by chance alone. Most women who have had two or more consecutive miscarriages are anxious to be investigated and reassured that there is no underlying cause. However, it is important to remember that after three consecutive miscarriages, there is still a 55–75% chance of success. This implies that recurrent miscarriage is unlikely to be a random event and that it is necessary to seek a cause.

Management

Examination of the patient should include gentle vaginal and speculum examination to ascertain cervical dilatation. If there is pyrexia, a high vaginal swab should be taken for bacteriological culture.

Some women may prefer not to be examined because of apprehension that the examination may promote miscarriage, and their wishes should be respected. Management in dedicated early pregnancy assessment units (EPAUs) reduces the need for hospital admission and length of stay. An ultrasound scan is valuable in deciding if the fetus is alive and normal. One effect of the routine use of scans in early pregnancy is that the diagnosis of miscarriage may be established before there is any indication that the pregnancy is abnormal. It is sometimes preferable to repeat the scan a week later than proceed to immediate medical or surgical uterine evacuation, to enable the mother to come to terms with the diagnosis.

Non-sensitized Rhesus (Rh)-negative women should receive anti-D immunoglobulin for all miscarriages and ectopic pregnancies managed surgically.

Anti-D immunoglobulin does not need to be given for women who have had only medical or expectant management for miscarriage or ectopic pregnancy, who have a threatened miscarriage or who have a pregnancy of unknown locations.

Threatened miscarriage

Women with bleeding in early pregnancy and a confirmed intrauterine pregnancy with a fetal heartbeat should be advised to return if bleeding gets worse or persists for more than 14 days but otherwise to continue with routine antenatal care.

Missed or incomplete miscarriage

Miscarriage may be complicated by haemorrhage and severe pain, and may necessitate blood transfusion and relief of pain with opiates. If there is evidence of infection, antibiotic therapy should be started immediately and adjusted subsequently if the organism identified in culture is not sensitive to the prescribed antibiotic.

> ❗ Septic miscarriage complicated by endotoxic shock is treated by massive antibiotic therapy and adequate, carefully controlled fluid replacement.

> ❗ If there is evidence of 'cervical shock' any products of conception protruding through the cervical os should be removed by grasping them with tissue-holding forceps.

> ✔ There is no evidence that bed rest improves the prognosis in cases of threatened miscarriage, although it may be beneficial in prolonging pregnancy in women at high risk of second-trimester loss or where there is prolapse of membranes into the cervical canal as a result of cervical weakness.

Expectant management

This is the favoured option for the first 7–14 days for women with confirmed miscarriages unless the woman is at increased risk of bleeding (e.g. late first trimester) or she is at an increased risk of the effects of bleeding or there is evidence of infection. Medical or surgical management may be a more acceptable option for some women and should be offered as an alternative. Success rates depend on similar factors to those for medical management, but patients should be warned that it may take 1–2 weeks for complete miscarriage to occur. If pain and bleeding resolve within 7–14 days the woman should be advised to take a repeat urinary pregnancy test and return for review if this remains positive. A repeat scan should be organized if bleeding has not started or persists after 14 days of expectant management.

Medical management

When the uterine contents have not begun to be expelled naturally, the process can be expedited by the use of a prostaglandin analogue such as misoprostol. Passage of the products will normally be accomplished in approximately 48–72 hours, but bleeding may continue for up to 3 weeks. Success rates of medical treatment vary between 13% and 96% depending on the type of miscarriage, sac size and dose of prostaglandin. Higher success rates occur in incomplete miscarriage treated with high-dose prostaglandins given vaginally. The advantages of medical management are that a general anaesthetic

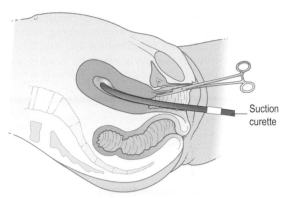

Suction curette

Fig. 18.4 Evacuation of retained products of conception.

is avoided, as are the potential complications of evacuation. Patients undergoing medical management should have 24-hour direct access to hospital services for advice or admission and should be advised to take a urinary pregnancy test 3 weeks after treatment and return for review if this remains positive to exclude molar or ectopic pregnancy.

Surgical management

Surgical evacuation of retained products of conception involves dilatation of the cervix and suction curettage to remove the products (Fig. 18.4). This is the modality of choice when there is heavy bleeding or persistent bleeding, if the vital signs are unstable or in the presence of infected retained tissue. Serious complications of surgical treatment occur in 2% of cases and include perforation of the uterus, cervical tears, intra-abdominal trauma, intrauterine adhesions and haemorrhage. Intrauterine infection may result in tubal infection and tubal obstruction with subsequent infertility. Screening for infection, including *Chlamydia trachomatis*, should be considered and antibiotic prophylaxis given if clinically indicated. If uterine perforation is suspected and there is evidence of intraperitoneal haemorrhage or damage to the bowel, a laparoscopy or laparotomy should be performed.

Whichever method is chosen, products should be sent for histological examination if possible, as a small number will prove to be gestational trophoblastic disease (GTD).

Sensitive disposal of fetal tissues

A woman or couple should be made aware that information on disposal options is available if they wish to have access to it. The cremation regulations do not apply to fetuses under 24 weeks' gestation, but cremation authorities may cremate them at their discretion. There is no legal duty under burial legislation to bury (or cremate) babies born dead before 24 weeks' gestation, but nothing to prevent either option. Communal burial is permitted for fetal tissue.

There is also the option for women or couples to bury at home, provided that certain criteria have been fulfilled.

Any baby, irrespective of gestational age, who is born alive and then dies immediately afterwards is a live birth and neonatal death and should be treated as such in terms of registration and disposal.

> Medical and expectant management is an effective alternative to surgical treatment in confirmed miscarriage.

Recurrent miscarriage

Women with a history of recurrent miscarriage should be offered referral to a specialist clinic. The karyotype of both parents and, if possible, any fetal products should be tested. Maternal blood should be examined for LA and aCL on at least two occasions 12 weeks apart. Women with recurrent second-trimester miscarriage should be screened for thrombophilias, including factor V Leiden, factor II gene mutation and protein S. An ultrasound scan should be arranged to assess ovarian morphology for PCOS and the uterine cavity. Suspected uterine anomalies (Fig. 18.5) may require further investigation such as hysteroscopy or laparoscopy. Women with persistent LA and aCL should be considered for treatment with low-dose aspirin and heparin during subsequent pregnancies. Treatment with low-dose heparin may also improve pregnancy outcomes in women with inherited thrombophilias where these are associated with second-trimester miscarriage. Couples with karyotypic abnormalities should be referred to a clinical geneticist. Cervical cerclage carried out at 14–16 weeks in cases of cervical incompetence reduces the incidence of pre-term delivery but has not been shown to improve fetal survival. An alternative approach to the use of prophylactic cerclage is serial ultrasound measurement of the length of the cervical canal with treatment only if this drops below 25 mm. There is increasing evidence that progesterone (which has anti-inflammatory properties) is effective in prolonging high-risk pregnancies. Bacterial vaginosis has been associated with second-trimester losses and pre-term delivery. Treatment of this condition with clindamycin (not metronidazole) does appear to reduce the risk of pre-term delivery, but there is no evidence to support empirical antibiotic use in women with second-trimester loss or for other infections. It is important to remember that no cause will be identified in a significant proportion of women with recurrent miscarriage. The prognosis with supportive care alone in these women is generally good, and there is no evidence to suggest that empirical treatment with hormonal, aspirin, heparin or immunotherapy treatment improves the outcome.

> Genetic abnormalities are the commonest cause of isolated miscarriage but a relatively uncommon cause of recurrent pregnancy loss.

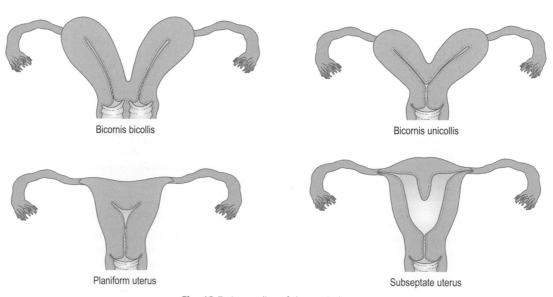

Bicornis bicollis

Bicornis unicollis

Planiform uterus

Subseptate uterus

Fig. 18.5 Anomalies of the genital tract.

Psychological aspects of miscarriage !

In Western Europe most women confirm their pregnancies considerably earlier than in previous generations. A spontaneous miscarriage is often regarded medically as not serious and is rarely investigated when it occurs for the first time. Follow-up is often left in primary care, and few women receive gynaecological attention or an explanation of their loss. Although there is no evidence to associate miscarriage with an overall increased risk of psychiatric morbidity, almost half of all women are considerably distressed at 6 weeks following miscarriage and often feel angry, alone and guilty. Women who have had a previous miscarriage and no live child, women who have had a previous termination of pregnancy and those with a previous psychiatric history are most at risk of becoming depressed in the months that follow miscarriage. Women who have had many miscarriages are particularly vulnerable and should probably receive gynaecological support and counselling.

Ectopic pregnancy

The term *ectopic pregnancy* refers to any pregnancy occurring outside the uterine cavity.

The most common site of extrauterine implantation is the Fallopian tube, but it may occur in the ovary as an ovarian pregnancy, in the abdominal cavity as an abdominal pregnancy, in the cervical canal as a cervical pregnancy or at the site of a previous caesarean section as a caesarean scar pregnancy (CSP) (Fig. 18.6).

Tubal pregnancy occurs in 11 in 1000 pregnancies in the UK, although this incidence varies substantially in different populations. Ectopic pregnancy remains an important cause of maternal mortality (0.2 per 1000 cases) in the first trimester, with 10–12 women dying every 3 years from the condition in the UK. Sadly, there is evidence of substandard care in two-thirds of these cases. Tubal pregnancy may occur in the ampulla, the isthmus and the interstitial portion of the tube, and the outcome will depend on the site of implantation.

Predisposing factors (Table 18.1)

The majority of cases of ectopic pregnancy have no identifiable predisposing factor, but a previous history of ectopic pregnancy, sterilization, pelvic inflammatory disease and/or subfertility increases the likelihood of an ectopic pregnancy. The increased risk for an intrauterine device (IUD) applies only to pregnancies that occur despite the presence of the IUD. Because of their effectiveness as contraceptives, ectopic rates per year in IUD users are lower than in women not using contraception.

Clinical presentation

Acute presentation

The classical pattern of symptoms includes amenorrhoea, lower abdominal pain and uterine bleeding. The abdominal pain usually precedes the onset of vaginal bleeding and may start on one side of the lower abdomen but rapidly becomes generalized as blood loss extends into the peritoneal cavity. Subdiaphragmatic irritation by blood produces referred shoulder tip pain, and syncopal episodes may occur.

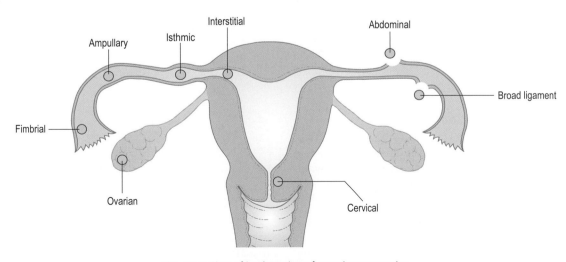

Fig. 18.6 Sites of implantation of ectopic pregnancies.

Table 18.1 Risk factors for ectopic pregnancy

	Relative risk
Previous history of PID	4
Previous tubal surgery	4.5
Failed sterilization	9
IUD in situ	10
Previous ectopic pregnancy	10–15

IUD, Intrauterine device; *PID*, pelvic inflammatory disease.

The period of amenorrhoea is usually 6–8 weeks but may be longer if implantation occurs in the interstitial portion of the tube or in abdominal pregnancy. Clinical examination reveals a shocked woman with hypotension, tachycardia and signs of peritonism, including abdominal distension, guarding and rebound tenderness. Pelvic examination is usually unimportant because of the acute pain and discomfort and should be undertaken with caution. This type of acute presentation occurs in no more than 25% of cases.

Case study: Subacute presentation

A 22-year-old woman, para 0, was admitted with vaginal bleeding after 8 weeks of amenorrhoea. She had had a positive home pregnancy kit test and described passing some tissue per vaginam. Ultrasound scan showed an empty uterus, although serum b-hCG was still positive. A presumptive diagnosis of incomplete miscarriage was made, and evacuation of the uterus carried out uneventfully. She was discharged the following day but readmitted that night with lower abdominal pain; a ruptured ampullary ectopic pregnancy was found at laparotomy. Some days later, histology of the original curettage was reported as 'decidua with Arias–Stella type reaction, no chorionic villi seen'.

Subacute presentation

After a short period of amenorrhoea, the patient experiences recurrent attacks of vaginal bleeding and abdominal pain. Patients may present with non-gynaecological symptoms such as breast tenderness, gastrointestinal symptoms (pain of defecation), urinary symptoms, dizziness or syncope. Any woman who develops lower abdominal pain following an interval of amenorrhoea should be considered as a possible ectopic pregnancy. In its subacute phase, it may be possible to elicit tenderness or feel a mass in one fornix

---

Case study: Acute presentation

An 18-year-old woman, para 0, was brought into casualty collapsed with lower abdominal pain. On admission, she was shocked with a blood pressure of 80/40, a pulse of 120 beats/min and a tender, rigid abdomen. Vaginal examination revealed a slight red loss, bulky uterus and marked cervical excitation with a tender mass in the right fornix. At laparotomy, 800 mL of fresh blood was removed from the peritoneal cavity and a ruptured right tubal ectopic pregnancy was found. Subsequently, a history of recurrent pelvic infections and irregular periods was elicited.

Other findings on examination may include an enlarged uterus with cervical motion tenderness, pallor or lower abdominal tenderness.

Pathology

Implantation may occur in a variety of sites, and the outcome of the pregnancy will depend on the site of implantation. Abdominal pregnancy may result from direct implantation of the conceptus in the abdominal cavity or on the ovary, in which case it is known as *primary abdominal pregnancy*, or it may result from extrusion of a tubal pregnancy with secondary implantation in the peritoneal cavity, which is known as *secondary abdominal pregnancy*. Implantation may occur at the site of previous uterine surgery, most commonly previous caesarean section, or in the interstitial portion of the Fallopian tube as a cornual pregnancy. Implantation of the conceptus outside of the uterus still results in hormonal changes that mimic normal pregnancy. The uterus enlarges, and the endometrium undergoes decidual change. Implantation within the fimbrial end or ampulla of the tube allows greater expansion before rupture occurs, whereas implantation in the interstitial portion or the isthmic part of the tube presents with early signs of haemorrhage or pain (Fig. 18.7).

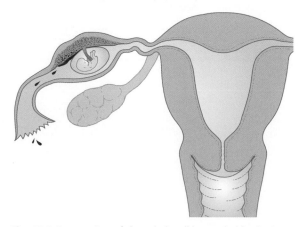

Fig. 18.7 Penetration of the tubal wall by trophoblastic tissue.

Trophoblastic cells invade the wall of the tube and erode into blood vessels. This process will continue until the pregnancy bursts into the abdominal cavity or into the broad ligament or the embryo dies, thus resulting in a tubal mole. Under these circumstances, absorption or tubal miscarriage may occur. Expulsion of the embryo into the peritoneal cavity or partial miscarriage may also occur with continuing episodes of bleeding from the tube.

Diagnosis

> **!** Ectopic pregnancy should always be suspected where early pregnancy is complicated by pain and bleeding.

Whilst the diagnosis of the acute ectopic pregnancy rarely presents a problem, diagnosis in the subacute phase may be much more difficult. It may be mistaken for a threatened or incomplete miscarriage. It may also be confused with acute salpingitis or appendicitis with pelvic peritonitis. It may sometimes be confused with rupture or haemorrhage of an ovarian cyst.

If sufficient blood loss has occurred into the peritoneal cavity, the haemoglobin level will be low and the white cell count will be usually normal or slightly raised. Serum hCG measurement will exclude ectopic pregnancy if negative with a specificity of greater than 99%, and urinary hCG with modern kits that can be used on the ward will detect 97% of pregnancies. In the presence of a viable intrauterine pregnancy, the serum hCG will double over a 48-hour period in 85% of cases (compared to 15% of ectopic pregnancies). A normal intrauterine pregnancy will usually be visualized on scan where the serum hCG level is more than 1000 IU/L (the discriminatory zone). Serial measurements of serum hCG levels in conjunction with ultrasound diagnosis can distinguish early intrauterine pregnancy from miscarriage or ectopics in up to 85% of cases. Ultrasound scan of the pelvis may demonstrate tubal pregnancy in 2% of cases (Fig. 18.8) or suggest it by other features, such as free fluid in the peritoneal cavity, but is mainly of help in excluding intrauterine pregnancy (Table 18.2). Intrauterine pregnancy can usually be identified by transabdominal scan at 6 weeks' gestation and somewhat sooner by transvaginal scan at 5–6 weeks gestation. Occasionally, there may be no clinical signs of an ectopic pregnancy, but if curettings submitted for histopathology show evidence of decidual reaction and the Arias–Stella phenomenon, then it is advisable to consider laparoscopy.

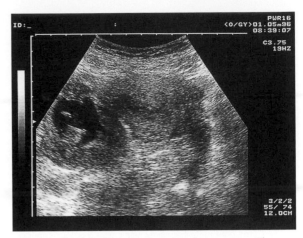

Fig. 18.8 Ultrasound image of an ectopic pregnancy. The uterus and endometrial cavity can be seen centrally. A fetal pole can be seen in the cavity to the left of the uterus.

Table 18.2 Features of intrauterine and ectopic pregnancy on transvaginal scan

Intrauterine pregnancy	Ectopic pregnancy
Intrauterine gestation sac (4–5 weeks)	Empty uterus
Yolk sac (5–6 weeks)	Poorly defined tubal ring with fluid in pouch of Douglas
Double decidual sign (5 weeks)	Pseudo-sac in uterus
Fetal heartbeat (7 weeks)	Tubal ring with extrauterine heartbeat

Management

Ideally management of haemodynamically stable patients with suspected ectopic pregnancy should take place in a dedicated EPAU or equivalent with access to point-of-care ultrasound. Patients who are haemodynamically compromised should be referred urgently to an emergency department and blood taken for urgent cross-matching and transfusion. Surgery should be performed as soon as possible with removal of the damaged tube.

Non-sensitized Rh-negative women should receive anti-D immunoglobulin in any ectopic pregnancy, regardless of the mode of treatment.

Performing a urinary pregnancy test

Although the exact configuration of the various home kits varies, the principal steps are as follows: (Fig. 18.9)

A. A sample of the patient's urine is placed on the sample area (a).
B. The urine is drawn along the kit by capillary action towards an area containing mouse immunoglobulin, which binds to the hCG molecule if present in the urine. These antibodies are also conjugated to an enzyme that catalyzes a colour change.
C. Bound and unbound mouse antibodies are drawn up the kit by capillary action to a second area containing fixed polyclonal antibodies to hCG and dye (b). Any mouse antibodies bound to hCG will be trapped here, and the enzyme conjugated to them will cause a colour change (a positive result).
D. Any remaining unbound antibodies will carry on past this area to the control strip zone (c), where they will be trapped by anti-mouse antibodies and catalyze a colour change (this will occur whether the urine contains hCG or not but helps to show that the test is working properly and that a negative result in the first area is due to an absence of hCG).

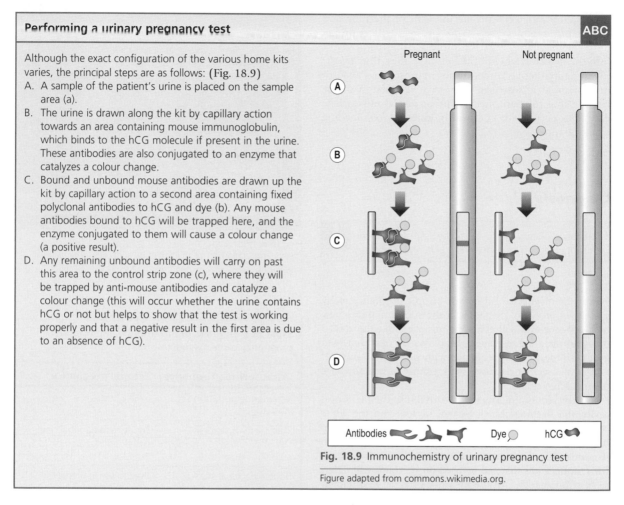

Fig. 18.9 Immunochemistry of urinary pregnancy test

Figure adapted from commons.wikimedia.org.

Surgical management

Once the diagnosis is confirmed, the options for treatment are:

1. *Salpingectomy* – If the tube is badly damaged or the contralateral tube appears healthy, the correct treatment is removal of the affected tube. If implantation has occurred in the interstitial portion of the tube, it may be necessary to resect part of the uterine horn in addition to removing the tube.
2. *Salpingotomy* – Where the ectopic pregnancy is contained within the tube, it may be possible to conserve the tube by removing the pregnancy and reconstituting the tube. This is particularly important where the contralateral tube has been lost. The disadvantage is the persistence of trophoblastic tissue requiring further surgery or medical treatment in up to 6% of cases.

Subsequent intrauterine pregnancy rates are similar after both types of treatment, although the risk of recurrent ectopic pregnancy is greater after salpingotomy. Both can be carried out as an open procedure or laparoscopically.

The laparoscopic approach is associated with quicker recovery time, shorter stay in hospital and less adhesion formation, and is the method of choice if the patient is stable and is now the expected standard of care.

Medical management

Medical treatment of an ectopic pregnancy involves the administration of methotrexate, either systemically or by injection into the ectopic pregnancy by laparoscopic visualization or by ultrasound guidance. Medical treatment is not suitable for all cases of ectopic pregnancy. It can be offered as first-line treatment where there is no significant pain, the ectopic is less than 35 mm in size with no visible heartbeat and there is no evidence of viable intrauterine pregnancy. Ideally the hCG level should be less than 1500 IU/L, although treatment can be offered as an alternative to surgery for levels up to 5000 IU/L, provided the other conditions are met and the woman understands that the chance of requiring further intervention is increased and there is a need to return urgently if her condition deteriorates. Following treatment the serum hCG should be repeated 4 and 7 days later and then weekly until a negative result is obtained. Systemic side effects occur in 20% of cases and abdominal pain in 75%. Tubal rupture requiring surgery occurs in 5–10% of cases.

After an ectopic pregnancy treated by any method, 85–90% of subsequent pregnancies will be intrauterine, but only 60% of women will manage to conceive spontaneously, reflecting global tubal disease.

Pregnancy of unknown location

This is defined as a positive pregnancy test where there are no signs on ultrasound of either an intrauterine or ectopic pregnancy or retained products of conception, and it occurs in 10% of pregnancies. This may represent an intrauterine pregnancy that is too small to see on ultrasound but requires follow-up to exclude ectopic pregnancy. Conservative management with serial hCG measurement and repeat ultrasound is safe for asymptomatic women. A serum progesterone level of less than 20 nmol/L is predictive of pregnancy failure but does not help in predicting pregnancy location.

Management of other forms of extrauterine pregnancy

Abdominal pregnancy

Abdominal pregnancy presents a life-threatening hazard to the mother. The placenta implants outside the uterus and across the bowel and pelvic peritoneum. Any attempt to remove it will result in massive haemorrhage, which is extremely difficult to control. The fetus should be removed by laparotomy and the placenta left in situ to reabsorb or extrude spontaneously.

Cervical pregnancy

Cervical pregnancy often presents as the cervical stage of a spontaneous miscarriage. Occasionally, it is possible to remove the conceptus by curettage, but haemorrhage can be severe, and in 50% of cases it is necessary to proceed to hysterectomy to obtain adequate haemostasis.

Cornual (interstitial) pregnancy

This occurs when implantation occurs in the interstitial portion of the tube. Previous salpingectomy, rudimentary horns and proximal intraluminal admissions are predisposing factors.

Rupture can be associated with significant bleeding, and diagnosis can be difficult, but if recognized before rupture occurs, medical treatment with methotrexate is an option. For pregnancies that have ruptured or are >5 cm in size, the traditional treatment has been wedge resection of the cornua via laparotomy or even hysterectomy, but laparoscopic cornuostomy has been increasingly used.

Caesarean scar pregnancy

This occurs when implantation takes place within the fibrous scar tissue at the site of a previous caesarean section. It is a rare but potentially life-threatening condition accounting for 6% of all ectopic pregnancies and affecting 0.15% of women with previous caesarean section. Diagnosis is usually made on ultrasound detection of enlargement of the caesarean section scar with an attached gestational sac or mixed mass. Treatment can be medical if the patient is stable with local or systemic methotrexate, or surgical with wedge resection of the gestational mass.

Gestational trophoblastic disease

Abnormality of the early trophoblast may arise as a developmental anomaly of placental tissue and results in the formation of a mass of oedematous and avascular villi. The placenta is replaced by a mass of grape-like vesicles known as a **hydatidiform mole** (Fig. 18.10). Hydatidiform moles can be classified as complete or partial. The latter usually contain embryonic or fetal material.

Malignant change occurs in 0.5–4% of partial moles and 15–25% of complete moles and is known as **choriocarcinoma**.

Other types of GTD include **persistent GTD, placenta site trophoblastic tumours** and **epithelioid trophoblast tumour.**

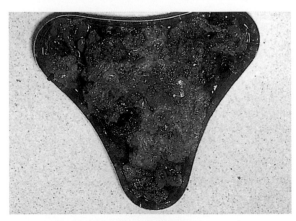

Fig. 18.10 Vesicles of a hydatidiform mole.

Incidence

The overall prevalence of this condition is about 1.5 in 1000 pregnancies in the UK but is much higher in Asia and Southeast Asia. It is more common at the extremes of reproductive age.

Pathology

Molar pregnancy is thought to arise from fertilization by two sperm and can be diploid with no female genetic material (complete mole) or may exhibit triploidy (partial mole). Benign mole remains confined to the uterine cavity and decidua. The histopathology exhibits a villous pattern (see Fig. 18.11). Choriocarcinoma comprises plexiform columns of trophoblastic cells without villous patterns. Widespread blood-borne metastases are a feature of this disease, which, until recently, carried a very high mortality rate. Metastases may occur locally in the vagina but most commonly appear in the lungs. Theca lutein cysts occur in about one-third of all cases as a result of high circulating levels of hCG. These regress spontaneously with removal of the molar tissue. Fifty percent of cases of choriocarcinoma are not associated with molar pregnancy.

Clinical presentation

Molar pregnancy most commonly presents as bleeding in the first half of pregnancy, and spontaneous miscarriage often occurs at about 20 weeks' gestation. Occasionally, the passage of a grape-like villus heralds the presence of a mole. The uterus is larger than dates in about half the cases, but this is not a reliable sign, as it may sometimes be small for dates. Severe hyperemesis, pre-eclampsia and unexplained anaemia are all factors suggestive of this disorder. The diagnosis can be confirmed by ultrasound scan and by the presence of very high levels of hCG in the blood or urine.

Management

Once the diagnosis is established, the pregnancy is terminated by suction curettage. Adequate replacement of blood loss is essential. Although there is an increased risk of blood loss, there is a theoretical concern over the routine use of oxytocic agents because of the potential to disseminate trophoblastic tissue through the venous system. If possible, these should be commenced once the evacuation has been completed. Occasionally repeat evacuation may be required if there is persistent bleeding or a raised serum hCG, but routine second evacuation is not helpful. All cases of molar pregnancy in the UK should be registered with one of the trophoblastic disease screening centres, who will arrange follow-up. All patients are followed up with serial hCG measurements (details vary between countries) for at least 6 months.

If the histological evidence shows malignant change, chemotherapy with methotrexate and actinomycin D is employed and produces good results. In the UK, management of these cases is concentrated in specialized centres. Some states in Australia and New Zealand have registries.

>
> It must be remembered that choriocarcinoma sometimes can occur following a miscarriage or a normal-term intrauterine pregnancy.

Pregnancy is contraindicated until 6 months after the serum hCG levels fall to normal. Oestrogen-containing oral contraceptives and hormone replacement therapy (HRT) can be used as soon as hCG levels are normal. The risk recurrence in subsequent pregnancies is 1 in 70, and serum hCG levels should be checked 6 weeks after any subsequent pregnancy.

Case study: Trophoblastic disease

A 27-year-old primigravid woman attended the clinic with a history of 12 weeks of amenorrhoea, complaining of bright vaginal blood loss and lower abdominal discomfort. Abdominal examination revealed that the uterine fundus was 16 weeks in size. There was fresh blood in the vagina, and the cervical os was closed. There was a high titre of hCG in the urine, and an ultrasound scan showed a snowstorm appearance with the uterine cavity filled with echoes but no evidence of fetal parts (Fig. 18.11). Suction evacuation of molar tissue was performed the following day, and recovery was uneventful.

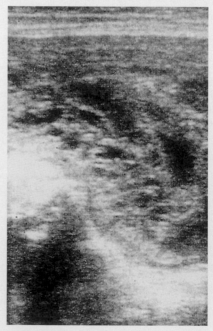

Fig. 18.11 Hydatidiform mole. The typical snowstorm appearance of molar tissue is apparent.

Vomiting in early pregnancy

Nausea and vomiting are common symptoms in early pregnancy (affecting 80% and 50% of women, respectively), usually starting between 4 and 10 weeks' gestation and resolving before 20 weeks. Symptoms persist beyond 20 weeks in 13% of cases, but new symptoms appearing after the twelfth week should not be attributed to hyperemesis. *Hyperemesis gravidarum* is defined as persistent pregnancy-related vomiting associated with weight loss of more than 5% of body mass and ketosis. Affecting 0.3–3% of all pregnant women, this is associated with dehydration, electrolyte imbalance and thiamine deficiency.

Aetiology

The aetiology of hyperemesis is uncertain, with multifactorial causes such as endocrine, gastrointestinal and psychological factors proposed. Hyperemesis occurs more often in multiple pregnancy and hydatidiform mole, suggesting an association with the level of hCG. Although transient abnormalities of thyroid function are common, this does not require treatment in the absence of other clinical features of hyperthyroidism. Infection with *Helicobacter pylori,* the organism implicated in gastric ulcers, may also contribute. Women with a previous history of hyperemesis are likely to experience it in subsequent pregnancies.

Diagnosis

It is important to ask about the frequency of vomiting, trigger factors and whether any other members of the family have been affected. A history of vomiting in a previous pregnancy or outside pregnancy should be sought. Smoking and alcohol can both exacerbate symptoms and should be enquired of. If this pregnancy resulted from fertility treatment or there is a close family history of twins, a multiple pregnancy is more likely. Early pregnancy bleeding or a past history of trophoblastic disease may point to a hydatidiform mole.

The clinical features of dehydration include tachycardia, hypotension and loss of skin turgor. Causes of vomiting not due to pregnancy, such as thyroid problems, urinary tract infection or gastroenteritis, need to be excluded, so the abdomen should be palpated for areas of tenderness, especially in the right upper quadrant, hypogastrium and renal angles. A dipstick analysis of the urine for ketones, blood or protein should be performed.

Routine investigations should include full blood count, electrolytes and liver and thyroid function tests. Elevated haematocrit, alterations in electrolyte levels and ketonuria are associated with dehydration. Urine should be sent for culture to exclude infection and an ultrasound arranged to look for multiple pregnancy or GTD.

Management

If the vomiting is mild to moderate and not causing signs of dehydration, usually reassurance and advice will be all that is necessary.

Simple measures include:
- Taking small carbohydrate meals and avoiding fatty foods
- Powdered ginger root or pyridoxine (vitamin B_6)
- Avoiding large-volume drinks, especially milk and carbonated drinks
- Raising the head of the bed if reflux is a problem

A history of persistent, severe vomiting with evidence of dehydration requires admission to hospital for assessment and management of symptoms.

Hypovolaemia and electrolyte imbalance should be corrected by intravenous fluids. These should be balanced electrolyte solutions or normal saline.

> Overly rapid rehydration with 5% dextrose can result in water intoxication or central pontine myelinolysis.

Thromboprophylaxis with compression stockings and low-molecular-weight heparin should be considered. Most women will settle in 24–48 hours with these supportive measures. Once the vomiting has ceased, small amounts of fluid, and eventually food, can be reintroduced.

Anti-emetic therapy is reserved for those women who do not settle on supportive measures or who persistently relapse. The use of anti-emetics in pregnancy received widespread publicity when links were found between thalidomide and severe malformations of children born to mothers who had taken the drug for morning sickness. Currently antihistamines such as cyclizine are the recommended pharmacological first-line treatment for nausea and vomiting, with no anti-emetic being approved for treatment. Dopamine antagonists (metoclopramide) and phenothiazines (prochlorperazine) have not been shown to be teratogenic in man (though metoclopramide is in animals). 5HT-selective serotonin antagonists, such as ondansetron, have been used, although patient safety data are limited, because it can be given as a wafer and provides an alternative to parenteral administration in patients unable to tolerate other oral therapy.

Vitamin supplements, including thiamine, should be given, particularly where hyperemesis has been prolonged. If vomiting continues and the history is suggestive of severe reflux or ulcer disease, endoscopy can be very valuable. It is a safe technique in pregnancy. If severe oesophagitis is confirmed, appropriate treatment with alginates and metoclopramide can be given. Ulcer disease will require H2 antagonist treatment (ranitidine) or, if very severe, omeprazole, though there is limited experience of this in pregnancy.

Very occasionally, women do not settle with a combination of these measures. Some of these women may improve with steroid therapy, though trials are still ongoing. Women in whom there is liver function derangement may benefit particularly. H2 antagonists must be given in conjunction with the steroid treatment. Parenteral nutrition is necessary for some who develop severe protein-calorie malnutrition. Specialized nutrition units can be very helpful in this setting.

If hyperemesis is left untreated, the mother's condition worsens. Wernicke's encephalopathy is a complication associated with a lack of vitamin B_1 (thiamine). Coma and death have been reported because of hepatic and renal involvement. Termination of pregnancy may reverse the condition and has a place in preventing maternal mortality. Hyperemesis persisting into the third trimester should be further investigated, as it may be symptomatic of serious illness such as acute fatty liver of pregnancy.

Essential information

Miscarriage

- Pregnancy loss before 24 weeks
- Complicates 10–20% of pregnancies
- Commonly associated with chromosome abnormalities
- Does not always require surgical treatment

Recurrent miscarriage

- Defined as three consecutive pregnancy losses
- Investigations should include screening for antiphospholipid antibodies, chromosome abnormalities and PCOS
- Chances of a successful subsequent pregnancy more than 60% without any treatment
- Women with antiphospholipid antibodies should be offered treatment with low-dose aspirin and heparin

Ectopic pregnancy

- 1% of pregnancies are ectopic
- Most important cause of maternal death in early pregnancy
- Atypical presentations are common

- Commonest site for ectopic pregnancy is the ampullary region of the Fallopian tube
- Can be accurately diagnosed by a combination of ultrasound and hCG measurement
- Laparoscopic treatment is associated with lower morbidity

Trophoblastic disease

- Affects 1 in 650 pregnancies in the UK
- Partial moles are triploid, complete moles diploid
- Treated initially by surgical evacuation of the uterus
- 50% of choriocarcinomas occur without a history of molar pregnancy
- Requires follow-up with serial hCG measurement

Hyperemesis gravidarum

- Persistent vomiting starting before 20 weeks in pregnancy associated with weight loss and ketosis
- Usually resolves in second trimester
- May lead to encephalopathy, renal and hepatic failure
- Hospital admission is indicated where there is evidence of dehydration or electrolyte imbalance

Chapter | 19 |

Sexual and reproductive health

Roger Pepperell

LEARNING OUTCOMES

After studying this chapter you should be able to:

Knowledge criteria

- Describe the methods of contraception in terms of efficiency, benefits, risks and side effects.
- Describe the surgical and medical options for termination of pregnancy.
- Discuss the ethical and legal issues relating to fertility control.
- Describe the aetiology, diagnosis, prevention and management of the common sexually transmitted infections, including HIV.
- Describe the aetiology, investigation and management of the common disorders of male and female sexual dysfunction.

Clinical competencies

- Take a history in relation to contraceptive and sexual health needs.
- Explain the benefits, risks and side effects of different forms of contraception.
- Counsel a woman about using the combined oral contraceptive pill.
- Counsel a woman and her partner about permanent contraception.
- Counsel a woman about emergency contraception.
- Plan appropriate investigation of men and women presenting with genital tract infections.
- Counsel a client about safe sexual behaviour.

Professional skills and attitudes

- Reflect on the sexual health care needs of vulnerable groups, e.g. the young, commercial sex workers and drug abusers.
- Reflect on the psychosocial impact of sexually transmitted infections and unplanned pregnancy.
- Recognize the need to respect cultural and religious beliefs as well as sexual diversity.

Contraception and termination of pregnancy

The ability to control fertility by reliable artificial methods has transformed both social and epidemiological aspects of human reproduction. Family size is determined by a number of factors, including social and religious customs, economic aspirations, knowledge of contraception and the availability of reliable methods to regulate fertility.

Artificial methods of contraception act predominantly by the following pathways:

- inhibition of ovulation
- prevention of implantation of the fertilized ovum
- barrier methods of contraception, whereby the spermatozoa are physically prevented from gaining access to the cervix

The effectiveness of any method of contraception is measured by the number of unwanted pregnancies that occur during 100 women-years of exposure, i.e. during 1 year in 100 women who are normally fertile and are having regular coitus. This is known as the *Pearl index* (Table 19.1).

Barrier methods of contraception

These techniques involve a physical barrier that reduces the likelihood of spermatozoa reaching the female upper genital tract. Barrier methods also offer protection against sexually transmitted infections (STIs). The relative risk of an STI-induced pelvic inflammatory disease (PID) is 0.6 for women using these methods. Women who use another method of contraception to prevent pregnancy are often advised to use a condom as well to reduce an otherwise-increased risk of STI.

Male condoms

The basic condom consists of a thin, stretchable latex film, which is moulded into a sheath, lubricated and packed in a foil wrapper. The sheath has a teat end to collect the

Table 19.1 Failure rates per 100 women for different methods of contraception

	U.S. DATA USED BY WHO: % OF WOMEN HAVING AN UNINTENDED PREGNANCY WITHIN THE FIRST YEAR OF USE[a]		OXFORD/FPA STUDY (ALL WOMEN MARRIED AND AGED ABOVE 25)[b]		
	Typical use*	Perfect use[†]	Overall (any duration)	Age 25–34 (≤2 years use)	Age 35+ (≤2 years use)
Sterilization					
Male (after azoospermia)	0.15	0.1	0.02	0.08	0.08
Female (Filshie clip)	0.5	0.5	0.13	0.45	0.08
Subcutaneous implant Nexplanon	0.05	0.05	–	–	–
Injectable (DMPA)	3	0.3	–	–	–
Combined pills					
50 µg oestrogen	8	0.3	0.16	0.25	0.17
<50 µg oestrogen	8	0.3	0.27	0.38	0.23
Evra patch	8	0.3	–	–	–
NuvaRing	8	0.3	–	–	–
Cerazette progestogen-only pill (POP)		0.17[‡]	–	–	–
Old-type POP	8	0.3	1.2	2.5	0.5
Intrauterine device (IUD) Levonorgestrel-releasing intrauterine system (LNG-IUS)	0.2	0.2	–	–	–
T-Safe Cu 380 A	0.8	0.6	–	–	–
Other >300 mm copper-wire IUDs (Nova-T 380, Multiload 375, Flexi-T 300)	≈1[‡]	≈1[‡]	–	–	–
Male condom	15	2	3.6	6.0	2.9
Female condom	21	5	–	–	–
Diaphragm (all caps believed similar, not all tested)	16	6	1.9	5.5	2.8
Withdrawal	27	4	6.7	–	–
Spermicides alone	29	18	11.9	–	–
Fertility awareness	25	5	15.5	–	–
Standard days method	–	3–4	–	–	–
Ovulation (mucus) method	–		–	–	–
Persona	6[‡]		–	–	–
No method, young women	80–90		–	–	–
No method at age 40	40–50		–	–	–
No method at age 45	10–20		–	–	–
No method at age 50 (if still having menses)	0–5				

Table 19.1 Failure rates per 100 women for different methods of contraception—cont'd

From [a]Trussell J (2007) Contraceptive efficacy. In: Hatcher RA, Trussell J, Nelson AL, et al. (eds). Contraceptive Technology: nineteenth revised edition. Ardent Media, New York.
Other Notes (1) Note influence of age: all the rates in the fifth column being lower than those in the fourth column. Lower rates still may be expected above age 45. (2) Much better results also obtainable in other states of relative infertility, such as lactation. (3) Oxford/FPA users were established users at recruitment – greatly improving results for barrier methods (*Qs 1.19, 4.9*). (4) The Nexplanon, Cerazette and Persona results come from pre-marketing studies by the manufacturer, giving an estimate of the Pearl 'method-failure' rate.
[b]Vessey M, Lawless M, Yeates D (1982) Efficacy of different contraceptive methods. Lancet 1(8276):841–842.
*Typical use: Among typical couples who initiate use of the method (not necessarily for the first time), the percentage who experience an accidental pregnancy during the first year if they do not stop use for any other reason.
[†]Perfect use: Among typical couples who initiate use of the method (not necessarily for the first time) and who then use it *perfectly* (both consistently and correctly), the percentage who experience an accidental pregnancy during the first year if they do not stop use for any other reason.
[‡]Data not available from Trussell, so best alternative data given, e.g. from manufacturer's studies.
(This table was published in Guillebaud J, MacGregor A (2013) Contraception, 6th edn. ©Elsevier. Reproduced from Trussell J, Wyn LL (2008) Reducing unintended pregnancy in the United States. Contraception 77(1): 1–5, with permission.)

ejaculate. The disadvantages of sheaths are that they need to be applied before intercourse and they reduce the level of sensation for the male partner. The advantages are that they are readily available, are without side effects for the female partner and provide a degree of protection against infection. They have an efficiency of 97–98% with careful use, although typical failure rates can be as high as 15 pregnancies per 100 women-years. Common reasons for failure are leakage of sperm when the penis is withdrawn, putting the condom on after genital contact, use of lubricants that cause the latex to break and mechanical damage. Condoms should be unrolled completely on to the penis before genital contact occurs and held when the penis is withdrawn to avoid leakage. The penis needs to be withdrawn from the vagina before the erection is lost, or sperm will inevitably be lost from it.

Female condoms

Female condoms are less widely used than the male equivalent but have a similar failure rate and give similar protection against infection. They are made of polyurethane and, like the male condom, are suitable for a single episode of intercourse only.

Diaphragms and cervical caps

The modern vaginal diaphragm consists of a thin latex rubber dome attached to a circular metal spring. These diaphragms vary in size from 45 to 100 mm in diameter. The size of the diaphragm required is ascertained by examination of the woman. The size and position of the uterus are determined by vaginal examination, and the distance from the posterior vaginal fornix to the pubic symphysis is noted. The appropriate measuring ring, usually between 70 mm and 80 mm, is inserted. When in the correct position, the

anterior edge of the ring or diaphragm should lie behind the pubic symphysis and the lower posterior edge should lie comfortably in the posterior fornix (Fig. 19.1).

The woman should be advised to insert the diaphragm either in the dorsal position or in the kneeling position while bending forwards. The diaphragm can be removed by simply hooking an index finger under the rim from below and pulling it out. The diaphragm should be smeared on both sides with a contraceptive cream, and it is usually advised that it be inserted dome down. However, some women prefer to insert the diaphragm with the dome upwards.

The diaphragm must be inserted prior to intercourse and should not be removed until at least 6 hours later. The main advantage of this technique is that it is free of side effects to the woman, apart from an occasional reaction to the contraceptive cream. The main disadvantages are that the diaphragm must be inserted before intercourse and typical failure rates are between 6 and 16 pregnancies per 100 women-years. The main reason for failure is probably that the diaphragm size chosen is actually too small and when orgasm occurs in the woman, when the vaginal size can increase dramatically, the diaphragm no longer fits adequately.

There are a variety of vault and cervical caps, which are of much smaller diameter than the diaphragm. These are suitable for women with a long cervix or with some degree of prolapse but otherwise have no particular advantage over the diaphragm.

Spermicides and sponges

Spermicides are only effective, in general, if used in conjunction with a mechanical barrier. Pessaries or suppositories have a water-soluble or wax base and contain a spermicide. They must be inserted approximately 15 minutes before

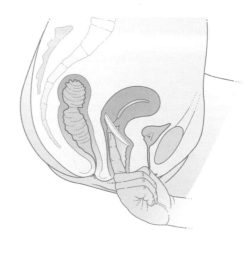

Fig. 19.1 Insertion of a vaginal diaphragm to cover the cervix and anterior vaginal wall.

intercourse. Common spermicides are nonoxynol-9 and benzalkonium. Creams consist of an emulsified fat base and tend not to spread. Care in insertion is essential so that the spermicide covers the cervix.

Jellies or pastes have a water-soluble base that spreads rapidly at body temperature. They therefore have an advantage over creams, as they spread throughout the vagina.

Foam tablets and foam aerosols contain bicarbonate of soda so that carbon dioxide is released on contact with water. The foam spreads the spermicide throughout the vagina. Pregnancy rates vary with different agents but average around 9–10 per 100 women-years.

Sponges consist of polyurethane foam impregnated with nonoxynol-9. The failure rate is between 9% and 32%, and their use in isolation is therefore not recommended. They are inserted at least 15 minutes before intercourse and can be left in for a maximum of 12 hours.

Intrauterine contraceptive devices

Intrauterine contraception is used by 6–8% of women in the UK. A wide variety of intrauterine devices (IUDs) have been designed for insertion into the uterine cavity (Fig. 19.2). These devices have the advantage that, once inserted, they are retained without the need to take alternative contraceptive precautions. It seems likely that they act mainly by preventing fertilization. This is a result of a reduction in the viability of ova and the number of viable sperm reaching the tube.

The first device to be widely used was the **Grafenberg** ring, which was made of a silver–copper alloy. Introduced in the 1930s, it ran into considerable difficulties with haemorrhage, infection, miscarriages and uterine perforation. Later, inert plastic devices such as the Lippes loop were associated with a significant increase in menstrual blood

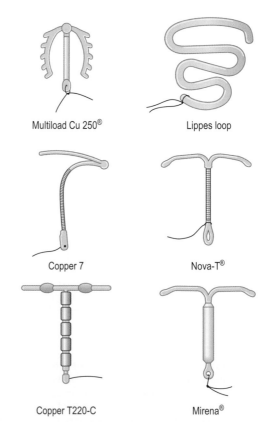

Multiload Cu 250®   Lippes loop

Copper 7   Nova-T®

Copper T220-C   Mirena®

Fig. 19.2 Some intrauterine contraceptive devices; on the right, the levonorgestrel intrauterine system.

flow in many users. The development of copper IUDs has been associated with improved contraceptive efficacy and a lessening of excess menstrual blood loss.

Types of devices

The devices are either inert or pharmacologically active.

Inert devices

Lippes loops, Saf-T-coils and Margulis spirals are plastic or plastic-coated devices. They have a thread attached that protrudes through the cervix and allows the woman to check that the device is still in place. Inert devices tend to be relatively large. They are not now available but may still be found in situ in some older users.

Pharmacologically active devices

The addition of copper to a contraceptive device produces a direct effect on the endometrium by interfering with endometrial oestrogen-binding sites and depressing uptake of thymidine into DNA. It also impairs glycogen storage in the endometrium. Examples of such devices are the Copper-T or Copper-7 (first generation), the Multiload Copper-250 (second generation) and the Copper-T 380 (third generation).

Devices containing progestogen

The levonorgestrel-releasing intrauterine system, or Mirena, contains 52 mg of levonorgestrel (see Fig. 19.2) which suppresses the normal buildup of the endometrium so that, unlike most IUDs, it causes a reduction in menstrual blood loss. However, there is a high incidence of irregular scanty bleeding in the first 3 months after insertion of the device. Unlike previous progestogen-containing devices, it does not appear to be associated with a higher risk of ectopic pregnancy. The superior efficacy of third-generation copper IUDs and the levonorgestrel-releasing system means that these are now considered the devices of choice.

Lifespan of devices

The Copper-T 380 is licensed for 8 years in the UK and Australia (and 13 in the United States). Other copper devices and the Mirena are licensed for 5 years. However, IUDs do not need to be replaced in women over the age of 40 years. They should be left in place until 2 years after menopause if this occurs under age 50 and for 1 year otherwise.

Insertion of devices

The optimal time for insertion of the device is in the first half of the menstrual cycle. With postpartum women, the optimal time is 4–6 weeks after delivery. Insertion at the time of therapeutic abortion is safe and can be performed when motivation is strong. It is unwise to insert IUDs following a miscarriage because of the risk of infection. Devices may be inserted within a few days of delivery, but there is a high expulsion rate.

Ideally, the woman should be placed in the lithotomy position. A cervical **human papilloma virus (HPV) assessment test or cervical Pap smear** should be taken and a swab taken for culture if there is any sign of infection. The uterus is examined bimanually, and its size, shape and position are ascertained. The cervix is swabbed with an antiseptic solution, and a vulsellum can be applied to the anterior lip of the cervix, although this is not essential and may cause discomfort.

The passage of a uterine sound will indicate the depth and direction of the uterine cavity, and the dimensions of the cavity may be assessed by devices known as cavimeters, which measure its length and breadth. Many IUDs are available in different sizes, and cavimeters help in choosing the appropriate IUD.

Insertion devices vary in construction but generally consist of a stoppered plastic tube containing a plunger to extrude the device, which may be linear or folded. The device is inserted in the plane of the lumen of the uterus, and care must be taken not to push it through the uterine fundus.

Attempts at insertion of a device where the cervical canal is tight may result in vagal syncope. Acute pain following insertion may indicate perforation of the uterus. The woman should be instructed to check the loop strings regularly and to notify her doctor immediately if the strings are not palpable.

Complications

The complications of IUDs are summarized in Figure 19.3.

Pregnancy rates

Pregnancy rates vary according to the type of device used, from 2 to 6/100 women-years for non-medicated IUDs and 0.5 to 2/100 for early-generation copper devices to less than 0.3/100 women-years for third-generation copper and levonorgestrel IUDs. If pregnancy does occur with an IUD in situ and its strings are easily grasped, it is sensible to remove it to reduce the incidence of a septic miscarriage, there being a high incidence of miscarriage in such pregnancies. If the strings are not accessible, the IUD should be left and removed at the time of delivery, although the risk of a miscarriage or premature rupture of the membranes would be increased. The risk of failure of the IUD diminishes with each year after insertion.

Perforation of the uterus

About 0.1–1% of devices perforate the uterus. In many cases, partial perforation occurs at the time of insertion and

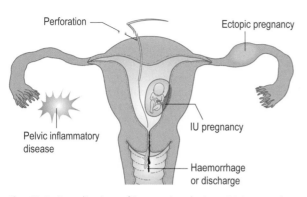

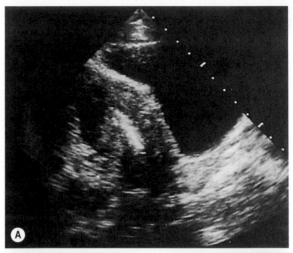

Fig. 19.3 Complications of intrauterine devices. *IU*, Intrauterine.

later migration completes the perforation. If the woman notices that the tail of the device is missing, it must be assumed that one of the following has occurred:

- The device has been expelled.
- The device has turned in the uterine cavity and drawn up the strings.
- The device has perforated the uterus and lies either partly or completely in the peritoneal cavity.

If there is no evidence of pregnancy, an ultrasound examination of the uterus should be performed. If the device is located within the uterine cavity (Fig. 19.4A), unless part of the loop or strings is visible, it will generally be necessary to remove the device with formal dilatation of the cervix under general or local anaesthesia. If the device is not found in the uterus, a radiograph of the abdomen will reveal the site in the peritoneal cavity (Fig. 19.4B). It is advisable to remove all extrauterine devices by either laparoscopy or laparotomy. Inert devices can probably be left with impunity, but copper devices promote considerable peritoneal irritation and should certainly be removed.

Pelvic inflammatory disease

Pre-existing PID is a contraindication to this method of contraception. There is a small increase in the risk of acute PID in IUD users, but this is largely confined to the first 3 weeks after insertion. If PID does occur, antibiotic therapy is commenced, and if the response is poor, the device should be removed. If the infection is severe, it is preferable to complete 24 hours of antibiotic therapy before removing the device. It is not uncommon to find evidence of *Actinomyces* organisms in the Pap smear routinely collected in an asymptomatic woman who has an IUD in place. This is generally not due to an actinomycotic pelvic infection, but due to the presence of these organisms on the surface of the IUD. There is no absolute consensus of what should be done if such organisms are found in the Pap smear. Some would remove the IUD, repeat the smear in 3 months and reinsert another IUD if the smear is clear, whereas others would leave the IUD in place but give a 2-week course of penicillin therapy.

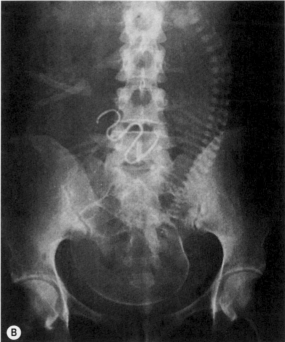

Fig. 19.4 (A) Ultrasound diagnosis of a plastic intrauterine device (IUD). (B) Radiography of the abdomen showing an IUD and a full-term pregnancy.

Abnormal uterine bleeding

Increased menstrual loss occurs in most women with an inert or copper IUD, but this can be tolerated by the majority. However, in 15% of such women, it is sufficiently severe to necessitate removal of the device. It can be controlled by drugs such as tranexamic acid or mefenamic acid. Intermenstrual bleeding may also occur, but if the loss is slight, it does not constitute a reason for IUD removal. Amenorrhoea occurs in at least 20% of women using the Mirena, and average menstrual blood loss is reduced by 90%.

Pelvic pain

Pain occurs either in a chronic low-grade form or as severe dysmenorrhoea. The incidence is widely variable, with up to 50% of women suffering some pain. However, the pain may be acceptable if it is not severe, and this is a decision that has to be made by the patient in relation to the convenience of the method.

Vaginal discharge

Vaginal discharge may be due to infection, but most women with an IUD develop a slight watery or mucoid discharge.

Ectopic pregnancy

Compared with women having unprotected intercourse, the incidence of pregnancy is lower in women with an IUD in situ (1.2/100 women years). However, should pregnancy occur, there is a higher risk (10%) of the pregnancy being extrauterine. It is therefore essential to think of this diagnosis in any woman presenting with abdominal pain and irregular vaginal bleeding who has an IUD in situ.

 Ectopic pregnancy should be excluded in any woman who conceives with an IUD in situ.

Hormonal contraception

Oral contraception is given as a **combined oestrogen and progestogen pill (OCP)** or as progestogen only.

Combined pill

Most of the current combined pills contain 20–30 μg of ethinyl oestradiol and 150–4000 μg of progestogen. The progestogens used are derived from 17-hydroxyprogesterone or 19-norsteroids (Box 19.1).

The pill is usually taken for 21 days, followed by a 7-day pill-free interval during which there is a withdrawal bleed. Everyday (ED) preparations include seven placebo pills that are taken instead of a pill-free week. The concentration of the hormones may be the same throughout the 21 days (monophasic preparations) or vary across the cycle (biphasic and triphasic preparations) in order to reduce breakthrough bleeding.

If the woman concerned is keen to avoid having periods altogether, she could be advised to take the combined hormone preparation every day, rather than having 7 hormone-free days each month, meaning that she will take the hormone tablets every day for up to 6 continuous months. This will often result in amenorrhoea during that time,

---

> **Box 19.1 Progestogen content of contraceptive pills**
>
> **Combined**
> Norethisterone
> Norgestrel
> Levonorgestrel
> Desogestrel
> Gestodene
> Cyproterone
> Drospirenone
> Dienogest
>
> **Progestogen only**
> Norethisterone
> Levonorgestrel

although some women do have irregular bleeding and are then usually advised to have only 3–4 months of continuous therapy thereafter.

Progestogen-only pill

Progestogen-only pills contain either norethisterone or levonorgestrel and are taken continuously on the basis of one tablet daily. Because of the low dose, they should be taken at the same time every day.

Mode of action of the contraceptive pills

Combined and triphasic pills act by suppressing gonadotrophin-releasing hormone (GnRH) and gonadotrophin secretion and, in particular, suppressing the luteinizing hormone peak, thus inhibiting ovulation. The endometrium also becomes less suitable for nidation, and the cervical mucus becomes hostile. Progesterone-only pills act predominantly to reduce the amount and character of the cervical mucus, although they do alter the endometrial maturation as well. Ovulation is completely suppressed in only 40% of women.

Contraindications

There are various contraindications to the pill, with some being more absolute than others.

The absolute contraindications include pregnancy, previous pulmonary embolism or deep vein thrombosis, sickle cell disease, porphyria, current active liver disease or previous cholestasis (particularly where it is associated with a previous pregnancy), migraine associated with an aura or carcinoma of the breast. It is necessary to maintain a high level of vigilance in women with varicose veins, diabetes, hypertension, renal disease and chronic heart failure, but

Table 19.2 Minor side effects of combined oral contraception

Oestrogenic effects	Progestogenic effects
Fluid retention and oedema	Premenstrual depression
Premenstrual tension and irritability	Dry vagina
Increase in weight	Acne, greasy hair
Nausea and vomiting	Increased appetite with weight gain
Headache	Breast discomfort
Mucorrhoea, cervical erosion	Cramps of the legs and abdomen
Menorrhagia	Decreased libido
Excessive tiredness	
Vein complaints	
Breakthrough bleeding	

none of these conditions constitute an absolute contraindication, and in some cases, the adverse effects of a pregnancy may substantially outweigh any hazard from the pill. Women who smoke and are also over the age of 35 years have a significantly increased risk of coronary artery and thromboembolic disease.

The occurrence of migraine for the first time, severe headaches or visual disturbances or transient neurological changes are indications for immediate cessation of the pill. A series of minor side effects may sometimes be used to advantage or may be offset by using a pill with a different combination of steroids (Table 19.2).

Other therapeutic uses of the combined oral contraceptive pill

Therapeutic uses other than contraception include the treatment of menorrhagia, premenstrual syndrome, endometriosis and dysmenorrhoea.

Major side effects

The risk of venous thrombosis is increased from 5/100,000 to 15/100,000 women per year and is further increased in smokers and women with a previous history of venous thrombosis. This compares to a risk of venous thrombosis in pregnancy and the puerperium of 60/100,000 women. Several studies have suggested that so-called *third- and fourth-generation* combined pills containing desogestrel, gestodene or drospirenone are associated with a twofold greater risk of venous thrombosis than those containing other progestogens, although the risk of venous thrombosis was lower in these studies than had previously been reported.

There is an increase in arterial disease, with a 1.6- to 5.4-fold increase in stroke and 3- to 5-fold increase in myocardial infarction (although there is no significant increase in women under 25 or in non-smokers). However, both these conditions are rare in women under the age of 35 years so the overall risk remains low, with deaths from venous thrombosis attributable to the combined pill of no more than 1–2/million women-years.

Although some reports have suggested there is a small increase in the relative risk of breast cancer (relative risk 1.24) and cervical cancer (relative risk 1.5–2) in pill users, especially if it is commenced before a first pregnancy, the increased risk breast cancer is not definitely proven, and the cervical cancer risk is probably due to the incidence of HPV infection and not the taking of the OCP.

There is an increase in gallstone formation and cholecystitis and an increase in glucose intolerance.

The progestogen-only pill has a higher failure rate and is more likely to be associated with irregular bleeding. If it fails, there is also a higher risk of ectopic pregnancy.

Beneficial effects

In addition to the prevention of unwanted pregnancy, the use of the combined pill is associated with a 30% reduction in blood loss at menstruation, a lower incidence of ectopic pregnancy (0.4/1000) and some protection against PID and benign ovarian cysts. Pill users also have a reduced risk of both endometrial and ovarian cancer of up to 50%, depending on the length of use, with this benefit lasting for up to 10 years after the OCP therapy has been ceased.

Practical care of a patient requesting to use the combined OCP ABC

It is important to obtain a complete general history and examination before prescribing the pill and to perform annual check-ups and cervical cytology or HPV assessment. A large number of compounds are commercially available, and some pills are marketed by different companies but contain the same compounds at the same concentrations. The history taken must exclude the contraindications detailed earlier. Examination should include breast examination, blood pressure assessment and, except in women who have never been sexually active, speculum examination, Pap smear or HPV testing and PV assessment. An appropriate pill for that particular patient should then be chosen, and counselling then given along the following lines.

Practical care of a patient requesting to use the combined OCP—cont'd   ABC

Which pill should you choose?

In general a 30-μg ethinyl oestradiol–containing pill is usually chosen first because of its effectiveness and low cost. The 20-μg–containing preparations are much more expensive but preferred by many women, and the side effects are usually less, except that breakthrough bleeding during the first few months of treatment is more common. If the woman had evidence of androgen excess, hirsutism or clinical polycystic ovarian syndrome (PCOS), the OCP Diane 35 should be given because its progestogen is cyproterone acetate, an anti-androgen. If the woman has fluid retention problems, an OCP containing drospirenone is usually advisable.

If the woman has used the OCP previously and had major problems with breakthrough bleeding, has conceived when taking the pill correctly or is on treatment with an anti-epileptic medication, it is safer to advise them to take an OCP containing 50 μg of ethinyl oestradiol.

When should it be commenced?

It is best commenced on day 2–3 of the next period but can be commenced at any time. Many combined pills include 7 days of placebo ('sugar') tablets so that the user takes a pill every day of the month and so reduces the risk of forgetting when to restart the pill after the normal 7 'pill-free' days each cycle (sometimes labelled 'ED' or everyday preparations). Each tablet, including the placebos, is labelled with a day of the week in these calendar packs, with the placebos being a different colour (Fig. 19.5). With these pills a woman should start taking the pill on the first day of her next period starting with the inactive tablet corresponding to the current day of the week. When changing from a higher- to a lower-dose pill preparation women should be advised to start taking the active tablets of the new pill immediately on completing the last tablet of her previous pill, omitting the normal 7-day gap.

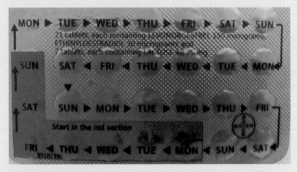

Fig. 19.5 The ED combined oral contraceptive pill.

When will it achieve its contraceptive effect?

When seven active hormone tablets have been taken on successive days.

What to do if a pill is missed or nausea, vomiting or diarrhoea occurs?

If the missed pill is not discovered until more than 12 hours after it was meant to be taken, that pill should not be taken, but the original course continued and alternative contraception used for the next 7 days. If discovered <12 hours after the time it was meant to have been taken, take that pill now, and continue the cycle taking the next one at the appropriate time. When the missed pill is close to the time the hormone tablets were due to be ceased and sugar tablets given, the original course can be stopped and a new pack commenced about 5–6 days later. There is no need for additional contraception under such circumstances.

What are the potential side effects, including the common ones of breakthrough bleeding, and what to do if such bleeding occurs?

The main nuisance side effect is breakthrough bleeding where generally light bleeding occurs despite the hormone tablets still being taken. This usually settles spontaneously within 3 months of starting the OCP, but if it persists a higher-dose pill should be given.

When is further review needed and why?

She should be reviewed in 2–3 months to check if any problems have occurred and to check that blood pressure has not become elevated. Further reviews, when blood pressure, breast examination and gynaecological assessment including Pap smear or HPV testing should be done, are generally done annually.

Table 19.3 Interaction of various drugs with oral contraceptives

Interacting drug	Effects of interaction
Analgesics	Possible increased sensitivity to pethidine
Anticoagulants	Possible reduction of effect of anticoagulant – increased dosage of anticoagulant may be necessary
Anticonvulsants	Possible decrease in contraceptive reliability
Tricyclic antidepressants	Reduced antidepressant response; increase in antidepressant toxicity
Antihistamines	Possible decrease in contraceptive reliability
Antibiotics	Possible decrease in contraceptive reliability. Possibility of breakthrough bleeding (this is most likely with rifampicin)
Hypoglycaemic agents	Control of diabetes may be reduced
Anti-asthmatics	Asthmatic condition may be exacerbated by concomitant oral contraceptive
Systemic corticosteroids	Increased dosage of steroids may be necessary

Interaction between drugs and contraceptive steroids

Many drugs affect the contraceptive efficacy of the pill, and therefore additional precautions should be taken (Table 19.3). Vomiting and diarrhoea also result in loss of the pill and hence the return of fertility – particularly with the low-dose pills now widely in use. Progestogen-only pills must be taken every day if they are to be effective.

Failure rates

The failure rate of combined pills is 0.27–5/100 women-years, with the higher end of this rate generally believed to be due to a failure of the woman to take the pill correctly, having a gastrointestinal disorder affecting its absorption or being on antibiotic therapy reducing its absorption. The failure rate for progestogen-only preparations is higher and varies between 0.3 and 8/100 women-years.

The pill and surgery

The pill increases the risk of deep vein thrombosis and should therefore be stopped at least 6 weeks before major surgery. It should not be stopped before minor procedures – particularly before laparoscopic sterilization procedures. The risk of an unwanted pregnancy occurring before admission is substantially greater than the risk of thromboembolism.

The pill and lactation

Combined preparations tend to inhibit lactation and are therefore best avoided. The pill of choice at this time is the progestogen-only pill, as it has minimal effect on lactation and may indeed promote it.

Injectable compounds

There are currently two main types: Depo-Provera and Implanon. Depo-Provera contains 150 mg of medroxyprogesterone acetate and is given as a 3-monthly intramuscular injection. Implanon is a single Silastic rod containing etonogestrel that is inserted subdermally in the upper arm and is effective for up to 3 years. An earlier type of implant, the levonorgestrel-releasing Norplant Silastic rod, has been discontinued, but some women may still have this in place. Each of these injectable preparations works by making the cervical mucus hostile and the endometrium hypotrophic and by suppressing ovulation.

Failure rates are low, at less than 0.1/100 women-years in the first year rising to 3.9/100 over 5 years. Failures mostly relate to women already pregnant at the time of injection of the Depo-Provera or insertion of the Implanon device, so it is essential that these methods are commenced at the time of a pregnancy termination or within the first 5 days of menstruation, with pregnancy excluded by a plasma beta human chorionic gonadotropin (β-hCG) pregnancy test if the last menstrual period was not entirely normal.

Parenteral progestogen-only contraceptives are long-acting but easily reversible, are effective, avoid first-pass-effect liver metabolism, require minimal compliance and avoid the side effects associated with oestrogens. However, they may cause irregular bleeding or amenorrhoea, which can be a source of anxiety because of the possibility of pregnancy. Removal of the implants may be difficult and should only be carried out by a doctor trained in the procedure. Some women will experience systemic progestogenic effects such as mood changes and weight gain or develop symptoms of oestrogenic deficiency.

Newer methods of hormonal contraception

In the last few years combined hormone transdermal patches and a vaginal contraceptive ring have been introduced. Each of these is as effective as the combined OCP, and there is good evidence that the actual hormone levels achieved with either of these is less variable than that seen with oral therapy, and lower overall. The transdermal contraceptive patches are changed weekly for 3 weeks, and the fourth week is then patch free. For the NuvaRing, the device is left in the vagina for 3 weeks, then removed for 1 week, then a new vaginal ring inserted. With each of these methods, as with the OCP, the period occurs during the hormone-free week.

Emergency contraception

After unprotected intercourse, a missed combined pill or a burst condom, a single 750-mg levonorgestrel tablet is taken within 72 hours of intercourse, followed by a second dose exactly 12 hours later. The levonorgestrel-only method has fewer side effects than the previously used combined OCP method and, in some countries, is available to women over the age of 16 years directly from pharmacists. Side effects include mild nausea, vomiting (an additional pill should be taken if vomiting occurs within 2–3 hours of the first dose) and bleeding. The woman should be advised that:

* Her next period might be early or late.
* She needs to use barrier contraception until then.
* She needs to return if she has any abdominal pain or if the next period is absent or abnormal.

If the next period is more than 5 days overdue, pregnancy should be excluded. Emergency contraception prevents 85% of expected pregnancies. Efficacy decreases with time from intercourse.

If the woman concerned does not attend until more than 72 hours after the sexual activity occurred, levonorgestrel therapy is ineffective; however, an IUD can be inserted if it is still before the time implantation of any embryo produced would have occurred.

Non-medical methods of contraception

The most fertile phase of the menstrual cycle occurs at the time of ovulation. In a 28-day cycle, this occurs on day 13 or 14 of the cycle. The fertile phase is associated with changes in cervical mucus that a woman can learn to recognize by self-examination and hormone changes that can be measured by home urine testing kits. Avoidance of the fertile period can be an extremely effective method in well-motivated couples.

Natural methods of family planning include the following:

* The *rhythm method*: Avoiding intercourse mid-cycle and for 6 days before ovulation and 2 days after it. The efficacy of this method depends on being able to predict the time of ovulation. If a regular 28-day cycle occurs, ovulation is predicted for day 14, and abstinence should be from days 8 to 16. If the cycles are highly variable, varying between 24 and 32 days, the earliest ovulation would be on day 10 and the latest on day 18, so abstinence would be required between days 4 and 20.

* The *ovulation method*: This method takes into account the ability of a woman to recognize the increase in vaginal wetness due to cervical mucus production in the phase before ovulation and abstaining from sex during that time and for 2 days after the peak wetness has been observed. This method is much better than the rhythm method, but many women only get 4 days advanced warning of the time of ovulation, so intercourse on the preceding 2 days can result in a pregnancy.

* *Coitus interruptus (withdrawal):* A traditional and still widely used method of contraception that relies on withdrawal of the penis before ejaculation. It is not a particularly reliable method of contraception, because the best sperm often reach the tip of the penis before the male experiences the imminent ejaculation, or he forgets in the 'heat' of the moment.

* *Lactational amenorrhoea method:* Breast-feeding has historically been the most important means of family 'spacing'. Ovulation resumes, on average, 4–6 months later in women who continue to breast-feed. During the first 6 months after birth, this is an effective method of contraception in mothers providing they are fully breast-feeding, not giving the baby any non-breast milk or other food AND have remained amenorrhoeic, with failure rates as low as 1/100 women being seen if all of these features exist.

Sterilization

Contraceptive techniques have the major advantage that they are easily reversible and provide a high level of protection against pregnancy. They have the disadvantage that they require a conscious act on behalf of the individual before intercourse. When family size is complete or there is a specific medical contraindication to continuing fertility, sterilization becomes the contraceptive method of choice. Around 30% of couples use sterilization for contraception, and this increases to 50% in those over the age of 40 years.

Counselling

It is essential to counsel both partners about the nature of the procedures and their implications and to discuss whether it is better for the male or female partner to be sterilized. In many cases, only one partner will be seeking sterilization, in which case only one point of view needs to be considered. It is important, however, to ensure that there is a full discussion of the alternatives.

Counselling should include reference to the intended method and its risks and failure rates (1/200 for female sterilization, 1/2000 for male sterilization). Women should be warned of the increased risk of ectopic pregnancy in the event of failure.

Remember that the reported failure rate for third-generation/levonorgestrel IUDs is comparable to that of sterilization, but male sterilization has a significantly lower failure rate.

   With the improvements brought about by microsurgery, it is no longer acceptable to say that sterilization is irreversible, and the patient should be counselled according to the technique to be used. The partner to be sterilized will be a matter of choice and motivation. If one partner has a reduced life expectancy from chronic illness, then that partner should be sterilized.

   Women should be advised to continue to use other contraception until the period occurs following the sterilization procedure. Men should be advised to use alternative contraception until they have had two consecutive semen analyses showing azoospermia 2–4 weeks apart, with these analyses not done until at least 10 ejaculations have occurred.

Timing of sterilization

The operation can be performed at any time in the menstrual cycle but is best done in the follicular phase of the cycle. A pregnancy test should be performed preoperatively if a woman has a late or missed period or thinks she may be pregnant.

Techniques

Female sterilization

The majority of procedures involves interruption of the Fallopian tubes but may vary from the application of clips on the tubes to total hysterectomy. In general terms, the more radical the procedure, the less likely there is to be a failure. However, very low failure rates can now be achieved using methods with high reversibility prospects and these should be the methods of choice.

   Laparoscopic sterilization. The use of the laparoscope for sterilization procedures has substantially reduced the duration of hospital stay. This is the method of choice in most developed countries, but an open approach through a mini-laparotomy may be more appropriate in countries where endoscopic facilities or training is limited.

- **Tubal clips.** This is the most widely used method of sterilization in the UK and Australia. The clips are made of plastic and inert metals and are locked on to the tube (Fig. 19.6). They have the advantage of causing minimal damage to the tube, but their disadvantage is a higher failure rate. Failures may be due to application on the wrong structure, extrusion of the tube from the clip and recanalization or fracture of the clip so that it falls off the tube. The *Filshie clip,* which has a titanium frame lined by silicone rubber, has the lowest failure rate (0.5%) and is easier to apply. *Yoon* or *Fallope rings* are applied over a loop of tube and are similar to a Madlener procedure (see later). This technique is associated with considerably greater abdominal pain postoperatively, and the failure rates vary between 0.3% and 4%. The rings are not suitable for application to the tubes in the puerperium when the tube is swollen and oedematous.
- **Tubal coagulation and division.** Sterilization is effected by either unipolar or bipolar diathermy of the tubes in two sites 1–2 cm from the uterotubal junction.

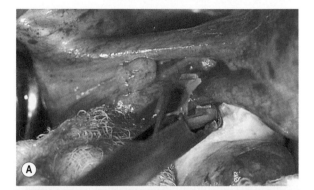

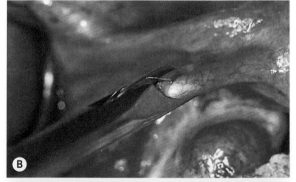

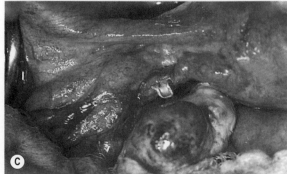

Fig. 19.6 Sterilization by clip occlusion. (A) The right Fallopian tube is grasped with the clip. (B) The clip is closed and the tube is crushed. (C) The Filshie clip is closed and locked across the Fallopian tube.

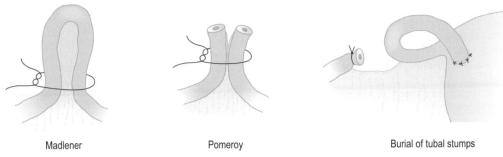

Madlener   Pomeroy   Burial of tubal stumps

Fig. 19.7 Sterilization by tubal ligation.

A considerable amount of tube can be destroyed with this technique. Division of the diathermied tube is said to reduce the risk of ectopic pregnancy. The failure rate depends on the length of tube destroyed. Because of the risk of thermal bowel injury with subsequent leakage and faecal peritonitis, diathermy should not be used as the primary method of sterilization unless mechanical methods of tubal occlusion are technically difficult or fail at the time of the procedure.

Tubal ligation (Fig. 19.7). These procedures are usually performed through a small abdominal incision (mini-laparotomy) or at the time of caesarean section. They are less widely used with the increase in laparoscopic procedures. Even when laparoscopy is contraindicated for some reason, it is still more common now to use clips to occlude the tubes.

The most basic form of the procedure involving simple ligation of the tube is known as the *Madlener procedure,* but the failure rate may be up to 3.7%. The *Pomeroy technique* is the same, but the loop of tube is excised and absorbable suture material is used for the ligation. There are several variations of this technique, including the separation of the cut ends of the tubes on contralateral sides of the broad ligament. The excised segments should be examined histologically to confirm that the tube has been excised.

The Essure procedure. This procedure consists of insertion of a small device into each tube at the time of a hysteroscopic examination, with this device resulting in fibrosis and ultimate occlusion of the tube on each side. This insertion can often be done without anaesthesia and does not require a laparoscopy. The device has a stainless steel coil, which holds the device in position in the proximal portion of the tube, and inner polyethylene terephthalate fibres, which induce the benign fibrotic reaction over the succeeding 3 months. Adequacy of tubal blockage is often checked by the performance of a hysterosalpingogram. Recent reports had detailed an increased failure rate with this technique of sterilization so it may be withdrawn from use in the near future.

Complications. Apart from the complications of laparoscopy, if it was performed to enable sterilization, the

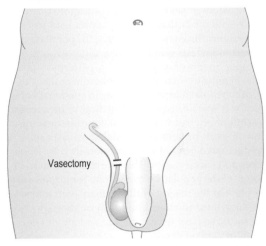

Fig. 19.8 Vasectomy involves excision of a segment of the vas deferens.

longer-term complications of any tubal sterilization are tubal recanalization and pregnancy, ectopic pregnancy, menstrual irregularity and loss of libido.

Vasectomy

This procedure is generally performed under local anaesthesia. Two small incisions are made over the spermatic cord and 3–4 cm of the vas deferens is excised (Fig. 19.8). The advantage of the technique is its simplicity. The disadvantages are that sterility is not immediate and should not be assumed until all spermatozoa have disappeared from the ejaculate. On average, this takes at least 10 ejaculations, and its effectiveness should be confirmed by a semen analysis before any unprotected intercourse is resumed.

The procedure is more difficult to reverse than most forms of female sterilization, and even when satisfactory re-anastomosis is achieved, only about 50% of patients will sire children, because of the adverse effect of the production of sperm-immobilizing and sperm-agglutinating antibodies. The failure rate is about 1/2000.

313

Failures may follow spontaneous recanalization and exclusion of an inadequate length of vas deferens. The excised segments should always be examined histologically to confirm that the vas has been excised. Complications of the operation include haematoma formation, wound infection and epididymitis. Also a painful granuloma may form at the cut end of the vas as a result of a foreign body reaction induced by spermatozoa.

Psychological implications of sterilization

Sterilization in women has acquired the reputation of leading to psychiatric problems and a deterioration in sexual function. Modern studies do not confirm this reputation. Apart from the fact that modern studies tend to use prospective standardized methodologies, the population being sterilized in the 21st century is very different to that of 40 years ago. Sterilization used to be performed predominantly on older women in poor gynaecological health, with large numbers of children and living in conditions of social adversity. It was carried out on medical recommendation, frequently shortly after childbirth, abortion or some other gynaecological procedure. Nowadays, sterilization is a widely accepted form of contraception used by women of all ages and social classes. They are therefore more representative of the population as a whole. Sterilization usually takes place at the request of the woman as an interval procedure unrelated to either childbirth or abortion. Women being sterilized have fewer children and are in better general health than previously.

The rate of psychiatric disorder following sterilization is, in general, no higher than that in the general female population. However, for women who are sterilized immediately following childbirth, there is an increased risk of suffering from postnatal depression. A previous psychiatric history and ambivalence or uncertainty about sterilization are risk factors for psychiatric disorders. Postpartum status, previous psychiatric history, ambivalence and marital discord are also risk factors for deterioration of psychosexual functioning and regret. Some authors have also suggested that in cultures where femininity is strongly associated with fertility and where there is guilt and shame about contraception, great care should be exercised to ensure that patients are properly prepared for sterilization. Regret, often measured by a request for reversal of sterilization, appears to be most strongly predicted by marital breakdown and subsequent remarriage.

Termination of pregnancy

In the UK this is carried out in approved centres under the provisions of the Abortion Act 1967. This requires that two doctors agree that either continuation of the pregnancy would involve greater risk to the physical or mental health

---

Box 19.2 Indications for termination

A. Risk to the life of the mother would be greater if the pregnancy continues
B. To prevent permanent harm to mental or physical health of the mother
C. Risk to mother's health greater* if the pregnancy continues
D. Risk to other children in the family* if the pregnancy continues
E. Risk of serious disability in the child

*Only if less than 24 weeks.

---

of the mother or her other children than termination or that the fetus is at risk of an abnormality likely to result in it being seriously handicapped (Box 19.2). The most recent amendment to the act (1991) set a limit for termination under the first of these categories at 24 weeks, although in practice the majority of terminations are carried out prior to 20 weeks.

All terminations carried out in the UK must be notified. Annual abortion numbers peaked in the UK in 1990 at 170,000 and declined after that until the scare over the risk of venous thrombosis with the 'third-generation' pills in 1996.

The availability and legality of pregnancy termination in Australia vary from state to state, and the rules in each state must therefore be defined and followed carefully before any such procedure is performed.

Methods

All women undergoing termination of pregnancy should be screened for STIs and/or offered antibiotic prophylaxis. Following termination, anti-D immunoglobulin should be given to all Rhesus-negative women. All women should be offered a follow-up appointment to check that there are no physical problems and that contraceptive measures are in place.

The rate of infection with *Chlamydia* spp. is 12% of women requesting termination of pregnancy. In these women there is a 30% risk of PID if appropriate antibiotic treatment is not given at the time of a surgical termination.

Surgical termination

This is the method most commonly used in the first trimester of pregnancy. The cervix is dilated by a number of millimetres equivalent to the gestation in weeks and the conceptus is removed using a suction curette. A variation involving piecemeal removal of the larger fetal parts with forceps (dilatation and evacuation) allows the method to be used for later second-trimester pregnancies. Although most procedures are carried out under general anaesthesia in the UK, local anaesthesia is widely used in many countries for terminations before 10 weeks and reduces the time the patient needs to stay in the hospital or clinic.

 Cervical dilation can be made easier by administration of prostaglandin pessaries before the operation.

Medical termination

This is the method most commonly used for pregnancies after 14 weeks and is increasingly being offered as an alternative to surgical termination in first-trimester pregnancies up to 9 weeks' gestation. The standard regimens for first-trimester termination use the progesterone antagonist mifepristone (RU 486) given orally, followed 36–48 hours later by prostaglandins administered as a vaginal pessary. There are several different regimens, but all have a success rate of greater than 95%. Second-trimester terminations can also be performed using vaginal prostaglandins given 3-hourly or as an extra-amniotic infusion through a balloon catheter passed through the cervix. Pretreatment with mifepristone significantly reduces the time interval from the administration of the prostaglandin preparation to abortion. After delivery of the fetus, an examination under general anaesthetic may be necessary to remove the placenta.

Complications

Early complications include bleeding, uterine perforation (with possible damage to other pelvic viscera), cervical laceration, retained products and sepsis. All the procedures also have a small failure rate (overall rate 0.7/1000). Late complications include infertility, cervical incompetence, isoimmunization and psychiatric morbidity. Adequate counselling (supported by written information) and explanation of the procedures and their risks are essential.

Psychological sequelae of termination

The majority of women who find themselves with an unwanted pregnancy are very distressed. Despite this, evidence shows that the majority of women do not experience medium- to long-term psychological sequelae, nor is there any evidence of an increase in the rate of psychiatric morbidity. The available evidence is that the rate of psychiatric morbidity following termination of pregnancy is less than if the pregnancy was allowed to proceed.

Risk factors for adverse sequelae of first-trimester abortion

Being married and having children prior to a termination can lead to problems of guilt and regret. Women in such circumstances need careful counselling before proceeding with the termination. Ambivalence, coercion, previous termination of pregnancy, past psychiatric history and termination associated with sterilization are risk factors for psychiatric morbidity.

Later terminations of pregnancy

The number of women having terminations of pregnancy after 12 weeks for psychosocial reasons is falling. Second-trimester terminations now account for fewer than 8% of all therapeutic terminations of pregnancy. A minority of these women are having a therapeutic abortion for psychosocial reasons; the majority for fetal abnormality.

Unlike first-trimester abortions, later terminations of pregnancy are associated with both marked psychological distress and an increased rate of psychiatric disorder. Some 39% of women having an abortion for fetal abnormality are depressed at 3–9 months postoperatively, although the rates fall to normal at 1 year. For women undergoing this procedure for psychosocial reasons, the cause for the increased rate of distress and morbidity is likely to be found in the delay in presenting for termination. The very young, the mentally handicapped and the chronically mentally ill may be found in this group, as well as those who have experienced marked ambivalence about their pregnancies.

The situation for women having a termination of pregnancy because of fetal abnormality is different. These are often older women who have a much-wanted pregnancy and whose problem has been diagnosed either because of a previous experience or as the result of screening. The decision to terminate the pregnancy is usually reached only after much thought and anguish. The consequence of termination is therefore very much like the spontaneous loss of a more advanced pregnancy, that is to say, a grief reaction. Their psychosocial recovery may be assisted by granting them the dignity of a naming and burial. Most late terminations of pregnancy involve the induction of labour and a prolonged process of giving birth. This can be a distressing and traumatic experience, and psychological recovery will be improved by sensitive and compassionate handling by the doctor and nursing staff.

Contraception following termination

Referral for termination should also be an opportunity to discuss future contraception and to ensure that adequate provision is made for this after the termination. The procedure can be combined with sterilization. This has the advantage of preventing further terminations for the woman who is certain that she has completed her family. There is little evidence that this is associated with an increase in the rate of complications or later contraceptive failure. However, because of the increase in the 'regret rate' for the sterilization, an interval procedure is generally recommended. IUD insertion can be carried out at the same time as termination and is not associated with an increased risk of perforation or failure. If the oral contraceptive is being used, this can be started on the same or following day.

Criminal abortion

Miscarriage induced by a variety of techniques makes up a substantial percentage of miscarriage in some countries, particularly in under-developed countries where legal abortion is not available. Where the indications for legal miscarriage are liberal, criminal abortion is infrequent, but in many countries, it contributes to a high percentage of apparently spontaneous miscarriages. The World Health Organization estimates that 250,000 women per year in the world die as a result of abortions, most of which are illegal. Mortality from abortion in the UK has fallen from a rate of 37/million maternities to 1.4/million since 1967. There have been no deaths from illegal abortion in the UK since 1982.

Genital tract infections

The female genital tract provides direct access to the peritoneal cavity. Infection may extend to any level of the tract and, once it reaches the Fallopian tubes, is usually bilateral.

The genital tract has a rich anastomosis of blood and lymphatic vessels that serve to resist infection, particularly during pregnancy.

There are other natural barriers to infection:
- The physical apposition of the pudendal cleft and the vaginal walls.
- Vaginal acidity – the low pH of the vagina in the sexually mature female provides a hostile environment for most bacteria; this resistance is weakened in the prepubertal and postmenopausal female.
- Cervical mucus that acts as a barrier in preventing the ascent of infection.
- The regular monthly shedding of the endometrium.

Taking a sexual history   ABC

Taking an accurate sexual history is essential to the management of genital tract infections, and aspects of sexual history are relevant to a range of other presentations, including subfertility, pelvic pain and disorders of sexual function. A concise sexual history will help to:
- identify specific risk behaviours
- assess symptoms to guide examination and testing
- identify anatomical sites for testing based on risk
- assess other related sexual health issues such as pregnancy risk and contraceptive needs
- inform the counselling process, health education required and contact tracing

Patients (and students!) are often anxious so it is important to create a relaxed and friendly environment and have a respectful and a non-judgemental attitude. Introducing self and role, maintaining eye contact and having appropriate body language are important aspects of good communication when obtaining a sexual history. The confidential nature of the consultation should be explained. It is important to use language that is understandable and does not use labels or make judgements. Ask general questions first, using open-ended questions. Move on to the exploration of reasons for presentation and more closed-ended questions (see later). Explain there are some 'universal' questions that are explicitly asked of everyone to assess risk, and avoid making assumptions about sexual orientation based on appearance.

Specific questions

Reason for attendance: the problem/issue, including symptoms
Direct questions about symptoms may include:
- duration and severity of symptoms
- urethral and vaginal discharge: amount, colour, odour, character
- abnormal vaginal or rectal bleeding
- genital and extra-genital rashes, lumps or sores
- itching and/or discomfort in the perineum, peri-anal and pubic region
- lower abdominal pain or dyspareunia
- difficulties/pain with micturition, defecation or during intercourse
Sexual behaviour risk assessment:
- last sexual intercourse (LSI)
- history of unprotected intercourse
- number and gender of sexual contacts in last 3–12 months (all men should be asked if they have ever had sex with another man in the past)

Lower genital tract infections

The commonest infections of the genital tract are those that affect the vulva and vagina. Infections that affect the vagina also produce acute and chronic cervicitis.

Symptoms

Swelling and reddening of the vulval skin is accompanied by soreness, pruritus and dyspareunia. When the infection is predominantly one of vaginitis, the symptoms include vaginal discharge, pruritus, dyspareunia and often dysuria. Cervicitis is associated with purulent vaginal discharge, sacral backache, lower abdominal pain, dyspareunia and dysuria. The proximity of the cervix to the bladder often results in co-existent trigonitis and urethritis, particularly in the case of gonococcal infections.

Chronic cervicitis is present in about 50–60% of all parous women. In many cases, the symptoms are minimal. There may be a slight mucopurulent discharge, which is not sufficient to trouble the woman and may simply present as an incidental finding that does not justify active treatment. In the more severe forms of the condition, there is profuse vaginal discharge, chronic sacral backache, dyspareunia and occasionally postcoital bleeding. Bacteriological culture of the discharge is usually sterile. The condition may cause subfertility because of hostility of the cervical mucus to sperm invasion.

Signs

These will depend on the cause. The appearance of the vulval skin is reddened, sometimes with ulceration and excoriation. In the sexually mature female, the vaginal walls may become ulcerated, with plaques of white monilial discharge adherent to the skin or, in protozoal infections, the discharge may be copious with a greenish-white, frothy appearance.

Bartholin's glands are sited between the posterior part of the labia minora and the vaginal walls, and these two glands secrete mucus as a lubricant during coitus. Infection of the duct and gland results in closure of the duct and formation of a Bartholin's cyst or abscess. The condition is often recurrent and causes pain and swelling of the vulva. Bartholinitis is readily recognized by the site and nature of the swelling.

In cervicitis the cervix appears reddened and may be ulcerated, as with herpetic infections, and there is a mucopurulent discharge as the endocervix is invariably involved. The diagnosis is established by examination and taking cervical swabs for culture.

Common organisms causing lower genital tract infections

Vaginal candidiasis

Candida albicans is a yeast pathogen that occurs naturally on the skin and in the bowel. Infection may be asymptomatic

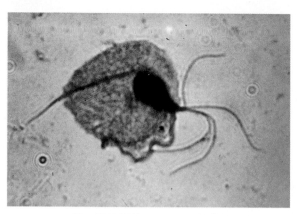

Fig. 19.9 *Trichomonas vaginalis.*

or associated with an increased or changed vaginal discharge associated with soreness and itching in the vulva area. There is no evidence of male-to-female sexual transmission. White curd-like collections attached to the vaginal epithelium may be seen on speculum examination, although these are not present in all cases.

Candidal infections are particularly common during pregnancy, in women taking the contraceptive pill and in underlying conditions involving immunosuppression, e.g. HIV infection, diabetes or long-term steroids. In each instance, vaginal acidity is increased above normal and bacterial growth in the vagina is inhibited in such a way as to allow free growth of yeast pathogens, which thrive well in a low-pH environment. *Candida* hyphae and spores can also be seen in a wet preparation and can be cultured.

Trichomoniasis

Trichomonas vaginalis is a flagellated, single-celled protozoal organism that may infect the cervix, urethra and vagina. In the male the organism is carried in the urethra or prostate and infection is sexually transmitted. The organisms are often seen on the Pap smear even in the absence of symptoms. The commonest presentation is with abnormal vaginal bleeding, but other symptoms include vaginal soreness and pruritus. The vaginal pH is usually raised above 4.5. A fresh wet preparation in saline of vaginal discharge will show motile trichomonads (Fig. 19.9). The characteristic flagellate motion is easily recognized, and the organism can be cultured.

Genital herpes

The condition is caused by herpes simplex virus (HSV) type 2 and, less commonly, type 1. It is a sexually transmitted disease. Primary HSV infection is usually a systemic infection with fever, myalgia and occasionally meningism. The local symptoms include vaginal discharge, vulval pain, dysuria and inguinal lymphadenopathy.

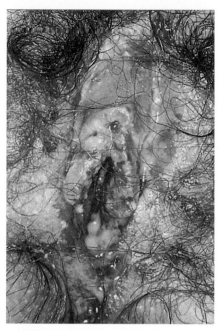

Fig. 19.10 Herpetic vulvitis. Lesions can also occur in the cervix and in the perivulvar region.

The discomfort may be severe enough to cause urinary retention. Vulval lesions include skin vesicles and multiple shallow skin ulcers (Fig. 19.10). The infection is also associated with an increased risk of cervical dysplasia. Partners may be asymptomatic, and the incubation period is 2–14 days.

The diagnosis is made by sending fluid from vesicles for viral culture or antigen detection. After the initial infection the virus remains latent in the sacral ganglia. Recurrences may be triggered by stress, menstruation or intercourse but are normally of shorter duration and less severe than the primary episode. Serum antibodies are raised in well-established lesions.

Bacterial vaginosis

This is due to an overgrowth of a number of anaerobic organisms, including *Gardnerella* spp. It is not sexually transmitted. It may be asymptomatic or cause a smelly vaginal discharge and vulval irritation. It is associated with an increased risk of PID, urinary tract infection and puerperal infection. Diagnosis is made by finding three of the following:

- An increase in vaginal pH of more than 4.5
- A typical thin homogenous vaginal discharge
- A fishy odour produced when 10% potassium hydroxide is added to the discharge
- Clue cells on Gram-stained slide of vaginal fluid (Fig. 19.11)

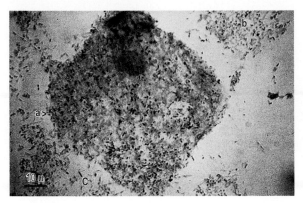

Fig. 19.11 Clue cells in bacterial vaginosis. These are epithelial squamous cells with multiple bacteria adherent to their surface. *a>*, Clue Cell; *b,* Normal epithelial cell; *C,* bacteria.

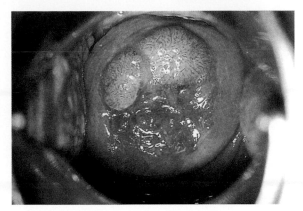

Fig. 19.12 Papilloma virus infection of the cervix: condylomata acuminata.

Gonococcal and chlamydial vulvovaginitis

These organisms can result in extensive pelvic infection (see later) but may also be asymptomatic or indicated merely by vaginal discharge and dysuria. *Chlamydia* is the commonest STI seen today.

Syphilis

The initial lesion appears 10–90 days after contact with the spirochaete *Treponema pallidum*. The primary lesion or chancre is an indurated, firm papule, which may become ulcerated and has a raised firm edge. This lesion most commonly occurs on the vulva but may also occur in the vagina or cervix. The primary lesion may be accompanied by inguinal lymphadenopathy. The chancre heals spontaneously within 2–6 weeks.

Some 6 weeks after the disappearance of the chancre, the manifestations of secondary syphilis appear. A rash develops which is maculopapular and is often associated with alopecia. Papules occur, particularly in the anogenital area and in the mouth, and give the typical appearance known as *condylomata lata*.

Swabs taken from either the primary or secondary lesions are examined microscopically under dark-ground illumination, and the spirochaetes can be seen. The serological tests have been described in Chapter 7.

The disease then progresses from the secondary phase to a tertiary phase. It may mimic almost any disease process and affect every system in the body, but the common long-term lesions are cardiovascular and neurological.

Genital warts (condylomata acuminata)

Vulval and cervical warts (Fig. 19.12) are caused by HPV. The condition is commonly, although by no means invariably, transmitted by sexual contact. The incubation period is up to 6 months. The incidence had risen significantly over the last 15 years, particularly in women aged 16–25 years, but since the introduction of quadrivalent HPV vaccination the incidence has fallen considerably.

The warts have an appearance similar to those seen on the skin in other sites, and in the moist environment of the vulval skin are often prolific – particularly during pregnancy. There is frequently associated pruritus and vaginal discharge. The lesions may spread to the peri-anal region and in some cases become confluent and subject to secondary infection. Diagnosis is usually made by clinical examination.

> Vaginal discharge in a child may also be associated with the presence of a foreign body, and this possibility should always be excluded.

Treatment of lower genital tract infections

When the diagnosis has been established by examination and bacteriological tests, the appropriate treatment can be instituted. The treatment for *Chlamydia* and gonorrhoea is discussed later under infections of the upper genital tract. Whenever a diagnosis of STI is made, it is essential to screen patients (and their partners) for other infections.

Vulval and vaginal monilial infections can be treated by topical or oral preparations. These include a single dose of clotrimazole given as a pessary or fluconazole taken orally. Recurrent infections can be treated by oral administration of ketoconazole and fluconazole. The patient's partner should be treated at the same time, and any predisposing factors such as poor hygiene or diabetes should be corrected.

Trichomonas infections and bacterial vaginosis are treated with metronidazole 400 mg taken twice a day for 5 days, which must be taken by both sexual partners if recurrence of the infection is to be avoided. Metronidazole may be administered as a single dose of 2 g, but high-dose therapy should be avoided in pregnancy. Topical treatment with metronidazole gel or clindamycin cream is also effective for bacterial vaginosis.

319

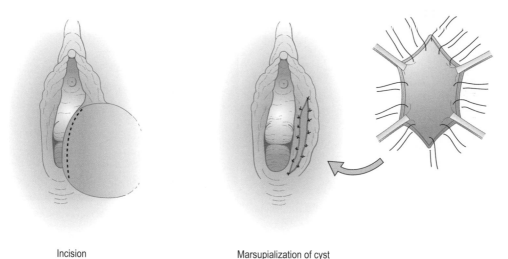

Incision   Marsupialization of cyst

Fig. 19.13 Marsupialization of a Bartholin's cyst or abscess. The incision is made over the medial aspect of the cyst *(left),* and the lining is sutured to the skin *(right).*

If a patient is asymptomatic and there is no evidence of vaginitis on clinical examination but trichomonal or monilial organisms are identified in a routine Pap smear, treatment of these patients is usually not required.

Non-specific vaginal infections are common and are treated with vaginal creams, including hydrargaphen, povidone–iodine, di-iodohydroxyquinoline or sulphonamide creams.

Syphilis is treated in the first instance with penicillin, and if this fails, for example in the case of co-infection with penicillin-resistant strains of the gonococcus, doxycycline hydrochloride or other antibiotics can be used.

Infections of the vagina associated with menopausal atrophic changes are treated by the appropriate hormone replacement therapy using an oral or vaginal oestrogen preparation, or lactic acid pessaries when oestrogens are contraindicated. The same therapy may be used, with the local application of oestrogen creams, in juvenile vulvovaginitis.

Infections of Bartholin's gland are treated with the antibiotic appropriate to the organism. If abscess formation has occurred, the abscess should be 'marsupialized' by excising an ellipse of skin and sewing the skin edges to result in continued open drainage of the abscess cavity (Fig. 19.13). This reduces the likelihood of recurrence of the abscess.

Vulval warts are treated with either physical or chemical diathermy using podophyllin applied directly to the surface of the warts. Any concurrent vaginal discharge should also receive the appropriate therapy.

Herpetic infections are notoriously resistant to treatment and highly prone to recurrence. The best available treatment is acyclovir administered in tablet form 200 mg five times daily for 5 days or locally as a 5% cream.

Acute cervicitis usually occurs in association with generalized infection of the genital tract and is diagnosed and treated according to the microbiology. Medical treatment is rarely effective in chronic cervicitis because it is difficult to identify an organism, and antibiotics do not penetrate the chronic microabscesses of the cervical glands. If the cervical swab is negative, the next most effective management is diathermy of the endocervix under general anaesthesia. Following diathermy, an antibacterial cream should be placed in the vagina, and the woman should be advised that the discharge may increase in amount for 2–3 weeks but will then diminish. She should also be advised to avoid intercourse for 3 weeks, as coitus may cause a secondary haemorrhage.

Upper genital tract infections

Acute infection of the endometrium, myometrium, Fallopian tubes and ovaries are usually the result of ascending infections from the lower genital tract causing PID.

However, infection may be secondary to appendicitis or other bowel infections, which sometimes give rise to a pelvic abscess. Perforation of the appendix with pelvic sepsis remains a common cause of tubal obstruction and subfertility. Pelvic sepsis may also occur during the puerperium and after pregnancy termination or after operative procedures on the cervix. Retained placental tissue and blood provide an excellent culture medium for organisms from the bowel, including *Escherichia coli, Clostridium welchii* or *C. perfringens, Staphylococcus aureus* and *Streptococcus faecalis.*

PID affects approximately 1.7% of women between 15 and 35 years of age per year in the developed world. Up to 20% of women with PID will have a further episode within 2 years. The disease is most common between the ages of 15 and 24 years, and particular risk factors include multiple sexual partners and procedures involving transcervical instrumentation. PID is an important cause of infertility. After a first episode, 8% of women will have evidence of tubal infertility; subsequent episodes approximately double this figure. Women with a past history of PID are four times more likely to have an ectopic pregnancy when they conceive.

 Forty per cent of women who have had three or more episodes of PID have tubal damage.

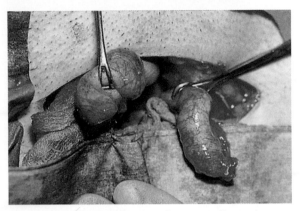
Fig. 19.14 Acute salpingitis: the tubes are swollen and engorged.

Symptoms and signs

The symptoms of acute salpingitis include:

- Acute bilateral lower abdominal pain: Salpingitis is almost invariably bilateral; where the symptoms are unilateral, an alternative diagnosis should be considered
- Deep dyspareunia
- Abnormal menstrual bleeding
- Purulent vaginal discharge
  However, many women shown to have chlamydial infection have no symptoms at all.
  The signs include:
- Signs of systemic illness with pyrexia and tachycardia.
- Signs of peritonitis with guarding, rebound tenderness and often localized rigidity. (It should be noted that guarding and rigidity rarely are seen if blood is in the peritoneal cavity, such as due to an ectopic pregnancy, whereas tenderness and release tenderness are seen even in the absence of peritonitis.)
- On pelvic examination, acute pain on cervical excitation and thickening in the vaginal fornices, which may be associated with the presence of cystic tubal swellings due to pyosalpinges or pus-filled tubes; fullness in the pouch of Douglas suggests the presence of a pelvic abscess (Fig. 19.14).
- An acute perihepatitis occurs in 10–25% of women with chlamydial PID, which may cause right upper quadrant abdominal pain, deranged liver function tests and multiple filmy adhesions between the liver surface and the parietal peritoneum, and is known as the *Fitz–Hugh–Curtis syndrome.*
- A pyrexia of 38°C or more, sometimes associated with rigors.

Common organisms

PID is thought to be the result of polymicrobial infection with primary infection by *Chlamydia trachomatis* or *Neisseria*

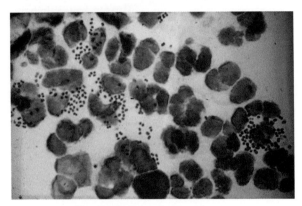
Fig. 19.15 *Neisseria gonorrhoeae.*

gonorrhoeae (or both) allowing opportunistic infection with other aerobic bacteria and anaerobes.

Chlamydia

C. trachomatis is an obligate, intracellular, Gram-negative bacterium. It is the commonest bacterial STI in Europe, Australia and North America and is thought to be the causative agent in at least 60% of cases of PID in those areas. Prevalence rates vary from 11% to 30% in women attending genitourinary medicine clinics, with the peak incidence in the UK in women aged 20–24 years. The main sites of infection are the columnar epithelium of the endocervix, urethra and rectum, but many women remain asymptomatic. Ascent of infection to the upper genital tract occurs in about 20% of women with cervical infection.

Gonorrhoea

N. gonorrhoeae is a Gram-negative, intracellular diplococcus (Fig. 19.15). Infection is commonly asymptomatic or associated with vaginal discharge. In cases of PID it spreads across the surface of the cervix and endometrium and causes tubal infection within 1–3 days of contact. It is the principal cause for 14% of cases of PID and occurs in combination with *Chlamydia* in a further 8%.

Differential diagnosis

It is often difficult to establish the diagnosis of acute pelvic infection with any degree of certainty. The predictive value of clinical signs and symptoms when compared to laparoscopic diagnosis is 65–90%. The differential diagnosis includes the following:

- **Tubal ectopic pregnancy:** Initially pain is unilateral in most cases. There may be syncopal episodes and signs of diaphragmatic irritation with shoulder tip pain. The white cell count is normal or slightly raised, but the haemoglobin level is likely to be low depending on the amount of blood lost, whereas in acute salpingitis, the white cell count is raised and the haemoglobin concentration is normal.
- **Acute appendicitis:** The most important difference in the history lies in the unilateral nature of this condition. Pelvic examination does not usually reveal as much pain and tenderness, but it must be remembered that the two conditions sometimes co-exist, particularly where the infected appendix lies adjacent to the right Fallopian tube.
- **Acute urinary tract infections:** These may produce similar symptoms but rarely produce signs of peritonism and are commonly associated with urinary symptoms.
- **Torsion or rupture of an ovarian cyst.**

Investigations

When the diagnosis of acute salpingitis is suspected, the woman should be admitted to hospital. After completion of the history and general examination, swabs should be taken from the vaginal fornices and cervical canal and sent to the laboratory for culture and antibiotic sensitivity. A midstream specimen of urine should also be sent for culture to exclude a possible urinary tract infection. An additional endocervical swab urine sample should be taken for detection of *Chlamydia* by polymerase chain reaction (PCR). Urethral swabs may identify chlamydial infection not detected by endocervical swabs. PCR assays of urine samples have a similar or better sensitivity (90%) compared to genital tract swabs and offer a potential means for screening for chlamydial infection in asymptomatic women.

Examination of the blood for differential white cell count, haemoglobin estimation and C-reactive protein may help establish the diagnosis. Blood culture is indicated if there is a significant pyrexia. The diagnosis of mild to moderate degrees of PID on the basis of history and examination

findings is unreliable and, where the diagnosis is in doubt, laparoscopy is indicated.

Negative swabs do not exclude the possibility of PID.

Management

When the patient is unwell and exhibits peritonitis, high-grade fever, vomiting or a pelvic inflammatory mass, she should be admitted to hospital and managed as follows:

- Fluid replacement by intravenous therapy – vomiting and pain often result in dehydration.
- When PID is clinically suspected, antibiotic therapy should be commenced. Antibiotic therapy initially prescribed for clinically diagnosed PID should be effective against *C. trachomatis*, *N. gonorrhoeae* and the anaerobes characterizing bacterial vaginosis. If the woman is acutely unwell, treatment should be started with an antibiotic such as cefuroxime and metronidazole given intravenously with oral doxycycline until the acute phase of the infection begins to resolve. Treatment with oral metronidazole and doxycycline should then be continued for 7 and 14 days, respectively.
- Pain relief with non-steroidal anti-inflammatory drugs.
- If the uterus contains an IUD, it should be removed as soon as antibiotic therapy has been commenced.
- Bed rest – immobilization is essential until the pain subsides.
- Abstain from intercourse.

Women who consulted after 3 days of symptoms had almost threefold increased risk of impaired infertility after PID compared with those who consulted promptly.

Patients who are systemically well can be treated as outpatients, with a single dose of azithromycin and a 7-day course of doxycycline, reviewed after 48 hours.

In all cases of confirmed STI, it is important to treat the partner and arrange appropriate contact tracing.

Indications for surgical intervention

In most cases, conservative management results in complete remission. Laparotomy is indicated where the condition does not resolve with conservative management and where there is a pelvic mass.

In most cases, the mass will be due to a pyosalpinx or tubo-ovarian abscess. This can either be drained or a salpingectomy can be performed.

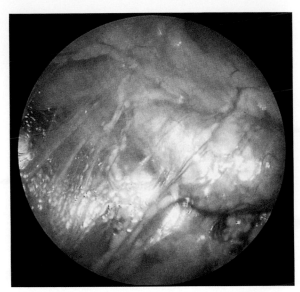

Fig. 19.16 Chronic pelvic inflammatory disease: a sheet of fine adhesions covering the tubes and ovary, which is buried beneath the tube.

Chronic pelvic infection

Acute pelvic infections may progress to a chronic state with dilatation and obstruction of the tubes forming bilateral hydrosalpinges with multiple pelvic adhesions (Fig. 19.16).

Symptoms and signs

Symptoms are varied but include:
- chronic pelvic pain
- chronic purulent vaginal discharge
- epimenorrhagia and dysmenorrhoea
- deep-seated dyspareunia
- infertility.

Chronic salpingitis is also associated with infection in the connective tissue of the pelvis known as parametritis.

On examination, there can be a purulent discharge from the cervix. The uterus is often fixed in retroversion, and there is thickening in the fornices and pain on bimanual examination.

Chronic pelvic pain occurs in 25–75% of women with a past history of PID.

Management

Conservative management of this condition is rarely effective, and the problem is only eventually resolved by clearance of the pelvic organs. Women with a history of PID are eight times more likely to have a hysterectomy than the general population. If the problem is mainly infertility due to tubal disease, the best treatment is in vitro fertilization (IVF). Tubal removal prior to IVF is usually indicated if hydrosalpinges are present because this improves the pregnancy rate achieved.

Human immunodeficiency virus

HIV-1 and HIV-2 are RNA retroviruses characterized by their tropism for the human CD4+ (helper) T lymphocyte. The proportion of cells infected is initially low, and there is a prolonged latent phase between infection and clinical signs. Transmission occurs by sex, infected blood products, shared needles, breast-feeding and at the time of delivery. Risk groups include intravenous drug abusers and their partners, the partners of bisexual men, haemophiliacs, prostitutes and immigrants from high-risk areas. Although HIV infection is more common in men in the developed world, anonymous testing shows that 0.3% of pregnant women in London are infected, and it is now the most common cause of death in African American females aged 24–35 years in the United States. In parts of sub-Saharan Africa, 20–30% of all pregnant women are HIV positive. Vertical transmission rates can be reduced from 40% to less than 1% by antenatal treatment with the modern antiretroviral drugs, delivery by elective caesarean section and avoidance of breast-feeding. Although HIV infection was a life-ending sentence for most people in the past, as most developed AIDS as an end result within a few years of becoming infected with HIV, with modern continuous therapy, most infections are able to be controlled and progression to AIDS is much less common.

The main clinical states can be identified as:
- a 'flu-like' illness 3–6 months after infection, associated with seroconversion
- asymptomatic impaired immunity
- persistent generalized lymphadenopathy
- AIDS-related complex with pathognomonic infections or tumours.

Common opportunistic infections include *Candida*, HSV, HPV, *Mycobacterium* spp., *Cryptosporidium* spp., *Pneumocystis carinii* and cytomegalovirus. Non-infective manifestations include weight loss, diarrhoea, fever, dementia, Kaposi's sarcoma and an increased risk of cervical cancer.

The diagnosis is made by detecting antibodies to the virus, although these may take up to 3 months to appear.

Disorders of female sexual function

Disorders of sexual function are reported by up to a third of women. Sometimes they are accompanied by awareness of the underlying disturbance, but often, as with other emotional difficulties, the link between cause and effect is obscure even to the sufferer. Sexual problems may therefore appear in the guise of mental or physical illness or disturbances of behaviour and relationships and thus form a part of the working experience not only of doctors but of anyone in the 'caring' professions. Lack of knowledge about sex and the anatomy of the genital tract remain common and a source of anxiety.

The commonest complaints are:
- painful sex (dyspareunia)
- vaginismus
- loss of desire (libido)
- orgasmic dysfunction.

Pay attention to the non-verbal communication during the consultation and examination.

Dyspareunia

Dyspareunia is defined as painful intercourse. It is predominantly but not exclusively a female problem. The aetiology is divided on the basis of whether the problem is superficial (at the entrance to the vagina) or deep (only occurs with deep penile insertion), and it is therefore particularly important to obtain a concise history.

Superficial dyspareunia

Pain felt on penetration is generally associated with a local lesion of the vulva or vagina from one of the following causes:
- **Infection:** Local infections of the vulva and vagina commonly include monilial and trichomonal vulvovaginitis. Infections involving Bartholin's glands also cause dyspareunia.
- **Narrowing of the introitus** may be congenital, with a narrow hymenal ring or vaginal stenosis. It may sometimes be associated with a vaginal septum. The commonest cause of narrowing of the introitus is the over-vigorous suturing of an episiotomy wound or vulval laceration or following vaginal repair of a prolapse.
- **Menopausal changes:** Atrophic vaginitis or the narrowing of the introitus and the vagina from the effects of oestrogen deprivation may cause dyspareunia. Atrophic vulval conditions such as lichen sclerosus can also cause pain.
- **Vulvodynia:** This is a condition of unknown aetiology characterized by persisting pain over the vulva.
- **Functional changes:** Lack of lubrication associated with inadequate sexual stimulation and emotional problems will result in dyspareunia.

Deep dyspareunia

Pain on deep penetration is often associated with pelvic pathology. Any woman who develops deep dyspareunia after enjoying a normal sexual life should be considered to have an organic cause for her pain until proved otherwise. The common causes of deep dyspareunia include:
- **Acute or chronic pelvic inflammatory disease:** including cervicitis, pyosalpinx and salpingo-oophoritis (see Fig. 19.16). The uterus may become fixed. Ectopic pregnancy must also be considered in the differential diagnosis in this group.
- **Retroverted uterus and prolapsed ovaries:** If the ovaries prolapse into the pouch of Douglas and become fixed in that position, intercourse is painful on deep penetration.
- **Endometriosis:** Both the active lesions and the chronic scarring of endometriosis may cause pain.
- **Neoplastic disease of the cervix and vagina:** At least part of the pain in this situation is related to secondary infection.
- **Postoperative scarring:** This may result in narrowing of the vaginal vault and loss of mobility of the uterus. The stenosis commonly occurs following vaginal repair and, less often, following repair of a high vaginal tear. Vaginal scarring may also be caused by chemical agents such as rock salt, which, in some countries, is put into the vagina in order to produce contracture.
- **Foreign bodies:** Occasionally, a foreign body in the vagina or uterus may cause pain in either the male or female partner. For example, the remnants of a broken needle or partial extrusion of an IUD may cause severe pain in the male partner.

Apareunia

Apareunia is defined as the 'absence' of intercourse or the inability to have intercourse at all. The common causes are:
- congenital absence of the vagina
- imperforate hymen.

Treatment

Accurate diagnosis is dependent on careful history taking and a thorough pelvic examination. The treatment will therefore be dependent on the cause. Congenital absence of the vagina can be successfully treated by surgical correction (vaginoplasty), and removal of the imperforate hymen is effective.

Medical treatment for deep dyspareunia includes the use of antibiotics and antifungal agents for pelvic infection, and the use of local or oral hormone therapy for postmenopausal atrophic vaginitis. Treatment for endometriosis is discussed in Chapter 16. Surgical treatment includes

---

Box 19.3 **Drugs that may impair libido**

- Antiandrogens – cyproterone
- Anti-oestrogens – tamoxifen and some contraceptives
- Cytotoxic drugs
- Sedatives
- Narcotics
- Antidepressants
- Alcohol and illegal drug misuse

---

correction of any stenosis and excision of painful scars where appropriate, and reassurance and sexual counselling are necessary in functional disorders.

Vaginismus

Vaginismus is the symptom resulting from spasm of the pelvic floor muscles and adductor muscles of the thigh, which prevents or results in pain on attempted penile penetration. A physical barrier may be present but is not necessarily causative. The woman may be unable to allow anyone to touch the vulva. Primary vaginismus is usually due to fear of penetration. Secondary vaginismus is more likely to be the result of an experience of pain with intercourse after infection, sexual assault, a difficult delivery or surgery. Even after the condition has improved, fear of further pain may lead to involuntary contraction of the vaginal muscles, which is in itself painful, completing the vicious circle. Encouraging the patient to explore her own vagina and feel for herself that there is no abnormality or pain can help break this cycle. Resort to surgery is likely to confirm the patient's fears of abnormality and often leaves the presenting problem unchanged.

Loss of libido

Loss of desire is the commonest symptom in women complaining of sexual dysfunction. If it has always been present, it may be a result of a repression of sexual thoughts as a result of upbringing or religious belief or a feeling that sex is dirty or unsuitable in some way. It may represent differences between the expectations of the couple. Loss of desire in a relationship that was previously satisfactory is more likely to be due to:

- major life events – marriage, pregnancy
- being ill, depressed or grieving
- endocrine or neurological disorders
- pain on intercourse
- medication (Box 19.3)
- menopause
- fear of pregnancy or infection
- stress or chronic anxiety.

Treatment

Helping the couple to look at the underlying reasons involved helps to identify what they might do to correct the situation. Relationship therapy may be an option for suitably motivated couples. Where loss of libido is a feature of menopausal symptoms, this will occasionally respond to low-dose testosterone therapy, along with conventional oestrogen hormone replacement therapy.

Orgasmic dysfunction

About 5–10% of women have not experienced orgasm by the age of 40 years. Orgasmic dysfunction is often linked to myths about it being the responsibility of the man to bring the woman to orgasm. The problem can be helped by breaking down inhibitions about self-stimulation and encouraging better communication during foreplay and intercourse.

Disorders of male sexual function

Normal male sexual function is largely mediated through the autonomic nervous system. Erection occurs as a result of parasympathetic (cholinergic) outflow causing vasocongestion. Orgasm and ejaculation are predominantly sympathetic (adrenergic). Emission occurs by the sequential expulsion of fluid from the prostate gland, vas deferens and seminal vesicles into the posterior urethra. Emission and closure of the vesical neck are mediated by alpha-adrenergic systems, while opening of the external sphincter (to allow antegrade ejaculation) is mediated through the somatic efferent of the pudendal nerve. Ejaculation is stimulated by the dorsal nerve of the penis and involves contractile activity of the bulbocavernous and ischiorectal muscles as well as the posterior urethra. These responses are easily inhibited by cortical influences or by impaired hormonal, neural or vascular mechanisms.

The principal features of sexual dysfunction in men are:
- failure to achieve erection
- problems with ejaculation
- loss of libido.

All or any of these may be present from adolescence or have their onset at any time of life after a period of healthy sexuality. The causes of loss of libido have been previously described under female sexual dysfunction.

Erectile dysfunction

Erectile dysfunction or impotence, the inability in the male to achieve erection for satisfactory penetration of the vagina, is the most common problem seen.

It is now recognized that a high proportion (50%) of such men, especially those over the age of 40 years, have an underlying organic cause. Of these, diabetes is the commonest as a result of damage to the large and small blood vessels and neuropathy. Neurological impotence may also be caused by injuries to the spinal cord, brain and prostate and multiple sclerosis. Hyperprolactinaemia is associated with erectile dysfunction as well as with loss of libido. While androgens are not essential for erection, they influence it through their effects on libido and nitrogen oxide release in the cavernosum. Recreational drugs such as alcohol are known to cause erectile failure, and more than 200 prescription drugs are known to have it as a side effect. The most common of these are antihypertensive and diuretic agents. Others include antidepressant and sedative medications.

In the younger age group, the cause is more likely to be psychogenic. Depression, reactive or endogenous, is an important aetiological or concomitant condition. The stress provoked by timing intercourse with ovulation may result in erectile dysfunction in couples undergoing treatment for infertility.

Treatment

Mild psychogenic cases will usually respond to simple measures such as counselling, sex therapy and sensate focusing exercises.

Treatment with bromocriptine may restore sexual function in cases where prolactin levels are raised.

Intracavernous injection of prostaglandin E_1 is effective in patients with both psychogenic and organic causes of erectile dysfunction, although pain and the fear of injection cause some patients to stop treatment. Sildenafil is an effective orally administered alternative, with up to 70% of attempts at intercourse being successful compared with 22% with placebo. It promotes erection by potentiating the effect of nitric oxide on vascular smooth muscle, thus increasing blood flow to the penis. Concurrent use in patients taking nitrate therapy for myocardial ischaemic disease causes significant hypotension.

Ejaculatory problems

Ejaculatory dysfunction encompasses premature, retarded, retrograde and absent ejaculation. Anejaculation and premature ejaculation are more often seen in younger patients. Retrograde ejaculation is often a result of an organic cause or after surgery, e.g. prostate operations. The diagnosis is usually made on the presenting history.

Treatment

For premature ejaculation, the squeeze technique described by Masters and Johnson involves application of pressure to the top of the penis. This diminishes the urge to ejaculate, although the success rate is poor. Alternative approaches include the use of a local anaesthetic and selective serotonin-reuptake inhibitors. Anejaculation and retarded ejaculation can be treated by teaching masturbation techniques, couple counselling and sensate focus exercises. Retrograde ejaculation is regarded mainly as a fertility problem. Treatment may involve surgery or drug therapy with alpha-adrenoceptor agonists.

Essential information

IUDs

- Prevent implantation and fertilization
- Inert or pharmacologically active
- Best for older multiparous women
- Can be inserted at time of delivery
- Replace after 3–5 years
- Failure rate 0.2–0.8/100 women-years
- Complications: perforation, PID, abnormal bleeding, ectopic pregnancy

Combined OCP

- Suppress gonadotrophins, but have other effects as well
- Oestradiol and progestogen
- Pregnancy, thromboembolism and liver disease contraindicate
- 1.3/100,000 mortality
- Failure rate 0.3/100 women-years

Sterilization

- 1/200 failure rate (female)
- Increased risk of ectopic pregnancy if procedure fails
- Permanence
- Risks of surgery
- Alternatives

Termination of pregnancy

- Methods:
  - surgical
  - medical
- Complications:
  - bleeding
  - infection
  - infertility
  - retained tissue
  - regret

Essential information—cont'd

Vulvovaginitis

- Commonest infection of genital tract
- Presents as pruritus, dyspareunia or discharge
- Common causes are *Trichomonas,* bacterial vaginosis and *Candida*
- Predisposing factors include pregnancy, diabetes, contraceptive pill
- Can be diagnosed by examination of fresh wet preparation of vaginal discharge

Herpes genitalis

- Caused by HSV
- Presents with pain, bleeding and vesicles or shallow ulcers on the vagina/vulva
- Associated with cervical dysplasia
- Tends to be recurrent but with decreasing severity
- Can be transmitted to the neonate during vaginal delivery if active

Infections of the cervix

- Acute (associated with generalized infection) or chronic
- Discharge, dyspareunia, low abdominal pain or backache, urinary symptoms and postcoital bleeding
- Can cause subfertility
- Difficult to isolate an organism when chronic
- Treatment includes appropriate antibiotics and cautery

Upper genital tract infection

- Usually from ascending lower genital tract infection
- Can follow abortion, normal delivery or an operative procedure on the cervix
- Commonly due to *C. trachomatis* or *N. gonorrhoeae* when sexually transmitted
- Presents as pain, fever, discharge and irregular periods

- Bilateral pain on cervical excitation and raised white cell count
- Differential diagnosis includes ectopic pregnancy, urinary tract infection and appendicitis
- Management includes fluid replacement, antibiotics, analgesia and rest
- Surgery (laparoscopy or laparotomy) is indicated to confirm diagnosis if in doubt, for drainage of pelvic mass and to clear pelvis in unresponsive chronic disease
- Major cause of infertility worldwide, resulting in tubal obstruction in 40% of cases after three or more attacks

HIV infection

- Retrovirus infection of T-helper cells and central nervous system
- Transmitted by sex, blood transfusion or to offspring (delivery or due to breast-feeding)
- Diagnosis by serology, differential lymphocyte count or opportunistic infection
- Can be asymptomatic, cause generalized malaise and lymphadenopathy or AIDS
- Rates of vertical transmission can be reduced by drug treatment, elective caesarean section and avoiding breast-feeding
- Incidence in heterosexuals increasing
- With current retroviral therapy, progressing to AIDS is rare

Disorders of sexual function

- Dyspareunia:
  - often caused by infection, atrophic conditions or lack of lubrication
  - deep dyspareunia indicates pelvic pathology
- Vaginismus and loss of libido are often psychogenic
- Failure to achieve erection – organic (50%) or psychogenic

Chapter | 20 |

Gynaecological oncology

Hextan Y. S. Ngan and Karen K. L. Chan

LEARNING OUTCOMES

After studying this chapter you should be able to:

Knowledge criteria

- Understand the epidemiology, aetiology, diagnosis, management and prognosis of gynaecological cancer
- Describe the aetiology, epidemiology and presentation of the common neoplasms of the female genital tract, including:
  - Vulval and cervical intraepithelial neoplasia
  - Vulval and vaginal carcinoma
  - Cervical carcinoma
  - Endometrial hyperplasia
  - Endometrial carcinoma
  - Malignant ovarian tumours
- Discuss the role of minor procedures and diagnostic imaging procedures in the management of gynaecological cancers, including:
  - Cervical and endometrial sampling
  - Ultrasound
  - Laparoscopy
  - Hysteroscopy
  - Magnetic resonance imaging and computerized tomography
- List the short- and long-term complications of medical and surgical therapies for gynaecological cancer
- Discuss the role of screening and immunization in the prevention of female genital tract malignancy

Clinical competencies

- Counsel a woman about screening for the preclinical phase of squamous cell carcinoma of the cervix
- Plan initial investigation of women presenting with symptoms of genital tract malignancy
- Communicate sensitively with a woman and her family about the diagnosis of gynaecological cancer

Professional skills and attitudes

- Discuss the principles of palliative care in gynaecological cancers

Lesions of the vulva

Vulval intraepithelial neoplasia

Vulval intraepithelial neoplasia (VIN) is a condition characterized by disorientation and loss of epithelial architecture extending through the full thickness of the epithelium. In the past, the World Health Organization classified VIN into VIN-1, 2 and 3 based on the extent to which normal epithelium is replaced by abnormal dysplastic cells. However, since VIN-1 mainly corresponds with condyloma that is not a precancerous lesion, the term VIN-1 has been abandoned, and VIN now refers to the previous VIN-2 and 3 in the latest classification of the International Society for the Study of Vulvar Disease.

VIN is categorized into usual VIN (classic VIN or Bowen's disease) and differentiated VIN (d-VIN) based on the distinctive pathological features (Box 20.1). Usual VIN often occurs in young women between 30 and 50 years and is associated with cigarette smoking and human papilloma virus (HPV) infection. Patients can be asymptomatic, or they may complain of pruritus, pain, dysuria and ulceration. Lesions can be white, pink or pigmented in the forms of plaques or papules. They are most frequently found in the labia and posterior fourchette; 3–4% of usual VIN may progress to invasive disease.

d-VIN occurs in postmenopausal women and accounts for only 2–10% of all VIN. It is associated with squamous hyperplasia, lichen sclerosus and lichen simplex chronicus

---

Box 20.1 Vulval intraepithelial neoplasia (VIN)

Squamous VIN
Usual VIN (formerly classic VIN or Bowen's disease)
Differentiated VIN (formerly 'simplex' VIN)
    Non-squamous VIN
Paget's disease

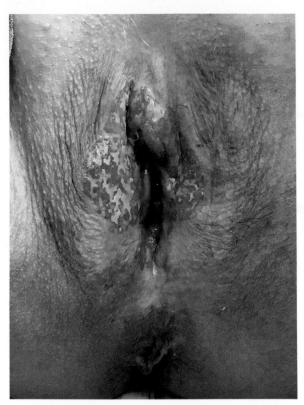

Fig. 20.1 Paget's disease of the vulva.

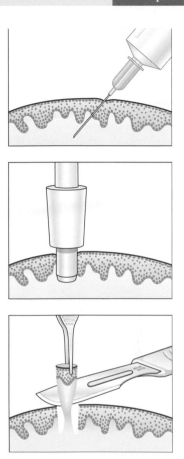

Fig. 20.2 Diagnosis of vulval skin lesions using Keye's punch biopsy under local anaesthetic.

and is considered the precursor of most HPV-negative invasive keratinizing squamous cell carcinomas (SCC). Patients have similar symptoms as with lichen sclerosus. Grey, white, red nodules, plaques or ulcers may be found. It is found in up to 70–80% of adjacent cancer and has a higher malignant potential than usual VIN. It is hence important to exclude malignancy when d-VIN is found.

Unlike VIN, which arises from squamous epithelium, extramammary Paget's disease arises from apocrine glandular epithelium. The appearance of the lesions is variable, but they are papular and raised; may be white, grey, dull red or various shades of brown; and may be localized or widespread (Fig. 20.1). These conditions are rare, with an incidence of 0.53/100,000, and commonly occur in women over the age of 50 years. Paget's disease is associated with underlying adenocarcinoma or primary malignancy elsewhere in 20% of cases, mainly breast and bowel.

Management

It is important to establish the diagnosis by biopsy (Fig. 20.2) and to search for intraepithelial neoplasia in other sites like the cervix and vagina, particularly when usual VIN is found. Treatment of usual VIN includes imiquimod, an immune modifier,

laser therapy and superficial excision of the skin lesion. There is no role for medical treatment in d-VIN, and surgical excision tends to be more radical than that for usual VIN. Recurrence is common, and because there is a risk of malignant progression, especially in d-VIN, long-term follow-up is essential.

Cancers of the vulva

Carcinoma of the vulva accounts for 1–4% of female malignancies: 90% of the lesions are SCCs, 5% are adenocarcinomas, 1% are basal carcinomas and 0.5% are malignant melanomas. Carcinoma of the vulva most commonly occurs in the sixth and seventh decades.

Vulvar cancer has two distinct histological patterns with two different risk factors. The more common basoloid/warty types occur mainly in younger women and are associated with usual VIN and HPV infection, sharing similar risk factors as cervical cancer. The keratinizing types occur in older women and are associated with lichen sclerosus. As noted earlier, there may be foci of d-VIN adjacent to the main tumour.

Symptoms

The patient with vulval carcinoma experiences pruritus and notices a raised lesion on the vulva, which may ulcerate and bleed (Fig. 20.3). Malignant melanomas are usually single, hyperpigmented and ulcerated. Vulval carcinoma most frequently develops on the labia majora (50% of cases) but may also grow on the prepuce of the clitoris, the labia minora, Bartholin's glands and in the vestibule of the vagina.

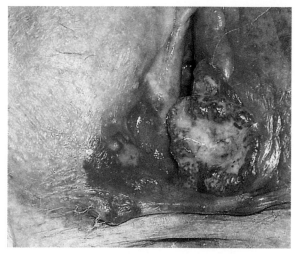

Fig. 20.3 Ulcerative squamous cell carcinoma of the vulva.

Mode of spread

Spread occurs both locally and through the lymphatic system. The lymph nodes involved are the superficial and deep inguinal nodes and the femoral nodes (Fig. 20.4). Pelvic lymph nodes, except in primary lesions involving the clitoris, have usually only secondary involvement. Vascular spread is late and rare. The disease usually progresses slowly, and the terminal stages are accompanied by extensive ulceration, infection, haemorrhage and remote metastatic disease. In some 30% of cases, lymph nodes are involved on both sides. Stages are defined by the International Federation of Obstetrics and Gynaecology (FIGO) on the basis of surgical rather than clinical findings (Table 20.1).

Treatment

Stage IA disease can be treated by wide local excision. Stage IB lesions that are at least 2 cm lateral to the midline are treated by wide local excision and unilateral groin node dissection. All other stages are treated by wide radical local excisions or radical vulvectomy and bilateral groin node dissection. Sentinel node dissection may replace conventional node dissection in centres with experience in the technique. Postoperative radiotherapy has a role in patients where the tumour extends close to the excision margin or there is involvement of the groin

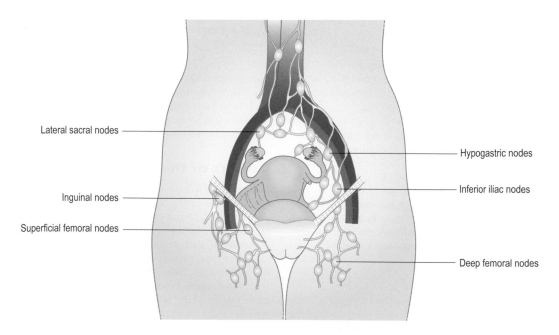

Lateral sacral nodes

Inguinal nodes

Superficial femoral nodes

Hypogastric nodes

Inferior iliac nodes

Deep femoral nodes

Fig. 20.4 Lymphatic drainage of the vulva.

Table 20.1 FIGO staging of vulval cancer (2009)

Stage I	Tumour confined to the vulva: *Stage IA*: Lesions ≤2 cm in size, confined to the vulva or perineum and with stromal invasion ≤1.0 mm*, no nodal metastasis *Stage IB*: Lesions >2 cm in size or with stromal invasion >1.0 mm*, confined to the vulva or perineum, with negative nodes
Stage II	Tumour of any size with extension to adjacent perineal structures (lower third of urethra, lower third of vagina, anus) with negative nodes
Stage III	Tumour of any size with or without extension to adjacent perineal structures (lower third of urethra, lower third of vagina, anus) with positive inguinofemoral lymph nodes: *Stage IIIA*: (i) With 1 lymph node metastasis (≥5 mm) or (ii) 1–2 lymph node metastasis(es) (<5 mm) *Stage IIIB*: (i) With 2 or more lymph node metastases (≥5 mm) or (ii) 3 or more lymph node metastases (<5 mm) *Stage IIIC*: With positive nodes with extracapsular spread
Stage IV	Tumour invades other regional (upper two-thirds of urethra, upper two-thirds of vagina) or distant structures: *Stage IVA:* Tumour invades any of the following: (i) upper urethral and/or vaginal mucosa, bladder mucosa, rectal mucosa or fixed to pelvic bone or (ii) fixed or ulcerated inguinofemoral lymph nodes *Stage IVB:* Any distant metastasis, including pelvic lymph nodes

*The depth of invasion is defined as the measurement of the tumour from the epithelial stromal junction of the adjacent most superficial dermal papilla to the deepest point of invasion.
Reproduced with permission from Pecorelli S & FIGO Committee on Gynecologic Oncology (2009). International Journal of Gynecology & Obstetrics, 105(2):103–104.

nodes. Preoperative radiotherapy, with or without chemotherapy, may be used in cases of extensive disease to reduce the tumour volume. Complications of radical vulvectomy and groin node dissection include wound breakdown, lymphocyst and lymphoedema (30%), secondary bleeding, thromboembolism, sexual dysfunction and psychological morbidity. Response to chemotherapy is generally poor. Patients are followed up at intervals of 3–6 months for 5 years.

Prognosis

Prognosis is determined by the size of the primary lesion and lymph node involvement. The overall survival rate in operable cases without lymph node involvement is 90% and is up to 98% where the primary lesion is less than 2 cm in size. This falls to 50–60% with node involvement and is less than 30% in patients with bilateral lymph node involvement. Malignant melanoma and adenocarcinoma have a poor prognosis, with a 5-year survival of 5%.

Neoplastic lesions of the vaginal epithelium

Vaginal intraepithelial neoplasia

Vaginal intraepithelial neoplasia (VAIN) is usually multicentric and tends to be multifocal and associated with similar lesions of the cervix. A two- instead of three-tiered grading classification comprising low-grade squamous intraepithelial lesion (LSIL) and high-grade squamous intraepithelial lesion (HSIL) replacing that of VAIN I–III was introduced in 2012 in the United States. The condition is asymptomatic and tends to be discovered because of a positive smear test or during colposcopy for abnormal cytology, often after hysterectomy. There is a risk of progression to invasive carcinoma, but the disease remains superficial until then and can be treated by surgical excision, laser ablation or cryosurgery.

Vaginal adenosis

This is the presence of columnar epithelium in the vaginal epithelium and has been found in adult females whose mothers received treatment with diethylstilboestrol during pregnancy. The condition commonly reverts to normal squamous epithelium, but in about 4% of cases the lesion progresses to vaginal adenocarcinoma. It is therefore important to follow these women carefully with serial cytology.

Vaginal malignancy

Invasive carcinoma of the vagina may be a squamous carcinoma or, occasionally, an adenocarcinoma. Primary lesions arise in the sixth and seventh decades but are rare in the UK. The incidence of adenocarcinoma, typically clear cell, associated with in utero exposure of diethylstilboestrol has declined since this drug was withdrawn from use in pregnancy.

Table 20.2 Clinical staging of vaginal carcinoma	
Stage 0	Intraepithelial carcinoma
Stage I	Limited to the vaginal walls
Stage II	Involves the subvaginal tissue but has not extended to the pelvic wall
Stage III	The tumour has extended to the lateral pelvic wall
Stage IV	The lesion has extended to involve adjacent organs (IVA) or has spread to distant organs (IVB)

Secondary deposits from cervical carcinoma and endometrial carcinoma are relatively common in the upper third of the vagina and can sometimes occur in the lower vagina through lymphatic spread.

Symptoms

The symptoms include irregular vaginal bleeding and offensive vaginal discharge when the tumour becomes necrotic and infection supervenes. Local spread into the rectum, bladder or urethra may result in fistula formation. The tumour may appear as an exophytic lesion or as an ulcerated, indurated mass.

Method of spread

Tumour spread, as previously stated, occurs by direct infiltration or by lymphatic extension. Lesions involving the upper half of the vagina follow a pattern of spread similar to that of carcinoma of the cervix. Tumours of the lower half of the vagina follow a similar pattern of spread to that of carcinoma of the vulva.

Treatment

The diagnosis is established by biopsy of the tumour. Staging is made before commencing treatment (Table 20.2).

The primary method of treatment is by radiotherapy – both by external beam therapy and brachytherapy.

Surgical treatment can also be considered in selected patients. For example, radical hysterectomy or vaginectomy and pelvic lymph node dissection can be considered in patients with stage I disease in the upper vagina, radical vulvectomy may be needed in stage I disease in the lower vagina and pelvic exenteration may be considered in patients with localized invasion to the bladder or rectum without parametrial or lymph node metastasis.

Prognosis

Results of treatment depend on the initial staging and on the method of therapy. Stages I and II have a 5 year survival of around 60% but this figure falls to 30–40% for stages III and IV. Adenocarcinoma of the vagina, which often occurs in young females, also responds well to irradiation.

Lesions of the cervix

Cervical cancer

Cervical cancer is the fourth most common female cancer worldwide. Incidence varies across the world. In many low-resource countries, this is the most common cause of death from cancer in women. In the UK, cervical cancer is the fourteenth most common, with about 3200 new cases per year, with the highest incidence rates in the 25–29 age group between 2013 and 2015. Cervical cancer has several histological types, of which SCC accounts for about 70–80%, while adenocarcinoma accounts for about 10–25%. Other subtypes, such as adenosquamous, neuroendocrine and undifferentiated carcinomas, are uncommon. The most important risk factor for cervical cancer is persistent HPV infection. Factors leading to higher risk for persistent HPV infection are risk factors for cervical cancer, e.g. early age of first intercourse, number of partners, smoking, low socio-economic status and immunosuppression.

HPV infection and cervical cancer

Almost all cases of cervical cancer (over 99%) are caused by high-risk HPV infection. There are more than 100 subtypes of HPV infection. HPV infection can infect genital and non-genital sites. The subtypes are classified as high risk or low risk. High-risk subtypes are associated with cancer, while the low-risk types cause warts. Amongst the 14 high-risk subtypes, HPV 16 and 18 cause about 70% of cervical cancer. HPV infection is mainly transmitted via close skin-to-skin contact, such as genital-to-genital contact and anal, vaginal and oral sex. It is a very common infection, where the majority of sexually active women would have been infected sometime during their lifetime. However, most infections are transient and are cleared by the body's natural immunity. Only persistent infections lead to cancer. Apart from cervical cancer, HPV infection also causes other cancers such as vulval, vaginal, anal and oropharyngeal cancers.

Pathophysiology

The squamocolumnar junction (SCJ) is the junction between the squamous epithelium of the ectocervix and the columnar epithelium in the endocervix. The SCJ moves in relation to the anatomical external cervical os. Changes in oestrogen during puberty, pregnancy or while on the combined oral contraceptive pill move the SCJ outwards, exposing columnar epithelium to the lower pH of the vagina. This reacts by undergoing transformation back to squamous epithelium by a process of squamous metaplasia. The area that lies between the current SCJ and that is reached as it moves outwards across the ectocervix is the *transformation zone*, and it is here that most preinvasive lesions occur.

Cervical cancer prevention

The natural history of cervical cancer is now well understood. HPV infects the cervical epithelium. Persistent HPV infection leads to premalignant changes in the cervical epithelium, known as *cervical intraepithelial neoplasia (CIN)*. CIN describes the changes in the squamous epithelium characterized by varying degrees of loss of differentiation and stratification and nuclear atypia (Fig. 20.5). It may extend below the surface of the cervix but does not extend beyond the basement membrane. In the UK, CIN is graded as mild (CIN-1), moderate (CIN-2) or severe (CIN-3), depending on the proportion of the epithelium replaced by abnormal cells. Twenty-five per cent of CIN-1 will progress to higher-grade lesions over 2 years, and 30–40% of CIN-3 to carcinoma over 20 years. Around 40% of low-grade

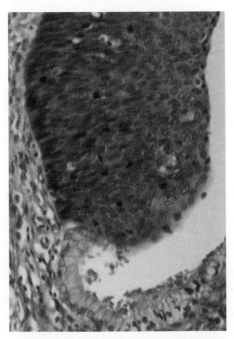

Fig. 20.5 Histological appearance of CIN-3.

lesions (CIN-1) will regress to normal within 6 months without treatment, especially in the younger age group. Similar to VAIN, a two-tier instead of three-tier grading of LSIL and HSIL, replacing that of CIN 1–3, is used in Australia and New Zealand. The process of progression from low-grade to high-grade lesions can be over 3–10 years. Since the progression from low-grade lesions to invasive cancer can take 10–20 years, this gives us a window of opportunity to screen and treat the premalignant lesions, thus preventing the development of invasive cancers.

Primary prevention – HPV vaccination

Since we now know that the main cause for cervical cancer is HPV infection, preventing HPV infections would be the best primary preventive measure. Prophylactic HPV vaccines have been developed. Bivalent and quadrivalent vaccines have been in the market for about a decade. The bivalent vaccine targets the two high-risk subtypes, HPV 16 and 18, while the quadrivalent vaccine covers HPV 16 and 18 as well as two low-risk subtypes, HPV 6 and 11, which cause genital warts. The prevention of HPV 16 and 18 infections could theoretically prevent more than 70% of cervical cancer cases, and indeed evidence from Australia after a decade of use has shown a 77% reduction in high-risk HPV serotypes in women aged 18–24 and 30–50% reaction in HSIL with a 90% reduction in genital warts. These vaccines are most effective when given before any exposure to the virus, i.e. before sexual debut. Vaccination using the quadrivalent vaccine was introduced for girls in Australia in 2007. In the UK, a national vaccination programme against HPV 16 and 18 infections was introduced in 2008. Since 2012, girls aged 12–13 years have been routinely offered the quadrivalent vaccine, with the first HPV vaccination given when they are in school year 8, and the second dose is offered 6–12 months after the first. In some other countries, e.g. Australia, the vaccination programme has extended to boys. Although boys do not get cervical cancer, they benefit from protection from other HPV-related cancers and genital warts, and their vaccination helps reduce the risk of transmission to their future partners by increasing her immunity to the virus. The HPV vaccine has been shown to offer protection for at least 10 years, and it is likely that the protection will be lifelong. Recently, a new nanovalent vaccine has been introduced. In addition to HPV 16 and 18, the nine-valent vaccine protects against five other oncogenic types (31, 33, 45, 52, 58) which, together with 16 and 18, account for nearly 90% of cervical cancers.

Secondary prevention – screening for premalignant lesions

The aim of cervical screening programmes is to detect the non-invasive precursor of cervical cancer, CIN, in the

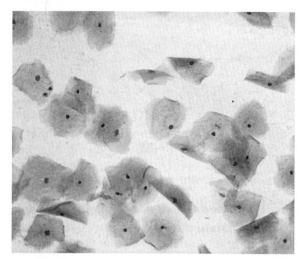

Fig. 20.6 Normal cervical smear showing superficial (pink) and intermediate (blue/green) exfoliated cervical cells (low-power magnification).

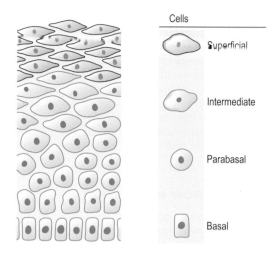

Fig. 20.7 Cell layers in the stratified squamous epithelium of the cervix and vagina.

asymptomatic population in order to reduce mortality and morbidity. The National Health Service (NHS) national cervical screening programme was introduced in England and Wales in 1988, and by 1991, 80% of all women between the ages of 20 and 65 were being tested on a 5-yearly basis. Since then mortality from cervical cancer has fallen by 7% a year. Currently all women aged between 25 and 49 are invited for screening every 3 years, and those between 50 and 64 are invited every 5 years. Conventionally, cervical cytology is taken from the cervix. This is often referred to as a *cervical smear* or a *Pap smear*, named after the inventor of the test, Georgios Papanicolaou. Conventional smears involve taking cells from the cervix on the whole of the transformation zone with a 360-degree sweep using an Ayres or Aylesbury spatula and smeared onto a glass slide. In recent years, liquid-based cytology (LBC) has largely replaced the conventional smears. For LBC, the cells from the transformation zone are taken with a plastic cervical brush. The brush is rotated in the same direction for five turns and transferred into a container of transport medium (see Chapter 15). LBC allows automated processing of the smears, and it reduces the rate of unsatisfactory smears. The sample can also be used for additional tests such as HPV testing. Cervical cytology (Figs 20.6 and 20.7) is primarily for screening for squamous lesions and cannot reliably exclude endocervical disease. In 2017 screening in Australia was changed to an HPV-based test collected in the same way as the Pap smear support by LBC only in women identified as being positive for one of a number of high-risk HPV serotypes. As in the UK screening begins at age 25; if negative, it is repeated at 5-year intervals until age 75.

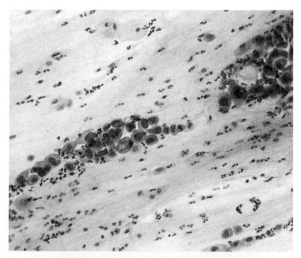

Fig. 20.8 Moderate dyskaryosis. The cells are smaller and the nuclear:cytoplasmic ratio is higher when compared with normal cells.

Classification of cervical cytology

The terminology used in the UK for reporting cervical smears was introduced by the British Society for Clinical Cytology in 1986 and updated in 2013. The term *dyskaryosis* is used to describe those cells that lie between normal squamous and frankly malignant cells and exhibit degrees of nuclear changes before malignancy (Fig. 20.8). Cells showing abnormalities that fall short of dyskaryosis are described as borderline. Atypical glandular cells may represent premalignant disease of the endocervix or endometrium.

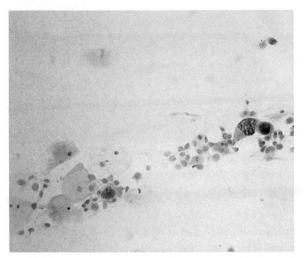

Fig. 20.9 Carcinoma cells. Note the large nuclei and abnormal distribution of chromatin.

Malignant cells show nuclear enlargement at the expense of cytoplasmic mass (Fig. 20.9). The nuclei may assume a lobulated outline. There is increased intensity of staining of the nucleus and an increase in the number of mitotic figures.

The Bethesda system of classification used in the United States (Table 20.3) differs by combining moderate and severe dyskaryosis as HSIL and using the term *atypical squamous cells of undetermined significance (ASCUS)* instead of borderline. In the current edition of the classification system, the emphasis is to try and separate out borderline cases that may potentially be a high-grade lesion. This group of borderline lesions is called *atypical squamous cells, cannot exclude high-grade intraepithelial lesion (ASC-H)*. A modified version of this classification is used in Australia and New Zealand with HSIL and LSIL, but the terms *possible low-grade squamous intraepithelial lesions (PLSIL)* and *possible high-grade squamous intraepithelial lesions (PHSIL)* are being used instead of ASCUS and ASC-H, respectively.

HPV testing

High-risk HPV testing has a sensitivity of about 90% for high-grade CIN, which is 25% more sensitive than cytology. One of the most commonly used HPV tests is the Hybrid Capture II (HCII) test, which tests for a pool of 13 high-risk HPV subtypes. Some HPV tests can not only test for the presence of any high-risk HPV subtypes (similar to the HC II) but also give individual results for HPV 16 and 18, which carry a particularly high risk for a high-grade lesion. HPV testing in conjunction with cervical cytology (co-test) or as a stand-alone test as a primary screening method has been evaluated. Co-testing is recommended

Table 20.3 Classification of cervical smears

UK system (2013)	U.S. Bethesda system (2014)
Negative	Negative for intraepithelial lesion
Borderline change in squamous cells	Atypical squamous cells of undetermined significance (ASC-US), ASC-H (cannot exclude HSIL)
Borderline change in endocervical cells	Atypical endocervical, endo-metrial or glandular (NOS or specify in comments) Atypical endocervical, endome-trial or glandular cells, favour neoplastic
Low-grade dyskaryosis	Low-grade SIL
High-grade dykaryosis (moderate)	High-grade SIL
High-grade dyskaryosis (severe)	High-grade SIL
High-grade dyskaryosis ? invasive squamous cell carcinoma	Squamous cell carcinoma
? Glandular neoplasia of endocervical type ? Glandular neoplasia (non-cervical)	Endocervical carcinoma in situ Adenocarcinoma – endocervi-cal, endometrial extrauterine, NOS

ASC-H, Atypical squamous cells (high-grade); *ASCUS*, atypical squamous cells of undetermined significance; *NOS*, not otherwise specified; *SIL*, squamous intraepithelial lesion.

in the United States for women over the age of 30, while HPV testing alone is recommended for women over age 25. High-risk HPV testing also has a very high negative predictive value, which allows a longer screening interval for women with a negative test, and it may be a more appropriate primary screening test for vaccinated women. However, high-risk HPV tests have lower specificity, since not all HPV infection would cause premalignant changes. Without a good triage system for high-risk HPV-positive results, more women would need to be referred for colposcopy (see later section) and result in more unnecessary interventions. Therefore, some areas in the UK have adopted the HPV test as the primary cervical screening method, and this would be gradually introduced across the country. Women testing positive for high-risk HPV would have cytology triage (i.e. have an LBC done). If the woman has a positive high-risk–positive test and an abnormal cytology result (borderline or worse), she would be referred for colposcopy. In Australia,

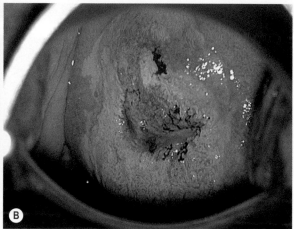

Fig. 20.10 Colposcopic appearance of a high-grade lesion before (A) and after (B) application of acetic acid. Note acetowhite appearance after the application of acetic acid.

the primary HPV test with genotyping for 16 and 18 has replaced cytology in its cervical screening programme (see earlier section).

Management of abnormal screening results

Abnormal cytology and positive HPV tests are screening tests. To get a diagnosis, a biopsy of the abnormal area is needed. A colposcopic examination helps identify the abnormal areas. Colposcopy is examination of the cervix and lower genital tract with a low-power binocular microscope with a light source (a colposcope). It is an outpatient procedure performed using a speculum to expose the cervix. Detailed protocols for referral to colposcopy after an abnormal screening test vary in different countries. In general, if a screening test is suggestive of a high possibility of a significant lesion, the patient should be referred to colposcopy for a biopsy. In the UK, women with high-grade dyskaryosis (moderate or severe) or suspicions for invasive carcinoma in her cytology should be referred for colposcopy. Women with borderline changes or low-grade dyskaryosis would have a reflex high-risk HPV test done. If high-risk HPV positive, they should be referred to colposcopy; if negative, they would return to routine recall. For women who undergo HPV testing instead of cervical smear as their primary screening methods, referral criteria would be more complicated. As many high-risk HPV infections would regress spontaneously and would not cause any premalignant changes, referring all high-risk HPV results would lead to many unnecessary colposcopies. Therefore a second test to triage those who are really at risk of a high-grade lesion is needed. This triage test can be a cytology test or can be genotyping for HPV 16 and 18, which are

particularly associated with high-grade lesions. For example, in Australia the woman would be referred for colposcopy if she is high-risk HPV positive and her cervical smear shows HSIL or she tests positive specifically for HPV 16 or 18, regardless of the results of the cytology

Principles of colposcopy

At colposcopy, the colposcopist adds acetic acid, followed by Lugol's iodine, to identify the most abnormal areas to take biopsies. Neoplastic cells have an increased amount of nuclear material in relation to cytoplasm and less surface glycogen than normal squamous epithelium. They are associated with a degree of hypertrophy of the underlying vasculature. When exposed to 5% acetic acid, the nuclear protein will coagulate, giving the neoplastic cells a characteristic white appearance (Fig. 20.10). Small blood vessels beneath the epithelium may be seen as dots (punctation) or a crazy paving pattern (mosaicism) due to the increased capillary vasculature. The neoplastic cells do not react with Lugol's iodine (Schiller's test), unlike the normal squamous epithelium that will stain dark brown (Fig. 20.11). Early invasive cancer is characterized by a raised or ulcerated area with abnormal vessels, friable tissue and coarse punctation with marked mosaicism. It feels hard on palpation and often bleeds on contact. In more advanced disease, the cervix becomes fixed or replaced by a friable warty-looking mass (Fig. 20.12).

Treatment of high-grade preinvasive lesions

If the colposcopic-directed biopsy shows a low-grade lesion, only regular surveillance would be required in most cases. However, if the biopsy shows a high-grade lesion, treatment

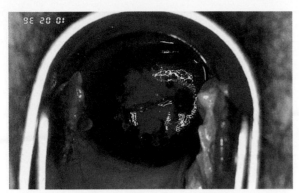

Fig. 20.11 Colposcopic appearances of CIN-2. The abnormal epithelium fails to stain with iodine.

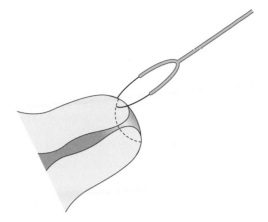

Fig. 20.13 Large loop excision of the cervix.

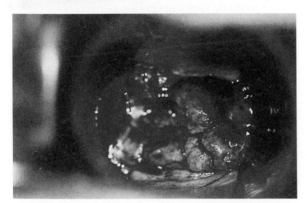

Fig. 20.12 Colposcopic appearance of invasive carcinoma of the cervix.

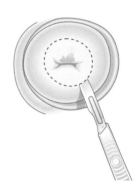

Fig. 20.14 Cone biopsy of the cervix.

by excision or destruction of the affected area (usually the whole of the transformation zone) is required.

Destructive/ablative methods such as laser ablation, cryocautery and coagulation diathermy are only suitable when the entire transformation zone can be visualized, there is no evidence of glandular abnormality or invasive disease and there is no major discrepancy between the cytology and histology results. Excision instead of ablation is the preferred treatment because the excised specimen can be sent for a histological diagnosis to confirm the biopsy result. The commonest excisional method is the large loop excision of the transformation zone (LLETZ) (Fig. 20.13), which is excision with a diathermy wire loop, which can be done under local anaesthetic in the outpatient clinic. When the SCJ cannot be seen or a lesion of the glandular epithelium is suspected, a deeper 'cone' biopsy is required to ensure that all of the endocervix is sampled (Fig. 20.14). About 5% of women will have persistent or recurrent disease following treatment; therefore, follow-up is important. Follow-up protocols vary in different countries. For example, in the UK, women are usually invited to return for repeat cytology ± HPV test as a test of cure 6 months later. If both cytology and high-risk HPV are negative, the woman can return in 3 years. If high-risk HPV is positive, she will need to have colposcopy again. If HPV is not available, then she needs to have repeat cytology.

Cervical cancer

Pathology

There are two types of invasive carcinoma of the cervix. Approximately 70–80% of lesions are SCC and 20–30% adenocarcinomas. Histologically, the degree of invasion determines the stage of the disease (Table 20.4).

The spread of tumour

Cervical carcinoma spreads by direct local invasion and via the lymphatics and blood vessels. Lymphatic spread occurs in approximately 0.5% of women with stage IA1 disease, rising to 5% for stage IA2 and 40% of women with stage II disease. Preferential spread occurs to the external iliac,

Table 20.4 FIGO classification of cervical cancer (2009)

Stage I	Carcinoma is strictly confined to the cervix (extension to the corpus would be disregarded): *Stage IA*: Invasive carcinoma that can be diagnosed only by microscopy, with deepest invasion ≤5 mm and largest extension ≤7 mm *Stage IA1*: Measured stromal invasion of ≤3.0 mm in depth and extension of ≤7.0 mm *Stage IA2*: Measured stromal invasion of >3.0 mm and not >5.0 mm with an extension of not >7.0 mm *Stage IB*: Clinically visible lesions limited to the cervix uteri or preclinical cancers greater than IA* *Stage IB1*: Clinically visible lesion ≤4.0 cm in greatest dimension *Stage IB2*: Clinically visible lesion >4.0 cm in greatest dimension
Stage II	Cervical carcinoma invades beyond the uterus but not to the pelvic wall or to the lower third of the vagina: *Stage IIA*: Without parametrial invasion *Stage IIA1*: Clinically visible lesion ≤4.0 cm in greatest dimension *Stage IIA2*: Clinically visible lesion >4.0 cm in greatest dimension *Stage IIB*: With obvious parametrial invasion
Stage III	The tumour extends to the pelvic wall and/or involves lower third of the vagina and/or causes hydronephrosis or non-functioning kidney:** *Stage IIIA*: Tumour involves lower third of the vagina with no extension to the pelvic wall *Stage IIIB*: Extension to pelvic wall and/or hydronephrosis or non-functioning kidney
Stage IV	The carcinoma has extended beyond the true pelvis or has involved (biopsy proven) the mucosa of the bladder or rectum. A bullous oedema, as such, does not permit a case to be allotted to stage IV: *Stage IVA*: Spread of the growth to adjacent organs *Stage IVB*: Spread to distant organs

Reproduced with permission from Pecorelli S & FIGO Committee on Gynecologic Oncology (2009). International Journal of Gynecology & Obstetrics, 105(2):103–104.

*All macroscopically visible lesions – even with superficial invasion – are allotted to stage IB carcinomas. Invasion is limited to a measured stromal invasion with a maximal depth of 5.0 mm and a horizontal extension of not >7.0 mm. Depth of invasion should not be >5.0 mm taken from the base of the epithelium of the original tissue – squamous or glandular. The depth of invasion should always be reported in millimetres, even in those cases with 'early (minimal) stromal invasion' (≈1 mm). The involvement of vascular/lymphatic spaces should not change the stage allotment.

**On rectal examination, there is no cancer-free space between the tumour and the pelvic wall. All cases with hydronephrosis or non-functioning kidney are included, unless they are known to be due to another cause.

internal iliac and obturator nodes. Secondary spread may also occur to inguinal, sacral and aortic nodes. Blood-borne metastases occur in the lungs, liver, bone and bowel.

Clinical features

Stage IA disease is usually asymptomatic at the time of presentation and is detected at the time of routine cervical cytology. The common presenting symptoms from invasive carcinoma of the cervix include postcoital bleeding, foul-smelling discharge which is thin and watery and sometimes blood-stained, and irregular vaginal bleeding when the tumour becomes necrotic. Lateral invasion into the parametrium may involve the ureters, leading eventually to ureteric obstruction and renal failure. Invasion of nerves and bone causes excruciating and persistent pain, and involvement of lymphatic channels may result in lymphatic occlusion with intractable oedema of the lower limbs.

The tumour may also spread anteriorly or posteriorly to involve the bladder or rectum, respectively. Involvement of

the bladder produces symptoms of frequency, dysuria and haematuria; if the bowel is involved, tenesmus, diarrhoea and rectal bleeding may occur. The neoplasm may initially grow within the endocervix, producing a cylindrical, barrel-shaped enlargement of the cervix with little external manifestation of the tumour.

The exophytic tumour grows over the vaginal portion of the cervix and appears as a cauliflower-like tumour. The tumour eventually sloughs and replaces the normal cervical tissue and extends on to the vaginal walls.

Investigation

The diagnosis is established histologically by biopsy of the tumour, which should be greater than 5 mm in depth to distinguish between microinvasive and invasive disease. Diagnostic LLETZ may be necessary. Examination under anaesthesia in tense patients by vaginal and rectal examination, with or without cystoscopy is generally recommended except in stage IA1 disease. Magnetic resonance imaging

(MRI) of the abdomen and pelvis is performed for assessment of the parametrium and lymph node status. Computed tomography (CT) of the thorax may also be needed if lung metastasis is suspected. Positron emission tomography (PET)-CT may be considered in advanced disease to assess for distant spread.

Treatment of invasive carcinoma

Treatment is by surgery or radiotherapy/chemoradiation or a combination of both methods.

Local excision by cone biopsy is an option for patients with stage IA lesions who wish to preserve fertility. Simple hysterectomy suffices for stage IA1 disease for those who have completed family.

Extended hysterectomy or radiotherapy can be used to treat stage IB–IIA. The cure rate is similar for both surgery and radiotherapy, but the former is generally associated with less long-term morbidity from vaginal stenosis. Surgery can also preserve ovarian function for those premenopausal women. Stage II–IV disease is usually treated with chemoradiation with weekly platinum-based chemotherapy and intracavity and external beam radiotherapy.

Surgery – radical hysterectomy and pelvic lymph node dissection

Radical hysterectomy (Fig. 20.15) includes removal of the uterus, parametrium and upper third of the vagina. The ovaries may be conserved. This method of treatment, together with internal and external iliac and obturator lymph node dissection, is appropriate for patients with stage IB1 and early-stage IIA1 diseases. Complications include haemorrhage, infection, pelvic haematomas, lymphocyst/lymphoedema, bladder dysfunction and damage to the ureters or bladder, which may result in fistula formation in 2–5% of cases. However, the incidence of vaginal stenosis is less than after radiotherapy, and so coital function is better preserved, making it the treatment of choice in the younger woman. Radical trachelectomy with pelvic lymph node dissection and prophylactic cervical cerclage can be considered in small-stage IB1 tumour (less than 2 cm) if preservation of fertility is desired.

Radiotherapy/chemoradiation

This is to treat other stages of cervical cancer and those patients with bulky stage IB disease or who are unfit for surgery. Survival stage-for-stage in early forms of the disease is similar to that for surgery. Adjuvant chemoradiotherapy is also used for those patients who have been found to have lymph node involvement at the time of surgery.

Chemotherapy is platinum based and given weekly in conjunction with radiotherapy.

Radiotherapy is administered by local insertion of a source of radium, cesium-137 and iridium-192 into the uterine cavity and the vaginal vault and by external beam radiation to the pelvic side wall. Complications include the effects of excessive radiation on normal tissues and may lead to radiation cystitis or proctitis, as well as fistula formation and vaginal stenosis.

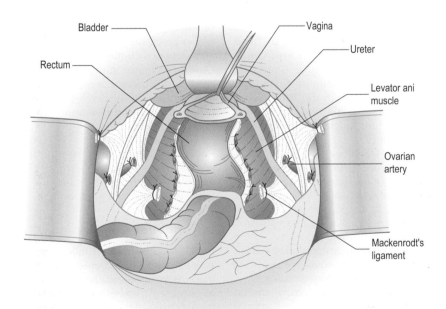

Fig. 20.15 Radical hysterectomy involves excision of the uterus, parametrium and upper third of the vagina.

Prognosis

This depends mainly on the stage at diagnosis and lymph node status. The results for 5-year survival are:
- stage I: 85%
- stage II: 60%
- stage III: 30%
- stage IV: 10%.

Recurrent cervical lesions occur in a third of cases and have a poor prognosis.

Where local recurrence involves the bladder or rectum but does not extend to other structures, curative excision may occasionally be achieved by radical excision or exenteration, including total cystectomy and removal of the rectum.

Malignant disease of the uterus

Endometrial carcinoma

In developed countries, endometrial adenocarcinoma is one of the commonest female cancers. In the UK, it is the fourth most common female cancer, accounting for 5% of all female cancers (2015). Over the last decade, the incidence has increased by 21%. It mainly affects postmenopausal women. The incidence peaks in women aged 65–69.

Specific factors are associated with an increased risk of corpus carcinoma, such as nulliparity, late menopause, diabetes and hypertension. It can also be hereditary. Women with hereditary non-polyposis colorectal cancer (HNPCC) syndrome have increased risk of endometrial and ovarian cancers, as well as colorectal cancer. However, the most important risk factors are associated with a hyperoestrogenic state:
- **Obesity:** The ovarian stroma continues to produce androgens after menopause, which are converted to oestrone in adipose tissue. This acts as unopposed oestrogen on the endometrium, resulting in endometrial hyperplasia and malignancy.
- **Exogenous oestrogens:** Unopposed oestrogen action, e.g. having oestrogen alone without progestogen for hormonal replacement, is associated with an increased incidence of endometrial carcinoma. The addition of a progestogen for at least 10 days of each month can reduce this risk, and the combined oral contraceptive pill reduces the incidence of the disease.
- **Endogenous oestrogens:** Oestrogen-producing ovarian tumours, such as granulosa cell tumours, are associated with an increase in the risk of endometrial cancer.
- **Tamoxifen in breast cancer:** Breast cancer patients on tamoxifen have a slightly increased risk of endometrial cancer, but most of these are detected in early stages and have good prognosis.
- **Endometrial hyperplasia:** Prolonged stimulation of the endometrium with unopposed oestrogen may lead to hyperplasia of the endometrium with periods of amenorrhoea followed by heavy or irregular bleeding. Endometrial hyperplasia can be classified into those with or without atypia. Women with atypical hyperplasia have an up to 50% chance of concurrent carcinoma and 30% chance of future progression to carcinoma. These women are usually treated by hysterectomy and bilateral salpingo-oophorectomy (BSO). The risk of carcinoma in those with hyperplasia without atypia is much lower (<5%). The majority of these women can be treated conservatively by progestogen therapy.

Symptoms

The commonest symptom is postmenopausal bleeding. However, in the premenopausal woman, endometrial carcinoma is associated with irregular vaginal bleeding and increasingly heavy menses. Endometrial cancer should also be suspected in elderly patients with pyometra. These women usually present with purulent vaginal discharge.

Pathology

Endometrial carcinoma can be divided into two types. Type I refers to endometrioid adenocarcinoma. This type is related to the hyperoestrogenic state and hence all the risk factors associated with hyperoestrogenism, such as obesity, diabetes, unopposed oestrogen, etc. Type II represents other histological types, such as serous papillary and clear cell subtypes. These tend to be aggressive tumours with poorer prognosis. Work is underway to better classify them according to their molecular profiles.

Most endometrial cancer is endometrioid (type I) cancer. The microscopic appearances include changes in the architecture with the development of closely packed polyhedral cells with dark-staining nuclei and considerable numbers of mitoses.

Endometrial cancer grows locally (Fig. 20.16). The tumour spreads by direct invasion into the myometrium and then transcervically, transtubally and by spillage of carcinomatous material. There can also be lymphatic spread to the pelvic and para-aortic nodes

Investigations

Initial investigations include a transvaginal ultrasound scan to assess the endometrial thickness and an endometrial aspirate to obtain endometrial tissue for histological assessment. An endometrial thickness of less than 5 mm on transvaginal ultrasound in a postmenopausal woman indicates a very low risk of endometrial cancer. However, using endometrial thickness is less reliable in premenopausal or

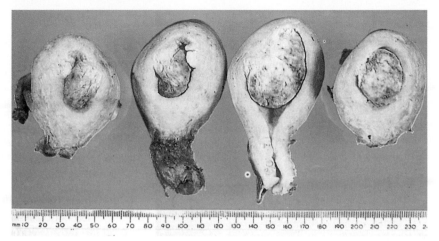

Fig. 20.16 Endometrial adenocarcinoma. Multiple sections showing a large endometrial carcinoma invading the substance of the myometrium.

perimenopausal women because the endometrial thickness varies with the menstrual cycle. In women over 40 years old who have abnormal vaginal bleeding, an endometrial aspirate should be the first-line investigation to assess the endometrium. Endometrial aspirate can be done with various endometrial samplers such as the Pipelle sampler. The Pipelle is a transparent plastic cannula with a very small diameter, e.g. 3 mm, that can be passed through the cervical os without dilation and can be done in the office without anaesthesia. However, if the endometrial aspirate is unsuccessful or inconclusive or symptoms persist despite a negative endometrial aspirate result, a diagnostic hysteroscopy and biopsy are required. These can be carried out as outpatient procedures or under general anaesthesia. During a diagnostic hysteroscopy, a hysteroscope, which is a narrow, rigid telescope, is passed through the cervical os and the uterine cavity is distended by either gas or fluid. This allows direct visualization of the uterine cavity, and directed biopsies of any endometrial lesions can be taken. The risk of this procedure is small, but complications can occur, such as uterine perforation, cervical laceration, pelvic infection and reaction to distension media. The diagnosis of endometrial cancer is established histologically by the endometrial biopsy result.

Treatment

The mainstay of treatment is total hysterectomy and BSO. The value of routine pelvic and para-aortic lymphadenectomy for all patients is controversial. Preoperative investigations include full blood count, renal and liver function test and a chest X-ray, as well as any additional investigations depending on individual health status such as electrocardiogram (ECG), blood sugar levels, etc.

Cancer (or carbohydrate) antigen 125 (CA-125) may be raised in advanced disease, and a preoperative baseline value can be useful for subsequent disease monitoring. Risk factors for extrauterine disease include high-grade lesions, unfavourable histological subtypes (e.g. serous or clear cell histology), tumour size and depth of myometrial invasion. The grading and histological subtypes can be assessed by endometrial biopsy. The tumour size and myometrial invasion can be assessed by preoperative imaging such as ultrasound, CT or MRI. Currently, MRI is the most widely used technique. It helps to assess myometrial invasion, cervical invasion and lymph node involvement. Nonetheless, MRI has limited accuracy and may not be cost-effective for all patients. Total hysterectomy can be done by open laparotomy, laparoscopically or vaginally. Patients should be individually assessed to determine the best route.

Adjuvant radiotherapy is often given to patients with high risk of recurrence. Vaginal brachytherapy can reduce local vault recurrence. External beam pelvic irradiation can be given to those with risk of pelvic recurrence. Chemotherapy should be considered for patients with high risk of distal recurrence. Patients with advanced disease are treated by debulking the tumour followed by chemotherapy with or without radiotherapy.

Prognosis

Endometrial cancer is surgically staged (Table 20.5). Prognosis largely depends on the stage of the disease as well as other prognostic factors that include age, histological subtype and grading. For stage I grade I, the 5-year survival can be over 90% for those with superficial myometrial invasion, but for those with deep myometrial

Table 20.5 FIGO staging for endometrial cancer (2009)

Stage I*	Tumour confined to the corpus uteri: *Stage IA*: No or less than half myometrial invasion *Stage IB*: Invasion equal to or more than half of the myometrium
Stage II*	Tumour invades cervical stroma but does not extend beyond the uterus**
Stage III*	Local and/or regional spread of the tumour: *Stage IIIA*: Tumour invades the serosa of the corpus uteri and/or adnexae# *Stage IIIB*: Vaginal and/or parametrial involvement# *Stage IIIC*: Metastases to pelvic and/or para-aortic lymph nodes# *Stage IIIC1*: Positive pelvic nodes *Stage IIIC2*: Positive para-aortic lymph nodes with or without positive pelvic lymph nodes
Stage IV*	Tumour invades bladder and/or bowel mucosa, and/or distant metastases: *Stage IVA*: Tumour invasion of bladder and/or bowel mucosa *Stage IVB*: Distant metastases, including intra-abdominal metastases and/or inguinal lymph nodes

*Either G1, G2 or G3.
**Endocervical glandular involvement only should be considered stage I and no longer stage II.
#Positive cytology has to be reported separately without changing the stage.
Reproduced with permission from Pecorelli S & FIGO Committee on Gynecologic Oncology (2009). International Journal of Gynecology & Obstetrics, 105(2):103–104.

invasion and grade III disease, the 5-year survival is only about 60% even if the disease is still confined to the uterus. For stage II, III and IV diseases, the 5-year survival is about 70–80%, 40–50% and 20%, respectively. Serous papillary and clear cell carcinomas have poorer prognosis, with 5-year survival rates of 50% and 35%, respectively.

Malignant mesenchymal tumours of the uterus

Non-epithelial tumours account for only 3% of uterine malignancies. In general, they arise from either myometrial smooth muscle (leiomyosarcomas) or stroma of the endometrium (stromal sarcomas). Mixed müllerian duct or carcinosarcomas contain malignant elements from both the endometrial epithelium and stroma and are considered variants of endometrial cancer.

Endometrial stromal sarcomas

These tumours, arising from the stroma of the endometrium, account for less than 10% of uterine sarcomas and about 1% of all uterine malignant tumours. They are classified as endometrial stromal nodule (ESN), low-grade endometrial stromal sarcoma (LGESS), high-grade ESS (HGESS) or undifferentiated uterine sarcoma (UUS). ESN is benign, while the others are malignant. HGESS is more aggressive and is associated with more recurrences and higher mortality than LGESS, and UUS has the worst prognosis. They tend to present in a younger age group (45–50 years) than other uterine tumours with vaginal discharge and bleeding. Endometrial stromal sarcoma is found in association with adenomyosis and endometriosis. The standard treatment is by total hysterectomy and BSO. Retention of the ovaries in young women with stage 1 disease may be an option. LGESS is usually positive for oestrogen and progesterone receptors, and hormonal treatment, such as progestins and aromatase inhibitors, is commonly given for advanced disease. HGESS and UUS have a high risk of recurrence. Chemotherapy is often given, although it is not clear if any form of adjuvant treatment would improve survival.

Leiomyosarcoma

These smooth muscle tumours arise in the myometrium of the uterus and account for only 1.3% of uterine malignancies. They are uncommon (0.7/100,000), with a peak incidence at the age of 52 years, about 10 years later than the peak incidence for fibroids. Between 5% and 10% arise in existing fibroids, although the risk of malignant change occurring in a fibroid is small (0.3–0.8%). Leiomyosarcomas are classified according to the degree of differentiation. They may present with pain, postmenopausal bleeding or a rapidly growing 'fibroid' but are often asymptomatic and diagnosed following hysterectomy for fibroids. Treatment is by hysterectomy. Adjuvant radiotherapy and/or chemotherapy are sometimes considered to reduce the risk of recurrence, but their role in improving survival is unknown.

Carcinosarcoma

These tumours (Fig. 20.17) consist of both epithelial and mesenchymal elements. The epithelial elements are usually endometrioid but can be squamous or a mixture. The stromal elements are either heterologous (chondroblastoma, osteosarcoma, fibrosarcoma) or homologous (leiomyosarcoma, presarcoma). They are managed in a similar way to that of a high-grade endometrial cancer. The mean age at presentation is 65 years. An enlarged, irregular uterus with tumour protruding through the cervical os is a common finding at examination. Extrauterine spread occurs early, and only 25% of patients have disease limited to the endometrium at the time of diagnosis.

Lesions of the ovary

Ovarian enlargement is commonly asymptomatic, and the silent nature of malignant ovarian tumours is the major reason for the advanced stage of presentation. Ovarian tumours may be cystic or solid, functional, benign or malignant. There are common factors in the presentation and complications of ovarian tumours, and it is often difficult to establish the nature of a tumour without direct examination.

Symptoms

Tumours of the ovary that are less than 10 cm in diameter rarely produce symptoms. The common presenting symptoms include:

- Abdominal enlargement – in the presence of malignant change, this may also be associated with ascites.
- Symptoms from pressure on surrounding structures such as the bladder and rectum.
- Symptoms relating to complications of the tumour (Fig. 20.18). These include:

- **Torsion:** Acute torsion of the ovarian pedicle results in necrosis of the tumour; there is acute pain and vomiting followed by remission of the pain when the tumour has become necrotic.
- **Rupture:** The contents of the cyst spill into the peritoneal cavity and result in generalized abdominal pain.
- **Haemorrhage** into the tumour is an unusual complication but may result in abdominal pain and shock if the blood loss is severe.
- **Hormone-secreting tumours** may present with disturbances in the menstrual cycle. In androgen-secreting tumours, the patient may present with signs of virilization. Although a greater proportion of the sex-cord stromal type of tumour (see later) are hormonally active, the commonest type of secreting tumour found in clinical practice is the epithelial type.

Signs

On examination, the abdomen may be visibly enlarged. Percussion over the swelling will demonstrate central dullness and resonance in the flanks. These signs may be obscured by gross ascites. Small tumours may be detected on pelvic examination and will be found by palpation in one or both fornices, although tumours smaller than 5 cm are often not palpable. As the tumour enlarges, it assumes a more central position. Most ovarian tumours are not tender on palpation; if they are painful, the presence of infection or torsion should be suspected. Benign ovarian tumours may be palpable separately from the uterine body and are usually freely mobile.

Benign ovarian tumours

Functional cysts of the ovary

These cysts occur only during menstrual life and rarely exceed more than 6 cm in diameter.

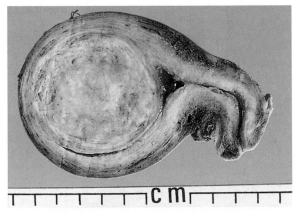

Fig. 20.17 Large mixed müllerian tumour.

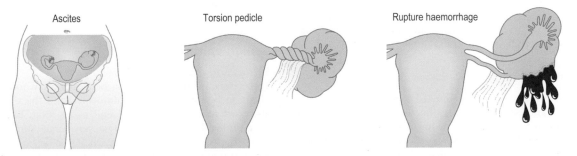

Fig. 20.18 Common complications of ovarian tumours that precipitate a request for medical advice.

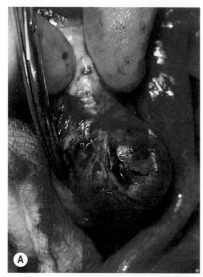

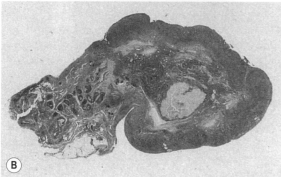

Fig. 20.19 (A) Small follicular cyst near mid-cycle. (B) Histological features.

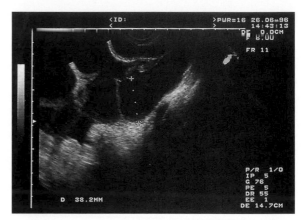

Fig. 20.20 Pelvic ultrasound showing ovarian hyperstimulation with multiple follicles.

Follicular cysts

Follicular cysts (Fig. 20.19) are the commonest functional cysts in the ovary and may be multiple and bilateral. The cysts rarely exceed 4 cm in diameter, with the walls consisting of layers of granulosa cells and the contents of clear fluid, which is rich in sex steroids. Most are asymptomatic and resolve spontaneously within a few months. These cysts may occur during ovarian stimulation with clomiphene or human menopausal gonadotrophin (Fig. 20.20).

Lutein cysts

There are two types of luteinized ovarian cysts:

- **Granulosa lutein cysts**, functional cysts of the corpus luteum, may be 4–6 cm in diameter and occur in the second half of the menstrual cycle. Persistent production of progesterone may result in amenorrhoea or delayed onset of menstruation. These cysts often give rise to pain and therefore present a problem in terms of differential diagnosis, as the history and examination findings mimic tubal ectopic pregnancy. Occasionally, haemorrhage occurs into the cyst, which may rupture and lead to a haemoperitoneum. The cysts usually regress spontaneously and require surgical intervention only when they give rise to symptoms of intra-abdominal haemorrhage.

- **Theca lutein cysts** commonly arise in association with high levels of chorionic gonadotrophin and are therefore seen in cases of hydatidiform mole. The cysts may be bilateral and can on occasion give rise to haemorrhage if they rupture. Once the cysts have been formed, they can be detected by ultrasound. They usually undergo spontaneous involution, but surgical intervention may be necessary if there is significant haemorrhage from the ovaries.

Benign neoplastic cysts

These tumours may be cystic or solid and arise from specific cell lines in the ovary. The full World Health Organization classification of ovarian tumours illustrates the complexity of tumours arising from the ovary; only the commoner ones will be discussed in this section.

Benign epithelial tumours

Serous and mucinous cystadenomas

These cysts are the commonest benign ovarian tumours. They can be unilocular or multilocular, and the size can also vary. Mucinous tumours tend to be more likely to be multilocular and can become very large, sometimes filling the peritoneal cavity (Fig. 20.21). When cut open, serous tumours contain serous fluid, while thick mucinous fluid is seen in mucinous tumours. The diagnosis is

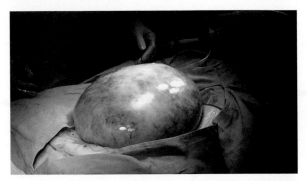

Fig. 20.21 Large benign mucinous cystadenoma occupying the abdominal cavity.

made histologically – the cells lining a serous cystadenoma resemble those from the Fallopian tube, while those lining a mucinous cyst are similar to cells in the endocervix or the gastrointestinal tract. Since these cysts tend to occur in women of reproductive age and they are benign, removal of the cyst by ovarian cystectomy is usually sufficient. Laparoscopy is the preferred route unless the cyst is very large.

> ⚠ Care should be taken to avoid rupture of the cysts because mucinous epithelium may implant in the peritoneal cavity, giving rise to a condition known as *pseudomyxoma peritonei*. Huge amounts of gelatinous material may accumulate in the peritoneal cavity.

Endometriotic cysts

Endometriomas contain chocolate-coloured fluid representing the accumulation of altered blood and have a thick fibrous capsule (see Fig. 16.13). The lining may consist of endometrial cells, but in old cysts these may disappear. Treatment is usually by ovarian cystectomy. (Also refer to section on endometriosis in Chapter 16.)

Sex cord stromal tumours

This is an uncommon group of tumours arising from the cells surrounding the oocytes. They can be benign or malignant. They can be pure sex cord tumours, such as granulosa cell tumours; pure stromal tumours, such as fibromas and thecomas; or they can have a mixed sex cord and stromal components, e.g. Sertoli–Leydig cell tumours. Granulosa cell tumours are generally considered malignant, while about 25% of Sertoli–Leydig cell tumours are malignant, and these would be discussed under the malignant section.

Fibroma

This is the commonest sex cord stromal tumour. Fibromas are benign solid tumours found mainly in postmenopausal women. They are not hormonally active. Treatment is by

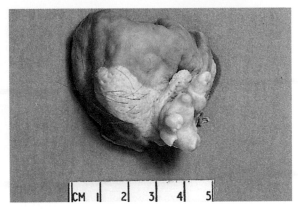

Fig. 20.22 Dermoid cyst (benign cystic teratoma) containing teeth and hair.

salpingo-oophorectomy. Meig's syndrome refers to the condition where the ovarian fibroma is associated with ascites or pleural effusion. Usually, the ascites and pleural effusion would resolve with removal of the mass.

Thecoma

Thecomas or theca cell tumours arise from the spindle-shaped thecal cells but are often mixed with granulosa cells. They are usually benign, solid tumours found mostly in postmenopausal women. They may produce oestrogen, which may in turn lead to abnormal vaginal bleeding or postmenopausal bleeding and endometrial hyperplasia. In postmenopausal women, total abdominal hysterectomy (TAH) BSO can be considered. In young women, unilateral salpingo-oophorectomy (USO) with endometrial sampling is the treatment of choice.

Germ cell tumours

Tumours of germ cell origin may replicate stages resembling the early embryo. These tumours can be benign or malignant.

Mature cystic teratoma (dermoid cyst)

Benign cystic teratomas account for 12–15% of ovarian neoplasms. They contain a large number of embryonic elements such as skin, hair, adipose and muscle tissue, bone, teeth and cartilage (Fig. 20.22). Some of the components can be recognized on imaging.

These tumours are often chance findings, as they are commonly asymptomatic unless they undergo torsion or rupture. They are bilateral in 12% of cases. Sometimes, one specialized element becomes predominant, e.g. in struma ovarii, thyroid tissue dominates. This may occasionally induce a state of hyperthyroidism. Treatment is by ovarian cystectomy while taking care not to rupture the cyst during the operation. Spillage of the cyst contents, such as the sebaceous material, may cause chemical peritonitis.

345

Dermoid cysts are the commonest solid ovarian neoplasm found in young women.

Ovarian malignancy

Ovarian cancer is the sixth most common cancer in females in the UK and is the fourteenth most common cause of death from malignant disease in women in the UK (2014). Although it is the second most common gynaecological cancer after endometrial cancer, it is the commonest cause of gynaecological cancer deaths. The lifetime risk of developing ovarian cancer was about 1 in 52 women in the UK in 2014. The incidence increases with age, with 80% being diagnosed in women over the age of 50 years. The poor survival is partly attributable to late diagnosis, as many women present late due to lack of obvious symptoms.

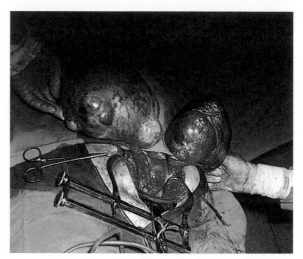
Fig. 20.23 Bilateral multicystic malignant ovarian tumours.

Aetiology

The exact aetiology of ovarian cancer is still under investigation. Different histological subtypes may have different aetiologies. In recent years, there is increasing evidence that the high-grade serous subtypes originate from precursors found in the Fallopian tube.

Genetic

About 10–20% of ovarian cancers are hereditary. Germline mutation of the *BRCA1* and *BRCA2* genes is the commonest genetic cause. It is inherited via an autosomal-dominant pattern. Women carrying the *BRCA1* and *BRCA2* mutations will have an average cumulative risk of 45% and 12%, respectively, in the development of ovarian cancer. Many other genes have also been found to be associated with the increased risk of ovarian cancers.

Parity and fertility

Multiparous women are at 40% less risk than nulliparous women of developing ovarian cancer, whereas women who have had unsuccessful treatment for infertility seem to be at increased risk. The use of the contraceptive pill may produce up to a 60% reduction in the incidence of the disease.

Pathology

Primary ovarian carcinoma

The distribution of histological types of ovarian cancers is as follows.

Epithelial type

This makes up 85% of cases of ovarian malignancy. Epithelial tumours include the following subtypes:

- **Serous cystadenocarcinoma** is the most common histological type of ovarian carcinoma (40%) and is usually unilocular. They may be bilateral. These tumours are more likely to contain solid areas than their benign counterparts.
- **Mucinous cystadenocarcinomas:** These multicystic tumours (Fig. 20.23) are characterized by mucin-filled cysts lined by columnar glandular cells and may be associated with tumours of the appendix.
- **Endometrioid cystadenocarcinomas** resemble endometrial adenocarcinomas and are associated with uterine carcinomas in 20% of cases.
- **Clear-cell cystadenocarcinoma** is the most common ovarian malignancy found in association with ovarian endometriosis. The unilocular thin-walled cysts are lined by epithelium with a typical hobnail appearance and clear cytoplasm.
- **Brenner's or transitional cell cystadenocarcinoma** is often found in association with mucinous tumours but has a better prognosis than similar tumours arising from the bladder.

Tumours of low malignant or borderline potential account for 10–15% of primary epithelial carcinomas. They are commonly serous or mucinous tumours. There are cytological changes of malignancy, including cellular atypia, with increased mitosis and multilayering but without invasion. They have a significantly better prognosis than invasive disease, with a 5-year survival of more than 95% for stage I lesions, but there is a 10–15% incidence of late recurrence.

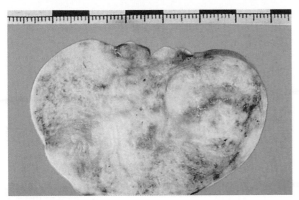

Fig. 20.24 Granulosa cell/theca cell tumour. This shows haemorrhagic areas in the solid white surface of the cut tumour.

Malignant sex cord stromal tumours

These tumours are relatively rare, as they make up only 6% of primary ovarian malignancy.

Granulosa cell tumours

Arising from ovarian granulosa cells, these tumours (Fig. 20.24) usually present as a unilateral, large, solid mass. Histologically, granulosa cells have the 'coffee bean' grooved nuclei, and these tumours are characterized by the presence of Call–Exner bodies where cells are arranged in small clusters around a central cavity. The majority of these tumours are slow growing but some exhibit aggressive behaviour. About 95% of the adult granulosa cell tumours that occur in middle-aged women and the remaining 5% are juvenile granulosa cell tumours, which affect young girls, usually before puberty, and they are usually more aggressive than the adult type. These tumours are the commonest oestrogen-secreting tumours. As granulosa cell tumours can present at any age, the symptoms depend on the age of occurrence. Tumours arising before puberty produce precocious sexual development, and in women of reproductive age, prolonged oestrogen stimulation results in endometrial hyperplasia and irregular and prolonged vaginal bleeding. Around 50% of cases occur after menopause and present with postmenopausal bleeding. Treatment is by total hysterectomy and BSO. Fertility-sparing surgery with USO may be feasible in young patients with disease confined to the ovary. However, if hysterectomy is not done, it is prudent to proceed with a hysteroscopy and endometrial sampling to exclude endometrial hyperplasia.

Sertoli–Leydig cell tumours (androblastomas)

These are tumours of Sertoli–Leydig cells. Approximately 25% of these tumours are malignant. They are rare androgen-secreting tumours that occur most frequently between 20 and 30 years of age. They present with symptoms of androgen excess, such as increasing facial and body hirsutism, deepening of the voice and enlargement of the clitoris. The diagnosis is established by the exclusion of virilizing adrenal tumours and the identification of a tumour in one ovary. The condition is treated by excision of the affected ovary.

Malignant germ cell tumours

- **Dysgerminomas:** These solid tumours may be small or large enough to fill the abdominal cavity. The cut surface of the tumour has a greyish-pink colour, and microscopically, the tumour consists of large polygonal cells arranged in alveoli or nests separated by septa of fibrous tissue.
- **Immature teratomas:** The malignant or immature form of teratoma is most commonly solid, unilateral and heterogenous with multiple tissue elements. These tumours may produce human chorionic gonadotrophin and alpha-fetoprotein.
- **Endodermal sinus or yolk sac tumours:** Although these tumours make up only 10–15% of germ cell tumours, they are the most common germ cell tumour in children. They are solid, encapsulated tumours containing microcysts lined by flat mesothelial cells. These tumours produce alpha-fetoprotein.

Secondary ovarian carcinomas

The ovaries are a common site for secondary deposits from primary malignancies in the breast, genital tract, gastrointestinal system and haematopoietic system.

Krukenberg's tumours are metastatic deposits from the gastrointestinal system. They are solid growths that are almost always bilateral. The stroma is often richly cellular and may appear to be myomatous. The epithelial elements occur as clusters of well-marked acini, with cells exhibiting mucoid change, known as *signet ring cells*.

Staging of ovarian carcinoma

Spread of primary ovarian tumours can be by direct extension, lymphatics or via the bloodstream. Ovarian cancer is surgically staged according to the FIGO staging system (Table 20.6). A staging procedure includes total hysterectomy with BSO, omentectomy and careful inspection and sampling of peritoneal surfaces and retroperitoneal (pelvic and para-aortic) lymph node dissection. Staging of ovarian carcinoma is important in determining both prognosis and management.

Diagnosis

Early ovarian carcinomas are mostly asymptomatic. The commonest symptoms are abdominal discomfort or distension. Clinically, a pelvic mass may be detected, and there may be ascites. A transvaginal ultrasound scan can exclude

Table 20.6 FIGO classification of ovarian carcinoma 2014

Stage		Characteristics
I		Tumour confined to ovaries
	IA	Tumour limited to one ovary
	IB	Tumour limited to both ovaries
	IC	Tumour limited to one or both ovaries, with any of the following:
	IC_1	Surgical spill
	IC_2	Capsule ruptured before surgery or tumour on ovarian surface
	IC_3	Malignant cells in ascites or peritoneal washing
II		Tumour with pelvic extension (below pelvic brim)
	IIA	Extension on uterus or Fallopian tubes or ovaries
	IIB	Extension to other pelvic intraperitoneal tissues
III		Tumour spread to peritoneum outside pelvis ± metastasis to retroperitoneal node
	$IIIA_1$	Positive retroperitoneal node only
	$IIIA_2$	Microscopic extrapelvic peritoneal involvement
	IIIB	Macroscopic peritoneal metastasis ≤2 cm
	IIIC	Macroscopic peritoneal metastasis >2 cm
IV		Distant metastasis

From Prat J & FIGO Committee on Gynecologic Oncology (2015) FIGO's staging classification for cancer of the ovary, fallopian tube, and peritoneum: abridged republication. J Gynecol Oncol 26(2): 87–89. Open access.

other causes of pelvic mass such as fibroids, and it is also useful in assessing features suggestive of malignancy, such as bilateral lesions, multilocular cysts, solid areas, papillary projections, metastases, ascites and increased blood flow (Doppler). CA-125 is a glycoprotein shed by 85% of epithelial tumours and can be used as a tumour marker for ovarian cancer. A cut-off level of 35 u/L is commonly used for postmenopausal women. CA-125 lacks sensitivity and specificity if used alone. It is only raised in 50% of early-stage ovarian cancers, and false-positive results occur in other malignancies (liver, pancreas) and many benign conditions such as endometriosis, pelvic inflammatory disease and early pregnancy. A risk of malignancy index (RMI) can be calculated based on the menopausal status, ultrasound features and CA 125 levels. RMI = U × M × CA125, where U represents the ultrasound score and M represents the menopausal status. The ultrasound result is scored 1 point for each of the following features: multilocular cysts, solid areas, metastases, ascites and bilateral lesions.

U = 0 for ultrasound score of 0, U = 1 for score of 1 and U =3 for score of ≥ 5. Menopausal status is scored as M = 1 for premenopausal women and M = 3 for postmenopausal women. Women with a pelvic mass with an RMI more than 200 should be referred to gynaecological oncologists for further workup and management. Other scoring systems such as the Risk of Malignancy Algorithm (ROMA) or the International Ovarian Tumor Analysis (IOTA) classification can also be used. ROMA is a formula for classifying whether the cyst is likely to be malignant by combining the two tumour marker levels: CA 125 and a new tumour marker, HE4 (human epididymis protein 4). IOTA classification is based on ultrasound appearances. Further imaging such as CT or MRI of the abdomen and pelvis or PET-CT can be done to assess for any metastases (Fig. 20.25) and a chest X-ray to look for lung metastases and pleural effusions. The diagnosis is made by histological assessment of the surgical specimens.

Management

Surgery is the mainstay of treatment of ovarian cancer, followed by chemotherapy. For early disease confined to the ovary, a staging laparotomy (see earlier) is done. In advanced disease, the aim is to remove all macroscopic disease (complete debulking). Subsequent prognosis is proportional to the amount of disease remaining after primary surgery. Surgery is often followed by adjuvant chemotherapy. In selected advanced cases, neoadjuvant chemotherapy before primary surgery can decrease morbidity of surgery with higher chance of achieving optimal removal of tumour. Germ cell tumours tend to occur in young women. Fertility-sparing surgery, e.g. USO with preservation of the uterus and the other ovary, should be considered even in the presence of metastatic disease because the tumour is highly chemosensitive.

Chemotherapy

Patients with high risk for recurrence, e.g. those with high-grade, poor histological subtypes or stage IC or above, are often given adjuvant chemotherapy. The platinum-based drugs cisplatin and carboplatin are currently the mainstay of treatment. The main side effects are marrow suppression, neurotoxicity and renal toxicity. Carboplatin has now largely replaced cisplatin due to its better side effect profile, and it is often combined with paclitaxel, another active agent for ovarian cancer. The overall response rate is up to 80%

Target therapy

The use of an anti-angiogenetic agent such as bevacizumab improves the progression-free survival but not overall survival. The use of poly (ADP- ribose) polymerase (PARP) inhibitor in *BRCA*-mutated ovarian cancer can

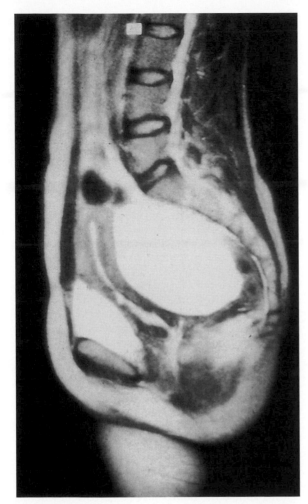

Fig. 20.25 Magnetic resonance image of a large ovarian cyst. The tumour can be seen distending the uterus and elongating the endometrium.

Table 20.7 Survival rates for ovarian cancer

Stage	5-year survival (%)
Stage I	89
Stage II	66
Stage III	34
Stage IV	18

examination. Imaging can be arranged if there is suspicion of recurrence. Chemotherapy is the mainstay of treatment for recurrence. Debulking of the tumour may be feasible if it is localized and there is a long interval to recurrence. In platinum-sensitive patients, i.e. those that recur after 6 months (partially sensitive) and 12 months from completion of primary treatment, rechallenge with first-line chemotherapy (carboplatin based) is recommended. Otherwise, there are wide ranges of second-line chemotherapy agents such as liposomal doxorubicin, gemcitabine and topotecan, but their response rates are only about 20–30%.

Prognosis

The 5-year survival figures depend on the stage and on whether the tumour has or has not been completely removed (Table 20.7).

Screening for ovarian cancer

Because the prognosis for early-stage disease is better than that for advanced disease, overall survival might be improved if the disease could be diagnosed earlier in asymptomatic women. However, the best screening strategy is unclear. The two main methods proposed are ultrasound and CA-125 measurement.

Transvaginal ultrasound is sensitive in picking up ovarian masses, but it is not accurate enough to differentiate between ovarian cancer and benign ovarian cysts. This leads to many unnecessary operations.

CA-125 lacks both sensitivity and specificity if used alone.

Combining transvaginal ultrasound with serial CA-125 has been investigated in large-scale randomized trials, e.g. the UK Collaborative Trial of Ovarian Cancer Screening (UKCTOCS). Whether screening can reduce mortality is still under investigation. Screening may be considered in women at high risk for ovarian cancer, such as *BRCA* carriers, to detect ovarian cancer at an earlier stage, but whether this would translate into improved overall survival is still not known.

also prolong progression-free survival. Many target therapies were undergoing trials, such as those targeting immunopathway, PD1 (programmed cell death protein 1) and PDL1 (programmed cell death ligand 1).

Borderline tumours

These can be treated by unilateral oophorectomy in young women wishing to preserve their reproductive capacity, although careful, long-term follow-up is required.

Follow-up and treatment of recurrence

Patients are followed up for any symptoms such as abdominal discomfort, tumour markers and clinical

Risk-reducing surgery for ovarian cancer

The most effective way to prevent ovarian cancer in *BRCA* carriers (see earlier) is risk-reducing salpingo-ophrectomy (RRSO) with an 80% decreased risk. The recommended age of RRSO is around 35–40. BSO can usually be done laparoscopically. Meticulous processing of the surgical specimen is needed to rule out occult cancer in the tube. With the discovery that many high-grade serous carcinomas arise from the tube, BSO has been proposed, but its exact effectiveness is still under investigation.

Principles of palliative care in gynaecological cancer

Despite optimal initial treatment, disease recurrence and progression are inevitable in a certain proportion of women with gynaecological cancer. In many of these situations, a cure is no longer a realistic option, but this by no means translates into withdrawal of the input from medical professionals. A multidisciplinary approach, with strong input from the palliative team to provide supportive care to the individual, is crucial. Palliative care aims to provide both physical and emotional support, as well as preparation for the eventual outcome of death. Quality of life and the patient's autonomy and dignity are the most important aspects in this final phase of life. Good communication and a trusting relationship between the patient and her carers are key to achieving these aims. Ideally, the concept of palliative care should be introduced in good time and not at a clinically critical moment so that the patient and her family can have time to develop acceptance and realistic expectations. The decision to either continue or stop anticancer treatment needs to take into account the overall benefit in quality of life, bearing in mind the additional stress and side effects arising from the treatment rather than the disease.

Uncontrolled symptoms can cause severe distress, and symptom control is one of the main areas for palliative care. Patients almost inevitably experience pain, which can be a result of the disease or the treatment. Pain is a subjective sensation; therefore, to achieve good control, it is important both to reduce the pain stimulus and to increase the personal pain threshold. Reducing pain stimulus requires careful assessment of the cause by taking a good history. Therapeutic measures can then be targeted at the mechanisms involved, e.g. non-steroidal anti-inflammatory drugs would be appropriate for pain arising from inflammation or antispasmodic agents for bowel spasms, while neuropathic pain can be relieved by tricyclic antidepressants or anticonvulsant drugs such as gabapentin.

Increasing the pain threshold involves good psychological support, possibly with the help of antidepressants and anxiolytics. The World Health Organization has developed a three-step 'ladder' for cancer pain relief. Administration of drugs should be in the following order: non-opioids (such as paracetamol and aspirin), mild opioids (codeine), then strong opioids such as morphine. At each step, 'adjuvant' agents can be added. Adjuvants are medications that have a primary indication other than pain control but can also help to relieve pain in certain situations, such as anticonvulsant and antidepressant agents. Opioids are very effective, but they need to be given at the right dose and at the right time. They should be given at regular intervals, and additional doses can be prescribed as required for breakthrough pain. Common opioid side effects include nausea, vomiting and constipation; therefore anti-emetics and regular laxatives should also be prescribed when starting opioids. Patients should be reassured that appropriate use of opioids would not cause addiction.

In women with extensive intra-abdominal disease, such as those in advanced ovarian cancer, bowel obstruction and ascites are common. Symptoms from bowel obstructions are difficult to deal with entirely. Surgical intervention can potentially give the best palliative effect but is often not feasible due to multiple sites of obstruction from extensive disease. Conservative management aims to reduce nausea and vomiting with anti-emetic ± nasogastric tube or gastrotomy and maintaining hydration by intravenous fluid. Occasionally, a trial of short-course corticosteroid drugs to decrease inflammatory oedema around the bowels may be effective in relieving the obstruction. Ascites from peritoneal disease can be effectively relieved by paracentesis, but they tend to re-accumulate, and often repeated paracentesis is required. Diuretics such as spironolactone can be tried to reduce the rate of re-accumulation.

Eventually, when the patient is very close to death, care plans should concentrate on providing a peaceful and dignified environment for the patient and her family. Futile medical interventions should be minimized, while distressing symptoms should be adequately controlled. Last but not least, it is important to be aware of the individual's cultural and spiritual preferences so that both the patient and her family can feel that she has come to a 'good end'.

Essential information

Malignant vulval lesions

- Commonest in sixth decade
- Majority are squamous (92%) or adenocarcinomas (5%)
- Present with pruritus, bleeding lesions
- Spreads by local invasion and via inguinal and femoral nodes
- Primary treatment by radical vulvectomy and groin node dissection with individual modification
- Good prognosis if confined to vulva at presentation

Malignant vaginal tumours

- Primary malignancy rare, squamous carcinomas arising in upper third
- Common site for spread from cervix and uterus
- Presents as pain, bleeding and fistula formation
- Spreads by local invasion and lymphatics
- Usually treated by radiotherapy

Cervical screening and vaccination

- Cytology 3–5-yearly intervals from 25 to 65 years of age
- HPV testing in screening every 5 years from 25 to 74
- Abnormal screening tests results require colposcopy and biopsy
- HPV 16 and 18 or nanovalent vaccination in girls (and in Australia boys) aged 12–13 years old

Cervical cancer

- Associated with HPV infection
- May be asymptomatic or present with vaginal bleeding, pain and bowel or bladder symptoms
- Spreads by local invasion and iliac/obturator nodes

- Treatment is radical hysterectomy and pelvic nodes dissection for early-stage disease, chemoradiotherapy otherwise
- 5-year survival varies from 10% to 90% depending on stage

Endometrial carcinoma

- Risk factors include obesity, nulliparity, late menopause, diabetes and unopposed oestrogens, HNPCC or Lynch's syndrome
- Commonly presents as abnormal vaginal bleeding or postmenopausal bleeding
- Spreads by direct invasion but tends to remain localized within the uterus initially
- Well-differentiated early-stage disease can be treated by surgery alone; more advanced lesions require chemotherapy and/or radiotherapy
- Has 90% 5-year survival if diagnosed early

Malignant ovarian tumours

- 75% of cases present with advanced disease
- Most cases are epithelial in type
- Prognosis depends on stage at diagnosis and extent of residual disease after initial surgery
- The primary treatment is surgery, followed by platinum-based chemotherapy
- 5-year survival 35–40%

Principles of palliative care

- Multidisciplinary approach for symptom control and relief, physical and emotional support
- Three-step ladder for pain relief with or without adjuvant
- Care plan for terminal stage and support to family

Chapter | 21 |

Prolapse and disorders of the urinary tract

Ajay Rane, Mugdha Kulkarni and Jay Iyer

LEARNING OUTCOMES

After studying this chapter you should be able to:

Knowledge criteria

- Describe the normal supports of the uterus and vagina.
- Describe the normal mechanisms that maintain urinary continence and the physiology of normal micturition.
- Describe the epidemiology, aetiology and clinical features associated with urinary incontinence, urinary frequency, urinary tract infections and genitourinary prolapse.
- Evaluate the common surgical and non-surgical treatments used in the management of urinary incontinence and genital prolapse, including catheterization, bladder retraining, pelvic floor exercises, medical therapies, vaginal repair with or without hysterectomy, sling procedures and colposuspension.

Clinical competencies

- Take a history from a woman presenting with bowel, bladder and sexual symptoms.
- Perform a pelvic examination to assess genitourinary prolapse and pelvic floor tone.
- Explain the investigations employed in the assessment of incontinence and prolapse, including microbiology, urodynamics, cystoscopy and imaging.

Professional skills and attitudes

- Consider the impact of urinary incontinence on women and the community.

Uterovaginal prolapse

The position of the vagina and uterus depends on various fascial supports and ligaments derived from specific thickening of areas of the fascial support (Figs 21.1–21.4). There has been a paradigm shift in our understanding of the anatomy of pelvic floor supports and with it the pathophysiology of development of pelvic organ prolapse. Three levels of pelvic organ support are clinically relevant and conceptually easier to grasp. The uterosacral ligaments responsible for providing level I support to the upper vagina and the cervix (and by extension to the uterus) have a broad attachment over the second, third and fourth sacral vertebrae arising posteriorly from the junction of the cervix and the upper vagina running on each side lateral to the rectum towards the sacral attachments. The other important structure is the arcus tendineus fasciae pelvis (ATFP; see Figs 21.3 and 21.5), also known as the *white line* – a condensation of pelvic cellular tissue on the pelvic aspect of the obturator internus muscle. The ATFP runs from the ischial spines to the pubic tubercle, and its terminal medial end is known as the *iliopectineal ligament* (Cooper's ligament), well known to general surgeons who operate on inguinal and femoral hernias. Extending medially from the white lines are condensed sheets of pelvic cellular tissue suspending the anterior and posterior vaginal walls and the

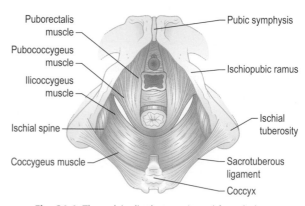

Fig. 21.1 The pelvic diaphragm viewed from below.

Puborectalis muscle — Pubic symphysis
Pubococcygeus muscle
Ilicoccygeus muscle — Ischiopubic ramus
Ischial spine — Ischial tuberosity
Coccygeus muscle — Sacrotuberous ligament
— Coccyx

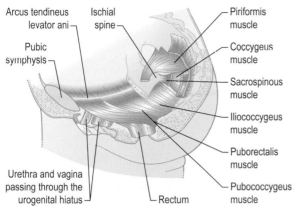

Fig. 21.2 Muscles of the pelvic floor, lateral view.

Labels (Fig. 21.2): Arcus tendineus levator ani; Ischial spine; Piriformis muscle; Pubic symphysis; Coccygeus muscle; Sacrospinous muscle; Iliococcygeus muscle; Puborectalis muscle; Urethra and vagina passing through the urogenital hiatus; Pubococcygeus muscle; Rectum.

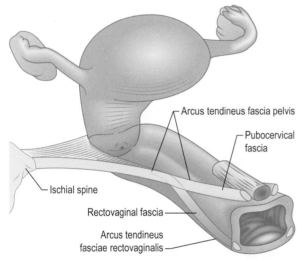

Fig. 21.3 The lateral attachments of the pubocervical fascia (PCF) and the rectovaginal fascia (RVF) to the pelvic sidewall. Also shown are the arcus tendineus fascia pelvis (ATFP), arcus tendineus fasciae rectovaginalis (ATFRV) and ischial spine (IS).

Labels (Fig. 21.3): Arcus tendineus fascia pelvis; Pubocervical fascia; Ischial spine; Rectovaginal fascia; Arcus tendineus fasciae rectovaginalis.

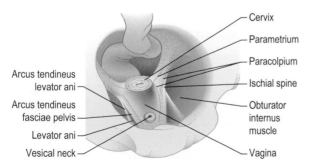

Fig. 21.4 Three-dimensional view of the endopelvic fascia. Notice the location of the cervix in the proximal anterior vaginal segment.

Labels (Fig. 21.4): Cervix; Parametrium; Paracolpium; Ischial spine; Obturator internus muscle; Vagina; Vesical neck; Levator ani; Arcus tendineus fasciae pelvis; Arcus tendineus levator ani.

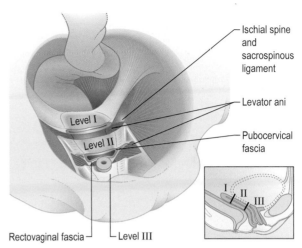

Fig. 21.5 The endopelvic fascia of a post-hysterectomy patient divided into DeLancey's biomechanical levels: level I, proximal suspension; level II, lateral attachment; level III, distal fusion. (Modified with permission from DeLancey JO (1992) Anatomic aspects of vaginal eversion after hysterectomy. Am J Obstet Gynecol 166:1717. © Elsevier.)

Labels (Fig. 21.5): Ischial spine and sacrospinous ligament; Levator ani; Pubocervical fascia; Level I; Level II; Level III; Rectovaginal fascia.

organs underlying these, namely the urinary bladder and the rectum providing level II support. The anterior support to the bladder was previously referred to as the *pubovesicocervical fascia* or *bladder pillars*, whereas the posterior support to the rectum was termed the *rectovaginal fascia*.

Level III support is provided by the perineal body posteriorly and the pubourethral ligaments anteriorly. The perineal body is a complex fibromuscular mass into which several structures insert. It is bordered cephalad by the rectovaginal septum (Dennonviller's fascia), caudal by the perineal skin, anteriorly by the wall of the anorectum and laterally by the ischial rami. The three-dimensional form has been likened to the cone of the red pine (*Pinus resinosa*), and it forms the keystone of the pelvic floor, a 4 cm × 4 cm fibromuscular structure providing support not just to the lower third of the vaginal wall (part of the genital hiatus) anteriorly but also to the external anal sphincter posteriorly. Attaching laterally to the perineal body are the superficial and deep perineal muscles.

The anterior vaginal wall is supported by the pubovesicocervical fascia, which extends from the ATFP on one side to the ATFP of the other, providing a hammock-like level II support. The posterior vaginal wall is supported by the fibrous tissue of the rectovaginal septum that is well defined only in the midline; laterally the hammock-like supports arise from the ATFP.

The uterus is supported indirectly by the supports of the vaginal walls but directly by the uterosacral ligaments. The round and broad ligaments provide weak, if any, support to the vagina and uterus. Indirect support of the lower third

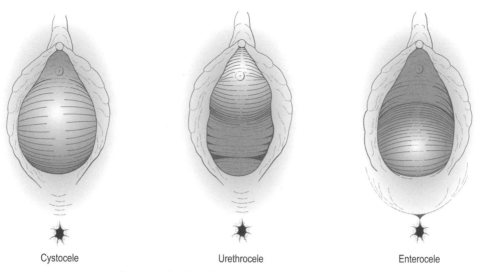

Cystocele Urethrocele Enterocele

Fig. 21.6 The clinical appearance of vaginal prolapse.

of the vagina and uterus is provided by the intact levator ani (pelvic floor). The role of the latter has always been in doubt, but the puborectalis portion of the levator ani plays a significant role in the distension of the genital hiatus in labour and delivery, making it very prone to injury. Injury to this muscle has been postulated to be the cause for vaginal prolapse later in life.

Definitions

Vaginal prolapse

Prolapse of the anterior vaginal wall may affect the urethra (*urethrocele*) and the bladder (*cystocele*, Fig. 21.6). On examination, the urethra and bladder can be seen to descend and bulge into the anterior vaginal wall and, in severe cases, will be visible at or beyond the introitus of the vagina. A urethrocele is the result of damage to level III (anterior) support, i.e. the pubourethral ligaments. Cystoceles usually result due to a loss of level II support and usually due to a midline defect in pubovesicocervical fascia. However, nearly half of anterior prolapses have apical defects as well. A *rectocele* is formed by a combination of factors: a herniation of the rectum through a defect in the rectovaginal fascia, as well as a lateral detachment of the level II support from the ATFP. This can usually be seen as a visible bulge of the rectum through the posterior vaginal wall. It is often associated with a deficiency and laxity of the perineum. This is the classical level III defect (posterior) affecting the perineal body.

An *enterocele* is formed by a prolapse of the small bowel through the rectouterine pouch, i.e. the pouch of Douglas, through the upper part of the vaginal vault (see Fig. 21.6). The condition may occur in isolation but usually occurs in association with uterine prolapse. An enterocele may also occur following hysterectomy when there is inadequate support of the vaginal vault. This represents damage to level I support.

Uterine prolapse

Descent of the uterus, which occurs when level I support is deficient, may occur in isolation from vaginal wall prolapse but more commonly occurs in conjunction with it. First-degree prolapse of the uterus often occurs in association with retroversion of the uterus and descent of the cervix within the vagina. If the cervix descends to the vaginal introitus, the prolapse is defined as second degree. The term *procidentia* is applied to where the cervix and the body of the uterus and the vagina walls protrude through the introitus. The word actually means 'prolapse' or 'falling' but is generally reserved for the description of total or third-degree prolapse (Fig. 21.7).

Symptoms and signs

Symptoms generally depend on the severity and site of the prolapse (Table 21.1).

> Mild degrees of prolapse are common in parous women and may be asymptomatic.

Some symptoms are common to all forms of prolapse; these include:

- A sense of fullness in the vagina associated with dragging discomfort

- Visible protrusion of the cervix and vaginal walls
- Lower backache is usually relieved on lying down

Symptoms are often multiple and related to the nature of prolapse. It is important to note that the symptoms (and signs) of prolapse are worse at the end of the day.

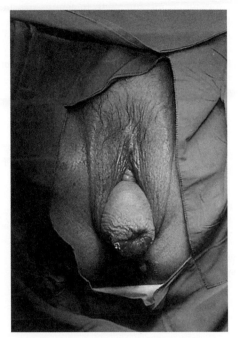

Fig. 21.7 Procidentia: a third-degree prolapse of the uterus and vaginal walls.

It is therefore of some value to schedule examination of patients who have typical symptoms of prolapse without its obvious signs a little later in the day.

Urethrocele and cystocele

Typically patients complain of 'something coming down' per vaginam. At times there may be incomplete emptying of the bladder, and this will be associated with double micturition, the desire to repeat micturition immediately after apparent completion of voiding. The patient may give a history of having to manually replace the prolapse into the vagina to void. Some patients may get recurrent urinary tract infections as a result of incomplete emptying of the bladder. Occasionally the patient may complain of occult stress incontinence, i.e. the involuntary loss of urine following raised intra-abdominal pressure that is not readily demonstrable on coughing but appears on reducing the prolapse.

The diagnosis is established by examination in the dorsal position. A single-bladed Sims' speculum can be used to visualize the anterior vaginal wall. When the patient is asked to strain, the bulge in the anterior vaginal wall can be seen and often appears at the introitus. It is important to culture a specimen of urine to exclude the presence of infection. The differential diagnosis is limited to cysts or tumours of the anterior vaginal wall and diverticulum of the urethra or bladder.

Rectocele

The prolapse of the rectum through the posterior vaginal wall is commonly associated with a deficient pelvic floor,

Table 21.1 Levels of supports with diagnosis and co-relation with symptoms

Level of pelvic organ support	Organ affected	Type of prolapse	Symptoms
Level I – uterosacral ligaments	Uterus/vaginal vault (post-hysterectomy)	Uterocervical/vault prolapse/enterocele	Vaginal pressure, sacral backache, 'something coming down', dyspareunia, vaginal discharge
Level II – arcus tendineus fascia pelvis (ATFP)	Urinary bladder	Cystocele	'Something coming down', double voiding, occult stress incontinence, recurrent urinary tract infection
	Rectum	Rectocele	'Something coming down', difficult defecation, manual digitation
Level III – anterior (pubourethral ligaments)	Urethra	Urethrocele	'Something coming down', stress incontinence
Level III – posterior (perineal body)	Lower third of the vagina/vaginal introitus/anal canal	Enlarged genital hiatus	Vaginal looseness, sexual dysfunction, vaginal flatus, needing to apply pressure to the perineum to evacuate faeces

disruption of the perineal body and separation of the levator ani. It is predominantly a problem that results from over-distension of the introitus and pelvic floor during parturition.

The symptoms of a rectocele include difficulty with evacuation of faeces with an occasional need to 'manually digitate'. Needless to say, the awareness of a reducible mass bulging into the vagina and through the introitus is often the presenting symptom.

Examination of the vulva usually shows a deficient perineum (measuring less than 3 cm in length) bringing the posterior fourchette in close apposition with the anterior anal verge. Patients can complain of vaginal looseness and sexual dysfunction as a result of this. Not uncommonly the symptom of vaginal 'flatus' can be uncovered on direct questioning.

Enterocele

Herniation of the pouch of Douglas usually occurs through the vaginal vault if the uterus has been removed. It is often difficult to distinguish between a high rectocele and an enterocele, as the symptoms of vaginal pressure are identical. Occasionally an examination in the standing position or a bidigital examination may reveal an enterocele in a woman with no obvious signs of prolapse but complaints of a dragging sensation in the pelvis or a low backache. Uncommonly the enterocele occurs anterior to the vaginal vault and may mimic a cystocele.

A large enterocele may contain bowel and may be associated with incarceration and obstruction of the bowel.

Uterine prolapse

Descent of the uterus is initially associated with elongation of the cervix and descent of the body of the uterus. Mostly the affected portion of the cervix is supravaginal, i.e. above the level of the vaginal fornices. The symptoms are those of pressure in the vagina and, ultimately, complete protrusion of the uterus through the introitus. At this stage, the prolapsed uterus may produce discomfort on sitting, and decubitus ulceration may result in bleeding. Sometimes patients with minor degrees of prolapse or with congenital prolapse may have infravaginal cervical elongation that often leads to confusion in staging the degree of prolapse, as it may appear to be in a more advanced stage than it actually is.

Urinary tract infection may occur because of compression of the ureters and consequent hydronephrosis due to incomplete emptying of the bladder. Not unusually, patients experience dyspareunia but are not very forthcoming with this symptom.

Staging/grading of prolapse

Baden–Walker halfway system (Fig 21.8 and Table 21.2)

This system was developed in an effort to introduce more objectivity into the quantification of pelvic organ prolapse. For example, measurements in centimetres are used instead of subjective grades. Nine specific measurements are recorded, as indicated in Figure 21.9.

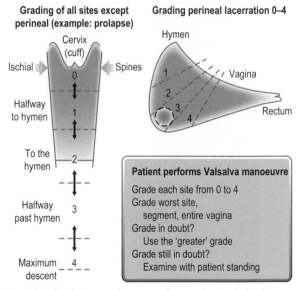

Fig. 21.8 Guidelines on how to assign grades in the Baden–Walker halfway system. (Reproduced with permission from Baden WF, Walker T (1992) Surgical repair of vaginal defects. Lippincott, Williams & Wilkins, Philadelphia.)

Table 21.2 Primary and secondary symptoms at each site used in the Baden–Walker halfway system

Anatomical site	Primary symptoms	Secondary symptoms
Urethral	Urinary incontinence	Falling out
Vesical	Voiding difficulties	Falling out
Uterine	Falling out, heaviness, etc.	
Cul-de-sac	Pelvic pressure (standing)	Falling out
Rectal	True bowel pocket	Falling out
Perineal	Anal incontinence	Too loose (gas/faeces)

Reproduced with permission from Baden WF, Walker T (1992) Surgical repair of vaginal defects. Lippincott, Williams & Wilkins, Philadelphia, p. 12.

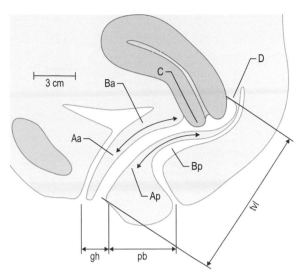

Fig. 21.9 Pelvic organ prolapse quantification system (POP-Q).

Pathogenesis

Prolapse may be:
- **Congenital:** Uterine prolapse in young or nulliparous women is due to weakness of the supports of the uterus and vaginal vault. There is a minimal degree of vaginal wall prolapse.
- **Acquired:** The commonest form of prolapse is acquired under the influence of multiple factors. This type of prolapse is both uterine and vaginal, but it must also be remembered that vaginal wall prolapse can also occur without any uterine descent. Predisposing factors include:
  - *High parity:* Uterovaginal prolapse is a condition of parous women. The pelvic floor provides direct and indirect support for the vaginal walls, and when this support is disrupted by laceration or over-distension, it predisposes to vaginal wall prolapse. Instrumental delivery employing forceps/ventouse, especially mid-cavity rotational forceps delivery, may play a contributory role in the causation of urinary incontinence and prolapse in later life.
  - *Raised intra-abdominal pressure:* Tumours or ascites may result in raised intra-abdominal pressure, but a more common cause is a chronic cough and chronic constipation.
  - *Hormonal changes:* The symptoms of prolapse often worsen rapidly at the time of menopause. Cessation of oestrogen production leads to thinning of the vaginal walls and the supports of the uterus. Although the prolapse is generally present before menopause, it is at this time that the symptoms become noticeable and the degree of descent visibly worsens. The age at first vaginal childbirth affects the incidence of prolapse and urinary incontinence in later life. It has been postulated that increased maternal age predisposes to levator trauma, making these women more prone to developing pelvic floor disorders.

Management

The management of prolapse can be conservative or surgical.

Prevention

Good surgical technique in supporting the vaginal vault at the time of hysterectomy reduces the incidence of later vault prolapse. Avoiding a prolonged second stage of labour and inappropriate or premature bearing-down efforts, encouraging pelvic floor exercises after delivery and the judicious use of instrumental delivery with appropriately individualized episiotomies may all help reduce the risk of prolapse in later life.

Conservative treatment

Many women have minor degrees of uterovaginal prolapse, which are asymptomatic. If the recognition of the prolapse is a coincidental finding, the woman should be advised against any surgical treatment.

Minor degrees of prolapse are common after childbirth and should be treated by pelvic floor exercises or the use of a pessary. Operative intervention is deferred for at least 6 months after delivery, as the tissues remain vascular and may undergo further spontaneous improvement.

Hormone replacement therapy may be used preoperatively to prepare the tissues but by itself is of limited benefit in alleviating symptoms.

Where short-term support is required or the general health of the woman makes operative treatment potentially dangerous, both vaginal wall and uterine prolapse can be treated by using vaginal pessaries. It is, however, necessary to have some pelvic floor support if a pessary is to be retained.

The most widely used pessaries (Fig. 21.10) are:
- **Ring pessary:** This pessary consists of a malleable plastic ring, which may vary in diameter from 60 to 105 mm. The pessary is inserted in the posterior fornix and behind the pubic symphysis. Distension of the vaginal walls tends to support the vaginal wall prolapse.
- **Hodge pessary:** This is a rigid, elongated, curved ovoid which is inserted in a similar way to the ring pessary and is principally useful in uterine retroversion.

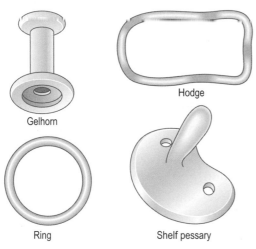

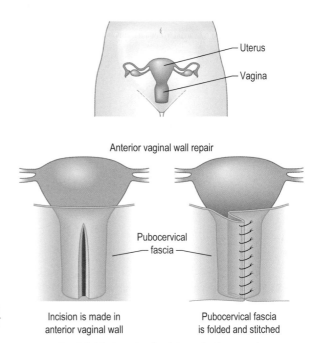

Fig. 21.10 Various types of vaginal pessaries used in the conservative management of uterovaginal prolapse.

- **Gelhorn pessary:** This pessary is shaped like a collar stud and is used in the treatment of severe degrees of prolapse.
- **Shelf pessary:** This is shaped like a coat hook and is used mainly in the treatment of uterine or vaginal vault prolapse.

The main problem with long-term use of pessaries is ulceration of the vaginal vault, and rarely a fistula may form, usually between the bladder and the vagina, if the pessary is 'neglected' or 'forgotten'. Pessaries should be replaced every 4–6 months, and the vagina should be examined for any signs of ulceration. In postmenopausal women it is considered good practice to prescribe vaginal oestrogen creams/tablets to prevent ulceration.

Pelvic floor physiotherapy

See the section on urinary incontinence.

Surgical treatment

The surgical management of uterovaginal prolapse has seen many changes in recent years. There was an increasing use of graft material and tissue anchors for increasing durability of the prolapse repair. Thus prolapse repairs can be classified into fascial repairs and graft-augmented repairs.

Fascial repairs

Classically surgical treatment of a cystocele is by anterior colporrhaphy (Fig. 21.11). The operation consists of dissection of the prolapsed viscus (the urinary bladder) off the vaginal flaps, buttressing the pubovesicocervical fascia with durable delayed absorbable sutures and closure of the vaginal skin. Current practice does not include excision of 'excess vaginal

Fig. 21.11 Anterior fascial repair of cystocele.

skin', as the vagina is expected to remodel and the perceived laxity all but disappears in 6–8 weeks' time.

Rectocele is repaired by again dissecting the prolapsing viscus (in this case the rectum) off the overlying vaginal skin and effecting a robust repair by apposing the torn ends of the rectovaginal fascia together with delayed absorbable sutures. Sometimes it is possible to identify the tears in the fascia, and often a reattachment of the torn ends suffices. Not uncommonly a rectocele is accompanied by a deficient perineal body where the perineal muscles are attenuated or retracted laterally, with the patient complaining of 'vaginal laxity' or sexual dysfunction. Intravaginal perineoplasty is the operation designed to treat these symptoms and involves lateral dissection to identify the retracted ends of the perineal muscles, apposing these in the midline and suturing the apposed muscles to the apex of the incision. This procedure helps re-create the perineal body and reduces the size of the genital hiatus, thus improving vaginal tone, and also corrects the vaginal axis. This operation is an improvement on the perineorrhaphy where the perineal skin is first incised and later excised but still fails to achieve the objectives stated earlier.

Where there is an enterocele, the procedure of choice is a McCall's culdoplasty. This involves the placement of delayed absorbable sutures through the cut ends of the uterosacral ligaments and the intervening peritoneum, hitching these successively to the vaginal vault. The aim of this operation is not just to treat the enterocele but also to prevent occurrence of vault prolapse.

The treatment of choice for uterine prolapse depends on the woman's preference for retaining her reproductive potential. If her family is complete, then a vaginal hysterectomy, usually with repair of the prolapsed vaginal walls, is the preferred approach. If preservation of reproductive function is required, then the uterus can be conserved by simply excising the elongated cervix that is fashioned to an appropriate length with suturing of the cardinal ligaments in front of the cervical stump. This procedure is known as a *Manchester* or *Fothergill repair*. The vaginal skin is then sutured into the cervical stump using circumferential sutures. Additionally the operating surgeon may elect to suspend the cervix by means of sutures taken through the sacrospinous ligament called *sacrospinous cervicopexy/hysteropexy*.

A similar procedure may be employed to treat vault prolapse occurring after hysterectomy; the procedure is then called *sacrospinous colpopexy* (*colpos* Gk: vagina).

Graft repairs

The earliest repairs using mesh have been to treat vault prolapse (Fig. 21.12). The prolapsed vaginal vault is treated by suspending the vaginal vault from the anterior longitudinal ligament of the sacrum using a synthetic mesh. This procedure is known as *sacrocolpopexy* – a procedure that can be performed laparoscopically, robotically or through a laparotomy. Needle-driven mesh kits were used for repair of vaginal prolapse. A Food and Drug Administration (FDA) report released in 2008 classified complications occurring

from these to be rare. However, with increasing use of vaginal mesh, this was changed in 2011 where the complications were no longer considered to be rare. Current literature suggests that most cases of pelvic organ prolapse could be treated without mesh, and there is no compelling evidence of greater success with mesh, particularly for vault and posterior compartment.

This evidence is mainly for older mesh, and there are no current randomized controlled trials (RCTs) about newer, lighter mesh. This does not apply to mesh used abdominally. Laparoscopic sacrocolpopexy is still considered a good option for level I prolapse.

Complications

Repairs, whether fascial or otherwise, can result in injury to the viscus being treated, i.e. bladder, small intestines, rectum or anal canal. The sigmoid colon or the ureters may additionally be injured when a McCall's culdoplasty is performed. The needle-driven devices were known to be rarely associated with damage to the deeper vessels in the pelvis and with more common occurrence of vaginal mesh exposure. Primary, reactionary and secondary haemorrhage may all occur with these procedures, as may infection. The immediate complications of vaginal hysterectomy include haemorrhage, haematoma formation, infection and, less commonly, urinary retention. The long-term complications are dyspareunia and reduced vaginal capacity, especially if vaginal skin is inappropriately excised. Fascial repairs, especially of the anterior compartment, may recur in about a third of cases. Posterior compartment fascial repairs perform better with only 20% recurrence. Inadequate support to the vaginal apex may result in recurrence of the prolapse of the vaginal vault. Mesh repairs were found to be more robust with lower rates of recurrence.

Urinary tract disorders

Structure and physiology of the urinary tract

The urinary bladder is a hollow muscular organ with an outer adventitial layer, a smooth muscle layer known as the *detrusor muscle* and an inner layer of transitional epithelium.

The innervation of the bladder contains both sympathetic and parasympathetic components. The sympathetic fibres arise from the lower two thoracic and upper two lumbar segments of the spinal cord, and the parasympathetic fibres from the second, third and fourth sacral segments.

The urethra itself begins outside the bladder wall. In its distal two-thirds, it is fused with the vagina, with which it shares a common embryological derivation. From the vesical neck to the perineal membrane, which starts at the

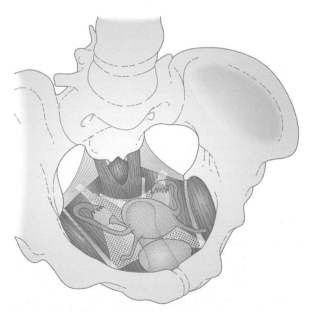

Fig. 21.12 Graft (mesh) used for vaginal prolapse repair (cystocele).

junction of the middle and distal thirds of the bladder, the urethra has several layers. An outer, circularly oriented skeletal muscle layer (urogenital sphincter) mingles with some circularly oriented smooth muscle fibres. Inside this layer is a longitudinal layer of smooth muscle that surrounds a very vascular submucosal venous plexus and non-keratinized squamous epithelium that responds to estrogenic stimulation. The continence mechanism is maintained by the urogenital sphincter, aided by the mucosal co-aptation of urethral epithelium and the 'bulking-up' effect provided by the submucosal venous plexus.

During micturition, the pressure in the bladder rises to exceed the pressure within the urethral lumen, and there is a fall in urethral resistance. The tone of muscle fibres around the bladder neck is reduced by central inhibition of the motor neurons in the sacral plexus. The bladder fills at 1–6 mL/min. The intravesical pressure remains low because of compliance of the bladder wall as it stretches and reflex inhibition of the detrusor muscle. At the same time the internal urethral meatus is closed by tonic contraction of the rhabdosphincter and the tone of the urethral mucosa. During rises in intra-abdominal pressure such as coughing or sneezing, continence is maintained by transmission of the pressure rise to the proximal urethra (which lies normally within the intra-abdominal space) and an increase in the levator tone.

The ureter is 25–30 cm long. It runs along the transverse processes of the lumbar spine, anterior to the psoas muscle, is crossed by the ovarian vessels and enters the pelvis anterior to the bifurcation of the common iliac vessels. From there it runs anterior to the internal iliac vessels to the ischial spines, where it turns medially to the cervix. It turns again anteriorly 1.5 cm lateral to the vaginal fornix, crossing below the uterine vessels to enter the posterior surface of the bladder.

> The ureters are particularly vulnerable to surgical damage at two sites in the pelvis. One is the point at which the ureter enters the pelvis under the lateral origin of the suspensory ligament. At the time of removal of a large ovarian tumour, clamping of the ligament may incorporate the ureter as the tumour is pulled medially and the ureter is lifted off the lateral pelvic wall. Second, during a hysterectomy the ureter may be damaged by clamping or dissection at the point where it passes under the uterine artery before entering the bladder.

Common disorders of bladder function

The common symptoms of bladder dysfunction include:
- urinary incontinence
- frequency of micturition
- dysuria

- urinary retention
- nocturnal enuresis.

Incontinence of urine

The involuntary loss of urine may be associated with bladder or urethral dysfunction or fistula formation. Types of incontinence are as follows:
- **True incontinence** is continuous loss of urine through the vagina; it is commonly associated with fistula formation but may occasionally be a manifestation of urinary retention with overflow.
- **Stress incontinence** is the involuntary loss of urine that occurs during a brief period of raised intra-abdominal pressure. It is usually related to injury to the continence mechanism described earlier and lack of estrogenic stimulation and usually manifests around menopause. Examination reveals the involuntary loss of urine during coughing usually accompanied by hypermobility of the urethra and descent of the anterior vaginal wall.
- **Urge incontinence** is the problem of sudden detrusor contraction with uncontrolled loss of urine. The condition may be due to idiopathic detrusor instability or associated with urinary infection, obstructive uropathy, diabetes or neurological disease. It is particularly important to exclude urinary tract infection.
- **Mixed urge and stress incontinence** occurs in a substantial number of women. Women with urge incontinence also have true stress incontinence, and it is particularly important to treat the detrusor instability prior to correcting stress incontinence. Failure to do so may lead to a worsening of the condition.
- **Overflow incontinence** occurs when the bladder becomes dilated or flaccid with minimal or no tone/function. It is not uncommon after vaginal delivery or when the bladder is 'neglected' after a spinal anaesthetic. A bladder scan usually reveals the presence of a residual of more than half the bladder capacity. The bladder then becomes 'lazy' and empties when it becomes full.
- **Miscellaneous types** of incontinence include infections, medications, prolonged immobilization and cognitive impairment and in certain situations may precipitate incontinence.

Urinary frequency

Urinary frequency is an insuppressible desire to void more than seven times a day or more than once a night. It affects 20% of women aged between 30 and 64 years and can be caused by pregnancy, diabetes, pelvic masses, renal failure, diuretics, excess fluid intake or habit, although the most common cause is urinary tract infection. The frequency may be diurnal (daytime) or nocturnal.

However, enhanced bladder contractility may occur without the presence of infection. Reduced bladder capacity may also result in frequency of micturition.

Dysuria

This symptom results from infection. Local urethral infection or trauma causes burning or scalding during micturition, but bladder infection is more likely to cause pain suprapubically after micturition has been completed. It is always advisable to perform a vaginal examination on any woman who complains of scalding on micturition because urethritis is associated with vaginitis and vaginal infection.

Urinary retention

Acute urinary retention is less of a problem in women. However, it can be seen:

- after vaginal delivery and episiotomy
- following operative delivery
- after vaginal repair procedures, particularly those operations that involve the posterior vaginal wall and perineum
- in menopause – spontaneous obstructive uropathy is more likely to occur in menopausal women
- in pregnancy – a retroverted uterus may become impacted in the pelvis towards the end of the first trimester
- when inflammatory lesions of the vulva are present
- as a result of untreated over-distension of the bladder (such as following delivery), neuropathy or malignancy.

Nocturnal enuresis or bed-wetting

This is urinary incontinence occurring during sleep and may have a psychological basis to it from childhood.

Diagnosis

The diagnosis is initially indicated by the history. Continuous loss of urine indicates a fistula, but not all fistulas leak urine continuously. The fistulous communication usually occurs between the bladder and vagina, *vesicovaginal fistula*, and the ureter and vagina, *ureterovaginal fistula*. Fistula formation results from:

- obstetric trauma associated with obstructed labour
- surgical trauma
- malignant disease
- radiotherapy.

There are other types of fistula with communications between bowel and urinary tract and between bowel and vagina, but these are less common.

Rectovaginal fistulas have a similar pathogenesis, with the additional factor of perineal breakdown after a third-degree tear.

Urinary fistulas are localized by:

- cystoscopy
- intravenous urogram
- instillation of methylene blue via a catheter into the bladder; the appearance of dye in the vagina indicates a vesicovaginal fistula.

The differential diagnosis between stress and urge incontinence is more difficult and is often unsatisfactory. Adequate preoperative assessment is important if the correct operation is to be employed or if surgery is to be avoided. It is important to assess patients with a validated patient questionnaire (the Modified Bristol Female Lower Urinary Tract Symptoms Questionnaire is a good example) with a 3-day urinary diary and a pad test. These help the clinician gain an insight into how the symptoms of urinary incontinence affect the patient on a day-to-day basis. The bladder and urethra are assessed in the laboratory by urodynamics. This procedure usually involves three basic steps:

1. *Uroflowmetry*: The patient is asked to pass urine into a specially designed toilet that measures voided volume, maximal and average urinary flow rates. Flow rates of >15 mL/sec are considered acceptable, and it is expected that a normal bladder will completely empty itself. Flow rates of <15 mL/sec are indicative of voiding dysfunction and in the female often indicate a 'functional obstruction' rather than an anatomical one. Occasionally a powerful detrusor may cause the bladder to contract against a closed internal urethral meatus resulting in dysfunctional voiding, a condition termed *detrusor–sphincter dyssynergia*.

2. *The cystometrogram* (Fig. 21.13): Pressure is measured intravesically and intravaginally or, less commonly, intrarectally because intravaginal pressure represents intra-abdominal pressure and is subtracted from the intravesical pressure to give a measure of detrusor pressure. The volume of fluid in the bladder at which the first desire to void occurs is usually about 150 mL. A strong desire to void occurs at 400 mL in the normal bladder. High detrusor pressure at a lower volume reflects an abnormally sensitive bladder associated with chronic infection. There should be no detrusor contraction during filling, and any contraction that occurs under these circumstances indicates *detrusor instability*. An underactive detrusor shows no contraction on complete filling and indicates an abnormality of neurological control. The average bladder has a capacity of 250–550 mL, but capacity is a poor index of bladder function. Thus, cystometry is a useful method for assessing detrusor muscle function or detrusor instability, which may result in urge incontinence. In the presence of urethral incompetence, there is low resting urethral pressure, no voluntary increase in urethral pressure, inability to stop midstream, decreased pressure transmission to the abdominal urethra and large volumes in the

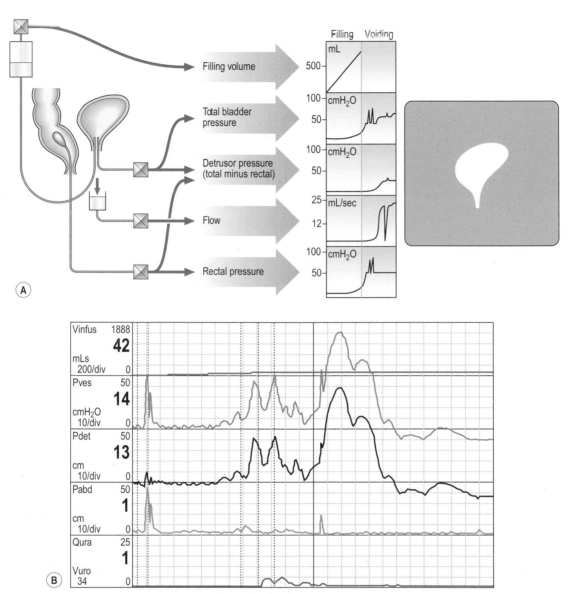

Fig. 21.13 (A) Bladder flow studies in the investigation of lower urinary tract symptoms. (B) Cystometrogram from a patient with idiopathic detrusor instability.

frequency/volume measurements. There is not always a clear-cut demarcation between the two conditions, as there may be a mixture of both stress and urge incontinence. Nevertheless, it is important to differentiate between the predominant influence of bladder neck weakness and stress incontinence and detrusor instability and urge incontinence.

3. *Urethral pressure profile*: This is performed at the very end of the cystometry and measures the pressure within the mid-urethra, in particular, the maximum urethral closure pressure (MUCP). This is of value in predicting the likelihood of surgical success after an anti-incontinence procedure. Pressures <20 cm of H_2O are predictive of poorer outcomes.

In some units an endoscopic view of the bladder called *cystoscopy* and an ultrasound scan of the pelvic floor are the additional procedures performed in the evaluation of the incontinent woman.

Management

Urinary tract fistula

In the developed world, most urinary tract fistulas result from surgical trauma. The commonest fistulas are vesico-vaginal or ureterovaginal and result from surgical trauma at the time of hysterectomy, or sometimes following caesarean section.

A vesicovaginal fistula will usually become apparent in the first postoperative week. If the fistula is small, closure may be achieved spontaneously.

The patient should be treated by catheterization and continuous drainage. If closure has not occurred after 2–3 months, the fistula is unlikely to close spontaneously, and surgical closure is recommended. The timing of further surgery is still a subject of controversy. Until recently, a delay of 6 months was recommended, but there is increasing evidence that good results can be obtained with early surgical intervention. However, the fistulous site should be free of infection.

Surgical closure may be achieved vaginally by meticulous separation of the edges of the fistula and closure in layers of the bladder and vagina. Postoperative care includes continuous catheter drainage for 1 week and antibiotic cover. An abdominal approach to the fistula can also be used and has some advantages, allowing the interposition of omentum in cases where there is a large fistula.

Ureterovaginal fistulas are usually treated by reimplantation of the damaged ureter into the bladder.

Stress incontinence

Stress incontinence should be managed initially by pelvic floor physiotherapy. Surgical treatment is indicated where there is a failure to respond to conservative management. In the presence of anterior vaginal wall prolapse, *anterior repair*, with the placement of buttressing sutures at the bladder neck, has the virtue of simplicity. It will certainly relieve the prolapse, but the results are variable as far as the stress incontinence is concerned, with relief in about 40–50% of cases. It is of no value in the absence of evidence of prolapse.

The following procedures are commonly used:
- Mid-urethral slings (Fig. 21.14):
  - **Retropubic sling:** Mid-urethral support can be achieved by placement of a tension-free vaginal tape. A polypropylene tape is inserted through a sub-urethral vaginal incision and guided via a needle paravesically to exit behind the symphysis pubis. This can be carried out under local, regional or general anaesthetic, and the tape is placed mid-urethrally in a tension-free manner. A cystourethroscopy is performed intraoperatively to rule out damage to the bladder and urethra. As this procedure is minimally

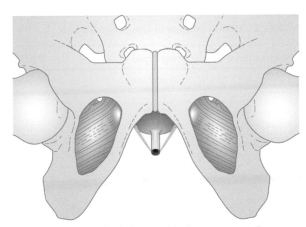

Fig. 21.14 Mid-urethral sling used in the treatment of stress incontinence.

invasive, most women are able to return to normal activity within 1–2 weeks. The long-term success rates are around 80%.
  - **Trans-obturator sling:** Less invasive compared to retropubic sling, performed by passing needles through the obturator foramina.
- Miscellaneous procedures still in vogue:
  - **Laparoscopic Burch colposuspension** involves bladder neck elevation by suturing the upper lateral vaginal walls to the iliopectineal ligaments under laparoscopic control. The success rates are around 60%, and the procedure results in voiding dysfunction in a significant majority of patients. This procedure was more or less invalidated by the more popular and safer mid-urethral slings but now is resurging due to the concerns around mesh.
  - **Transurethral injections:** Injectable bulking agents can be injected via a cystoscope into the mid-urethra. These are simple procedures with very little perioperative morbidity and have success rates of about 40–60%. These are useful adjuncts to the mid-urethral slings, especially in recurrences and in women with multiple failed operations. The commonest agents employed are collagen (glutaraldehyde cross-linked bovine collagen), silicon (macroparticulate silicon particles), Durasphere (pyrolytic carbon-coated beads), Bulkamid, etc.

The unstable bladder: overactive bladder syndrome (OAB)

The features of the unstable bladder are those of frequency of micturition and nocturia, urgency and urge incontinence. When confronted with this history, it is important to obtain some indication of the frequency as related to fluid intake and output. A chart should therefore be kept by the patient to clarify this aspect.

Table 21.3 Drug therapy of overactive bladder

Drug name	Drug type	Dosage	Available doses	Side effects
Oxybutynin	Antimuscarinic	2.5–5 mg PO tid	5-mg tablet, 5-mg/mL syrup	Dry mouth, constipation, dizziness, palpitations, anorexia, nausea, amblyopia
Oxybutynin (transdermal)	See earlier	3.9 mg/d; patch changed twice weekly	36-mg patch	
Tolterodine (short-acting)	M_3-selective antimuscarinic	1–2 mg PO bid	1-, 2-mg tablet	
Tolterodine (long-acting)	See earlier	2–4 mg PO once daily	2-, 4-mg capsule	
Trospium chloride	Antimuscarinic quaternary amine	20 mg PO bid	20-mg tablet	
Darifenacin	M_3-selective antimuscarinic	7.5–15 mg PO daily	7.5-, 15-mg tablet	
Solifenacin	M_3-selective antimuscarinic 5–10 mg PO once daily	5–10 mg PO once daily	5-, 10-mg tablets	
Imipramine hydrochloride	Tricyclic antidepressant, anticholinergic, adrenergic, antihistamine	10–25 mg PO bid-tid	10-, 25-, 50-mg tablets	
Mirabegron	B_3 agonist	25–50 mg once daily	25-, 50-mg tablet extended release	Palpitations, headache

The assessment of predisposing factors includes urine culture, urinary flow rates and urodynamic studies.

Treatment will obviously be directed at the cause, so the presence of urinary tract infection necessitates the administration of the appropriate antibiotic therapy. Postmenopausal women with atrophic vaginal epithelium and symptoms of urgency and frequency often respond to replacement therapy with low-dose oestrogens.

Detrusor instability of unknown aetiology

If the problem arises at a cerebral level, psychotherapeutic measures are indicated. Bladder drill involves a regimen of gradually increasing the voiding interval on a recorded pattern. This is effective in the short term, but the relapse rate is high.

The placebo response rate in detrusor instability is more than 40%, and spontaneous remissions occur.

Drug treatment

The alternative approach is to use anticholinergic drugs that act at the level of the bladder wall. These act on the muscarinic receptors on the bladder wall and cause relaxation. Some of these drugs are more specific and act on M_3 receptors. The more specific the drug, the less likely it is to cause side effects. The drugs listed in Table 21.3 are in increasing order of specificity and better side effect profile.

Botulinum toxin A (Botox): This drug is now being used effectively to manage OAB and neurogenic bladder. Botox can be injected under local, sedation or general anaesthesia. Each unit performing these needs to ensure they have a strict trial of void (TOV) protocol and back-up plan in case of voiding dysfunction.

Pelvic floor physiotherapy: pelvic floor muscle training

In women who have mild to moderate symptoms of urinary incontinence, pelvic floor muscle training (PFMT) may allow improvement, if not cure. Also known as *Kegel exercises*, PFMT entails voluntary contraction of the levator ani muscles. These need to be repeated several times a day up to 50 or 60 times to be of any clinical benefit.

The specifics are a bit variable, being very clinician specific and dependent on the clinical setting. Most patients find isolating the levator ani muscles most challenging and often contract their abdominal muscles instead. Therefore it is imperative that these exercises be demonstrated by a physiotherapist with a special interest in pelvic floor rehabilitation. To augment efficacy of these exercises, weighted vaginal cones or obturators may be placed into the vagina during Kegel exercises. These provide resistance against which pelvic floor muscles can work.

Electrical stimulation (interferential therapy)

As an alternative/adjunct to active pelvic floor contraction, a vaginal probe may be used to deliver low-frequency electrical stimulation to the levator ani muscles. Although the mechanism is unclear, electrical stimulation may be used to improve either stress urinary incontinence (SUI) or urge incontinence. With urge incontinence, traditionally a low frequency is applied, whereas higher frequencies are used for SUI.

Biofeedback therapy

Many behavioural techniques, often considered together as *biofeedback therapy,* measure physiological signals such as muscle tension and then display them to a patient in real time. In general, visual, auditory and/or verbal feedback cues are directed to the patient during these therapy sessions. These cues provide immediate performance evaluation to a patient. Specifically, during biofeedback for PFMT, a sterile vaginal probe that measures pressure changes within the vagina during levator ani muscle contraction is typically used. Readings reflect an estimate of muscle contraction strength. Treatment sessions are individualized, dictated by the underlying dysfunction and modified based on response to therapy. In many cases, reinforcing sessions at various subsequent intervals may also prove advantageous.

Dietary modifications

Patients are encouraged to avoid carbonated drinks and caffeine and commence cranberry tablets because these often help with reducing symptoms of urgency and frequency.

Timed voiding

Patients are encouraged to void 'by the clock' in an attempt to limit the waves of urgency that patients with OAB symptoms often experience. Over time the bladder is able to hold successively increasing volumes without resulting in leakage.

Vaginal oestrogen

Oestrogen has been shown to increase urethral blood flow and increase alpha-adrenergic receptor sensitivity, thereby increasing urethral coaptation and urethral closure pressure. In theory, **oestrogen** may increase collagen deposition and increase vascularity of the periurethral capillary plexus. These are purported to improve urethral coaptation. Thus, for incontinent women who are atrophic, administration of exogenous **oestrogen** is reasonable.

Bladder outlet obstruction

Primary bladder neck obstruction in the female probably results from the failure of the vesical neck to open during voiding and can be treated either with α-adrenergic blocking agents like tamsulosin, urethral dilatation or urethrotomy. Secondary outlet obstruction is usually associated with previous surgery for incontinence and may respond to urethral dilatation, but the results are not particularly good.

The neuropathic bladder

Loss of bladder function may be associated with a variety of conditions that affect the central nervous system. These conditions may also be associated with alteration in bowel function, sexual dysfunction and loss of function of the lower limbs.

Presentation

The neuropathic bladder is a reflection of dyssynergy between the activity of the detrusor muscle and the bladder sphincter. This results in a variety of disorders ranging from the 'automatic bladder' through retention with overflow at high or low pressure to total stress incontinence. It may also be associated with renal failure.

Aetiology

The causation may be suprapontine, such as a cerebrovascular accident, Parkinson's disease or a cerebral tumour. Infrapontine causes include cord injuries or compression, multiple sclerosis and spina bifida. Peripheral autonomic neuropathies that affect bladder function may be idiopathic or diabetic and, occasionally, secondary to surgical injury.

Diagnosis

The diagnosis is established by a systematic search for the cause involving cystometry, urinary flow rate studies, neurological screening, brain scan, pyelography and renal isotope scans.

Management

The management clearly depends on establishing the cause, but symptomatically it also involves non-surgical management using absorptive pads and clean intermittent self-catheterization. Anticholinergic drugs also have a place for some patients. Surgical treatment includes the use of artificial sphincters and sacral nerve stimulators. Palliative therapy can be in terms of suprapubic catheters.

Painful bladder syndrome

Chronic bladder pain in the absence of a known aetiology was known as interstitial cystitis (IC). Painful bladder syndrome and IC can be used interchangeably. The pathogenesis is poorly understood, and the aim of treatment is mainly towards symptom relief. It is usually diagnosed in the fourth decade of life, but symptoms in younger populations have been noted.

Diagnosis is made on the basis of history of specific symptoms and excluding other causes for the pain.

Management

A systematic approach with conservative medical therapies and/or bladder injections or instillations is considered.

Self-management and behaviour modification play an important role. Avoiding certain activities, foods and beverages that exacerbate symptoms can help. Analgesics in the form of oral, transdermal and bladder instillations can be done as well.

Amitriptyline, pentosan polysulphate sodium and antihistamines have been found to have a modest effect. Third-line therapy involves bladder distension and submucosal injection with steroids and local anaesthetic. Further management with sacral neuromodulation and cyclosporine is being studied.

Essential information

Prolapse

- May involve anterior or posterior vaginal wall with varying degrees of uterine descent
- Predisposing factors include high parity, chronically raised intra-abdominal pressure and hormonal changes
- Symptoms depend on degree of prolapse and whether bowel or bladder neck involved
- May undergo spontaneous improvement up to 6 months postpartum
- Treatment of choice is surgical repair ± hysterectomy
- No treatment required for asymptomatic minor degrees of prolapse

Stress incontinence

- Involuntary loss of urine causing social or hygienic problems and objectively demonstrable

- Commonly associated with prolapse of the anterior compartment
- Associated with detrusor instability in up to 30% of cases

Detrusor instability

- Presents as frequency, urgency, nocturia and incontinence
- Usually idiopathic but needs to be distinguished from obstructive uropathy, diabetes, neurological disorders and infection
- May present as stress incontinence
- Management includes bladder drill, anticholinergics and treatment of infection

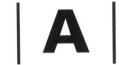

Appendix | A |

Principles of perioperative care

Stergios K. Doumouchtsis

LEARNING OUTCOMES

After studying this appendix you should be able to:

Knowledge criteria

- List the principles of infection control.
- Describe the appropriate use of blood and blood products.
- Discuss the general pathological principles of postoperative care.
- Describe the principles of fluid–electrolyte balance and wound healing.
- Understand aspects of surgical safety in the operating theatre.
- Describe principles of enhanced recovery.

Clinical competencies

- Plan perioperative care for a patient undergoing the common gynaecological procedures.
- Recognize the normal postoperative course.
- Interpret relevant postoperative investigations.
- Recognize symptoms and signs of common postoperative complications.
- Initiate a management plan for common/serious postoperative complications.

Preoperative care

Patient counselling and consent (see also Appendix C)

Selecting the appropriate procedure for the appropriate patient should include detailed counselling and informed consent. The patient should be informed about the proposed procedure and its risks and benefits, adverse events and other procedures that may become necessary; length of hospital stay; anaesthesia; recovery; tissue examination, storage and disposal; use of multimedia in records; teaching; and alternative therapies available, including no treatment. If there are any procedures that the patient would specifically not wish to be performed, this needs to be documented.

Risks should ideally be presented as a frequency or percentage and estimated according to individual risk factors. Consent should be obtained by someone who is capable of performing the procedure or has experience of the procedure and confirmed by the operating or supervising surgeon.

Preoperative assessment

Clinical history

Clinical history should include medical and surgical history, medications and allergies, as well as information related to the medical condition for which the procedure is planned; co-morbidities and factors related to risks of complications; personal or family history or risk factors for thromboembolism; and personal or family history of anaesthetic complications.

The preoperative medical assessment should also include questions on chest pain or breathlessness, history of angina or heart attack, stroke, epilepsy, neck or jaw problems, kidney liver or thyroid disease, asthma, diabetes, bronchitis and other respiratory conditions.

Clinical examination

Preoperative screening of medical conditions or risk factors should be followed by clinical examination, including cardiovascular and respiratory examination to evaluate fitness for anaesthesia. A complete pelvic examination should be performed preoperatively. A pelvic examination is often repeated under anaesthesia to confirm the previous findings.

Investigations

Preoperative blood investigations include full blood count; urea and electrolytes for screening for renal disease in patients with hypertension or diabetes and in women on diuretics; liver function tests for patients with a history of alcohol abuse or liver disease; and group and screen prior to procedures with risk of bleeding and cross-match if heavy bleeding is anticipated or antibodies are present. The availability of a cell saver should be considered if significant bleeding is anticipated.

Blood glucose tests and HbA1C are indicated to screen for diabetes and assess diabetic control. Routine coagulation screening is not necessary unless the patient has a known bleeding disorder or has been on medication that causes anticoagulation. A chest X-ray is indicated for patients with chest disease. A pregnancy test should be undertaken in all women of reproductive age. An electrocardiogram (ECG) is mandatory preoperatively in patients with cardiac disease, hypertension and advanced age.

Medications

Aspirin should be discontinued 7–10 days before surgery, as it inhibits platelet cyclooxygenase irreversibly, so platelet aggregation studies can be abnormal for up to 10 days. Non-steroidal anti-inflammatory drugs (NSAIDs) cause inhibition of cyclooxygenase, which is reversible.

Clopidogrel bisulphate, an oral antiplatelet agent, causes a dose-dependent inhibition of platelet aggregation and takes about 5 days after discontinuation for bleeding time to return to normal. Patients on oral anticoagulants need to be converted to low-molecular-weight heparin (LMWH). Management of these patients should be undertaken by a multidisciplinary team involving haematologists.

Women with risk factors for venous thromboembolism (VTE) should receive LMWH thromboprophylaxis. The combined oral contraceptive pill should be stopped 4–6 weeks prior to major surgery to minimize the risk of VTE, and alternative contraception should be offered. The progesterone-only pill is not known to increase the risk of VTE. Although hormone replacement therapy is a risk factor for postoperative VTE, this risk is small and it is not necessary to stop prior to surgery. On the day of surgery, patients should be advised which of their medications they should take.

Preoperative preparation

Management of anaemia

Iron-deficiency anaemia should be treated with iron therapy before surgery. Recombinant erythropoietin (Epo) can be used to increase haemoglobin concentrations. To be effective, iron stores must be adequate, and iron should be given before or concurrently with Epo. When significant blood loss is anticipated in women who will not accept blood products, Epo may be used to increase the haemoglobin concentration preoperatively.

Gonadotropin-releasing hormone agonists may be used preoperatively to stop abnormal uterine bleeding and increase haemoglobin concentrations.

Autologous blood donation avoids the risks of HIV or hepatitis infection and transfusion reactions.

Antibiotic prophylaxis

Antibiotic prophylaxis should be administered intravenously before the start of the procedure. In prolonged procedures or where the estimated blood loss is excessive, additional doses should be administered. Co-amoxiclav or cephalosporins with metronidazole are the commonly used antibiotics. For patients with known hypersensitivity, alternative broad-spectrum agents include combinations of clindamycin with gentamicin, ciprofloxacin or aztreonam; metronidazole with gentamicin; or metronidazole with ciprofloxacin. In patients with a known history of methicillin-resistant *Staphylococcus aureus* (MRSA) infection or colonization, addition of vancomycin is recommended. Preoperative screening is recommended in women at risk for sexually transmitted infections, and antibiotic cover for *Chlamydia* with doxycycline or azithromycin should be given.

Skin preparation with an antiseptic and a sterile technique reduces the risks of infection. Minor procedures do not require antibiotic prophylaxis.

Management of diabetes

Good glucose control in the perioperative period is important for the prevention of diabetic ketoacidosis and healing and infectious complications. Oral hypoglycaemics should be stopped on the day of surgery and replaced by an insulin sliding scale, except for minor procedures in a well-controlled patient. People with type 1 diabetes should have a sliding scale commenced on the day of surgery.

Surgical safety in the operating theatre

Standard systems should be in place in the operating theatre to prevent and identify potential errors and failures that may lead to adverse events. Common measures to reduce risk include introduction of all team members, review of the patient's informed consent, checklists and team briefings before and after surgery. Ensuring the correct procedure on the correct site, administration of the appropriate antibiotic prophylaxis, patient handling issues, availability of instruments and other equipment and use of imaging when required are essential parts of a checklist.

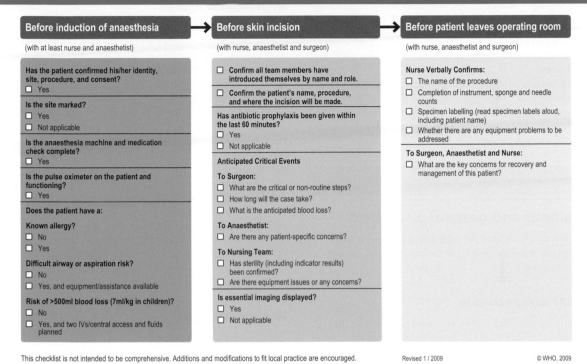

Fig. A1.1 The WHO Surgical Safety Checklist. (Reproduced with permission of the World Health Organization.)

A standardized checklist should be completed prior to the start of each procedure to ensure that all safety measures are followed. An example is the World Health Organization (WHO) surgical safety checklist (Fig. A1.1), which provides a set of checks to be done at three stages of a surgical procedure (sign in, time out and sign out).

The WHO Surgical Safety Checklist was developed with an aim to reduce errors and adverse events and increase teamwork and communication in surgery. The use of this checklist has been associated with significant reductions in both morbidity and mortality, as well as postoperative complications, and is now used by the majority of surgical settings worldwide.

Before surgery, a preoperative team briefing, or 'huddle', should be performed.

The entire team participates, including the surgeon(s), anaesthetist(s), circulating nurse(s) and scrub nurse. A preoperative briefing should include the following elements:

- Team introductions by names and roles
- Confirmation of patient identity and consent; the planned surgical procedure; and the site, side or level of surgery

- Identifying the patient's medical status and investigation results, with a management plan for medical co-morbidities
- Discussion of antibiotic administration
- Confirmation of VTE risk assessment and prophylaxis
- Ensuring blood group and save or blood product availability
- Determining ideal patient status monitoring and availability of equipment
- Verifying availability and proper functioning of all necessary surgical equipment and instruments and identifying any concerns
- Discussion of appropriate patient positioning, padding and skin preparation
- Ensuring team anticipation of critical or non-routine steps
- Discussion of postoperative plan (e.g. high-dependency or intensive care unit if appropriate)
- Invitation to all team members to ask questions and to speak up regarding any concerns

A debriefing postoperatively aims to establish that all steps have been completed, as well as to identify any problems or hazards and suggest improvements. A debriefing checklist includes:

- Completion of all documentation
- Checking of specimens and specimen forms for pathology
- Discussion of any equipment problems that may have been encountered
- Identification of any errors and issues on safety or efficiency
- Discussion of patient transfer and patient instructions after surgery

Errors and near-misses identified during debriefing are essential to be used in clinical governance and quality improvement processes.

Intraoperative complications

Regional and general anaesthesia

Complications related to regional and general anaesthesia include fluid overload, electrolyte disturbances and gas embolization.

Local anaesthesia

Serious adverse reactions are uncommon, but they are secondary to inadvertent intravascular injection, excessive dose and delayed clearance. Central nervous system side effects include mouth tingling, tremor, dizziness, blurred vision, seizures, respiratory depression and apnoea. Cardiovascular side effects are those of myocardial depression (bradycardia and cardiovascular collapse).

The adverse events associated with injectable local anaesthetic agents are reduced by attention to total dosage and avoidance of inadvertent intravascular administration.

Topical agents can also be associated with adverse events secondary to systemic absorption.

Complications secondary to patient positioning

Acute compartment syndrome

Compartment syndrome in the legs may occur due to the lithotomy position when the pressure in the muscle of an osteofascial compartment is increased, causing ischaemia followed by reperfusion, capillary leakage from the ischaemic tissue and further increase in tissue oedema resulting in neuromuscular compromise and rhabdomyolysis. Leg holders, pneumatic compression stockings, high body mass index and prolonged surgical time are risk factors.

Decompression techniques and early physiotherapy may reduce long-term sequelae.

Neurological injury

Injury to motor nerves arising from the lumbosacral plexus (femoral, obturator and sciatic nerves) and the sensory nerves (iliohypogastric, ilioinguinal, genitofemoral, pudendal, femoral, sciatic and lateral femoral cutaneous nerves) can occur with the lithotomy position and prolonged operative time.

Femoral neuropathy may occur secondary to excessive hip flexion, abduction and external hip rotation, which contribute to nerve compression. The sciatic and peroneal nerves are fixed at the sciatic notch and neck of the fibula, respectively. Flexion of the hip with a straight knee and excessive external rotation of the thighs cause stretch at these points. The sciatic nerve can be traumatized with excessive hip flexion. The common peroneal nerve is also susceptible to compression injury.

Ideal lithotomy positioning requires moderate flexion of the knee and hip, with limited abduction and external rotation. The surgeons and assistants should avoid leaning on the thigh of the patient.

Haemorrhage

Intraoperative haemorrhage is blood loss of more than 1000 mL or blood loss that requires blood transfusion. Massive haemorrhage is defined as acute loss of more than 25% of the patient's blood volume or a loss that requires a lifesaving intervention.

A loss of 30–40% of the patient's blood volume may result in cardiovascular instability. More than 40% blood loss is life threatening. Severe haemorrhage can lead to multiple organ failure and death unless resuscitation takes place within an hour.

The first step is pressure applied to the bleeding area. In laparoscopic surgery, pressure can be applied with an atraumatic laparoscopic grasper. In large-vessel bleeding, a laparotomy is usually required.

Diathermy, suturing or surgical clips can be used to control small-vessel bleeding. Vessels should be separated from surrounding structures before ligation to avoid inadvertent injury.

If initial attempts to arrest bleeding fail, bilateral internal iliac artery ligation should be considered but only performed by surgeons experienced with this procedure.

Topical haemostatic agents for control of diffuse, low-volume venous bleeding include Gelfoam/thrombin (Pfizer), an absorbable gelatine matrix; Surgicel (Ethicon), made of oxidized regenerated cellulose; FloSeal (Baxter), a haemostatic agent made from human plasma and constituted by mixing gelatine and thrombin; and Tisseel (Baxter), a mixture of thrombin and highly concentrated human fibrinogen.

The patient's haemodynamic status should be continuously monitored. Fluid replacement and transfusion of blood and blood products should be considered. Assistance of a second senior gynaecologist and anaesthetist, additional nursing and theatre staff and an additional surgeon with expertise in vascular surgery may be necessary. Blood should be cross-matched. Haemoglobin, platelet count, partial thromboplastin time (PTT) and activated partial thromboplastin time (aPTT) should be checked. If the PTT and aPTT exceed 1.5 times the control value, fresh frozen plasma should also be given. The ratio of red blood cells (RBCs) to fresh frozen plasma should be <2:1, as studies on trauma suggest that ratios of 1–1.5:1 are associated with reduced mortality. If fibrinogen is low, cryoprecipitate should be given and a haematologist involved.

Platelet transfusion is indicated if the platelet count is less than 50,000/mL. Acid–base balance and plasma calcium and potassium levels should be monitored.

A systolic blood pressure <70 mmHg, acidosis and hypothermia inhibit clotting enzymes and increase the risk of coagulopathy. Large volumes of fluids and transfusion of packed RBCs dilute the clotting factors and platelets and predispose to coagulopathy. Component therapy is used when there is clinical evidence of coagulopathy or microvascular diffuse bleeding.

If other measures fail to control bleeding, a pressure pack may be left in the pelvis for 48–72 hours. A pelvic drain will enable monitoring of continued bleeding. An indwelling urinary catheter allows urine output monitoring.

Ureteric and bladder injury

The incidence of ureteric and bladder injury during major gynaecological surgery is 2–6 per 1000 cases and 3–12 per 1000 cases, respectively.

Risk factors for bladder injury include endometriosis, infection, bladder over-distension and adhesions. In cases with adhesions, it is important to use sharp dissection of the bladder during a hysterectomy, as blunt dissection may result in injury. During laparoscopic surgery, the bladder should be empty to avoid injury with the trocars. Lateral rather than suprapubic trocar insertion will reduce the risk of bladder injury. Bladder thermal injury may be delayed and clinically manifest several days postoperatively.

Small defects less than 1 cm heal spontaneously and do not need to be repaired. A larger injury is closed in two layers using a running absorbable suture. The integrity of the bladder can be assessed by filling the bladder with indigo carmine or methylene blue dye. Ureteric patency is assessed using indigo carmine intravenously to demonstrate dye efflux from both ureters or by ureteric stenting. An indwelling catheter should be inserted for 7–14 days.

Ureteric trauma may be caused by transection, crush injury, de-vascularization or thermal injury. If ureteric injury is suspected, patency can be evaluated by intraoperative cystoscopy with dye or ureteric stenting. If there is doubt, a urologist should be consulted and, in case of confirmed injury, an end-to-end anastomosis or re-implantation can be undertaken.

Cystoscopy should be performed intraoperatively where possible after all prolapse or incontinence surgery to rule out bladder or ureteric injury. In undiagnosed ureteric injuries, patients present with symptoms of abdominal pain, fever, haematuria, flank pain and peritonitis.

Gastrointestinal injury

Gastrointestinal (GI) injury during gynaecological surgery occurs in between 0.05% and 0.33% of cases. Intraoperative GI injury has a mortality rate as high as 3.6%. Injury may occur during Veress needle or trocars insertion, adhesiolysis, tissue dissection, devascularization and electrosurgery. Previous abdominal surgery increases the risk of adhesions. In these cases, laparoscopy should be undertaken using an open (Hassan) technique or entry through the left upper quadrant (Palmer's point).

If an injury is suspected, the bowel should be examined and a surgeon's opinion should be sought if in doubt. Unrecognized injuries present 2–4 days postoperatively with nausea, vomiting, abdominal pain and fever.

Veress needle injuries do not usually need to be repaired in the absence of bleeding or a tear. For punctures of the large intestine without tearing, meticulous irrigation of the peritoneal cavity and antibiotic treatment are important, as the large intestine contents have a high bacterial load. Intestinal injury should be repaired in two layers. In extended lacerations, a segmental resection is recommended. Thermal injuries require wide resection due to the risk of tissue necrosis, which may take days to manifest clinically.

Injury to the rectosigmoid colon may be detected by proctosigmoidoscopy.

A diverting colostomy is indicated in extensive colon injuries or injuries involving the mesentery.

Gastric perforation during laparoscopy may occur in cases with prior upper abdominal surgery and an inadvertently gas-distended stomach following induction of anaesthesia. Small Veress needle punctures with no bleeding can be treated by irrigation. Larger defects such as trocar injuries require repair in two layers by a surgeon experienced in gastric surgery. The abdominal cavity should be irrigated to remove any gastric contents. Nasogastric suction usually is maintained postoperatively until normal bowel function returns.

Postoperative care

Analgesia

Analgesia should be planned preoperatively. Major abdominal surgery is likely to require an epidural or patient-controlled analgesia (PCA). This can then be gradually converted to regular paracetamol and an NSAID, with or without opioids for breakthrough pain. Anti-emetics and stool softeners should be prescribed with opioids.

Fluid and electrolyte balance

In the immediate postoperative period, it is important to maintain fluid balance and monitor serum electrolyte levels whilst a patient is on intravenous fluids. The normal fluid intake of approximately 2.5 L/24 hours requires additional replacement of fluid deficit due to intraoperative blood loss and insensible water losses. In cases of hyperkalaemia, an ECG is indicated for the assessment of cardiac rhythm, as well as calcium gluconate for prevention and management of arrhythmia and an insulin–dextrose infusion for the reduction of potassium levels. Hypokalaemia is treated by adding potassium in the intravenous fluids. Hyponatraemia is usually caused by excessive fluid intake, and hypernatraemia by dehydration. A fall in the urine output below 0.5 mL/kg/hour may indicate insufficient replacement. This can be confirmed with a fluid challenge of a colloid. Fluid challenges should be given with caution in elderly patients or those with cardiac disease, as this may exacerbate pulmonary oedema. If no improvement in urine output is seen, an assessment of cardiac and renal function is required.

Cardiovascular stability

Epidural analgesia, dehydration and bleeding are common causes of postoperative hypotension. This in turn can result in reduced tissue perfusion and impaired healing, cerebral infarction, renal failure and multiple organ failure. Unless the patient is stable, orientated, with pulse 50–100 beats/min, warm peripheries, capillary refill <2 seconds and a good urine output, further investigations to identify the cause are required.

Bladder care

An indwelling catheter in the postoperative period allows for accurate measurement of urine output and prevents urinary retention secondary to the general anaesthetic or pain. The catheter should be removed when the patient is able to mobilize. The trial of void involves measurement of the voided volume and estimation of the post-void residual volume using a portable bladder ultrasound scan. If greater than 150 mL, re-catheterization for 24–72 hours is indicated. With persistent voiding difficulty, the patient may need to go home with an indwelling catheter and return after 7–10 days for a trial without catheter or be taught intermittent self-catheterization until bladder function is normal, i.e. she has control of micturition.

Oral intake

Early postoperative oral hydration and feeding may reduce the length of patient stay without any increase in ileus. If there is vomiting, feeding should be delayed. With persistent vomiting, bowel obstruction should be excluded. Other symptoms include abdominal pain and an absence of passage of flatus or faeces. Signs include abdominal distension and tenderness with pronounced bowel sounds. An abdominal X-ray would show dilated loops of bowel. Management involves nil by mouth, intravenous fluids and insertion of a nasogastric tube. If there is no improvement, further contrast imaging is required to identify the site of obstruction for surgical intervention. In cases at high risk of paralytic ileus (excessive bowel handling or bowel injury), a nasogastric tube should be inserted with slower introduction of diet.

Postoperative complications

Postoperative haemorrhage

Signs of intra-abdominal bleeding include tachycardia, hypotension, abdominal distension, oliguria, confusion, sweating and abdominal pain. Minimal bleeding can be managed expectantly with monitoring, serial haemoglobin measurements and transfusion if indicated. Small retroperitoneal hematomas may eventually be reabsorbed. Patients with shock and increasing abdominal girth require immediate surgical exploration.

Pelvic arterial embolization can be considered for haemodynamically stable women with active arterial bleeding.

Pyrexia

An isolated episode of pyrexia >38°C within the first 24 hours will usually resolve with conservative measures, but persistent pyrexia or pyrexia after 24 hours is likely to represent infection. Identification of the source and early treatment aim to reduce morbidity. Examination of the chest, heart, abdomen, wound and legs should be followed by blood tests, including full blood count, C-reactive protein, urea and electrolytes and liver function tests. A mid-stream urine or catheter specimen should be sent for microscopy, culture and sensitivity along with blood and sputum cultures.

A chest X-ray enables investigation for pneumonia or atelectasis. Regular paracetamol will reduce pyrexia, and fluid administration is required to replace increased losses.

Surgical site infections

Surgical site infections (SSIs) can be caused by endogenous flora of the skin or vagina. Common organisms in SSIs of abdominal incisions are *S. aureus*, coagulase-negative staphylococci, *Enterococcus* spp. and *Escherichia coli*. SSIs of vaginal procedures include Gram-negative bacilli, enterococci, group B streptococci and anaerobes from the vagina and perineum. Postoperative pelvic abscesses are commonly associated with anaerobes.

Risk factors include diabetes, smoking, systemic steroid medication, radiotherapy, poor nutrition, obesity, prolonged hospitalization and blood transfusion. Surgical factors associated with SSIs include prolonged operating time, excessive blood loss, hypothermia, hair removal by shaving and surgical drains.

SSIs can be superficial incisional, deep incisional and involve organ or space, i.e. vaginal cuff cellulitis and pelvic abscess.

The most serious form of SSI is necrotizing fasciitis, often caused by a poly-microbial infection that can rapidly lead to necrosis of the surrounding tissue, sepsis and end-organ damage.

Laboratory investigations include a full blood count and culture from the incision or abscess discharge. When organ or space SSIs are suspected, computed tomography (CT) scan, magnetic resonance imaging (MRI) or ultrasonography is indicated to localize the site of infection.

Treatment

Patients with wound cellulitis can be treated as outpatients with oral antibiotics. Admission and intravenous antibiotic treatment are indicated in cases of pyrexia, peritonitis, intra-abdominal or pelvic abscess; inability to tolerate oral antibiotics; or other signs of sepsis. In a localized wound infection, incision and drainage are indicated. In the absence of an abscess, cuff cellulitis can be treated with oral antibiotics.

In case of deep incisional or organ/space infections, intravenous broad-spectrum antibiotics should be

continued until the patient is apyrexial and clinically well for at least 24–48 hours. If patients do not demonstrate systemic improvement and if there is no resolution of fever within 48 hours, repeat imaging and change of antibiotics following consultation with a microbiologist should be considered.

Septic pelvic thrombophlebitis should be ruled out in patients who are not responding to broad-spectrum antibiotics in the absence of an abscess or haematoma. Treatment includes antibiotics and intravenous heparin.

Superficial abscesses should be opened and drained. After debridement of necrotic tissue, wound healing may be facilitated with packing, wound vacuum or secondary closure after re-granulation. In deep incisional and organ/space infections, debridement and drainage are occasionally required.

Necrotizing fasciitis is life threatening and requires immediate, wide, local debridement and broad-spectrum intravenous antibiotics.

Cardiovascular and respiratory complications

Surgery and general anaesthesia increase the risk of myocardial infarction, especially in those with risk factors. An ECG and cardiac enzymes should be considered in a patient with chest pain. In cases of arrhythmia, differential diagnosis includes sepsis, hypovolaemia, electrolyte abnormalities and drug toxicity.

Respiratory complications include respiratory tract infection, atelectasis, pulmonary oedema and pulmonary embolism. A blood gas on air is required to determine the severity and adjust oxygen therapy. Assisted ventilation and admission to intensive care unit should be considered for patients with oxygen saturations <90% or a PO_2 <8.0 kPa.

Venous thromboembolism

If there is clinical suspicion of pulmonary embolism (PE), diagnostic imaging is required. If there is a delay in obtaining imaging, a treatment dose of LMWH should be administered.

If there is high clinical probability of a deep vein thrombosis (DVT) but a negative leg Doppler ultrasound, it may be appropriate to continue with treatment and repeat the scan after 1 week.

Computerized tomography pulmonary angiogram (CTPA) and isotope lung scanning after a chest X-ray are the recommended imaging investigations. In a positive diagnosis, a treatment dose of LMWH should be commenced and converted to oral anticoagulants once the patient is stable and the risk of bleeding is reduced. The patient should be referred to a haematologist and anticoagulation specialist.

Discharge from hospital

A discharge summary should provide information of the perioperative events, and the patient should be supplied with adequate analgesia and medications, as well as contact information in case of complications or concerns.

Enhanced recovery

Enhanced recovery is a care pathway that combines evidence-based elements of care pre-, intra-, and postoperatively to reduce physiological stress and organ dysfunction and enable patients to recover and resume activity earlier and to have a shorter hospital stay. Enhanced recovery pathways have been associated with reduced pain and nursing requirements and improved patient satisfaction and quality of life. These pathways should be individualized as indicated.

Patients undergoing elective gynaecological surgery with an overnight stay are potential candidates for enhanced recovery.

Enhanced recovery focuses on optimizing patient education and perioperative expectations, decreasing the perioperative fasting period, maintaining haemodynamic stability and normothermia, increasing mobilization, providing effective pain relief, nausea and vomiting prophylaxis and decreasing use of catheters and drains.

Preoperative enhanced recovery elements include assessment of the patient's health and fitness for a surgical procedure and optimization of any problems identified and preoperative patient preparation, as well as patient education (verbal and written instructions).

Intraoperative elements of enhanced recovery involve both the anaesthetists and surgeons. On the day of the surgical procedure, the period of starvation is reduced to 2 hours for clear fluids prior to anaesthetic to avoid dehydration. Interventions aim at perioperative pain control. Avoidance of long-acting sedative pre-medication is associated with earlier postoperative mobilization. Short-acting anaesthetic agents, ventilation measures, prophylaxis for postoperative nausea and vomiting and avoidance (or early removal) of nasogastric tubes are intraoperative measures commonly applied in enhanced recovery pathways. The use of minimal access techniques is strongly encouraged.

Postoperative enhanced recovery measures focus on early feeding, reducing intravenous fluid infusions, pain management, bowel function and mobilization. After gynaecological procedures, patients are usually discharged within 1–2 days.

Criteria for discharge include ability to eat and drink, ambulation and pain management with oral analgesia. Patients should be provided written advice on recovery and expected return to normal function, as well as emergency contact information.

Appendix 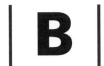 B

Governance, audit and research

Tahir Mahmood and Sambit Mukhopadhyay

LEARNING OUTCOMES

After studying this appendix you should be able to:

Knowledge criteria

- Understand the principles of storage, retrieval, analysis and presentation of data.
- Discuss the range of uses of clinical data, its effective interpretation and associated confidentiality issues.
- List the basic principles of the Data Protection Act.
- Describe the audit cycle as applied to obstetrics and gynaecology locally and nationally (specifically related to maternal and perinatal mortality).
- Discuss the role of guidelines, integrated care pathways and protocols, e.g. National Institute for Health and Clinical Excellence and the Royal College of Obstetricians and Gynaecologists guidelines.
- Describe the elements of clinical effectiveness, including evidence-based practice, types of clinical trial, evidence classification and grades of recommendation.
- Describe the principles of risk management, including incident reporting.
- Contrast the differences between audit and research.

Professional skills and attitudes

- Consider the principles behind good research design and critical analysis of research, including statistics and ethical issues.

Data collection in the National Health Service (NHS)

Patients connect with their doctors either in the primary care or in the hospital setting. The first interface usually occurs in the primary care setting, and that accounts for 80% of contact between the patient and the health system.

In the hospital setting, patients are seen either in outpatient clinics or as an emergency through acute admission units. A small proportion of patients will eventually be admitted to inpatient beds, either for further diagnostic workup or requiring surgical or medical intervention. At each stage of the patient's journey, information is collected either in paper form (case notes) or entered into electronic data systems (paperless notes).

The challenge for health care planners is first to ensure that the information collected at the primary and secondary interfaces can then be linked to national databases to define trends in disease patterns, population needs and future health service planning.

The second challenge is to assure that data sets are robust and 'clean' in such a format which can be easily analyzed. These data help in carrying out epidemiological studies such as maternal mortality rates. These data also allow international comparisons such as the World Health Organization (WHO) report on Maternal Mortality and regional comparisons in caesarean section and hysterectomy rates in England. Third, local quality improvement projects and cost efficiency heavily depend upon the accuracy of these data. NHS Right Care, a division of NHS England, provides data to commissioners for potential cost improvement in delivery of health care.

Sources of data collection and computing systems

General practitioner consultations and registrations

All patient interfaces with primary care are captured so that a picture can evolve on why patients are making contact with their general practitioners (GPs), such as diagnosis of depression, upper respiratory tract infection, arthritis, minor injuries, vaginal bleeding, contraceptive require-ments, etc. Furthermore these data can also be used to meet national quality targets by setting alert signals, for example:

- That >90% of women eligible for cervical cytology have been screened

Registration of births and deaths

Since 1838 there has been an enforced system of registra-tion of birth and deaths in England and Wales. As a junior doctor, you may be asked to complete a death certificate. It is important to follow the instructions carefully and make correct entries. A death certificate has two sections:
1. A direct cause of death
2. Contributory factors to the cause of death

It is a legal requirement to register all births irrespective of the place of birth. Therefore, it is possible to accurately know what proportion of babies have been born at home or in obstetric units.

Using these data, it is also possible to study in detail the changes in birth rates and death rates per 1000 population. Subtraction of the death rates from the birth rates gives the annual growth rate of a population.

Hospital Episode Statistics

Hospital Episode Statistics (HES) collects inpatient admin-istrative and clinical data transcribed from patients' case notes. The clinical data include the principal condition causing admission, other relevant conditions and the description and date of any operation performed. The administrative data include the date the patient was put on the waiting list, the source and date of admission, the spe-cialty, the date of discharge or death and the destination on discharge or transfer. The data provide overall activity data such as number of operations performed such as hysterec-tomies and caesarean sections, and this information can be used in the planning of hospital services such as local needs for maternity beds.

Mortality rates statistics

These are calculated from hospital admissions. The maternal mortality data in the UK have been reported through a triennial report since 1952. These reports tell us that major postpartum haemorrhage, hypertensive disease of pregnancy, infection and venous embolic dis-ease remain the major causes for maternal deaths. How-ever, since 2012, the maternal mortality report is now published on an annual basis and addresses one particu-lar theme making a bigger contribution towards mater-nal deaths. The *National Confidential Enquiry into Patient Outcome and Death* (NCEPOD) annual report analyzes

data on perioperative deaths and has reported that only 22% of the high-risk group were cared for in a critical care unit, thus receiving suboptimal care leading to their deaths.

Data on perinatal mortality rates (PNMRs) are collected annually. They include the number of stillbirths during pregnancy and deaths in the first week of life per 1000 live births. These data include all fetuses after 20 weeks of gestation or 500 g. Pre-term births are the most com-mon cause of perinatal death, followed by birth defects and small-for-gestation babies. PNMR is a major marker used to compare the quality of health care delivery among maternity units within a country and to compare quality of care worldwide. The Royal College of Obstetricians and Gynaecologists (RCOG) has been funded to study all still-births in depth to identify underlying cause(s) in each case to see if antenatal or intrapartum policy changes within obstetric units can reduce these losses. The RCOG pub-lishes an annual report, Every Baby Counts, which is acces-sible at www.rcog.org.uk.

Morbidity rates statistics

Hospital admissions data are utilized to look at the morbid-ity data related to specific diseases: for example, pregnancy-related morbidity data are captured by calculating the incidence of major postpartum haemorrhage (blood loss >2.5 L), admission to intensive care unit following delivery, stroke during pregnancy, pulmonary embolism and deep vein thrombosis, etc. In Scotland all cases of severe mater-nal morbidity are reported to NHS Quality Improvement Scotland, and an annual report (near-miss survey) is pub-lished showing comparative data for all the obstetric units.

Research and data linkage

Linkage of records gives us a picture of the full course of ill-ness and of the different illnesses occurring in the life of an individual. It is also possible to use record linkage between different databases to develop quality indicators such as patients' re-admission rates within 28 days with a diagnosis of deep vein thrombosis or the number of patients having a re-operation.

Data Protection Act

The Data Protection Acts in the UK and Australia seek to strike a balance between the rights of the individual and the sometimes-competing interests of those legitimate reasons for using personal information. Staff who hold or process personal data must abide by the following principles.

Personal information must be:
- Fairly and lawfully processed
- Processed for limited purposes

- Adequate, relevant and not excessive
- Accurate and up to date
- Not kept longer than necessary
- Processed in accordance with the individual's rights
- Kept secure at all times
- Not transferred to other countries unless the country has adequate protection for individuals

General Data Protection Regulations, 2018

The previous data protection laws were put in place during the 1990s and have not been able to keep pace with the levels of technological change. The General Data Protection Regulations (GDPR) were introduced on 25 May 2018 to update personal data rules. It is a mandatory regulation in EU law on data protection and privacy for all individuals within the European Union and European Economic Area (EEA). It also addresses export of personal data outside the EEA and EU. Therefore even companies and organizations registered outside the EEA and EU but operating within Europe must comply with this regulation.

Essentially the GDPR offers new rights for people to access the information companies/organizations hold about them, and there are obligations for organizations for better management of data or to risk a new regimen of fines.

The two key terms in the GDPR involve personal and sensitive data. Personal data can be anything that allows a *living* person to be identified directly or indirectly. This may be name, address or even an IP address. It includes automated personal data and anonymized data if a person can be identified.

Sensitive personal data include special categories of information. These involve sexual orientation, religious beliefs, political opinions, racial information, etc.

Under GDPR, personal data use must be:
- Fair (defined as good-faith approach to data use)
- Lawful (requires compliance with any applicable law)
- Transparent (this includes the notification and related communication obligation)
- Legal basis – data processing should have one of the following conditions: consent, contract, legal obligation, vital interests, public task and legitimate interest
- In addition, where the personal data relate to health, another legal basis must apply. The most relevant of these will be:
  - The provision of health care
  - Explicit consent
  - Protection of vital interests of an individual where they cannot consent

The GDPR also specifies data subject rights. Patients have new rights over their data.

- The right to be informed, usually covered by privacy notices
- The right of access to case notes, whether electronic or paper
- The right to rectification
- The right to erasure
- The right to restrict processing
- The right to data portability
- The right to object
- Rights in relation to automated decision-making and profiling

The GDPR also advises using reliable methods for transmitting data. If transmitting data over the Internet, an encrypted communication protocol should be used. Fax machines should be used as a last resort, and fax machines should only be accessible to people with legitimate rights.

The good old postal system is still considered to be more reliable.

Caldicott principles

In the UK the Caldicott Report (1997) recommended the appointment of a Caldicott Guardian in each NHS organization and that staff who handle patient-identifiable information ensure that the Caldicott principles are met whenever information is transferred, i.e. by word of mouth, written, by electronic or any other means.

When you consider undertaking a clinical audit which would require review of case notes, you must seek permission from the Caldicott Guardian of your hospital. This process ensures that you observe the principles of information governance and the data extracted are anonymized. You must not store data on your private computer. You can only use authorized encrypted USB drives.

Social media

Social media forms an important part in today's practice. The most familiar social media networks are Facebook, Twitter, Instagram and Snapchat. Within each platform there can be thematic networks like LinkedIn, Mumsnet, Patients Like Me, Metoo, blogs, video sharing, etc.

It is estimated that 60% of the UK adult population use some form of social media. The uptake amongst the younger population is higher. There are potential benefits and risks for doctors and health care professionals if they are engaging with social media. Whilst there are advantages of networking professionally and socially and the public accessing health-related information from professionals, challenges exist in maintaining confidentiality and professional and personal boundaries. It is therefore important that all doctors be aware of and adhere to the General Medical Council's guidance on the use of social media.

Evidence-based health care

Evidence-based practice is the process of systematically finding and using contemporaneous research findings as a basis for clinical decision-making and is an integral part of a clinical governance framework. In order to facilitate the development of evidence-based practice, the following processes need to be applied:

- Identify areas in practice from which clear clinical questions can be formulated.
- Identify the best related evidence from available literature such as guidelines.
- Critically appraise the evidence for validity and clinical usefulness.
- Implement and incorporate relevant findings into practice.
- Subsequently measure performance against expected outcomes or against peers.
- Ensure staff are supported and developed through adequate resourcing of evidence-based practice, education and training programmes.

Clinical audit

A clinical audit is the systematic and critical analysis of the quality of clinical care, including the procedures used for diagnosis and treatment, the associated use of resources and the resulting outcome for the patient. A clinical audit should seek to improve the quality and outcome of patient care through clinicians examining and modifying their practice according to standards of what could be achieved based on the best available evidence (Box B1.1).

Box B1.1 **Key facts about clinical audits**

- A clinical audit is not research but is focused on improving patient care.
- A clinical audit takes time and requires multi-professional involvement.
- A clinical audit should have a clearly defined question which needs to be addressed derived from the best evidence-based practice.
- A clinical audit requires adequate time for planning, engagement with stakeholders, collecting reliable data, analyzing and then presenting the results to the team.
- A clearly thought-out strategy is important to disseminate the best practice, implement it, monitor and demonstrate improvement in clinical care.

Four steps of a clinical audit

Defining best practice

The area identified must address important aspects of practice about quality of care, such as high infection rates following caesarean section.

The next stage is to describe current practice to illustrate the problem and identify areas for improvement. This can be done by looking at resources such as the RCOG Green Top Guidelines, Scottish Intercollegiate Guidelines Network (SIGN), National Institute of Health and Clinical Excellence (NICE), RANZCOG statements on women's health and the NHS evidence website.

Finally a particular area of interest is identified in the guideline that would help to define a 'standard' (a broad statement of good practice based on the best possible evidence) against which current practice can be measured (this is termed *criteria*). The criteria refer to resources used for the successful achievement of the standard (structure), the actions that must be undertaken (process) and the results (outcomes).

Preparing to monitor

The criteria should be easy to measure and to collect relevant data, and the collected data are useful clinically. Baseline data are collected first, which provides a starting point from which progress can be measured. The standard should be widely disseminated through newsletters and departmental meetings to the wards and the clinical staff to make them aware of the audit.

Monitoring your achievement

It is important to agree on a sample size and time frame with your clinical supervisor to complete the audit cycle. The hospital information system manager may have information about the number of patients with particular clinical conditions so that you can estimate how long it might take to collect your data. The next step would be to agree who will be collecting data and who will be recording it on an audit software package in order to generate timely feedback.

Planning for improvement

Once the audit data have been collected, the audit summary should be completed and the results carefully looked at in order to provide constructive feedback to the clinical team. The results should be discussed with the professional groups to ask for their comments for the interpretation of results and action planning. Areas of good practice are clearly highlighted, and areas that need to be addressed are clearly documented. A named individual should be identified so that appropriate changes in the policy can be implemented and monitored.

It is important to remember that a clinical audit is a continuing process, and one clinical audit quite often leads to a second clinical audit to demonstrate that the first audit cycle has made measurable changes leading to redefining unit policy or adopting new ways of delivering care to meet national standards. Therefore it is the responsibility of the doctor undertaking a clinical audit to write a detailed report and to make appropriate recommendations on how the next group of foundation doctors could continue with the same theme in order to ensure that the second or third audit cycle is completed.

National clinical audits

Maternal mortality and morbidity data are used as quality indicators for maternity services nationally and internationally. The maternal deaths are categorized as *direct causes* where there are obstetric causes and the death occurs during pregnancy or within the first 42 days following delivery. The commonest causes of direct maternal deaths are major postpartum haemorrhage, hypertensive disease of pregnancy, community-acquired infection and deep vein thrombosis. The *indirect causes* of death include non-obstetric causes such as suicide occurring within 1 year of childbirth. Every maternal death is analyzed in depth by a panel of experts. Similarly, perinatal mortality data are also collected. Their analyses provide data and trends on causes of perinatal deaths, and the main causes are unexplained stillbirths and deaths related to prematurity.

Clinical guidelines

Clinical guidelines have been defined as systematically developed statements to assist practitioners in patient management decisions about appropriate health care for specific clinical circumstances. The Green Top Guidelines of the RCOG are an excellent resource.

The development of clinical guidelines is a fairly time-consuming procedure and it can take between 18 and 24 months to develop the guideline from inception to completion of the task. At an earlier stage the clinical questions within a guideline are agreed. They provide the framework for the systematic review of the available evidence. The literature is synthesized and evidence is graded by using the Grading of Recommendations, Assessment, Development and Evaluation (GRADE) working group. It is also accepted that for many therapies, randomized controlled trials or systematic reviews of randomized controlled trials may not be available. In those instances observational data may provide better evidence, as is generally the case for their outcomes.

GRADE evidence levels: They are graded from level 1 (randomized controlled trials for a systematic review) to level 4 (expert opinion): more details are available at www.sign.ac.uk. Once the evidence has been collated for each clinical question, it is then appraised and reviewed.

Based on the level of evidence, recommendations are made within a clinical guideline.

Grading of recommendation: The recommendations for guidelines based on evidence are graded as Grade A (based on meta-analysis, systematic reviews or randomized controlled trials) to Good Practice point where clinicians make a consensus recommendation (www.rcog.org.uk).

Integrated care pathways have been described as the journey of a patient through all interfaces within the health care system and should take care of all the steps of patient journey from primary care to secondary and tertiary care. Each stage of an integrated care pathway should have a clearly defined checklist of recommended measures to ensure that the care providers have adhered to those recommendations and appropriate care has been provided.

The principles enshrined in a clinical guideline need to be adapted for local use (*local protocol*) so that a care pathway is developed for easy access to instructions on how to look after a patient within the local service provision and adherence to the local protocol can be monitored.

Research

The primary aim of research is to drive generalizable new knowledge, whereas the aim of an audit is to measure standards of care.

For clinical research, application is made for approval from a suitably constituted research ethics committee, whereas no such approval is normally required for a clinical audit.

There is a legal and a moral impetus to ensure that research is conducted with maximum respect for participants and their privacy, even if the research is not linked to clinical care. It is generally believed that explicit consent should be obtained to use identifiable personal data for medical research, particularly for multi-centre or secondary research where people who are not part of the clinical team need access to data. The skills, attitude and commitment of the people who manage and use a research database are important to protect the privacy of its data subjects.

Concern has been expressed regarding widespread misconduct in research. This dishonesty in publishing erroneous findings in order to promote careers or to get financial rewards has undermined public confidence in medical research.

379

Types of research studies

Descriptive studies

Descriptive studies provide information that can be used to test an aetiological hypothesis generated by other research methods. For example, the long-term toxic effects of tobacco and the relationship to the development of lung cancer were first discovered by epidemiological studies. Quite often descriptive studies have been used to substantiate suspicions arising from other sources, e.g. vaginal carcinoma in childhood resulting from maternal stilboestrol therapy, maternal hyperglycaemia during pregnancy associated with large-for-dates babies and pleural mesothelioma from asbestos exposure. Similarly, data on multiple sclerosis show that it occurs with the same degree of frequency in African Americans and Caucasians in the northern U.S. states. This observation suggests that environmental influences are critically important in determining whether the disease is common or rare.

Analytical studies

Two kinds of epidemiological observations are made in groups of individuals rather than populations and provide evidence that a particular event may be a cause of a particular disease. *Case control studies* compare people with the disease and those without it. *Cohort studies* compare people exposed to the suspected cause and those not exposed. The two types of studies answer two different questions.

To explain this, suppose that investigation is required to determine whether delivery by forceps and the accompanying trauma to the infant's head can result in brain damage, which can then manifest itself as childhood epilepsy.

A *case control study* would involve comparing the obstetric histories of a group of epileptic children with those of a control group of non-epileptic children. If it is found that the proportion of epileptic children with a history of forceps delivery exceeded the proportion of control children, this would suggest that forceps delivery may be a cause of epilepsy; but there are many other determinants of epilepsy so that among the group of epileptics only a small percentage of cases may be attributed to forceps delivery. This proportion can be calculated by using a mathematical formula.

A *cohort study* of the same problem would compare a group of children delivered by forceps with a group of children delivered normally. If it is found that the proportion of forceps-delivered children who developed epilepsy exceeded the proportion of normally developed children, this would suggest that forceps delivery is associated with and may be a cause of epilepsy. Forceps delivery does not invariably lead to epilepsy, which occurs in only a small percentage of children delivered in this way. By using mathematical calculations, it is possible to calculate the excess or attributable risk.

Clinical trials

Clinical trials are carried out in medical research and drug development to allow safety and efficacy data to be collected for health interventions. A clinical trial may be designed to:

- Assess the safety and effectiveness of new medication, e.g. antibiotics
- Assess the safety and effectiveness of a different dosage of medication than is commonly used, e.g. 5 IU of oxytocin instead of 10-IU dose for the third stage of labour
- Assess the safety and effectiveness of a surgical device, e.g. laparoscopic surgical instruments
- Compare the effectiveness of two or more already approved interventions, e.g. comparing medication 1 against medication 2

Clinical trials are usually conducted in three phases:

- *Phase 1* to test the treatment in a few healthy people to learn whether it is safe to take.
- *Phase 2* to test the treatment in a few patients to see if it is active against the disease in the short term.
- *Phase 3/4* trials to test the treatment on several hundred to several thousand patients, often at many different clinics or hospitals. These trials usually compare the new treatment with either a treatment already in use or occasionally with no treatment.

Randomized clinical trials can be:

- *Double blind*: The subjects and the researchers involved in the study do not know which study treatment they receive. This blinding is to prevent bias so that the physician should not know which patient was getting the study treatment and which patient was getting the placebo or, in a two-drug comparison study, whether it was drug A or drug B.
- *Placebo controlled*: The use of a placebo (fake treatment) allows the researchers to isolate the effects of the study treatment. It is important that the dummy treatment is closely matched to the active drug treatment. The patients in both study groups are monitored very closely for the impact of treatment and the side effects experienced by patients in both groups.

All clinical trials should be approved by the ethics committee and overseen by a panel of experts. It is important that before recruiting a patient into a clinical trial, an informed consent has been signed. The process of randomization is agreed to before the start of a clinical trial.

It is the responsibility of the clinical researcher to ensure that the safety of the subjects is closely monitored for any adverse outcomes. Therefore clinical trials of drugs are designed to exclude women of childbearing age, pregnant women and/or women who become pregnant during the study.

The results of the drug trials are sent to the appropriate national licensing authority.

Clinical governance

Clinical governance has been defined as a framework for the continual improvement of patient care by minimizing clinical risks (Box B1.2).

Risk management

Risk management simply means 'to develop good practice and reduce the occurrence of harmful or adverse incidents'. Clinical risk is defined as 'a clinical error to be at variance from intended treatment, care, therapeutic intervention or diagnostic result; there may be an untoward outcome or not'. For example, if patients in an obstetric unit develop wound infections following caesarean section, this results in an extended length of stay, increased patient discomfort and increased workload and cost for staff working in that unit. It is important to consider the broader issues surrounding this situation, such as ward cleanliness, lack of adherence to infection control policies, failure to follow national guidelines on sepsis prophylaxis and addressing education and training needs of the staff. Each unit should have a clinical risk strategy and a system in place for reporting, monitoring and evaluating

> **Box B1.2 Key attributes associated with promotion of a quality organization**
>
> - There is an integrated approach to quality improvement throughout the whole organization.
> - Leadership skills are developed in line with professional and clinical needs.
> - Infrastructures exist that foster the development of evidence-based practices.
> - Innovations are valued and good practices are shared within and without the organization.
> - Risk management systems are in place.
> - There is a proactive approach to reporting, dealing with and learning from untoward incidents.
> - Complaints are taken seriously and actions taken to prevent any recurrence.
> - Poor clinical performance is recognized, thus preventing potential harm to patients or staff.
> - Practice and professional development are aligned and integral to the clinical governance framework.

Clinical data are of the best quality and can be used effectively to monitor patient care and clinical outcomes (White Paper *The New NHS; Modern, Dependable (DH 1997)*.

clinical incidences and near-misses. *Near-misses* have been described as 'potentially harmful incident that could have adverse consequences for the patient/carer'. Similarly, there should be a system in place for *complaints reporting*, monitoring and learning from these complaints to improve patient care.

The National Clinical Negligence Scheme for Trusts (CNST) was established in 1995. With CNST specifically in obstetrics, each unit pays a premium based on the size of the unit and level achieved through CNST standards and receives a discount for managing clinical risks. There are three levels of CNST accreditation: the higher the level you achieve, the higher the discount. It has been recognized that the CNST standards have done much to advance risk management and reduce clinical risks.

Clinical incident reporting

Clinical incident reporting is required for staff and patients in highlighting any areas where an individual or organization fails to deliver the appropriate standard of care. Incident reporting offers a framework for the detection of untoward incidents and near-misses, which enable actions to be taken and lessons to be learned, practices to be reviewed and information to be shared to prevent any recurrence. Let us take an example of monitoring third- and fourth-degree perineal tears in an obstetric unit. These incidents are reported, and information is collated. Monthly reports will identify if the number of third- or fourth-degree tears are increasing following instrumental deliveries. That observation would call into question whether the doctors undertaking those procedures are appropriately skilled, trained and supervised.

Conclusion

It is important to appreciate that clinical governance is about assuring sustained, continuous quality improvement that can only be achieved by determined and conscious efforts by the clinical and non-clinical staff who have the appropriate support of their organization to deliver best practice. Quality improvement is based around the following robust systems and processes:
- clinical risk management and clinical audit
- continued practice and professional development
- implementing and continuing professional development within the NHS organization
- research and development
- evidence-based health care.

Appendix | C |

Medicolegal aspects of obstetrics and gynaecology

Roger Pepperell

LEARNING OUTCOMES

After studying this appendix you should be able to:

Knowledge criteria

- Discuss the issues of confidentiality and consent in under-16-year-olds (Fraser competency) and vulnerable adults.
- Outline the legal regulation of abortion, sexual offenders and assisted reproduction and the relative legal status of the fetus and the mother.
- Describe the principles of child protection.
- Describe the principles and legal issues surrounding informed consent.

Clinical competencies

- Obtain informed consent for the common procedures in obstetrics and gynaecology.

Professional skills and attitudes

- Be aware of the legal rights of and provisions for pregnant women.

Principles and legal issues around informed consent

When a woman agrees to a surgical procedure or a specific method of treatment, it is essential that the implications of benefits and risks are explained to her or informed consent to such treatment is obtained. Indeed, it is a fundamental law of medical and legal practice that a doctor must obtain consent from the patient for any medical or surgical treatment and that without appropriate consent, a procedure may constitute an act of assault or trespass against the person.

Second, the patient must receive sufficient knowledge of any proposed treatment to make a valid choice about whether to consent. The consent form provides evidence that consent has been given for a procedure, but it only has meaning if it is evident that the patient did understand the nature and implications of the procedure.

In explaining the nature of a procedure to any woman, it is important to explain the purpose of the operation and the potential complications. Given that there may be a range of complications for any operation, the question arises as to how far it is necessary to go in explaining all the potential complications, given that this may induce disproportionate anxiety about a series of very remote risks.

In general terms, a risk of more than a 1% chance should be explained to the patient, although this is a guideline rather than an absolute figure. Where the risk is well under 1% but is serious and would influence the quality of life subsequently if it occurred, this also needs to be explained in detail so that an informed decision can be made by the patient as to whether she wishes to proceed. However, the 2015 ruling on *Montgomery v. Lanarkshire* where a short-statured diabetic mother was not told about possible risk of shoulder dystocia and risk of hypoxic injury has brought in a new understanding of how risks should be explained and consent should be taken. The court ruled that whatever could be considered material risk to the patient should be explained to the patient rather than what the doctor thinks is the material risk that should be told. This would make counselling consent time consuming but more satisfying to the patient. Where non-surgical methods of treatment could be used instead of a surgical procedure, these also need to be explained to the patient.

A common example that addresses the issues of informed consent is the information given to patients before sterilization about potential failure rates. During the 1980s a substantial number of legal actions were based on alleged failure to inform patients that there was a significant risk of failure and that pregnancy could follow any of the commonly used sterilization procedures. The patient bringing a claim would generally allege that no advice was given about the risk of failure and subsequent pregnancy and that, had such advice been given, either the woman would not have had the operation or she would have continued to use contraception after the sterilization procedure. It is now standard practice to advise all patients, both female and male, that there is a risk of failure and to record a statement to the effect that such advice has been given. Regarding sterilization, the character of the menstrual cycle also needs to be borne in mind. Where the periods have been particularly heavy or irregular and have been controlled during treatment with the oral contraceptive pill (OCP), when the OCP is ceased after the sterilization, the abnormal periods will almost certainly return. If the patient is made aware of this likelihood, she may well decide to just continue the OCP rather than having the sterilization performed.

The failure of a sterilization procedure in either sex may result from a method failure or recanalization. In the female, a clip may be applied to the wrong structure, may transect the tube during application or may not remain closed. In each of these instances, pregnancy usually occurs within 6 months of the procedure. The second cause of failure is recanalization of the Fallopian tubes or, in men, the vas deferens. This may result in a pregnancy many years later and is an unavoidable risk of the procedure. Despite the signing of a consent form that records the risk of failure, errors of technique are generally indefensible.

> A consent form does not protect either the patient or the surgeon if performance of the procedure is faulty.

It is important that consent is obtained by a member of staff who is medically qualified and who signs the consent form with the patient after explaining both the nature of the procedure and the potential complications. Ideally the procedure should be performed in the follicular phase of the cycle or alternative contraception given in that cycle.

> Ideally, consent should be obtained by the surgeon who is performing the procedure. There are limitations as to what can be reasonably included in a consent form, and it is common practice to include a general statement, either in the text of the consent form or in the patient's records, that the risks and the intended purpose of the procedure have been explained to the patient. Such a general statement is often found to be inadequate when defending a medicolegal case, and it is much better if headings of the matters discussed are recorded on the consent form or within the medical record at the time the consent form is signed.

It is also important to ensure that the details concerning the patient's name and the description of the procedure to be performed are correct. For example, it is not sufficient to write 'sterilization' to describe the operation when the procedure may be tubal cautery, clip sterilization or tubal ligation. The actual procedure to be performed must be written on the consent form.

The consent form must always be available and must be checked at the time of admission to hospital and in theatre before any operation is commenced. The condition of the patient at that time, including the date and normality of the last menstrual period, should also be checked, where the procedure is being done more than 4 weeks after the previous review. The patient may have conceived in the interim and wish a change in the treatment previously proposed.

Litigation in obstetrics and gynaecology

Litigation in obstetrics and gynaecology has had a profound effect on the provision of maternity services. In the UK and Australia, the problem has been masked to some extent by Crown indemnity and its equivalent in Australia. The government provides insurance coverage for all doctors and midwives practising within the public health services. However, in countries such as the United States, closure of maternity units and the reduction of maternity services are common events because of the risk of litigation and the size of the costs to defend a case or settle the damages awarded. The costs of insurance must be passed on to the mothers, or the services cannot survive. The reality of the situation is that, regardless of the issues of fault, unless damages are capped, maternity services are often commercially uninsurable. Indeed, in many parts of the United States, obstetricians cannot purchase insurance coverage, as their specialty is too high risk.

When a patient decides to make a claim against her doctor, she will approach her solicitor. If the solicitor considers there is justification, she or he will advance the action by issuing a summons, seek access to the relevant case note records and then lodge an application for a hearing. If the case is to proceed, in England and Wales it will be heard in the High Court by Masters of the Queen's Bench Division. Cases may also be heard in the County Court if the costs are below a certain figure. In the UK, cases are heard before a judge and not a jury. In Australia, cases are usually heard before a judge and jury. The case usually commences with the barrister for the plaintiff outlining their perceived problem and the care given. This is generally reported widely in the daily press, often in large type on the first or second pages of the paper and often resulting in severe adverse publicity for the doctor or hospital concerned. If it is ultimately proven that the doctor or hospital was not at fault, it is rare for the press to detail these findings as widely, and the comments tend to be almost hidden in small type deep in the publication.

Medical litigation may occur soon after a problem has been perceived to have occurred by a patient but may be delayed for some years. Where the problem does not involve a child, the litigation process must generally be submitted to the Court involved within 7 years of the 'adverse' event occurring. Where the condition of the child is the reason for the litigation, the case should reach the Court within 7 years of that child reaching 'maturity' – in other words, the case can reach the Court any time in the 25 years after the 'adverse' event occurred. Because no one can remember exactly what happened 12 months ago, let alone 25 years ago, the documentation about any adverse event must be extensive and detailed. There also tends to be a long interval between the issuing of a summons and its hearing and between setting down a case for trial and the actual date of the trial.

Medical litigation is expensive, and it is not therefore surprising that most plaintiffs in the UK are supported by Legal Aid. In Australia, this is often not the case unless a large payout is expected. The Statement of Claim outlines the nature of the claim, and it is up to the defendant to respond and either acknowledge or refute the allegations. The legally aided litigant has considerable advantages, as the Legal Aid fund meets all costs and there is usually no penalty for failure of a claim.

> To speed up the resolution of disputes in the UK and in Australia, new regulations have been introduced through the Civil Procedures Rules and were implemented as guidance to expert witnesses from April 2002.
>
> The rules specify that the primary responsibility of an expert is to the Court and that this responsibility overrides any obligation to any other person from whom the expert has received instructions or payment.
>
> After providing a report, the format of which has now been standardized, the reports of the plaintiff's and defendant's experts are exchanged, and some Courts advise the various parties to put one list of written questions to the experts. These questions must be put within 28 days of service of the report, and the questions must be answered within a further 28 days.
>
> It is now common practice for the Court to order that the experts should also meet to discuss a common agenda submitted by the solicitors of both parties and to prepare a joint report outlining the extent of agreement and disagreement. The joint report should outline the reasons for any disagreements and should enable many cases to be resolved out of court, resulting in a substantial reduction in the legal costs involved.

The trial itself is an adversarial process, and the onus is on the plaintiff to prove that the staff failed to provide a reasonable level of care with the result that the patient suffered unnecessary injury.

During any trial, the major evidence tends to be drawn from the case records. As a resident medical officer, it is important to remember that case notes will be examined in detail and constitute a legal document. It is therefore important to record facts properly, and these guidelines should be followed:

- Entries into case notes must be clear, concise and factual and should detail the diagnosis, differential diagnoses, investigations arranged and plan of management to be instituted on that day.
- The details written on the next day should include the progress over the previous 24 hours, the results of investigations that are to hand, further investigations arranged (if any) and any change in the diagnosis or treatment to be given.
- All entries concerning intraoperative complications or problems should be detailed and preferably written by the most senior person in the operating theatre at the time.
- Entries should always be initialled and dated, and preferably timed. Although initialling should allow identification of the writer in the future, if required, it is better if the identification of the writer is printed or stamped in and the medical registration number included. Timing of the record writing is particularly important in the delivery suite, intensive care unit and emergency department where emergencies are more likely and the rapidity of care needs to be assessed.
- No attempt should be made to alter entries in case records without countersigning the alteration and indicating why it has been made. Retrospective information concerning an adverse event can be added to the medical record, providing it is dated, appropriately signed and factual.

If a letter is received from a solicitor asking for information with a view to initiating legal action, it is important to:
- Notify one's medical defence organization
- Notify the complaints officer in the hospital concerned, who will usually then notify the solicitors who represent them

Litigation commonly ensues when there are complications following a surgical procedure or where there is a perinatal death or the birth of a child who has brain dysfunction or skeletal or nerve injuries such as Erb's palsy.

> All the evidence available in the literature suggests that fewer than 10% of cases of cerebral palsy or mental retardation are related to the events that occur during labour. However, the difficulty that judges have is deciding whether, on the balance of probabilities, the adverse outcome could have been avoided or reduced in severity by more appropriate care during labour. If the judge decides in favour of the plaintiff, the quantum of the award will be assessed on the level of disability and the life expectancy of the child. This may amount to an award of several million pounds or dollars.

Shoulder dystocia resulting in damage to the brachial plexus is a common cause for litigation in obstetrics. The arguments proffered in such cases are that either the dystocia could have been avoided by predicting the likelihood of shoulder dystocia and delivering the child by caesarean section or delivering vaginally but at an earlier gestation when the baby was smaller, or that the damage to the brachial plexus could have been avoided by not using excessive traction and by changing the angle of entry of the pelvic brim by placing the patient in McRobert's position and exerting directed suprapubic pressure to deliver the anterior shoulder or using appropriate internal manoeuvres.

Other reasons for litigation against an obstetrician include:
- Inadequate screening for a possible fetal abnormality during the antenatal period because the patient would have requested termination had the abnormality been defined.
- Failure to recognize a baby was growth restricted and defining why.
- Failure to recognize a baby was going to die in utero and performing appropriate monitoring to prevent this.
- Failure to adequately assess the significance of a fetal heart rate abnormality seen on the cardiotocographic record obtained during labour.
- Allowing the second stage of labour to last too long, resulting in sphincter injury leading to bowel incontinence problems.
- Too long a delay between the time a decision was made to perform a caesarean section on the grounds of fetal distress and the actual time the baby was delivered, resulting in adverse outcome to the newborn.
- Not adequately treating a postpartum haemorrhage, resulting in the patient requiring a hysterectomy to control the life-threatening bleeding.

Litigations in gynaecology are often related to sterilization or contraception failure, complications occurring during or after gynaecological surgery (particularly when this has been performed laparoscopically) or failure or delay in diagnosing a malignancy in a patient.

Most obstetricians/gynaecologists will be the subject of a litigious claim during their professional careers, but the risk can be minimized by:
- Careful adherence to the principle of not undertaking procedures for which one is inadequately trained or supervised.
- Careful and considerate provision of information to the patient before any surgical procedure concerning the nature of the procedure and the possible complications.
- Prompt action if there are abnormal findings in any tests that necessitate intervention; for example, an abnormal fetal heart rate during labour demands a decision. The decision may be to continue observation, to

take a scalp blood sample for pH measurement or to deliver the baby. It is not acceptable to ignore the recording. The findings must be recorded in the notes as well as the decision concerning the further plan of care.

Patient confidentiality (including data protection)

The doctor normally has an ethical obligation to keep secret all details of a personal nature that may be revealed during consultation and treatment. The duty is not, however, absolute, as confidentiality may be breached under special circumstances. It must be remembered that unauthorized disclosure of information without the patient's consent is not a criminal offence, but it does expose the doctor to disciplinary procedures by the medical board or medical council of the country concerned. Disclosure may involve matters of public interest, particularly where the patient may constitute a risk of violence or transmission of infections such as AIDS to the public or to the immediate relatives.

Human immunodeficiency virus infection is not notifiable by statute, although in the UK, the General Medical Council (GMC) advises that doctors 'should make every effort to persuade a patient of the need for their General Practitioners and sexual partners to be informed of a positive diagnosis'.

Some acts of disclosure are compulsory by law, but do vary in different countries, and these include:
- Notification of births and deaths
- Notification of a treatment cycle of in vitro fertilization
- Notification of artificial insemination by donor

In all Australian States and Territories, HIV infections and AIDS-related deaths are notifiable conditions. The designated persons (doctors and pathologists) must notify their respective State or Territory health authorities who then forward coded data to the National HIV Surveillance Program. The notifier must provide the first 2 letters of the person's family name, the first 2 letters of the person's given name and the postcode. The full name or the address of the person diagnosed should not be provided.

Because of the time scales of possible legal action being taken against a doctor or hospital, it is necessary for all medical records to be stored for at least 7 years, or 25 years if the record includes pregnancy care, in case a problem occurs in the baby produced by that pregnancy".

The rules regarding abortion

The Abortion Act (1967) in the UK radically changed the availability of termination of pregnancy in the UK and had the effect of both legalizing and liberalizing abortion.

Under this law, termination of pregnancy can be performed under the following four conditions.

- That the pregnancy has not exceeded its twenty-fourth week and that continuance of the pregnancy would involve greater risk, than if the pregnancy were terminated, of injury to the physical or mental health of the pregnant woman or any existing children of her family
- That the termination is necessary to prevent grave permanent injury to the physical or mental health of the pregnant woman
- That the continuance of the pregnancy would involve risk to the life of the pregnant woman greater than if the pregnancy were terminated
- That there is a substantial risk that if the child were born it would suffer from physical or mental abnormalities to be seriously handicapped

Under the conditions of the Act, the decision to terminate a pregnancy must be agreed by two practitioners unless the practitioner 'is of the opinion, formed in good faith, that the termination is immediately necessary to save life or to prevent grave permanent injury to the physical or mental health of the pregnant woman'.

Termination of pregnancy must be carried out in a hospital vested by the Secretary of State for the purposes of his or her functions under the National Health Services Act (1977). In other words, premises must be licensed for termination of pregnancy. In addition, the need to ensure the fetus will not be born alive is a requirement where the pregnancy is terminated after 22 weeks of gestation. This often necessitates the injection of potassium chloride or other substances into the fetal heart under ultrasonic guidance to result in fetal death.

Notification is also a statutory requirement, first of the intention to perform an abortion and second of the performance of the termination and any complications during or after the event. This is perhaps why so much emphasis is still laid on notification when the Act itself is very liberal and in a legal framework that does not require notification of conception or sterilization.

In other countries, the rules concerning pregnancy termination and the availability of it vary dramatically. In some countries, abortion is not allowed, and any doctor performing an abortion or patient having an abortion can be convicted of a felony and punished appropriately. In Australia, there is no universal rule concerning abortion, although it is readily available in most, but not all, of the states. Those states that allow it do so under similar rules to those defined earlier in the UK. In Victoria, for many years, the Menhennitt ruling was applied, with this ruling being like the rules in the UK. Currently only the Australian Capital Territory and Victoria have decriminalized abortion.

Third trimester abortions are performed in some states in Australia, despite the existence of child destruction laws, presumably because they have satisfied the conditions

necessary for legal abortion. In public hospitals performing such procedures, the appropriateness of such an abortion is usually assessed and the procedure approved by a special medical and legal committee before it can be performed.

The use of assisted reproduction in infertility care

The Human Fertilisation and Embryology Act (1990) (which applies in the UK) provides the statutory authority that regulates all matters relating to assisted reproduction. The Act is long and complex and should be read by all personnel involved in these procedures. The Act is administered by the Human Fertilisation and Embryology Authority, which consists of:

- A chairman and deputy chairman
- Such numbers of other members as the Secretary of State appoints

The Human Fertilisation and Embryology Authority has the following duties:

- To keep under review information about embryos and any subsequent development of embryos and about the treatment services and activities governed by this Act and to advise the Secretary of State, if asked to do so, about these matters
- To publicize the services provided to the public by the Human Fertilisation and Embryology Authority or provided in pursuance of licenses
- To provide, to such extent as it considers appropriate, advice and information for persons to whom licenses apply or who are receiving treatment services or providing gametes or embryos for use for the purpose of activities governed by this Act or may wish to do so
- To perform such other functions as may be specified in the regulations

Overall, the Human Fertilisation and Embryology Authority has the power to license and supervise centres providing assisted reproduction and to decide which procedures are acceptable within the terms of reference of the Act. It also has wide-ranging powers under the clinical law, including, under warrant, the rights to enter premises 'using such force as is reasonably necessary' to take possession of whatever may be required as evidence of breach of the law and to take the necessary steps to preserve such evidence.

In other countries, similar bodies and legislation exist and control not only the availability of this treatment to appropriate 'couples' but also may include recommendations as to the number of embryos to be transferred to reduce the likelihood of multiple pregnancies and the place for pre-implantation genetic diagnosis and ensure that all patients having such treatment, whether donor gametes are required or not and who conceive, are appropriately registered for subsequent assessment by any child so produced. Any such child has a right to know how he or she was conceived and whose gametes were involved.

The relevant legal status of the fetus, the pregnant woman, the child and the pubertal girl

Although in some countries the fetus has legal rights as soon as conception occurs, in most the fetus has no legal rights in any trimester of the pregnancy but gets these as soon as it is born alive. It is therefore imperative that you are familiar with the law in the country in which you are working to understand what your responsibility is to the fetus when a woman is pregnant.

During the last few years in the United States, some Courts have been asked to decide whether a woman can be forced to allow a caesarean section to be performed on the grounds of an identified problem within the fetus but where she has refused such treatment, and in some instances caesarean section has been ordered. In others, the rights of the mother have been deemed to override those of the fetus and the pregnancy has been allowed to continue. In many other countries, the rights of the pregnant woman have clearly overridden those of the fetus, and Court applications allegedly on behalf of the fetus have not been made.

Once the child has been born, a Court will usually approve treatment of the child which has been refused by the mother, where that treatment may be lifesaving (such as blood transfusion for blood group immunization) or would reduce the likelihood of significant morbidity.

During childhood consent for treatment is usually given by the parents, with this generally accepted as being appropriate for most medical care, including serious illnesses, emergency care and for necessary operative procedures but *not* for sterilization. If the child is mentally disabled, again parental consent is appropriate for most treatment required. However, sterilization, abortion and the use of some forms of contraception such as an intrauterine device or Depo-Provera would usually require the approval of a Government Body, such as a Guardianship Board, which deals with the rights of a disabled child or adult.

Although by definition a child does not become an adult and achieve full adult's rights until the age of 18 years in most countries, thereby obtaining the ability to consent to treatment or the performance of operative procedures, a child younger than 18 years has been deemed mature enough to make such decisions under certain circumstances. These circumstances define Gillick competency or satisfaction of the Fraser Guidelines, which refer to a case in the UK in 1982 where a woman took a case to Court to prevent contraceptive advice or treatment being given to a child under the age of 16 years without parental consent. Ultimately, this case was settled in the House of Lords as follows: 'whether or not a child is capable of giving the necessary consent will depend on the child's maturity and understanding and the nature of the consent required. The child must be capable of making a reasonable assessment of the advantages and disadvantages of the treatment proposed, so the consent, if given, can be properly and fairly described as true consent.' In order to satisfy the Fraser guidelines, the doctor concerned must be satisfied that:
- The young person will understand the professional's advice
- The young person cannot be persuaded to inform their parents
- The young person is likely to begin, or to continue having, sexual intercourse with or without contraceptive treatment
- Unless the young person receives contraceptive treatment, their physical or mental health, or both, are likely to suffer
- The young person's best interests require them to receive contraceptive advice or treatment, with or without parental consent

The ramifications of this decision extend beyond that of the provision of contraception, because if the child is 'Gillick competent', he or she can prevent the parents from viewing his or her medical record.

Many countries have accepted the UK decision on Gillick competence, and this rule now applies in most developed countries.

The role of the doctor in child protection

All doctors have a role in child protection when the possibility of child abuse or neglect is defined. This abuse can be physical abuse, sexual abuse or the denial of appropriate and necessary therapy. Relevant information needs to be shared with other staff members of the institution concerned, including senior medical personnel and medical social workers, even where the child or their parent does not consent, or it is not possible or it is inappropriate to ask for such consent. A decision should then be made concerning the need for referral to external agencies, and an understanding of the roles, policies and practices of such agencies in the country concerned would be necessary.

OSCE stations: Questions

Paul Duggan

Format of and approach to OSCE stations

OSCE is the abbreviation used for objective structured clinical examination. The OSCE stations are written to comply with the '2 + 8' format. This involves 2 minutes' reading time and 8 minutes' performance per station.

OSCEs are used for assessment of clinical skills. Typically, a sound performance includes acquiring pertinent clinical information (history and/or examination), requesting and interpreting investigations and formulating and explaining your plan of management. The degree of emphasis on these components varies, and not all will necessarily be included in any particular station. You might during the performance also be required to answer questions posed by the patient/actor.

How is an OSCE performance assessed? Different organizations use different tools, but they all have in common that the performance criteria are linked to the learning outcomes for your course. Some marking systems categorize performance by domains, such as Professionalism, Knowledge, Reasoning and Clinical Practice.

How should you prepare for an OSCE? Know the subject; practise your skills as appropriate with patients, friends and colleagues; and read and answer the question!

Chapter 6

Setting: Outpatient clinic, general maternity unit
Role: Junior doctor (intern)
Scenario: Mary Maxwell is a 35-year-old woman in her third pregnancy attending her local maternity unit for a routine booking visit. Ms Maxwell works full time as a teacher and lives with her husband and their 4-year old child. This pregnancy is planned. Her current medications are atenolol 50 mg daily and folic acid 5 mg daily. She has no allergies.

Ms Maxwell has been weighed, her blood pressure (BP) has been recorded and urinalysis performed.

The results are:
Height, weight, body mass index (BMI): 160 cm, 88 kg, 34.4 kg/m^2
Blood pressure: 140/90 mmHg (large cuff)
Urinalysis: positive for glucose; negative for protein, ketones, white blood cells and nitrites
Tasks:
Take an **obstetric and medical history** from Ms Maxwell. (6 minutes)
Advise Ms Maxwell of the **next steps that you will arrange** in relation to her ongoing care in this pregnancy. (1 minute)
Answer any questions she might have. (1 minute)
Note: The actor might not have the stated physical characteristics.

Chapter 7

Setting: Outpatient clinic, general maternity unit
Role: Junior doctor (intern)
Scenario: Hilda Humphries is a 27-year-old woman at 7 weeks' gestation in her first pregnancy. She works full time as a cook and lives with her 32-year-old partner John Jamieson, who is a long-distance truck driver.

Hilda has a history of subfertility and polycystic ovarian syndrome. She conceived spontaneously after losing 10 kg in weight by dieting and with regular exercise. Her current weight is 82 kg (BMI 29.8 kg/m^2).

She wants to discuss with you the adjustments, if any, she should make to her diet and in her exercise routine at the gym during her pregnancy.
Tasks:
Take a **directed history** from Ms Humphries. (5 minutes)
Advise Ms Humphries regarding diet and exercise and any other matters you uncover that are relevant to optimizing her health and the outcome of her pregnancy. (2 minutes)
Answer any questions she might have. (1 minute)
Notes: The actor might not have the described physical characteristics. Assume the dates are certain.

Chapter 8

Setting: Assessment unit, general maternity unit
Role: Junior doctor (intern)
Scenario: Freda Fisher is a 33-year-old woman in her second pregnancy who has presented to the acute assessment unit at her local maternity unit with vaginal bleeding.

Ms Fisher is currently at 34 weeks' gestation.

The assessment unit midwife has recorded the following observations:

Pulse: 72 beats/min
Blood pressure: 130/70 mmHg
Abdominal palpation: soft abdomen, breech presentation
Symphysial fundal height: 34 cm
Fetal heart rate (hand-held Doppler device): 140 bpm
Urinalysis: positive for blood; negative for leukocytes, nitrites, protein, ketones
Tasks:
Take a **relevant history** from Ms Fisher. (6 minutes)
Explain to Ms Fisher the **next steps that you will arrange in the assessment unit.** (1 minute)
Answer any questions she might have. (1 minute)
Note: The actor might not have the stated physical characteristics.

Chapter 9

Setting: Prenatal counselling clinic, general maternity unit
Role: Junior doctor (intern)
Scenario: Mary Morris is a 33-year-old G_3P_1 woman referred to your clinic by her local doctor for prenatal counselling.

Ms Morris lives with her partner and their 4-year-old daughter. She is homozygous for the factor V Leiden gene mutation and has been taking warfarin on a daily basis for several years.

She and her partner want to have another child.

The patient's current BMI is 28 kg/m^2 and her blood pressure is 120/70 mmHg.
Tasks:
Take a **relevant history** from Ms Morris. (6 minutes)
Explain to Ms Morris the **next steps that you will arrange** in relation to her prenatal care. (1 minute)
Answer any questions she might have. (1 minute)
Note: The actor might not have the stated physical characteristics.

Chapter 10

Setting: Outpatient clinic, general maternity unit
Role: Junior doctor (intern)
Scenario: Alison Albright is a 39-year-old woman in her fourth pregnancy attending her local maternity unit for an antenatal visit.

Ms Albright is currently at 34 weeks' gestation (based on a dating scan at 8 weeks' gestation). She has not attended several routine clinic appointments. She has been caring for her ill mother and has been managing by herself a busy household comprising her three school-aged children. Her husband has been posted overseas on military service for 5 months now and is not due to return home for another month.

At the previous visit (30 weeks' gestation), routine observations included blood pressure 110/80 mmHg, breech presentation and symphysial–fundal height 28 cm.

At today's visit:
Blood pressure: 110/80 mmHg
Symphysial–fundal height: 28 cm
Breech presentation
Urinalysis: normal
Tasks:
Take a **brief directed history** from Ms Albright. (3 minutes)
Advise Ms Albright of the **investigations that you will arrange** today. (1 minute)
You will then be provided with some results. **Read the results.** (1 minute)
Explain the results to Ms Albright and **advise her of your plan of management.** (2 minutes)
Answer any questions she might have. (1 minute)
Note: The actor might not have the stated physical characteristics.

Chapter 11

Setting: Delivery suite seminar room, general maternity unit
Role: Junior doctor (intern)
Scenario: You are undertaking a 'teaching on the run' session with a first-year nursing student on a brief attachment to the unit.

Your student is Barbara Bain, who has not set foot in a maternity unit before. Ms Bain has asked you to explain to her the use of a partogram and cardiotography machine in the delivery suite. You will do this using one of the unit's teaching partograms and a supporting 20-minute section of a cardiotograph (CTG) trace taken in labour.

The clinical case synopsis:

G_1P_0, normal-term pregnancy.

Spontaneous onset of contractions with rupture of the membranes occurring at home 12 hours ago.

Admission to delivery suite with regular painful contractions 10 hours ago (partogram commenced).

Copy **ONLY** of the partogram is available during the reading time.

Equipment in room:

Copy of the partogram.

Reproduced image of 20-minute section of a de-identified CTG trace in labour.

Tasks:

Explain to Ms Bain, using the partogram and CTG trace provided:

- The indications for use of both items
- The normal and abnormal features shown on the partogram
- The normal and abnormal features shown on the CTG
- Your interpretation of the situation, including any intervention you believe is indicated

Answer any questions Ms Bain might have. (1 minute)

Chapter 12

Setting: Medical school tutorial room

Role: Junior doctor (intern)

Scenario: You are filling in at short notice for a colleague who had agreed to undertake a 'catch-up' tutorial for a medical student on an obstetrics rotation.

Your student is Fred Fallows, and the tutorial topic is assisted vaginal delivery.

The clinical case synopsis:

G_1P_0 normal-term pregnancy

Spontaneous onset of labour 2300 last night

Epidural inserted 8 hours ago

IV oxytocin infusion commenced 8 hours ago

Indwelling urinary catheter inserted 7 hours ago – draining copious clear urine

Fully dilated 4 hours ago

Pushing commenced 2 hours ago with slow progress

Fetal heart rate now showing deep variable decelerations and baseline tachycardia 170 bpm

Epidural now topped and fully functional

Abdominal examination: presenting part not palpable

Vaginal examination: full dilatation, station +2, position left occipitoanterior, caput and moulding positive

Equipment in room:

Vacuum extractor cup, tubing and pump model and type per local norms

Outlet forceps

Full-size model of term fetus

Tasks:

Explain to Mr Fallows:

- Your reason(s) for:
  - Advising assisted delivery now
  - The choice of instrument (1 minute)

Demonstrate to Mr Fallows (ask him to assist as required):

- The application of your preferred instrument to the fetal head.
- The direction of pull.
- Precautions, caveats and restrictions. (5 minutes total)

Answer any questions Mr Fallows might have. (1 minute)

Chapter 13

Setting: Postnatal ward of a maternity unit

Role: Junior doctor (intern)

Scenario: You have been paged by the postnatal ward midwife to provide advice on contraception for Wanda Warrington (G_1P_1), aged 31 years.

Ms Warrington is ready for discharge together with her 1-day-old son William.

William was born vaginally after spontaneous labour at 40 weeks' gestation. His birth weight was 3800 g and Apgar scores were 8 and 10 at 1 and 5 minutes, respectively.

William has been cleared for discharge by the neonatology team.

The pre-discharge midwifery check for Ms Warrington is normal.

Tasks:

Take a relevant history from Ms Warrington. (5 minutes)

Advise Ms Warrington regarding her options for contraception. (2 minutes)

Answer any questions Ms Warrington might have. (1 minute)

Chapter 14

Setting: Postnatal ward of a maternity unit

Role: Junior doctor (intern)

Scenario: You have been paged by the postnatal ward midwife to review Antonietta Allington (G_3P_2), aged 31 years.

The midwife is concerned about the mental health state of Ms Allington, who has in the last 24 hours appeared withdrawn and 'flat'.

Ms Allington delivered by emergency caesarean section 3 days ago following a presentation at 30 weeks' gestation with antepartum haemorrhage. Deep variable decelerations were observed on cardiotocography, and there was no time for antenatal corticosteroids. Andrew has required ventilation since birth and this morning has been diagnosed with a grade II intraventricular haemorrhage.

Ms Allington has a prior history of postnatal depression. She has a 3-year-old daughter, Aimee, who is currently being cared for by her grandmother. Ms Allington separated from her partner Anthony earlier this year. Anthony is the father of both children.

Tasks:

Take a relevant history from Ms Allington. (6 minutes)

Advise Ms Allington regarding her continuing management. (2 minutes)

Note: DO NOT perform a formal psychiatric evaluation.

Chapter 15

Setting: Medical school simulation suite

Role: Simulation suite demonstrator

Scenario: You are rostered to teach 1:1 a group of second-year medical students how to take a cervical sample for polymerase chain reaction (PCR) testing for *Chlamydia* and gonorrhoea.

Your student is Patrick Price.

Tasks:

Explain to Mr Price what you would tell a patient prior to undertaking this test. (2 minutes)

Demonstrate using the model and equipment provided the procedure for this test, including answering any questions Mr Price might pose whilst you do so. (6 minutes)

Chapter 16

Setting: General (family) practice

Role: First-year medical graduate on general practitioner (GP) rotation

Scenario: You are about to undertake a consultation for Eliza Etheridge, a 42-year-old woman who is known to the practice.

Ms Etheridge had been referred to the local hospital gynaecology unit for management of refractory heavy menstrual bleeding. They undertook hysteroscopy and insertion of a levonorgestrel intrauterine system 3 months ago.

This is the planned follow-up visit as requested by the gynaecology unit.

The synopsis of her medical record is:

Eliza Etheridge

Single, lives alone, works full time as personal assistant to chief partner of large legal firm.

Medications: levonorgestrel intrauterine device

Surgical: hysteroscopy – normal findings (biopsy result: disordered proliferative phase endometrium)

Obstetric: never pregnant

Gynaecological: heavy menstrual bleeding and Fe-deficiency anaemia. Unresponsive to courses of norethisterone, mefenamic acid and tranexamic acid.

Cervical screening test: normal and up to date

The practice nurse has just completed taking routine observations (normal weight and blood pressure). During this Ms Etheridge confided to the nurse that she has not been happy with the results of her management to date and was thinking about having a hysterectomy.

Tasks:

Take a directed history from Ms Etheridge. (4 minutes)

Discuss further management with Ms Etheridge. (3 minutes)

Answer any questions Ms Etheridge may have. (1 minute)

Chapter 17

Setting: General (family) practice

Role: First-year medical graduate on GP rotation

Scenario: You are 'parallel consulting' with your training supervisor. You are about to undertake a follow-up consultation for a couple who were seen by a locum practitioner 2 weeks ago.

This is the synopsis of the locum GP's consultations for this couple:

Jane Johnson age 32 years

Unable to get pregnant – trying for 18 months. Has never been pregnant.

Well, no medical history.

De facto (Robert Robertson, age 35) – have lived together last 4 years.

Medications: folic acid supplement

Surgical: nil

Investigation requested: pelvic ultrasound

Robert Robertson age 35 years

Well, no medical history.

De facto (Jane Johnson, age 32) – have lived together last 4 years

Medications: nil

Surgical: nil

Investigation requested: semen analysis

Results summary:

Pelvic ultrasound: normal

Semen analysis: sperm concentration 10 M/mL (normal ≥15 M/mL), normal morphology 3% (normal ≥4%), all other features normal.

The couple are anxious to learn the results of their tests and for assistance with their infertility.

Tasks:

Explain the test results to this couple. (1 minute)

Take additional history from the couple. (5 minutes)

Advise them of your plan of management and **answer any questions** they may have. (2 minutes)

Chapter 18

Setting: General hospital emergency department

Role: First-year medical graduate

Scenario: Elvira Evington, a 24-year-old woman, has been triaged to your list in the emergency department – your very first patient since graduation.

The record made by the triage nurse is:

Elvira Evington age 24 years

Self-referred walk-in

Lower abdominal pain since last night, onset 0400 vaginal bleeding – initially heavy with clots +++, now settled to very light bleeding

Pregnant, scan last week = 6 weeks

Observations: looks comfortable, pulse 72 bpm, BP 130/80 mmHg, O_2 sat 99%, point-of-care haemoglobin (Hb) 110 g/L

Urinary hCG: positive

Urinalysis: normal

Plan: intern review

Tasks:

Take a history from Ms Evington. (5 minutes)

Explain the examination you propose to undertake. (1 minute)

You will then be provided with some examination findings.

Read the information provided. (1 minute)

Inform Ms Evington of your provisional diagnosis and plan of management. (1 minute)

Chapter 19

Setting: General practice

Role: First-year medical graduate on rotation

Scenario: Felicity Farrington, a 32-year-old woman, has been allocated to your consultation list today. Your supervisor has asked you to manage her request for contraception.

Ms Farrington has been a patient of this practice for several years. The practice record includes:

Felicity Farrington age 32 years

Occupation: Teachers' aide at local primary school

Marital status: Married (Mordred McCallum)

Dependents: One child (Martin McCallum – current age 3 years; healthy)

Surgery: Caesarean section

Obstetric: G_1P_1 (unplanned – condom failure); emergency lower segment caesarean section (LSCS) at term for fetal distress

Medical: nil

Last visit to the practice: 6 months ago for routine health check

Tasks:

Take a relevant history from Ms Farrington. (5 minutes)

Discuss with Ms Farrington her options for contraception and **answer her questions.** (3 minutes)

Chapter 20

Setting: General practice

Role: First-year medical graduate on rotation

Scenario: Giana Giannopoulos, a 35-year-old woman, has been allocated to your consultation list today.

Ms Giannopoulos booked the appointment to discuss whether she should give consent for her 11-year-old daughter Haley to be vaccinated at school against human papilloma virus (HPV). Haley is completely healthy and is the only child of Ms Giannopoulos.

In addition, there is a 'red flag' alert in Ms Giannopoulos's records related to her non-attendance for routine cervical screening tests since she joined the practice 12 years ago.

Tasks:

Address Ms Giannopoulos' concerns regarding Haley's vaccinations. (4 minutes)

Discuss with Ms Giannopoulos her own participation in the cervical screening programme. (4 minutes)

Chapter 21

Setting: A general gynaecology outpatient clinic

Role: Junior doctor (intern)

Scenario: You are about to see a new patient referred by her local general practitioner.

This is the text of the referral letter:

Dear Doctor

Re: Olivia Oliphant, age 56 years

Thank you for seeing Ms Oliphant regarding long-standing urinary incontinence and vaginal prolapse. There has been no response to pelvic floor exercises. Is surgery appropriate?

Current medications: nil

Yours sincerely,

Dr B Local

These are the patient's booking details:

Age: 56 years
Marital status: single
Height: 160 cm
Weight: 90 kg
BMI: 31.1 kg/m^2
Parity: 0
Allergies: sticking plasters and surgical tape

Tasks:

Take a directed history from Ms Oliphant. (4 minutes)

Explain to Ms Oliphant the examination and investigations you require. (1 minute)

Read the available examination findings and investigation results. (1 minute)

Explain your proposed management. (1 minute)

Note: The actor might not have the stated physical characteristics.

Appendix A

Setting: A general gynaecology ward in a metropolitan hospital

Role: Junior doctor (intern)

Scenario: You are undertaking a scheduled (routine) postoperative ward round at 0800. The patient you are about to see is Ms Madeline McGrath, aged 42 years.

Ms McGrath had been admitted yesterday for laparoscopically assisted vaginal hysterectomy and anterior vaginal wall repair (anterior colporrhaphy) for heavy menstrual bleeding and POPQ stage 2 anterior compartment prolapse. The procedure was undertaken 23 hours ago. The patient is scheduled for discharge home following your review.

Ms McGrath will be lying propped up in a hospital bed (or barouche) and wearing hospital clothing.

This is the text of the operation note:

Madeline McGrath, age 42 years

Procedure summary: laparoscopically assisted vaginal hysterectomy, right salpingo-oophorectomy, left salpingectomy, anterior vaginal repair.

Findings: stage 2 anterior compartment prolapse, multiple uterine fibroids, uterus enlarged to 14 w size, 4 cm endometrioma right ovary – elected also to perform right oophorectomy.

Postoperative instructions: remove urinary catheter midnight. Discharge home per 23-hour policy following intern review.

The following is the synopsis of her postoperative observations:

Moderately uncomfortable night, requiring oxycodone 10 mg 6-hourly

Urinary catheter removed midnight; has not passed urine as of 0600
Pulse: 84 bpm
BP: 120/80 mmHg
Temperature: 37.4 °C

Tasks:

Take a directed history from Ms McGrath. (3 minutes)

Perform an abdominal examination. (1 minute)

Explain your proposed management. (3 minutes)

Answer Ms McGrath's questions. (1 minute)

Appendix C

Setting: A general gynaecology outpatient clinic in a metropolitan hospital

Role: Junior doctor (intern)

Scenario: You are consulting in an outpatient clinic. The woman you are about to see is Ms Zoe Xenophon, aged 52 years.

Ms Xenophon has been referred by her local gynaecologist for management of postmenopausal bleeding.

This is the text of the referral note:

Dear Doctor

re: Zoe Xenophon, age 52 years

Thank you for on-going management of Ms Xenophon. Her menopause was 3 years ago. For the past 3 months she has noticed irregular, period-like vaginal bleeding.

Pelvic ultrasound identified endometrial thickness of 1.5 cm. Cervical screening test and liquid-based cytology results are normal.

Current medications: nil

Allergies: nil

Medical: overweight, type 2 diabetes diet controlled

Social: married, works full time as cleaner

Surgical: LLETZ procedure age 32 for CIN2

Obstetric: 1 child now aged 24 years

I attempted hysteroscopy in my rooms. The attempt was abandoned due to patient discomfort (cervical stenosis). Unable to obtain endometrial sample.

Please see and treat.

Tasks:

Take a brief, directed history from Ms Xenophon. (2 minutes)

Explain to Ms Xenophon the procedure that is required to evaluate her problem, including risks, benefits and alternatives (if any). (4 minutes)

Answer any questions she might have. (2 minutes)

OSCE stations: Answers

Chapter 6

In this scenario, a pregnant woman of unstated gestational age is presenting for a booking visit. The woman is obese, is on treatment for hypertension and is taking high-dose folic acid. She is living with her husband with no mention of children. She is positive for glycosuria, which is a distractor.

You should establish from the history the gestational age, the details of her two past pregnancies, history of familial or inheritable disorders, general medical and surgical history and progress to date in the current pregnancy. Include open questions regarding any concerns the patient might have.

Treated hypertension is a key feature in this case. Establish how long the woman has been taking atenolol, the underlying cause of hypertension, if known, and what her recent blood measurements have been. Enquire regarding symptoms of poorly controlled hypertension, and consider pre-eclampsia if the gestational age is 20 weeks or more.

The second key feature is that the woman is taking high-dose folic acid. Ask her why she is taking this high dose. It might be related to neural tube defect in a previous pregnancy. Or it could indicate a thrombophilia.

The third key feature is that the woman is obese. This increases her risk of pregnancy complications, including gestational diabetes. Glycosuria is a distractor. Nevertheless, consider what screening or diagnostic tests for gestational diabetes and other pregnancy complications (pre-eclampsia, fetal anomalies, perturbation in fetal growth) are appropriate.

Synthesize the data you have acquired and explain to the actor your working diagnosis/diagnoses and plans for management. In addition to screening and/or diagnostic tests, this case is high risk and requires specialist management per local protocols.

Finally, be prepared for simple questions from the actor. These could be for clarification of diagnosis and management, safety of atenolol in pregnancy or related to a social issue such as appropriateness of her continuing to work full time in a stressful occupation.

Chapter 7

In this scenario, a woman is enquiring about adjustments during her pregnancy that she should make to her diet and exercise routine. The woman is overweight, has polycystic ovarian syndrome and has successfully lost weight through changes to her diet and with exercise.

The key requirements are to establish what her current diet and exercise habits are. This should include open questions regarding any concerns the woman has.

Evidence regarding what constitutes an adequate diet in pregnancy is limited in part due to the retrospective nature of most studies and the wide range of diets people have. However, some generalizations are likely to apply to your locale, including recommendations for routine pre-pregnancy supplementation with folic acid and routine antenatal supplementation with oral Fe regimens. A diet that consists largely of junk food and soft drinks increases the risk of pre-eclampsia and gestational diabetes. Other dietary factors include inadequate calcium and iodine intake (e.g. by avoidance of dairy foods and iodized salt). Some vegetarians might, without dietary supplementation, have inadequate vitamin B_{12} intake. The woman's occupation creates opportunities for overeating. Estimation of daily calorie intake should be covered in the enquiry.

In addition, enquire about intake of relevant non-food substances, including alcohol and cigarettes, and consider whether she has adequate sun exposure for sufficient vitamin D production.

Exercise in pregnancy appears to limit excessive weight gain, and aerobic exercise maintains or improves fitness. Exercise in combination with diet appears to reduce the risk of gestational diabetes and caesarean delivery. Unfortunately, there is insufficient evidence to tailor this general information to an individual's diet and exercise habits. However, there are pragmatic considerations, for example, does the woman have an existing condition such as low back pain or joint pain that might be exacerbated during pregnancy and impact her ability to exercise? If so, how would you address that in relation to her recommended calorie intake?

Be prepared to answer questions such as 'Should I eat for two?' 'Will continuing with my daily gym circuit harm the baby or bring labour on early?' and 'What exercises can I do later in pregnancy?'

Chapter 8

In this scenario, a woman in her second pregnancy presents with a third-trimester antepartum haemorrhage. The woman has been triaged by a midwife. She is clinically stable, the fetal heart rate is normal, abdomen soft and symphysial–fundal height is consistent with dates and with a breech presentation. The haematuria is likely explained by contamination of the sample.

Begin by forming an impression of the patient's state both physically and mentally by 'end of the bed' observations. Although this is not a real encounter, be alert to cues from the actor that might suggest the situation is more acute than indicated by the observations provided.

From your history, establish the onset and nature of the bleeding, associated or precipitating factors and whether this is the first or a recurrent episode. Antepartum haemorrhage is conventionally categorized as painful (suggesting placental abruption and/or pre-term labour) or painless (suggesting placenta praevia or a local cause of bleeding). Confirming dates is critical, as is enquiring about prior investigations such as previous placental location by ultrasound, and blood group and antibody status. The obstetric history must also be established. If the patient has had a prior lower segment caesarean delivery, consider placenta praevia accreta.

The next steps include repeating the abdominal examination, performing a speculum examination and arranging in the unit a cardiotograph (CTG) and relevant blood tests. It would be prudent also to request a formal urine microscopy and culture. Most acute assessment units will have a portable ultrasound, and this would be used to check the presentation and placental localization. All of this should be explained to the actor in clear lay terms. Include in your explanation the reasons for performing the additional examination and tests, i.e. say what you are looking to find or exclude. Local protocol might include that this patient be offered betamethasone and likely will

require her to be observed for a minimum period either in the assessment unit or admitted to the ward. However, as this is a high-risk situation, you should indicate that the patient will also be reviewed by a senior member of the medical staff.

Finally, the patient will be anxious about the bleeding and, if she has a child at home, about arrangements for that child's care whilst she remains under observation. In relation to fetal safety, cautious reassurance is appropriate whilst recognizing this is an unpredictable situation that might yet result in pre-term operative delivery. It is not safe at present for the woman to leave hospital, so child care arrangements will need to be made with that in mind.

Chapter 9

In this scenario, a woman with one child and two pregnancy losses is attending for prenatal counselling. She has thrombophilia (homozygous factor V Leiden), has been taking warfarin 'for several years' and is normotensive. She might have had recurrent thromboembolism.

As this is a prenatal presentation, establish what the woman's plans are. When does she want to become pregnant? The couple are probably using either barrier contraception or a levonorgestrel intrauterine system. Are there subfertility problems that need to be addressed? Are there any other health problems in the woman or in the family history that also must be considered? Are her vaccinations up to date?

Warfarin is teratogenic and will need to be replaced with a safer anticoagulant, such as enoxaparin, prior to conception. The woman should be well informed about her thrombophilia and its management and might have used enoxaparin in her last pregnancy. Use open questions such as 'Why you are taking warfarin?' and 'How was this problem managed in your last pregnancy?' Establish in detail the obstetric history, being mindful of the association with early pregnancy loss and intrauterine growth restriction in such cases. Were there complications in the last pregnancy requiring early delivery? What was the birth weight? Is the child healthy?

As this is an advanced topic, the next step in management requires engagement of an obstetrician or a multidisciplinary team per local protocols. However, you should also indicate what you expect will be done, including a managed change in the anticoagulation regimen, plus routine preventive health care, such as updated vaccinations where required and supplements to minimize risk of neural tube defect.

The actor is likely to ask only for clarification of your proposed management if that is required.

Chapter 10

In this scenario, a woman at 34 weeks' gestation (sure dates) and with limited antenatal care presents for a routine antenatal clinic review. There is a breech presentation and no change in the symphysial–fundal height in 4 weeks, suggesting intrauterine growth restriction (IUGR). The dates are accurate, and pre-eclampsia, although on the differential diagnosis of IUGR, appears unlikely in this case.

The history should be directed at establishing whether the woman has noticed anything wrong, enquiring about fetal movements and about risk factors for IUGR, including maternal smoking, chronic maternal disease, potentially harmful medications, results of screening for fetal anomalies, transplacental infection, antepartum haemorrhage and IUGR in previous pregnancies. Because time is short, the actor will be scripted to answer in the negative for most or all of these problems.

Prompt investigations are required to assess fetal wellbeing and rule in or rule out the provisional diagnosis. A CTG should be requested, as should formal ultrasound evaluation for assessment of fetal growth parameters, amniotic fluid volume and Doppler flow velocity (fetal umbilical artery plus or minus fetal middle cerebral artery per local protocol). Other investigations usually can be delayed pending these results. Explain the investigations – what they are and their purpose – using plain language.

You will then be provided with results in report form (some schools might expect you to interpret an unreported CTG). Explain your interpretation of these data to the actor. Conclude with an explanation of your management, including factoring in the significance of the breech presentation if confirmed. As this is a complicated case, input of an obstetrician is required.

The actor is likely to ask only for clarification of your proposed management.

Chapter 11

In this scenario, you are provided in the reading time with a 'teaching partogram' based on observations over 10 hours of a primigravid woman presenting with spontaneous labour at term. The pregnancy is uncomplicated. The partogram will indicate a common obstetric problem, most likely poor progress of labour associated with a persisting, deflexed occiput posterior (OP) position or a deep transverse arrest, with meconium liquor detected and subsequent application of a fetal scalp electrode for direct monitoring of the fetal heart rate. The CTG could be normal, or it might have an obvious abnormality such

as recurrent deep variable decelerations with a baseline tachycardia.

Your task is to recognize and explain in terms suitable for a novice student nurse (which should include technical terms with their explanation in lay language) how the recordings are done and what they mean.

The actor might ask for clarification of your proposed management or if you thought the labour could have been better managed and, if so, how. The latter question would only be asked if management was suboptimal in accordance with local protocol, e.g. in relation to use of intravenous (IV) oxytocin or use of analgesia.

Chapter 12

In this scenario, you are describing to an actor, or perhaps a real medical student, assisted vaginal (outlet) delivery in a case of prolonged second stage and with an abnormal fetal heart rate pattern.

Explain briefly why delivery is indicated, the abdominal and vaginal examination findings that indicate assisted vaginal delivery is safe and why the timing is now optimal (optimal analgesia, bladder empty).

The choice of instrument might be determined by local protocol. If so, usually vacuum extraction is preferred due to the lower risk of anal sphincter trauma. However, the vacuum cup is more likely to pull off. Individual operator skill is an important factor. Explain your choice of instrument with these factors in mind.

Then, demonstrate on the model of the fetus and with the aid of the student/actor the application to the fetal head of the instrument you prefer, and explain as you do so the precautions, caveats and restrictions in the use of this device.

The student/actor might ask for clarification of your proposed management, e.g. use of an episiotomy, what you would do if delivery was not achieved as you had anticipated or what form of fetal monitoring you would use.

Chapter 13

In this scenario, you are required to provide advice on contraception in the postnatal period. To do so effectively, establish antecedent use and preference, social and financial circumstances including whether she is in a current heterosexual relationship, relevant medical and family history, plans for breast-feeding and plans for future children.

Potential permutations include prior negative experience of certain methods, personal choice and preference, medical or family history that render some methods unsuitable (e.g. homozygous factor V Leiden), intention not to breast-feed, a split from her partner during the pregnancy or intention not to have more children.

The actor might ask for clarification of a recommendation, about when she can resume having sex or what she should do to prevent sexually transmitted infection.

Chapter 14

In this scenario, you are asked to assess a woman with known risk factors for depression and whose behaviour in the past 24 hours has changed and given cause for concern.

Your first task is to develop rapport with the actor, who has been instructed to answer your questions but with little expression or emotion and to avoid eye contact.

After introducing yourself, enquire about the woman's progress and that of her baby. Explain the purpose of the interview. Establish the following:
Medical, psychiatric, family and social history
Obstetric and sexual history, including risk of violence and abuse from her ex-partner
Risk of harm to self and her children

Although this appears to be a case involving evaluation of mental health and risk assessment for the woman and her children, consider also the possibility that there might be contributing medical conditions (e.g. hypothyroidism). You must indicate that you will involve senior medical staff, including the consultant obstetrician and neonatology team. Indicate that you will request an opinion from the on-call psychiatrist or mental health team. If Ms Allington and the children are at risk of violence from her ex-partner, indicate that you will involve a social services worker who will be able to arrange safe housing and emergency financial support. If you are concerned that Ms Allington might herself pose a risk to her children, you might be legally required to personally notify the local child welfare authorities. Open disclosure is required, but be careful and sensitive in manner and choice of words.

Chapter 15

In this scenario, you are teaching a junior medical student (or actor) pre-examination counselling and, using a model of a pelvis, the technique of taking a cervical sample for polymerase chain reaction (PCR) testing for *Chlamydia* and gonorrhoea.

You will be provided with a vaginal speculum and other relevant equipment. Although there is no live patient, to keep the simulation experience as authentic as possible, the recommended counselling should be patient focussed (use lay language).

Chapter 16

In this scenario, a 42-year-old woman, presenting 3 months after insertion of a levonorgestrel intrauterine system, has indicated that she is seeking hysterectomy, as she is unhappy with the outcomes of oral non-steroidal anti-inflammatory, anti-fibrinolytic and progestogen regimens and the intrauterine system.

Establish why she is unhappy with the levonorgestrel system and her reasons for considering hysterectomy as the next step. What is the nature of the bleeding problem? Are there associated symptoms that might indicate endometriosis? Although chronic pelvic infection seems unlikely given the endometrial biopsy result, check if she has abnormal vaginal discharge and if she has been screened for sexually transmitted infection (STI). Check her compliance with and duration of use of the prior regimens. Consider other reasons for treatment failure, in particular, clotting disorders – Does she bruise easily? Is there a family history of bleeding tendencies? Is she taking any over-the-counter substances that might contribute to abnormal uterine bleeding? Establish her sexual history, including whether she has any concerns about permanent loss of fertility from an intervention. Has she considered alternatives to hysterectomy, including waiting longer to establish the efficacy of the current treatment, continuous active tablets from an oral contraceptive pill regimen or endometrial ablation?

The actor might ask for clarification of a recommendation, for example, return to work after a surgical procedure.

Chapter 17

In this scenario, a couple with primary infertility are attending a follow-up visit to learn the results of a pelvic ultrasound and semen analysis. The semen analysis result is mildly abnormal. However, neither partner has had an adequate history documented, which you are to rectify prior to recommending management.

Establish the menstrual and sexual history, enquire regarding hyperandrogenism (acne, hirsutism), frequency and timing of sex, problems with erection or ejaculation, alcohol and drug use, risk factors for STI and consider other lifestyle issues (e.g. obesity).

Your management should aim to exclude tubal factor infertility and STI, lifestyle issues if present should be addressed, the semen analysis should be repeated after at least 3 days of abstinence and referral for specialist review should be discussed.

The actors might ask for clarification of a recommendation or for your views on a specific aspect of management such as laparoscopy or in vitro fertilization.

Chapter 18

In this scenario, you are asked to assess a woman who has presented in early pregnancy (≈7 weeks) with abdominal pain and vaginal bleeding. An intrauterine pregnancy has previously been confirmed, and the information provided indicates the woman is not currently on the verge of haemorrhagic shock.

Enquire regarding pain and bleeding to confirm the impression that the woman is clinically stable or improving. However, early pregnancy loss is emotionally distressing, regardless of physical impact, whether the pregnancy was planned or not. Acknowledge this and ask if the woman needs a support person to be contacted. Tactfully enquire if the pregnancy was planned. If this was the result of failure of contraception, do not assume that the pregnancy is not wanted. A brief medical history is also required, which in this age group is usually normal.

Abdominal and pelvic examination is required. The woman might not have had either type of examination before, so check this and explain how the examination is done and why it is indicated. You will then be provided with the results, which will guide you regarding the provisional diagnosis and to the next step: investigations. A typical scenario is that the cervical os admits a finger (i.e. is widely dilated), suggesting complete miscarriage. In most units this provisional diagnosis will be confirmed by ultrasound, and routine blood tests, including a full blood count, blood group and antibody screen, arranged. If products of conception are in the vagina, indicate that histopathological examination will be arranged and why. Be prepared to explain the local protocol for administration of anti-D immunoglobulin if relevant.

Chapter 19

In this scenario, you are asked to manage a request for contraception made by a 32-year-old woman.

First establish what the patient's goals are from this visit. Does she want reversible or permanent contraception? If she wants more children, what are her plans? If she has completed her family, what are the couple's views regarding vasectomy/tubal ligation? Are there any co-existing factors to be considered, e.g. menstrual, sexual or new medical problems?

Once you have an idea of what the woman wants, explain suitable options, including reliability, cost, other (non-contraceptive) benefits and key risks.

The actor might ask for clarification of a recommendation or for your views on a specific aspect of management such as prevention of STI.

Chapter 20

In this scenario, a woman is requesting information to help her decide whether her 11-year-old daughter should participate in a human papilloma virus (HPV) vaccination programme offered at school. In addition, the woman is not up to date with recommended cervical screening tests.

Start by establishing what the woman already knows about HPV, the HPV vaccination programme and what her concerns for her daughter are. You can anticipate that Ms Giannopoulos will be concerned about vaccination safety and effectiveness and, perhaps, perceived encouragement of precocious sexual experience. A more technical nuance could be a question regarding the alternative of self-funding a nonovalent vaccine if that is not yet available in the school-based programme in your region.

This part should segue naturally into the second task. Establish what the woman already knows about the cervical screening programme and her reasons for not responding to requests from the practice to participate in this programme. You can anticipate that she has been single and not sexually active for several years so felt there was no need to be tested and that her last test was painful and embarrassing, so she would prefer not to have another speculum examination. If so, be prepared to discuss patient self-collection as an alternative.

Chapter 21

In this scenario, a 56-year-old nulliparous woman presents with vaginal prolapse and urinary incontinence unresponsive to pelvic floor exercises. The referring doctor has questioned whether surgery is indicated.

Establish the details of the presenting symptoms, including severity, risk factors (noting nulliparity and obesity), sexual function, psychological health, medical and surgical history, treatments tried and fluid intake. Specifically enquire regarding chronic cough and, if present, the possible causes; diabetes, diuretic medications, behavioural polydipsia, depression, social isolation, prior pelvic surgery or radiotherapy and occupational issues (e.g. a job requiring heavy lifting). How did she learn and for how long has she been doing pelvic floor exercises?

The scenario is likely to be mixed urinary incontinence with no other lower urinary tract symptoms, normal bowel function and recent detection of a vaginal bulge whilst showering. She will not be in a sexual relationship and will have been taught the pelvic floor exercises by a physiotherapist and been fully compliant for 6 months, without benefit.

Explain in plain language to the actor the examination you propose to undertake. In a short station it is reasonable this be restricted to abdominal and vaginal (bimanual and speculum) examination, plus urinalysis. Explain what you will be looking for, e.g. descent of the uterus and vaginal walls and urinary leakage with 'bearing down'. The actor will then provide you with the available examination findings. A common scenario is visible loss of urine with Valsalva and a pelvic organ prolapse quantification system (POPQ) stage 2 anterior vaginal compartment prolapse.

Using plain language, explain the provisional diagnosis and the underlying cause(s) of the condition(s), if known, and advise the next stage in management. Bear in mind there has been no response to pelvic floor exercises and that the patient appears from the referral letter to have been primed to consider a surgical solution. For the examination findings described, surgery is a reasonable approach. However, there is no time to go into details. Indicate that referral to a specialist is required to consider further a surgical approach if you believe that is indicated.

Appendix A

In this scenario, you are to establish if a woman 23 hours following major gynaecological surgery is fit to be discharged home per preoperative planning. However, the performed procedure is different from the booked procedure due to the discovery of a right endometrioma managed by oophorectomy. Furthermore, the woman has not passed urine since removal of the urinary catheter several hours ago, and her pain is not well controlled with oxycodone at high dose.

Observe the woman from the end of the bed as you ask her how she is feeling. The actor will be instructed to look distressed and respond that she is not feeling well and that the procedure was more painful than she had anticipated. Establish the nature and location of pain, exacerbating and

relieving factors and whether she has been able to get up to pass urine or to use a bedpan.

Explain in plain language to the actor the abdominal examination you propose to undertake and seek permission to perform it, ensuring appropriate hand hygiene technique. Time is short, so the scenario will develop as a single postoperative complication, which could be urinary retention or an unexpected surgical injury, e.g. ureteric injury related to the dissection of the right ovary or peritonism related to postoperative bleeding or bowel injury (less likely, as tachycardia is difficult to emulate). The actor will also be instructed to mimic appropriate signs.

Explain in plain language your provisional diagnosis and plan of management, which should include review by an experienced doctor. The patient was not scheduled to have her right ovary removed. This might be the only 'positive' feature that you uncover and will need to be included in your explanation. If the woman expresses discontent with that aspect of her management, express regret that she is unhappy with the management and reassure that you will promptly draw this to the attention of the surgeon.

Appendix C

In this scenario, the diagnosis of exclusion is endometrial cancer in a 52-year-old woman presenting with postmenopausal bleeding and significantly increased endometrial thickness. Her referring gynaecologist has diagnosed cervical stenosis, probably secondary to cervical surgery for cervical intraepithelial neoplasia (CIN). Hysteroscopy and dilatation and curettage in a day-case operating theatre are now indicated.

Establish if there are any other major risk factors for endometrial cancer (mismatch repair gene, prior diagnosis of atypical endometrial hyperplasia would impact decision-making if the next hysteroscopy was also unsatisfactory) and confirm the nature and number of prior gynaecological procedures. Does the patient have a medical history that raises concern for anaesthesia or for preoperative cervical priming with misoprostol? Does the patient have any particular concerns? Does she need a support person present?

Explain in simple language the provisional diagnosis, acknowledging that this is provisional and that cancer is not a certainty but that it must be excluded. Explain the procedure in lay language and in sufficient detail for local requirements for informed consent. This should include that this is a diagnostic, not curative, procedure and that prompt follow-up will be required to give the results and plan further management. Risks of the procedure should not be exaggerated, but they include uterine perforation, creation of a false passage resulting in failure to complete the procedure satisfactorily, gut side effects from misoprostol if used for preoperative priming of the cervix and complications related to anaesthesia. You can anticipate that the actor will ask why she can't simply have a hysterectomy 'to get it all over and done with'. The response should include that the condition could be benign and not require hysterectomy and that some malignancies require surgical staging procedures that are more complex than a simple hysterectomy. Be sure to indicate that involvement of a senior doctor is required in such cases.

Self-assessment: Questions

Kevin Hayes

Chapter 1

1. What is the most appropriate description of the arterial supply of the pelvis?
   A. The external iliac artery arises at the level of the lumbosacral articulation and passes over the pelvic brim
   B. The anterior division provides the superior, middle and inferior vesical arteries that provide the blood supply for the bladder
   C. The uterine artery initially runs downward in the subperitoneal fat under the superior attachment of the broad ligament
   D. The uterine artery crosses the ureter approximately 0.5 cm from the lateral fornix of the vagina
   E. The ovarian arteries descend behind the peritoneum on the surface of the corresponding obturator internus muscle until they reach the brim of the pelvis

2. The vagina:
   A. Is closely related anteriorly to the trigone of the bladder and the urethra
   B. Has the rectum as its only direct relation posteriorly
   C. Is composed of striated muscle
   D. Has a pH in the sexually mature non-pregnant female of 2.0–3.0
   E. Is lined by glandular epithelium

3. In regard to the uterus and its supporting structures, which of the following statements is true?
   A. Posteriorly, the uterosacral ligaments and their peritoneal covering form the lateral boundaries of the rectouterine pouch (of Douglas)
   B. Laterally, the broad ligaments form an important supporting structure for the uterus
   C. In about 50% of women, the uterus lies in a position of retroversion in the pouch of Douglas
   D. In labour, the isthmus (lower segment) of the uterus plays a significant role in expulsion of the fetus
   E. The anterior ligaments and uterovesical folds play an important role in maintaining anteversion of the uterus.

4. The ovary:
   A. Lies in close relation to the internal iliac vessels
   B. Derives its blood supply from the ovarian artery, which arises from the internal iliac artery
   C. Is covered by ciliated columnar epithelium
   D. Is supported laterally by the suspensory ligament, which lies in close relation to the ureter
   E. Contains Graafian follicles, which are found only in the central medulla of the organ

5. With regard to the uterus, which one of the following is correct?
   A. Lymphatic drainage from the lower part of the uterus passes to the superficial inguinal and adjacent superficial femoral nodes
   B. Uterine pain is mediated through sympathetic afferent nerves passing up to T11–T12 and L1–L2
   C. The uterine artery lies beneath the ureter at the point where the ureter enters the bladder
   D. The blood supply of the uterus is derived entirely from the uterine artery
   E. The isthmus (lower segment) of the uterus is partly innervated by the pudendal nerve

Chapter 2

1. What is the most appropriate statement relating to spermatozoa?
   A. The tail contains a coiled helix of mitochondria that provides the 'powerhouse' for sperm motility
   B. During their passage through the Fallopian tubes, the sperm undergo the final stage in maturation (capacitation), which enables a more efficient transport along the last section of tube
   C. Seminal plasma has a high concentration of galactose, which is the major source of energy for the spermatozoa
   D. The sperm head fuses with the oocyte plasma membrane, and the sperm head and midpiece are engulfed into the oocyte by phagocytosis

E. Sperm migration is at a rate of 6 mm/min, nearly all due to sperm motility
2. Which one of the following best describes normal follicular growth occurring in a 25-year-old woman?
   A. About 100 ovarian follicles show obvious follicular growth in each menstrual cycle
   B. In most women one follicle is selected to become the dominant follicle on about day 5–6 of that cycle
   C. The dominant follicle grows by about 1 cm per day from days 6 to 14 of the cycle
   D. The follicle ruptures when it reaches about 4 cm in diameter
   E. A separate but adjacent follicle becomes the corpus luteum
3. Which one of the following statements about meiosis is correct?
   A. Meiosis is the mechanism of production of the 7 million germ cells found in the ovary at 6 months of fetal life
   B. The first meiotic division is completed prior to birth of the baby
   C. The second meiotic division commences at the time of attachment of the sperm to the oocyte
   D. Rearrangements of the genes within the chromosomes occur after the male zygote chromosomes have entered the nucleus and combine with those of the female zygote
   E. The delay between the end of the first meiotic division and the commencement of the second meiotic division is the cause of the increased chromosome abnormality rate seen in women who conceive after the age of 37 years
4. Which one of the following statements about the process of fertilization in the human female is correct?
   A. It usually occurs within the outer end of the Fallopian tube
   B. The female gamete determines the sex of a resulting fetus
   C. A twin pregnancy is due to failure of the normal inhibitory process, where further sperm are prevented from entering the oocyte following attachment of the first sperm to the zona pellucida
   D. Fertilization can occur up to 6 days after ovulation
   E. Sperm capacitation occurs within the seminiferous epithelium of the testis
5. Which one of the following facts about implantation is correct?
   A. Implantation usually occurs about 2 days after fertilization
   B. At the time of implantation the embryo is usually at the eight-cell stage
   C. Human chorionic gonadotropin (hCG) is produced by the implanting embryo soon after implantation has commenced

D. If the endometrial appearance at the time of implantation is proliferative, the pregnancy is lost as a spontaneous miscarriage
E. If implantation occurs, the period is always delayed, and a urinary pregnancy test performed 2–3 days after the day the period was expected will be positive

Chapter 3

1. What is the most appropriate statement regarding immunology in pregnancy?
   A. The villous trophoblast never expresses human leucocyte antigen (HLA) class I or class II molecules
   B. The extra-villous trophoblast never expresses HLA class I or class II molecules
   C. The main type of decidual lymphocytes are the uterine plasma cells
   D. The Th1:Th2 cytokine ratio shifts towards Th1 in pregnancy
   E. The thymus shows some reversible involution during pregnancy, apparently caused by the oestrogen-driven exodus of lymphocytes from the thymic cortex
2. Regarding the rise in cardiac output, which one of the following is correct?
   A. It occurs in late pregnancy
   B. It is entirely driven by a rise in stroke volume
   C. It is associated with a rise in afterload
   D. It can precipitate heart failure in women with heart disease
   E. It causes an increase in pulmonary arterial pressure
3. Considering respiratory function in pregnancy, which one of the following statements is correct?
   A. Progesterone sensitizes the adrenal medulla to CO_2
   B. Maternal P_aO_2 rises by $\approx 15\%$
   C. There is no increase in maternal 2,3-DPG
   D. Maternal oxygen-carrying capacity rises by $\approx 18\%$
   E. There is an 80% increase in minute ventilation
4. Considering renal function in pregnancy, which one of the following statements is correct?
   A. Most increase in renal size occurs in late pregnancy
   B. The ureters are floppy and toneless
   C. The rise in glomerular filtration rate (GFR) activates the renin–angiotensin system
   D. About 1800 mmol sodium is retained during pregnancy
   E. Urinary tract infections are less common in pregnancy
5. In relation to endocrine function in pregnancy, which one of the following statements is correct?
   A. Insulin resistance develops
   B. Glycosuria is not common

C. The thyroid involutes

D. The gut absorbs more calcium but less is lost in the urine

E. The increased skin pigmentation is caused by thyroid-stimulating hormone

Chapter 4

1. In early placental development, which one of the following is correct?
   A. The outer cytotrophoblast invades the endometrial cells and the myometrium
   B. Decidual cells do not support the invading trophoblasts
   C. With the placental invasion, large lacunae are formed and are filled with fetal blood
   D. Chorion frondosum forms the placenta
   E. Chorion laevae forms the placenta

2. Which one of the following is correct regarding the umbilical cord?
   A. It has two veins and one artery
   B. The arterial blood has more oxygen
   C. One artery and one vein are compatible with fetal growth and a live baby
   D. Cord artery has a systolic pressure of 120 mmHg
   E. The vessels are surrounded by a hydrophobic mucopolysaccharide called Wharton's jelly

3. Which one of the following is correct regarding placental transfer?
   A. Transfer of placental gases is by simple diffusion
   B. Transfer of glucose is by simple diffusion
   C. In active transport the concentration of the substrate transported in fetal blood is lower than on the maternal blood
   D. Low-molecular-weight substrates are transported by pinocytosis
   E. Amino acids are transferred by facilitated diffusion

4. Placental function includes all of the following except:
   A. Gaseous exchange
   B. Fetal nutrition
   C. Removal of waste products
   D. Endocrine function
   E. A barrier for infections

5. Regarding amniotic fluid, which one of the following is correct?
   A. Polyhydramnios is associated with fetal anomaly
   B. On average amniotic fluid volume at 38 weeks' gestation is 500–600 mL
   C. The only complication of long-standing severe oligohydramnios is postural deformities
   D. Most cases of intrauterine growth restriction have normal liquor volume

E. Amnio-infusion is a standard procedure for variable decelerations observed on the cardiotocography

Chapter 5

1. Which one of the following statements is true of perinatal mortality?
   A. Perinatal mortality is an indication of the wealth of the nation
   B. Perinatal mortality rate describes the number of stillbirths and early neonatal deaths per 105 total births
   C. It is an important indication of maternal health and the standard of maternal and neonatal care
   D. The World Health Organization has set targets of perinatal mortality for each country
   E. The World Bank gives financial incentives to countries that have the best perinatal mortality rates

2. Which one of the following statements is true of stillbirth?
   A. Stillbirths are the number of stillbirths per 105 total births.
   B. Using the Wigglesworth Classification, around 30% are classified as of unknown antecedent
   C. The most common cause of stillbirth is intrapartum stillbirth
   D. The region with the highest stillbirth rate in the world is in the Caribbean
   E. Using modern classifications, the most common cause of stillbirth is fetal growth restriction

3. Which one of the following statements is true of neonatal deaths?
   A. Low birth weight is a well-known direct cause
   B. In low-resource countries, tetanus remains one of the most important causes of neonatal deaths
   C. The neonatal death rates related to prematurity in developing countries have shown a significant fall
   D. In the UK (CMACE) extreme prematurity accounts for nearly half of the neonatal deaths
   E. The best investment to improve the neonatal death rates is to build more neonatal intensive care units

4. Which one of the following statements most accurately describes maternal deaths?
   A. Direct maternal deaths arise from complications or their management, which are unique to pregnancy, occurring during the antenatal, intrapartum or postpartum periods
   B. Coincidental causes occur when two or more causes are noted to cause a mother's death
   C. The maternal mortality rate in the UK is defined as the number of direct and indirect deaths per 100,000 live births

D. Maternal mortality rates reflect the state of antenatal care of a country
E. They can be reduced by increasing the number of doctors and midwives
5. Which one of these statements is true of maternal mortality?
  A. Group B streptococcus is a major cause of maternal mortality
  B. Cardiac disease is the leading cause of direct deaths in the UK
  C. Group A streptococcus sepsis is easily recognized and treated
  D. Group A streptococcus sepsis was the leading cause of maternal deaths in the UK between 2006 and 2008
  E. Venous thromboembolism is now a rare cause of death

Chapter 6

1. What is the most appropriate description of recognized physiological changes in pregnancy?
  A. Breast lumps are a physiological variant in pregnancy
  B. A reddish-brownish pigmentation over the cheeks should prompt the investigation of possible concomitant lupus (systemic lupus erythematosus [SLE])
  C. A reduction in Hb concentration is principally due to reduced red cell production
  D. The pelvic shape becomes more gynaecoid under the influence of hormonal change in pregnancy
  E. The pelvic inlet is bounded posteriorly by the sacral promontory and anteriorly by the superior pubic rami and upper margin of the pubic symphysis
2. In eliciting an obstetric history, which of the following is correct?
  A. Previous obstetric history is relatively unimportant, as management decisions are made on how the current pregnancy has progressed
  B. The first date of the last menstrual period (LMP) is a reliable indicator of the expected date of delivery (EDD)
  C. The pre-ovulatory period is fairly constant, whereas the post-ovulatory period shows a wide variation in a typical menstrual cycle
  D. Ultrasound scan in the third trimester accurately determines the gestational age
  E. Hormonal contraception may be associated with a delay in ovulation in the first cycle after discontinuation
3. Regarding symptoms of pregnancy, which one of following statements is most appropriate?

A. Nausea and vomiting commonly occur 10 weeks after missing the first period
B. Hyperemesis gravidarum is characterized by excessive vomiting in the third trimester
C. Increased frequency of micturition tends to worsen after the first 12 weeks of pregnancy as the uterus rises above the symphysis pubis
D. Plasma osmolality gradually increases with advancing gestation
E. There is an increased diuretic response after water loading when the woman is sitting in the upright position
4. During pregnancy, which of the following statements is correct?
  A. Blood pressure is recorded with the patient lying flat on her back to get the most accurate reading
  B. Blood pressure should be recorded on different positions during each antenatal visit, alternating the blood pressure cuff on different arms
  C. If inferior vena cava compression is not recognized for a prolonged period, fetal compromise may occur secondary to a reduction in uteroplacental circulation
  D. Diastolic pressure should be taken with the fourth Korotkoff's sound (i.e. fading of the sound)
  E. Benign 'flow murmurs' due to the hypodynamic circulation are common and are of no significance
5. In pelvic examination during pregnancy, which of the following is correct?
  A. Routine pelvic examination to confirm pregnancy and gestation at booking should be performed, even in settings where an ultrasound scan is freely available
  B. Digital vaginal examination is contraindicated in later pregnancy in cases of antepartum haemorrhage until placenta praevia can be excluded
  C. Routine antenatal radiological pelvimetry has been shown to be of value in predicting outcome of labour in primigravid women
  D. In a normal female or gynaecoid pelvis, because the sacrum is evenly curved, maximum space for the fetal head is provided at the pelvic outlet
  E. The diameter of the pelvic inlet is usually longer in the anteroposterior (AP) diameter than the transverse diameter

Chapter 7

1. Antenatal screening for infection is designed to provide the best outcome for the mother and the fetus/newborn. Which one of the following investigations is not recommended as part of routine antenatal care?
  A. Hepatitis B
  B. Cytomegalovirus

C. Syphilis

D. Rubella

E. HIV

2. What is the most appropriate statement regarding group B streptococcus?

   A. It is a Gram-negative bacteria

   B. It is not a commensal organism

   C. It is associated with an increased risk of pre-term birth

   D. Screening is routine in the antenatal period in all countries

   E. If group B streptococcus is found in urine culture, there is no need to treat subsequently in labour

3. There is an increased risk of gestational diabetes in all of the following except:

   A. Previous macrosomic baby weighing >4.5 kg

   B. Maternal body mass index (BMI) >35

   C. First-degree relatives with diabetes mellitus

   D. Gestational diabetes in previous pregnancy

   E. Maternal age <20

4. Extra folic acid supplementation is recommended in all of the following except:

   A. Previous child with neural tube defects

   B. Women on anti-epileptic medication

   C. Women with diabetes mellitus

   D. Maternal obesity with a body mass index (BMI) >35

   E. Mothers who had a previous Down's syndrome baby

5. Which one of the following is the most appropriate advice in pregnancy?

   A. Mothers are encouraged to reduce exercise and rest routinely

   B. Anti-D Ig is routinely administered after complete spontaneous miscarriage at 8 weeks' gestation

   C. Moderate alcohol consumption is not harmful in pregnancy and is reasonable

   D. Smoking is harmful to the fetus and should be stopped promptly

   E. Paracetamol is proven to be a safe drug in pregnancy

Chapter 8

1. With regard to an antepartum haemorrhage at 36 weeks, what is considered the commonest cause?

   A. Placenta previa

   B. Placental abruption

   C. Idiopathic

   D. A cervical gynaecological lesion

   E. Vasa previa

2. With regard to hypertension in pregnancy, which statement is most appropriate?

   A. Normal physiological change is for an increase in blood pressure from the first trimester onwards

   B. A diastolic reading of >90 mmHg is more significant than a systolic reading of >150 mmHg

   C. Pre-eclampsia is defined as the development of hypertension after 20 weeks

   D. The most important regulatory factor of maternal blood pressure in pregnancy is a fall in peripheral resistance

   E. The HELLP syndrome is a mild variant of pre-eclampsia

3. In twin pregnancy, what is the most appropriate statement?

   A. The prevalence of identical (monozygotic) twins varies from country to country

   B. The twin peak sign is most commonly seen on a first-trimester ultrasound in dizygotic twins

   C. Miscarriage is less common than in singleton pregnancies

   D. Pre-term delivery is increased by a factor of two with respect to a singleton pregnancy

   E. The feto-fetal (twin–twin) transfusion syndrome presents only after 24 weeks' gestation

4. The causes of an unstable lie include all of the following except:

   A. Placenta previa

   B. Polyhydramnios

   C. Subseptate uterus

   D. Primiparity

   E. Twin pregnancy

5. In prolonged pregnancy, which one of the following statements is correct?

   A. 'Postmaturity syndrome' refers to pregnancy beyond 294 days

   B. 'Postmaturity syndrome' is characterized by polyhydramnios

   C. Postmaturity is associated with an increased incidence of meconium in the amniotic fluid

   D. Is only associated with an increase in perinatal morbidity, not mortality

   E. It is managed by induction of labour at 40 weeks' gestation

Chapter 9

1. Anaemia in pregnancy is most frequently caused by:

   A. Sickle cell disease

   B. Folate deficiency

   C. B_{12} deficiency

   D. Thalassaemia

   E. Iron deficiency

2. Which of the following is not considered a causative hormone that can increase the risk of gestational diabetes?

   A. Cortisol

B. Glucagon

C. Human placental lactogen

D. Oestrogen

E. Progesterone

3. In acute venous thromboembolism in pregnancy, which one of the following statements is true?

A. Is more likely to occur in the right leg compared to the left

B. Can be diagnosed by the use of D-dimer measurements

C. Is two times more likely than in the non-pregnant state

D. Is a leading cause of maternal mortality in the developed world

E. Is treated by warfarin in the first instance

4. Which of the following infections is true regarding Zika virus in pregnancy?

A. Approximately 80% of women will be symptomatic

B. Pregnant women are more susceptible to infection than non-pregnant women

C. Routine antenatal testing of asymptomatic women in high-risk areas is recommended

D. The commonest method of transmission is sexual

E. The principal clinical concern in pregnancy is congenital abnormality

F. Similar efficacy of ultrasound screening

5. Concerning epilepsy and pregnancy, which of the following statements is true?

A. The majority of women will have an increase in seizure frequency in pregnancy

B. Women with epilepsy have a 25% chance of having a child who develops epilepsy

C. Neural tube defects and cardiac abnormalities are the commonest abnormalities seen with anti-epileptic medication

D. 400 μg of folic acid should be taken pre-conceptually and throughout the first trimester

E. Breast-feeding should be avoided

Chapter 10

1. Ultrasound of fetal anatomy at 20 weeks does not detect the majority of abnormalities in which of the following organ systems?

A. Cardiac

B. Central nervous system

C. Skeletal

D. Gastrointestinal

E. Urogenital

2. A woman aged 20 years (with a background risk of delivering a baby with Down's syndrome of 1:1500) has a first-trimester screening test for Down's syndrome which reports a risk of 1:150. Which of the following statements is true regarding this?

A. The positive predictive value of the screening test is high

B. The negative predictive value of the screening test is low

C. Her chances of having a baby with Down's syndrome are approximately 1350 times (1500–150=1350) greater than we would expect in someone of her age

D. There is less than 1% chance her baby has Down's syndrome

E. If she has a chorionic villus sampling (CVS), she will have about a 1 in 50 chance of miscarrying from the procedure

3. Which one of the following statements about assessment of fetal growth in pregnancy is not correct?

A. Ultrasound measurement of fetal abdominal circumference is the best single parameter to record fetal growth

B. The relative size of fetal head and abdominal circumferences measured by ultrasound is a useful measure in clinical practice

C. Serial symphysio-fundal height measurements during pregnancy will detect over 80% of small-for-dates fetuses

D. Identification of a small-for-dates fetus on ultrasound is an indication to confirm that fetal anatomy is normal

E. Identification of a small-for-dates fetus on ultrasound is an indication to assess blood flow in the umbilical artery with Doppler ultrasound

4. Which of the following tests used in the management of women with high-risk pregnancies have been shown to improve fetal outcome in randomized controlled trials?

A. Fetal cardiotocography

B. Umbilical artery blood flow recorded with Doppler ultrasound

C. Maternal fetal movement counting

D. Fetal biophysical profile testing

E. Ultrasound measurement of amniotic fluid volume

5. Which of the following chromosomal abnormalities is most commonly found on screening?

A. 45XO (Turner's)

B. Trisomy 21 (Down's)

C. 47 XXY (Klinefelter's)

D. Trisomy 18 (Edwards)

E. Trisomy 13 (Patau)

Chapter 11

1. Which one of the following is diagnostic of labour?

A. The appearance of 'show'

B. Rupture of membranes

C. Self-reported painful uterine contractions

D. Regular painful uterine contractions with cervical change
E. Backache and abdominal pain

2. Slow labour progress in the first stage of labour is most likely to be due to which one of the following.
A. Fetal weight of >4 kg
B. Incoordinate uterine contractions
C. Malposition of the fetal head
D. Gynaecoid pelvis
E. Primigravidity

3. Normal-term labour appears to be initiated by which of the following mechanisms?
A. Systemic progesterone withdrawal
B. Reduced prostaglandin secretion
C. Downregulation of fetal inflammatory response
D. Placental production of the corticotrophin-releasing hormone (CRH)
E. Infection of the amniotic membranes

4. The complications of epidural analgesia include all of the following except:
A. Blood-stained tap
B. Accidental dural tap
C. Hypertension
D. Total spinal blockade
E. Accidental nerve injury

5. Electronic fetal monitoring features that are reassuring for the fetal state are:
A. Accelerations of the fetal heart rate
B. Absence of accelerations
C. Presence of variable decelerations
D. Absent baseline variability
E. Presence of late decelerations

6. In the management of pre-term labour, which of the following is associated with a proven clinical benefit?
A. Terbutaline
B. Atosiban
C. Corticosteroids
D. Antibiotics
E. Glyceryl trinitrate (GTN)

7. Which one of the following is not an accepted indication for induction of labour?
A. Prolonged pregnancy
B. Diabetes in pregnancy
C. Macrosomic baby
D. Intrauterine growth restriction
E. Pre-eclampsia at term

8. The following are all known complications of induction of labour except:
A. Prematurity
B. Cord prolapse
C. Fetal distress
D. Uterine rupture
E. Less painful labour

Chapter 12

1. In normal delivery, which one of the following statements is correct?
A. The normal duration of the second stage of labour in a nulliparous woman who has received epidural analgesia is commonly regarded as lasting up to 2 hours
B. The fetal head is said to be engaged when the bony part of the vertex has descended to the level of the ischial spines
C. The mother experiences a sensation to bear down when the cervix becomes fully dilated
D. Continuous pushing throughout the duration of a contraction is the preferred method for maternal expulsion
E. The fetal head should be maintained in an attitude of flexion until it has passed through the introitus

2. In perineal injury and episiotomy, which one of the following statements is correct?
A. Mediolateral episiotomy compared to midline episiotomy is associated with more third- and fourth-degree perineal injuries
B. A third-degree perineal tear is diagnosed when the external anal sphincter is completely torn
C. A fourth-degree laceration has occurred when both the external and internal anal sphincters are disrupted
D. Instrumental delivery and persistent occipitoposterior (OP) position are risk factors for severe perineal tears
E. Failure to repair injury to the anal sphincter may result in short-term, but not long-term, incontinence of flatus and faeces

3. Regarding caesarean section, which one of the following statements is correct?
A. The rising caesarean section rate witnessed over recent years has resulted in a corresponding decrease in the instrumental delivery rate
B. Women who have had one previous lower segment caesarean section (LSCS) should not attempt vaginal delivery in a subsequent pregnancy
C. A previous LSCS carries a greater risk of scar dehiscence than a classical caesarean section because the lower segment is thinner
D. A persistent occiput posterior (OP) position of the fetus in the second stage of labour is a contraindication for forceps or vacuum-assisted delivery
E. Almost all babies with a face presentation in labour are delivered by caesarean section

4. Regarding operative vaginal delivery, which one of the following statements is correct?
   A. McRobert's manoeuvre alone is successful in about 50% of cases of shoulder dystocia
   B. Elective caesarean delivery of all macrosomic infants (>4500 g) will eliminate the majority of cases of shoulder dystocia
   C. The vacuum extractor is just as successful as the obstetric forceps for assisted vaginal delivery
   D. Forceps delivery compared with vacuum extraction is associated with more third- and fourth-degree perineal lacerations
   E. Vacuum extraction, but not forceps delivery, may be attempted when the cervix is not completely dilated and the fetal head position is not certain

5. Regarding postpartum haemorrhage (PPH), which one of the following statements is correct?
   A. Uterine atony is responsible for at least 75% of primary PPH obstetric cases
   B. Active management of the third stage of labour does not reduce the risk of postpartum bleeding
   C. Tranexamic acid within 3 hours of PPH will reduce mortality by 80%
   D. Ergometrine should not be administered intravenously despite continuing PPH because of the risk of vasoconstriction
   E. Intrauterine tamponade may increase postpartum bleeding by preventing effective contraction and retraction of the uterine muscle

Chapter 13

1. Physiological changes in the puerperium include:
   A. Increase in serum levels of oestrogen and progesterone
   B. Increase in clotting factors
   C. Decrease in prolactin levels in women who breast-feed
   D. Drop in platelet count
   E. Sudden decrease in cardiac output

2. Risk factors for anal sphincter injury include:
   A. Occipitoanterior position
   B. Second stage of an hour
   C. Epidural analgesia
   D. A baby weight less than 4 kg
   E. Multiparous pregnancy

3. In the UK, the most common overall direct cause of maternal death in 2016 was:
   A. Thromboembolism
   B. Cardiac disease
   C. Haemorrhage
   D. Sepsis
   E. Amniotic fluid embolism

4. With regard to postnatal anticoagulation for pulmonary embolism (PE), which one of the following statements is correct?
   A. Heparin is contraindicated in breast-feeding
   B. Warfarin is contraindicated in breast-feeding
   C. Warfarin cannot be commenced immediately postpartum
   D. Anticoagulant therapy should be continued for a total of at least 3 months
   E. Postnatal review for women who develop venous thromboembolism (VTE) during pregnancy should be with the general practitioner (GP)

5. In examination of the newborn, which one of the following statements is correct?
   A. Most commonly involves assuring normality
   B. The ideal time for this is at 7 days of age
   C. Jaundice in the first 24 hours is normal
   D. Umbilical hernias carry a risk of strangulation and need referral to the surgeon
   E. A high-pitch cry is normal

Chapter 14

1. Regarding psychiatric disorders of pregnancy and childbirth, which one of the following statements is true?
   A. They affect less than 5% of women in pregnancy
   B. Psychiatric medication should be stopped in the first trimester
   C. Pregnancy and childbirth are less likely to precipitate psychiatric disorders than other major life events
   D. It is a leading cause of direct maternal death
   E. Elevated incidence of severe mood disorders is associated with increased risk of suicide

2. Regarding depressive illness in pregnancy, all of the following statements are true except:
   A. Stopping medication will cause relapse in 50% of mothers
   B. Anxiety is a prominent feature
   C. Counselling and cognitive behavioural therapy are more effective than medication for mild to moderate depression and anxiety
   D. Commonly used antidepressants are selective serotonin reuptake inhibitors (SSRIs)
   E. Most women will be able to discontinue antidepressant therapy during pregnancy

3. In postpartum psychosis, which of the following statements is true?
   A. The overall incidence is greatest between 6 and 12 weeks postnatal
   B. Depression is the commonest antecedent psychiatric condition

C. Bipolar affective disorder, when stable, can usually be managed by the obstetric services

D. Symptoms and signs of the disease are commonly subtle

E. The chances of recurrence in a woman with previous postpartum psychosis is 50%

4. Selective serotonin reuptake inhibitors (SSRIs) are associated with all of the following except:
   A. No increase in congenital malformation in the fetus
   B. Increased pregnancy loss
   C. Intrauterine growth restriction
   D. Pulmonary hypertension in the newborn
   E. Neonatal hypoglycaemia

5. Regarding eating disorders in pregnancy and the puerperium, which of the following is correct?
   A. A consistent association between low birth weight and anorexia has been reported
   B. A consistent association between prematurity and anorexia has been reported
   C. Mother–baby relationships are recognized to be more difficult
   D. Eating disorders tend to be of the same severity in the antenatal and postnatal periods
   E. Most pregnant women with eating disorders disclose their illness

Chapter 15

1. In which of the following circumstances is it reasonable for a chaperone not to be present during vaginal examination?
   A. If the doctor performing the examination is known to the patient
   B. If the doctor is female
   C. If the examination is performed in the clinic with a nurse outside the room
   D. Where the patient has indicated that they do not wish a third person to be present
   E. If the patient is elderly

2. You are performing a pelvic examination on a 26-year-old woman who has presented with abnormal bleeding. Having explained the procedure and obtained verbal consent, you perform the examination, but as you insert the speculum the patient becomes distressed and asks you to stop. In addition to acknowledging her distress and apologizing for the discomfort which of the following would be the most appropriate response?
   A. Withdraw the speculum and proceed with bimanual pelvic examination
   B. Change to smaller speculum and try again
   C. Explain that without being to do the examination you will be unable to make a diagnosis and retry the

examination again after a few minutes
   D. Stop the examination, allow the patient to get dressed and discuss alternatives
   E. Explain that the examination will only take a few more seconds and complete the examination

3. On performing a speculum examination for a routine Pap smear for a 30-year-old multiparous woman on the contraceptive pill, you notice an area of epithelium surrounding the cervical os that appears darker red than the pink epithelium covering the rest of the cervix. There is no abnormal discharge, ulceration or contact bleeding. The Pap smear result is normal. You see her 2 weeks later to discuss the results. Which of the following would be the most appropriate action to take?
   A. Refer for colposcopic examination
   B. Ask her to return for a further Pap smear at the normal screening interval
   C. Take a punch biopsy from the area
   D. Request a first-pass urine sample for Chlamydia polymerase chain reaction (PCR)
   E. Organize for cryotherapy to the affected area

4. Which of the following findings on bimanual pelvic examination can be considered normal?
   A. Increased discomfort on movement of the cervix
   B. A 7-cm palpable mass in the right adnexal region
   C. A mobile retroverted uterus
   D. Nodularity in the posterior formix
   E. A uterus equivalent in size to a 12-week pregnancy in a non-pregnant patient

5. For which of the following is a Sims' speculum normally used in outpatient vaginal examinations?
   A. Taking a cervical smear
   B. Taking vaginal swabs
   C. Assessment of anterior vaginal wall prolapse
   D. Assessment of pelvic floor tone
   E. Insertion of an intrauterine device

Chapter 16

1. A 50-year-old premenopausal woman is referred to the gynaecology clinic following an ultrasound which indicates the presence of a 7-cm solitary leiomyoma in the posterior uterine wall. She is asymptomatic. Which one of the following would be the most appropriate management?
   A. Reassure her that no treatment is necessary unless she develops symptoms
   B. Uterine artery embolization (UAE)
   C. Laparoscopic myomectomy
   D. A 6-month course of gonadotrophin-releasing hormone (GnRH) analogues
   E. Hysterectomy

2. A 45-year-old multiparous woman presents with regular heavy periods. Pelvic examination and recent Pap smear are normal. She is sexually active but has completed her family and is using condoms for contraception. A full blood count shows that she is anaemic with a haemoglobin of 104 g/L and an iron-deficient picture. She smokes 10 cigarettes a day but is otherwise in good health with no significant past medical or family history. Which of the following would be the most appropriate management for her symptoms?
   A. Tranexamic acid 1 g qds during her periods
   B. Norethisterone 5 mg bd day 12–26 of each cycle
   C. Insertion of Mirena intrauterine device (IUD)
   D. Endometrial resection
   E. Laparoscopically assisted vaginal hysterectomy

3. A 22-year-old woman presents with a 2-year history of oligo-amenorrhoea and a negative pregnancy test. Examination is normal except that she has a body mass index (BMI) of 30. Pelvic ultrasound is normal. A day-21 serum progesterone level is consistent with anovulation. Results of other initial blood investigations are normal except for a marginally raised prolactin level and an increased free-androgen index. Which one of the following would be the most likely cause for her symptoms?
   A. Pituitary adenoma
   B. Premature ovarian failure
   C. Turner's syndrome
   D. Polycystic ovarian syndrome
   E. Functional hypothalamic amenorrhea

4. An 8-year-old girl is brought to her general practitioner (GP) after having had her first period. On examination she is on the 95th centile for her age in height, has stage 2 breast development and has some axillary and pubic hair development. Which of the following would be the most likely diagnosis?
   A. Idiopathic
   B. Central nervous system (CNS) tumour
   C. Congenital adrenal hyperplasia (non-classical)
   D. Granulosa cell tumour of the ovary
   E. Follicular cysts of the ovary

5. A 49-year-old woman with no significant past medical history except for a hysterectomy for heavy menstrual bleeding 2 years ago is requesting hormone replacement therapy (HRT) for hot flushes. Which of the following conditions would she be at increased risk of developing if she takes HRT?
   A. Ischaemic heart disease
   B. Colonic carcinoma
   C. Osteoporosis
   D. Endometrial cancer
   E. Deep venous thrombosis

Chapter 17

1. A couple are investigated, and the woman is found to have premature ovarian failure. Which biochemical pattern would support this?
   A. Elevated follicle-stimulating hormone (FSH), elevated luteinizing hormone (LH), suppressed oestradiol
   B. Suppressed FSH, suppressed LH, suppressed oestradiol
   C. Normal FSH, elevated LH, normal oestradiol
   D. Suppressed FSH, suppressed LH, normal oestradiol
   E. Normal FSH, normal LH, suppressed oestradiol

2. Which of the following is not a recognized cause of oligospermia?
   A. Sulfasalazine
   B. Mesalazine
   C. Cyclophosphamide
   D. Nandrolone
   E. Cannabis

3. Regarding in vitro fertilization, which one of the following statements is correct?
   A. The natural luteinizing hormone (LH) surge is used to induce final oocyte maturation
   B. The chance of a live birth after a single cycle of treatment at age 40 years is approximately 30%
   C. Gonadotropin medications are given from the start of the luteal phase of the cycle
   D. Embryos reach the blastocyst stage 2 days after fertilization
   E. Endometrial thickness on the day of embryo transfer should exceed 5 mm in order to give a good chance of implantation

4. Which of the following is not a feature of in vitro fertilization (IVF) ovarian hyperstimulation syndrome (OHSS)?
   A. Decreased capillary permeability
   B. Elevated serum oestradiol
   C. Pleural effusion
   D. Pericardial effusion
   E. Ascites

5. Which of the following is most appropriate regarding pre-implantation genetic screening (PGS)?
   A. The purpose of PGS is to look for single gene defects in known carriers
   B. The aim is to use PGS to select the best embryo for transfer.
   C. PGS should be used for aneuploidy screening in all cases of in vitro fertilization (IVF)
   D. PGS has been shown to increase the success of IVF cycles
   E. PGS has most utility with maternal age <35

Chapter 18

1. A 45-year-old woman has a miscarriage in her first pregnancy at 11 weeks' gestation. She has no other family or medical history of note. Which one of the following would be the most likely cause for the loss of her pregnancy?
   A. Isoimmunization
   B. Antiphospholipid antibody syndrome
   C. Cervical incompetence
   D. Bicornuate uterus
   E. Fetal chromosomal abnormality
2. When chromosomal abnormality is responsible for a sporadic miscarriage, what is the most likely karyotypic abnormality?
   A. 45-XO
   B. 47-trisomy 21
   C. 46XY/45XO mosaic
   D. 69-triploidy
   E. Unbalanced robertsonian translocation
3. A 26-year-old is admitted to the emergency department of a small local hospital with a 12-hour history of lower abdominal pain and vaginal bleeding. Her last period was 8 weeks ago, and she has a positive urinary pregnancy test. On examination she is pale and sweaty with a blood pressure of 70/40 and a pulse of 50. Her abdomen is soft on palpation with no evidence of guarding or rebound. After obtaining intravenous access and starting resuscitation, which of the following would be the most appropriate next step in treatment?
   A. Arrange an ultrasound scan to check for an intrauterine pregnancy
   B. Take her to theatre for laparoscopy to exclude ectopic pregnancy
   C. Perform a speculum examination to check for products of conception
   D. Prescribe misoprostol and arrange ultrasound scan for 2 days' time
   E. Arrange for transfer to the nearest hospital with a gynaecology department
4. Regarding uterine abnormalities and miscarriage, which one of the following uterine variations has the highest association with miscarriage?
   A. Arcuate
   B. Bicornuate
   C. Subseptate
   D. Unicornuate
   E. Didelphus
5. After diagnosis of an ectopic pregnancy in a woman with significant pain, what is the most appropriate statement regarding treatment?
   A. Urgent methotrexate administration is a reasonable management plan

   B. Salpingotomy is the preferred option if the contralateral tube is normal
   C. Recurrent ectopic pregnancy is more common after salpingotomy compared to salpingectomy
   D. Persistent trophoblastic disease is more common following salpingectomy
   E. Subsequent pregnancy rates are lower following salpingectomy compared to salpingotomy
6. Which of the following situations should be prescribed anti-D immunoglobulin prophylaxis?
   A. Threatened miscarriage
   B. Complete miscarriage
   C. Incomplete miscarriage with conservative management
   D. Ectopic pregnancy with laparoscopic salpingectomy
   E. Pregnancy of unknown location (PUL) with conservative management

Chapter 19

1. A 19-year-old attends a sexual health clinic because she is concerned she may have contracted a sexually transmitted infection (STI) following recent unprotected sexual intercourse. That partner has informed her he has chlamydia. She is asymptomatic, and examination is completely normal. What would be the most appropriate investigation to test for chlamydia?
   A. Low vaginal swab for culture
   B. High vaginal swab for culture
   C. IgM antibody testing
   D. IgG antibody testing
   E. Polymerase chain reaction (PCR)
2. A 25-year-old woman comes for advice about the effectiveness of various contraceptive methods, as she has a new partner. There are no contraindications to any method. Which one of the following would be considered to have the best efficacy in preventing an unwanted pregnancy?
   A. The combined oestrogen/progestogen oral contraceptive pill
   B. The Nuva vaginal contraceptive ring
   C. A desogestrel progesterone-only pill
   D. Three monthly injections of Depo-Provera
   E. The Implanon contraceptive rod
3. A 26-year-old woman, who has always had irregular periods, presents for contraceptive advice. Her body mass index (BMI) is 32, blood pressure is 120/80 mmHg and clinical examination is normal apart from some hirsutism. Which one of the following oral contraceptive pills (OCP) would be most appropriate to prescribe?
   A. An OCP containing 20 μg of ethinyl oestradiol and levonorgestrel

411

B. An OCP containing 30 μg of ethinyl oestradiol and levonorgestrel

C. An OCP containing 50 μg of ethinyl oestradiol and levonorgestrel

D. An OCP containing ethinyl oestradiol and cyproterone acetate

E. An OCP containing low-dose levonorgestrel only

4. Following insertion of a copper intrauterine contraceptive device (IUCD), the strings are not visible on first string check. Which of the following IUCD complications is not a possible cause of missing strings?
   A. Pregnancy
   B. Endometrial infection
   C. Expulsion
   D. Device inversion
   E. Perforation

5. Which of the following is most appropriate regarding deep venous thrombosis and combined oral contraceptive pill (COCP) use?
   A. The risk with the COCP is equivalent to that in pregnancy
   B. The relative risk is three times the general population risk
   C. The risk is equivalent, regardless of progestogen content
   D. The relative risk is around 15/100,000 women per year
   E. The risk is higher in COCP users who are younger

Chapter 20

1. Which of the following is commonly found with vulval cancer?
   A. Vulval intraepithelial neoplasia (VIN)
   B. Differentiated VIN
   C. Paget's disease
   D. Condyloma
   E. Herpes simplex infection

2. Regarding primary prevention of cervical cancer, which is the most appropriate statement?
   A. Cytological screening has been shown to be an effective primary prevention measure
   B. The bivalent vaccine targets the two high-risk subtypes: HPV 6 and 11
   C. The quadrivalent vaccine targets four high-risk subtypes
   D. Human papilloma virus (HPV) vaccination programmes have shown at least a 70% reduction in high-risk HPV
   E. HPV vaccines are of no efficacy after sexual debut

3. Which of the following is a predisposing factor for endometrial cancer?
   A. Oral contraceptive pills
   B. Multiparity
   C. Obesity
   D. Human papillomavirus infection
   E. BRCA carrier

Chapter 21

1. The uterosacral ligaments provide support to:
   A. The urinary bladder
   B. Rectum
   C. Upper vagina and cervix
   D. Urethra
   E. The external anal sphincter

2. A 58-year-old patient with a cystocele may commonly present with symptoms of:
   A. Postmenopausal bleeding
   B. Deep dyspareunia
   C. Incomplete bladder emptying
   D. Constipation
   E. Urinary urgency

3. A 22-year-old para 1 has symptoms of stress urinary incontinence. Which of the following would be the first step in management?
   A. Pelvic floor physiotherapy
   B. Advise a mid-urethral sling
   C. Arrange bladder pressure studies
   D. Oxybutynin
   E. Anterior colporrhaphy

4. A 29-year-old G_1P_1 presents with uterovaginal prolapse. She is planning to have further pregnancies. Which of the following would be the most appropriate management?
   A. Vaginal pessaries
   B. Manchester repair
   C. Fascial repairs of the vagina
   D. Graft (mesh) repairs of the vagina
   E. Arrange pelvic floor physiotherapy and advise her to delay surgery until her family is completed

5. Which of the following is least likely to be a cause of acute retention of urine in women?
   A. Vaginal tears during childbirth
   B. Impacted retroverted gravid uterus
   C. Inflammatory lesions of the vulva
   D. Vaginal repair of prolapse
   E. Radiotherapy for cervical cancer

Appendix A

1. Which of the following is not a routine preoperative investigation?
   A. Full blood count in an otherwise healthy patient
   B. Pregnancy test in a reproductive-age woman
   C. Coagulation screen in an otherwise healthy patient
   D. Electrocardiogram in patients of advanced age
   E. Urea and electrolytes in a woman on loop diuretics

2. Regarding World Health Organization (WHO) perioperative checks, which of the following is most appropriate?
   A. 'Sign in' is the final WHO stage of any procedure
   B. The preoperative 'huddle' should include administrative staff to reduce the risk of wrong patient identification
   C. 'Time out' is the first WHO stage of any procedure
   D. 'Sign out' should include swab and instrument count recording
   E. WHO checklists, whilst sensible, have not yet been shown to reduce morbidity and mortality

3. Which of the following medications should be avoided before major surgery to reduce the risk of thromboembolism?
   A. Progesterone-only pill
   B. Hormone replacement therapy (HRT)
   C. Combined oral contraceptive pill (OCP)
   D. Gonadotropin-releasing hormone (GnRH) agonists for abnormal uterine bleeding
   E. Antibiotic prophylaxis before the start of the procedure

4. Which of the following complications could be caused by an inappropriate lithotomy position?
   A. Gas embolization
   B. Skin necrosis
   C. Femoral hernia
   D. Ankle pain
   E. Acute compartment syndrome

5. Which of the following factors do not increase the risk of urinary tract injuries?
   A. Endometriosis
   B. Bladder overdistension
   C. Advanced age
   D. Suprapubic trocar insertion
   E. Urinary infection

6. Which of the following is not a common cause of postoperative hypotension?
   A. Dehydration
   B. Bleeding
   C. Renal failure
   D. Heart failure
   E. Epidural analgesia

7. Which one of the following statements is correct?
   A. Klebsiella is a common microorganism in surgical site injuries
   B. Postoperative pelvic abscesses are frequently caused by aerobic flora
   C. Diabetes is a risk factor for surgical site infections, while smoking is protective
   D. Hair removal by shaving is a protective factor
   E. Surgical drains are a risk factor for surgical site infections

8. Concerning enhanced recovery programmes for elective surgery, which one of the following statements is correct?
   A. Enhanced recovery pathways are associated with more initial pain due to increased mobilization
   B. Enhanced recovery pathways require more nursing time
   C. Enhanced recovery pathways are principally aimed at reducing the effects of intraoperative insult
   D. Enhanced recovery pathways are generic
   E. The period of starvation is reduced to 2 hours for clear fluids prior to anaesthetic to avoid dehydration

Appendix B

1. Which of the following is considered a potential disadvantage of using social media in a medical context?
   A. Patients accessing health information
   B. Professional networking
   C. Social networking
   D. Maintaining confidentiality
   E. Communicating with large numbers easily

2. Regarding General Data Protection Regulation (GDPR) data protection, which of the following statements is correct?
   A. GDPR was introduced in 2016
   B. GDPR is an EU data protection law
   C. GDPR has no remit outside the UK
   D. The key term in GDPR involves corporate data
   E. GDPR offers rights for people to have completely open access to the information companies/organizations hold about them

3. Regarding research and a clinical audit, which of the following statements is correct?
   A. A clinical audit and clinical research address similar questions in order to improve patient care
   B. A clinical audit seeks to improve the quality of patient care against agreed standards
   C. Clinical research critically appraises routine clinical practice to identify gaps in service provision
   D. A clinical audit should only be done if there is a national guideline
   E. Clinical research is usually funded by the pharma-

413

ceutical companies to test their drugs

4. Regarding clinical guidelines, which of the following statements is correct?
   A. Clinical guidelines are evidence-based statements to assist clinicians to make appropriate clinical decisions in order to improve patient care
   B. It is mandatory for all organizations to implement all clinical guidelines once they are published
   C. Guidelines are usually developed by clinicians working in the hospitals
   D. Different organizations developing clinical guidelines regularly consult each other and follow similar methodology
   E. The clinical guidelines recommendations are based on cost-effectiveness data

5. In research, which one of the following statements is correct?
   A. Descriptive studies provide information on disease prevalence in a population
   B. Case control and cohort studies compare people with the disease and those without it
   C. Randomized clinical trials involve allocation of different treatments (interventions) on good faith of the clinicians
   D. Clinicians are usually aware of whether their patients are being treated with an active or a dummy preparation
   E. Clinical trials of new drugs must exclude pregnant women and those who wish to become pregnant during the study

6. Regarding evidence-based health care, which of the following statements is correct?
   A. Evidence-based health care should ensure that risk management strategies are in place to reduce risk to all patients
   B. Clinical risk management strategies should only focus on cases of maternal and neonatal mortality
   C. Clinical incident reporting involves setting up investigation panels against all those involved in the care of a specific patient
   D. Patients should be encouraged to complain against staff, as it helps to improve care
   E. The investigations of near-misses within an organization should be privately conducted to reduce risk to the organization

Appendix C

1. A 49-year-old woman is admitted to hospital for the performance of a total abdominal hysterectomy and bilateral salpingo-oophorectomy. She has been fully investigated as an outpatient of the hospital and diagnosed with severe anaemia due to dysfunctional uterine bleeding (DUB). A blood transfusion has been given. You are the surgical registrar who will be performing the surgery, but you have not seen this patient previously. You have available a written document concerning the risks of such surgery; this has been produced by the College of Obstetrics and Gynaecology of the country concerned. Which one of the following statements regarding the obtaining of informed consent is correct?
   A. The consent form must have been discussed and witnessed by the consultant of the surgical unit
   B. Because she has been evaluated in the outpatient clinic, there is no need to discuss the care further
   C. There is no need for you to discuss any potential complications where the risk of these is under 1%
   D. You must discuss the possible alternatives to the proposed surgery, the complications which might occur during the surgery, the care required if such a complication occurred and the postoperative complications and care
   E. You must provide the written college statement concerning the possible complications of the surgery proposed to the patient

2. A 46-year-old woman had a total abdominal hysterectomy for uterine fibroids 10 days ago. The operation itself was apparently uncomplicated; however, a deep vein thrombosis occurred during the postoperative period. She is currently on treatment with warfarin, and this is planned to continue for at least 6 months. Which of the following rules regarding retention of the medical records of the woman should apply?
   A. Retention for 5 years
   B. Retention for 7 years
   C. Retention for 10 years
   D. Retention for 15 years
   E. Retention for 25 years

3. Which one of the following methods of evaluating the adequacy of a particular method of treatment of a specific condition is best?
   A. Expert opinion from a specialist in the field
   B. Occasional case reports
   C. Multiple case reports
   D. Retrospective case/control studies
   E. Randomized controlled clinical trials

4. A 34-year-old woman has just been delivered of a 4500-g baby. The head was delivered by a midwife, but when shoulder dystocia was defined, you were requested to complete the delivery and did so. Unfortunately, the baby has Erb's palsy. Which one of the following pieces of information must be included in the medical record you are completing immediately after the delivery in case the Erb's palsy does not resolve and litigation occurs against you or the hospital?
   A. The exact date and time the baby's head was delivered and by whom
   B. Detailed information of all of the techniques you and others used to effect delivery of the shoulders and the remainder of the baby and signed by you

C. The exact time the remainder of the baby was delivered
D. The Apgar score of the baby at the time of birth
E. All of the above

5. A 15-year-old girl attends your surgery because she wishes a prescription for the oral contraceptive pill (OCP) so that she can commence a sexual relationship with a 'wonderful man'. She has not been sexually active previously. He has indicated to her that he is not prepared to use condoms. She indicates that she does not wish her parents to be informed, as they would not allow such sexual activity. Which one of the following would be the most appropriate advice to give her?
   A. It is illegal to give her the contraceptive pill because of her age
   B. To give her the pill, she would need to give consent for her parents to be informed
   C. To give her the pill she would need to give consent for the appropriate health department to be informed
   D. To give her the pill more information about the male involved would need to be obtained
   E. She should just get her partner to use condoms

Self-assessment: Answers

Chapter 1

1. What is the most appropriate description of the arterial supply of the pelvis?

   B is correct. The internal iliac artery arises at the level of the lumbosacral articulation and passes over the pelvic brim, continuing downward on the posterolateral wall of the cavity of the true pelvis. The anterior division provides the superior, middle and inferior vesical arteries that provide the blood supply for the bladder. The uterine artery initially runs downward in the subperitoneal fat under the inferior attachment of the broad ligament. The uterine artery crosses over the ureter shortly before that structure enters the bladder approximately 1.5–2 cm from the lateral fornix of the vagina. The ovarian arteries descend behind the peritoneum on the surface of the corresponding psoas muscle until they reach the brim of the pelvis.

2. The vagina:

   A is correct. The vagina is a tube of smooth muscle lined by non-cornified squamous epithelium. Anteriorly, it is intimately related to the trigone of the urinary bladder and the urethra. Posteriorly, the lower third is separated from the anal canal by the perineal body, the middle third is related to the rectum and the upper third to the rectouterine pouch (pouch of Douglas). The pH of the vagina in the sexually mature non-pregnant female is between 4.0 and 5.0, which has an important antibacterial function in reducing the risk of pelvic infection.

3. Uterus and its supporting structures:

   A is correct. The anterior ligament is a fascial condensation which, with the adjacent peritoneal uterovesical fold, extends from the anterior aspect of the cervix across the superior surface of the bladder to the peritoneal peritoneum of the anterior abdominal wall. It has a weak supporting role. Likewise, the broad ligament plays only a minor supportive role. Posteriorly, the uterosacral ligaments play a major role in supporting the uterus and the vaginal vault, and these ligaments and their peritoneal covering form the lateral boundaries of the rectouterine pouch (of Douglas). In pregnancy, the isthmus of the uterus enlarges to form the lower segment of the uterus, which in labour becomes a part of the birth canal but does not contribute greatly to the expulsion of the fetus. (The incidence of uterine retroversion is about 10%.)

4. The ovary:

   D is correct. The ovary lies on the posterior surface of the broad ligament in close proximity to the external iliac vessels and the ureter on the lateral pelvic wall. It is attached to the pelvic brim by the suspensory ligament of the ovary. The surface of the ovary is covered by a cuboidal or low columnar type of germinal epithelium. The blood supply is derived from the ovarian artery, which arises directly from the aorta. The follicles are found in both the cortex and medulla of the organ.

5. Uterus:

   B is correct. The blood supply to the uterus comes largely from the uterine artery, but branches of this anastomose with branches of the ovarian vessels in the upper part of the broad ligament, assuring adequate collateral supply to the uterus even following internal iliac ligation. Lymphatic drainage follows the blood vessels. Uterine pain is mediated through sympathetic afferent nerves passing up to T11–T12 and L1–L2. The pudendal nerve (somatic nerve) supplies the vulva and pelvic floor.

Chapter 2

2. What is the most appropriate statement relating to spermatozoa?

   D is correct. The sperm head fuses with the oocyte plasma membrane, and the sperm head and midpiece are indeed engulfed into the oocyte by phagocytosis. The body contains a coiled helix of mitochondria that provides the 'powerhouse' for sperm motility. The tail consists of a central core of two longitudinal fibres surrounded by nine pairs of fibres that terminate at various points until a single ovoid filament remains. These contractile fibres propel the spermatozoa. During their passage through the Fallopian tubes, the sperm undergo the final stage in maturation (capacitation), which enables penetration of the zona pellucida. Seminal plasma has a high concentration of fructose, which is the major source of energy for the spermatozoa. Under favourable circumstances, sperm migrate at a rate of 6 mm/min. This is much faster than could be explained by the motility of the sperm and must therefore also be dependent on active support within the uterine cavity.

2. Normal follicular growth:
B is correct. In a normal ovulatory menstrual cycle, one follicle is selected to become the dominant follicle on day 5–6 of the cycle (B is therefore correct); however, up to 10 show obvious but lesser growth than the dominant follicle (A is therefore incorrect). The dominant follicle grows by 2 mm per day thereafter (C is therefore incorrect) and ruptures at about 2 cm in diameter (D is therefore incorrect), and this ruptured follicle becomes the corpus luteum after release of the oocyte (E is therefore incorrect).

3. Meiosis:
C is correct. The 7 million germ cells produced during fetal life are produced by mitosis, not meiosis (A is therefore incorrect). The first meiotic division commences in utero in the fetus but ceases in prophase. It does not recommence its division until the luteinizing hormone surge occurs in the particular menstrual cycle, and this first meiotic division is completed just prior to fertilization of the oocyte by the sperm (B is therefore incorrect). The attachment of the sperm results in the commencement of the second meiotic division (C is therefore correct). The crossover process between adjacent copies of the same chromosome occurs during prophase of meiosis I, not after meiosis I has been completed (D is therefore incorrect). The long delay between the cessation of prophase I in fetal life and the time when it recommences in the cycle concerned (which can be 40–45 years later) is the reason for the increased incidence of chromosomal abnormalities associated with advanced maternal age (E is therefore incorrect).

4. Regarding the process of fertilization in the human female:
A is correct. The female gametes only contain an X chromosome and therefore cannot determine the sex of the resulting fetus. This is determined by the male gamete, which will contain either an X or Y chromosome (B is therefore incorrect). Twin pregnancies occur due to division of the embryo (identical or monochorionic twin pregnancy) or if two separate oocytes are fertilized by two separate sperm (a dichorionic twin pregnancy; therefore C is incorrect). The exact time during which the oocyte can be fertilized after ovulation is uncertain, but it is believed fertilization does not occur if this time interval is in excess of 36 hours (D is therefore incorrect). Sperm capacitation to facilitate fertilization generally occurs within the genital tract of the woman (E is therefore incorrect).

5. Implantation:
C is correct. Implantation generally occurs 5–6 days after ovulation and fertilization (A is therefore incorrect), at which time the embryo is at the blastocyst stage (B is therefore incorrect). Human chorionic gonadotropin (hCG) is produced soon after the implantation process commences (C is therefore correct), and then the plasma levels double every 48 hours if the pregnancy is progressing normally. The endometrium must be secretory in type to allow implantation (D is therefore incorrect) and is then converted to the appearance of decidua. Implantation will not occur if the endometrium is proliferative in type so a pregnancy will not result. Implantation and hCG production can occur even where the embryo is very abnormal, under which circumstances the period occurs at the expected time and the woman concerned never knows she was actually pregnant in that cycle (E is therefore incorrect). A urinary pregnancy test performed 2–3 days after the period commenced will be negative.

Chapter 3

1. What is the most appropriate statement regarding immunology in pregnancy?
A is correct. Only two types of feto-placental tissue come into direct contact with maternal tissues: the villous and extra-villous trophoblast (EVT), and there are effectively no systemic maternal T- or B-cell responses to trophoblast cells in humans. The villous trophoblast, which is bathed by maternal blood, never expresses human leucocyte antigen (HLA) class I or class II molecules. EVT, which is directly in contact with endometrial/decidual tissues, does not express the major T-cell ligands, HLA-A or HLA-B, but does express the HLA class I trophoblast-specific HLA-G, which is strongly immunosuppressive, along with HLA-C and HLA-E. The main type of decidual lymphocytes is the uterine natural killer (NK) cells. The thymus shows some reversible involution during pregnancy, apparently caused by the progesterone-driven exodus of lymphocytes from the thymic cortex, and the Th1:Th2 cytokine ratio shifts towards Th2.

2. Regarding the rise in cardiac output:
   D is correct. The rise in cardiac output is seen from early pregnancy. The increase in cardiac output is brought about by increase in the stroke volume and the heart rate. It is associated with a fall in the afterload. The heart is already strained due to the need to pump an extra 40% of blood volume, and in those with heart disease it can tip the balance and cause heart failure, especially if they are anaemic or if they contract an infection. The pulmonary vasculature in a mother is able to accommodate the increased blood flow without causing pulmonary hypertension.

3. Considering respiratory function in pregnancy:
   D is correct. Progesterone sensitizes the medulla oblongata and not the adrenal medulla to CO_2. This causes some over-breathing, which reduces the CO_2 level that allows the fetus to offload its CO_2 to the maternal side. Not the maternal P_aO_2 but the oxygen-carrying capacity of blood increases by 18%. There is an increase in maternal 2,3-DPG that shifts the maternal oxygen dissociation curve to the right, thus facilitating the downloading of oxygen to the fetus. There is a 40% increase in minute ventilation due to increase in tidal volume from 500 to mL.

4. Considering renal function in pregnancy:
   C is correct. There is an increase in renal size of up to 70% due to an increase in size of the parenchyma in addition to the enlargement of the pelvicalyceal system and the ureter, but the increase is seen from early pregnancy. The ureters increase in size due to the influence of progesterone and increased urinary output, but they are not floppy and have good tone. Because of an increase in blood volume there is a 50% increase in glomerular filtration rate (GFR) that activates the renin–angiotensin system. About 900 and not 1800 mmol of sodium are retained during pregnancy. Because of ureteric dilatation and reflux of urine due to lack of sphincteric action at the point entry of the ureter into the bladder and higher incidence of urinary stasis, there is higher incidence of urinary tract infection in pregnancy.

5. In relation to endocrine function in pregnancy:
   A is correct. Insulin resistance develops with progress of pregnancy due to the change in the hormonal milieu. There is a significant increase in human placental lactogen after 28 weeks as a result of which some women develop gestational diabetes. Due to increased glomerular filtration rate, more glucose is presented to the kidneys, and in some mothers the quantity of glucose exposed for absorption exceeds the tubular maximal absorption capacity and hence presents as 'renal' glycosuria without a high blood glucose level. Because of increased metabolism, the thyroid increases in size. The gut absorbs more calcium but more is also lost in the urine and in areas of dietary deficiency, so calcium supplementation becomes necessary. Skin pigmentation is caused by an increase in melanocyte-secreting hormone.

Chapter 4

1. In early placental development:
   D is correct. The villi have an inner cytotrophoblast and an outer syncytiotrophoblast that invade the endometrium and myometrial layers. Decidual cells provide the initial nutrition for the invading trophoblasts. The spiral arterioles are invaded by the trophoblasts making large lacunae that are full of maternal blood, and the tertiary villi bathe in these lacunae to accomplish the respiratory, nutrition and excretory functions. Chorion frondosum forms the placenta. Chorion laevae is the layer surrounding the membranes, and it fuses with the uterine cavity.

2. Regarding the umbilical cord:
   C is correct. The umbilical cord has two arteries and one vein. The fetus pumps the blood through these arteries to the placenta to get more oxygen and excrete the carbon dioxide, and hence arterial blood has less oxygen compared with the vein. One in 200 babies has only one artery and one vein, and they grow normally and live birth is achieved. Cord arterial pressure is between 60 and 70 mmHg. The vessels are surrounded by a hydrophilic mucopolysaccharide known as *Wharton's jelly*.

3. Placental transfer:
   A is correct. Simple diffusion is according to the concentration gradients, and this facilitates transfer of oxygen and carbon dioxide in the right direction for the fetus. Glucose is transferred according to the gradient, but it needs energy, i.e. facilitated diffusion. Active transport needs energy for transport and to drive the substances against the gradient, and hence there could be cases where the concentration may be already higher in the fetal blood. This process occurs with amino acids and water-soluble vitamins. Higher-molecular-weight substrates are transferred by pinocytosis.

4. Placental function:
   E is correct. The placenta has multiple functions. It helps with gas exchange and is an important organ for transferring nutrition to the fetus and excreting waste products from the fetus. It produces a number of hormones – initially human chorionic gonadotrophin and later oestrogens and progesterones, which are all essential for maintenance of pregnancy. But it is a poor barrier against infections; thus the fetus is affected by malaria, syphilis, HIV, cytomegalovirus (CMV) and toxoplasmosis.

5. Amniotic fluid:

A is correct. Polyhydramnios may suggest fetal anomaly such as neural tube defects, anencephaly, gut atresia and several other known pathologies. The amniotic fluid volume increases rapidly in parallel with fetal growth and gestational age up to a maximum volume of around 1000 mL at 38 weeks. Postural deformities are one of the complications of long-standing severe oligohydramnios. A major problem with this situation is pulmonary hypoplasia. Adequate fluid is needed to push the alveoli and bronchioles to expand; if not, it results in lung hypoplasia. Most cases of intrauterine growth restriction would be associated with reduced amniotic fluid due to less urine production caused by less renal perfusion. Amnio-infusion may abolish the variable decelerations, but trials have shown no improvement in clinical outcome, and hence it is not a standard procedure.

Chapter 5

1. Perinatal mortality:

C is correct. Perinatal mortality rate describes the number of stillbirths and early neonatal deaths per 1000 total births (live births and stillbirths). This gives a picture of maternal health and the standard of care provided to mothers and their newborn babies. By improving socio-economic conditions, the quality of obstetric and neonatal care and an active screening programme for common congenital abnormalities, perinatal mortality rates can be significantly improved. The World Health Organization has two targets for assessing progress in improving maternal health (Millennium Development Goal [MDG] 5). These are reducing the maternal mortality ratio by 75% between 1990 and 2015 and achieving universal access to reproductive health by 2015.

2. Regarding stillbirths:

E is correct. Stillbirths are the number of stillbirths per 1000 total births. Until 2011, the Centre for Maternal and Child Enquiries has published annual perinatal reports for the UK. The report showed a significant reduction in both stillbirth rates and early neonatal deaths. Stillbirth rates indicate the quality of antenatal care and screening programmes and are the largest contributors to perinatal mortality. Most stillbirths occur antenatally. The traditionally used systems such as the Wigglesworth and the Aberdeen (Obstetric) classifications consistently reported up to two-thirds of stillbirths as being from unexplained causes. The ReCoDe (Relevant Condition at Death) system, which classifies the relevant condition present at the time of death, was developed in the UK. By using this system, the most common cause of stillbirth was fetal growth restriction (43%), and only 15.2% remained unexplained. The sub-Saharan regions of central Africa have the highest stillbirth rates.

3. Regarding neonatal deaths:

B is correct. Birth weight is no doubt an indication of maternal health and nutrition. Low birth weight, although not a direct cause of neonatal death, is an important association. Neonatal tetanus remains a common cause of neonatal death in settings where lack of hygiene and inadequate cord care are prevalent, as many women are not immunized against tetanus. Prematurity remains a significant contributor to perinatal mortality rates in developing countries, and improving maternal health and obstetric care is a more important step to improving the outcome than providing more neonatal intensive care units. In the UK, the neonatal classification used by the Confidential Enquiry into Maternal Deaths (CMACE) looked at the primary cause and associated factors for neonatal deaths. In the past, nearly half of the neonatal deaths were due to immaturity, but the new classification restricted extreme prematurity to only cases below 22 weeks' gestation, resulting in only 9.3% of neonatal deaths.

4. Regarding the description of maternal deaths:

A is correct. Direct maternal deaths are defined as those resulting from conditions or complications or their management that are unique to pregnancy, occurring during the antenatal, intrapartum or postpartum periods. Coincidental (fortuitous) deaths occur from unrelated causes which happen to occur in pregnancy or the puerperium. Definitions of maternal death can vary across the regions and between countries. As the UK has the advantage of accurate denominator data, including both live births and stillbirths, it has defined its maternal mortality rate as the number of direct and indirect deaths per 100,000 maternities as a more accurate denominator to indicate the number of women at risk. Maternities are defined as the number of pregnancies that result in a live birth at any gestation or stillbirths occurring at or after 24 completed weeks of gestation and are required to be notified by law. Improving the socio-economic status of women, coupled with improved maternal health and antenatal care, is key to the improvement of maternal mortality rates.

5. Maternal mortality:

D is correct. In the 2006–2008 UK Confidential Enquiry into Maternal Deaths Report, the leading cause of direct deaths was sepsis, particularly from group A streptococcus. This infection can occur at any time during the antenatal or postpartum period, and the onset can be insidious and non-specific. Cardiac diseases remained the leading cause of indirect deaths.

The reduction in the number of deaths from venous thromboembolism is due mainly to improved screening and thromboprophylaxis guidelines adopted by all maternity units in the UK. However, it remains an important and avoidable cause of death.

Chapter 6

1. Physiological changes in pregnancy:
   E is correct. Breast cancer during pregnancy is reportedly associated with rapid progression and poor prognosis. Hence, any complaint of a 'lump' in the breast should prompt a detailed breast examination. Many women develop a reddish-brownish pigmentation called *chloasma* over the cheeks, which is normal and needs no investigation in the absence of any other symptoms or signs. There is a physiological reduction in Hb concentration due to a relative haemodilution (plasma expansion is greater than red cell expansion). The pelvic shape remains unchanged in itself – it is what is from birth. The plane of the pelvic inlet or pelvic brim is bounded posteriorly by the sacral promontory, laterally by the iliopectineal lines and anteriorly by the superior pubic rami and upper margin of the pubic symphysis.

2. In eliciting an obstetric history:
   E is correct. Past obstetric history is pivotal to managing the index pregnancy, e.g. past history of diabetes, hypertensive or psychiatric illness would help us to plan management better. Many women do not remember the last menstrual period (LMP) accurately, and when facilities permit, the gestation is assessed by ultrasound in the first trimester and estimated date of delivery (EDD) is calculated based on the early scan. The post-ovulatory period is fairly constant and is about 14 days whether the cycle is long or short. Ultrasound for dating can be + or − 3 weeks if it is based on third-trimester scans, while it is + or − 1 week if it is based on a first-trimester scan. Hormonal contraception may delay the first ovulatory cycle after discontinuation of the method.

3. Regarding symptoms of pregnancy:
   E is correct. Nausea and vomiting can start within 2 weeks of the missed period, and it is believed to be secondary to the rise, at least partly, of human chorionic gonadotrophin (hCG). Severe and persistent vomiting leading to maternal dehydration, ketonuria and electrolyte imbalance is termed *hyperemesis gravidarum* and is typical in the first trimester only. The frequency of micturition is due to the increased urine production, which is due to an increased glomerular filtration rate following 40% expansion of the blood volume in addition to the pressure on the bladder by the gravid uterus. This pressure is relieved after 12 weeks when the uterus becomes an intra abdominal organ – hence the frequency lessens. Plasma osmolality reduces with advancing gestation due to increased intravascular volume and reduced plasma proteins. There is increased diuresis after water loading when the woman is sitting in an upright position, perhaps due to increased perfusion.

4. During pregnancy:
   C is correct. Blood pressure (BP) is recorded when the patient is sitting up or lying at a 45-degree incline and not whilst she is lying on her back because the venous return may be reduced, affecting the cardiac output and the reading. BP should be recorded in the same position during each visit using an appropriate size cuff – obese women would need a larger cuff. If inferior venocaval compression is prolonged, it is likely to affect the cardiac output of the mother and hence the uterine circulation, which could compromise the baby. Current recommendation is to consider the Korotkoff's fifth sound, and if the point at which the sound disappears cannot be identified, then use the Korotkoff's fourth sound. The flow murmurs are due to the hyper-dynamic circulation and are generally of no significance unless associated with symptoms or other worrying clinical features, where they should be differentiated from any murmur due to cardiac pathology.

5. In pelvic examination during pregnancy:
   B is correct. With the availability of first-trimester scanning, it is not essential to perform a routine pelvic examination. When there is painless bleeding in late pregnancy, placenta praevia should be excluded. Digital vaginal examination in cases of placenta praevia may cause torrential haemorrhage and require an emergency caesarean section; hence, it is contraindicated. Radiological examination of the pelvis is of little value in predicting labour outcome, as labour is a dynamic process with changes in dimensions occurring with flexion of the baby's head, moulding and pelvic 'give'. The gynaecoid pelvis is 'roomy' at all levels of the pelvis to allow cephalic descent. The diameter of the pelvic inlet is usually longer in the transverse diameter than the anteroposterior (AP) diameter.

Chapter 7

1. Regarding antenatal screening for infection:
   B is correct. Screening for hepatitis B is routinely carried out. Hepatitis B is easily transmitted to the fetus and then the newborn whilst it traverses the birth canal. If the mother has hepatitis B antigens, further

testing is required to confirm if they are positive for surface (s) antigens or core (e) antigens. Those who are positive for core antigens are considered to have active viruses and may have a high transmission rate of up to 85% to the fetus. In most countries newborns are given gamma globulins and the active vaccine if e positive and only the vaccine if they are s positive. If the infection is transmitted, there is a high possibility of liver cirrhosis followed by hepatocellular cancer, hence the need to actively immunize the newborn. No routine screening is done for cytomegalovirus (CMV), as re-infection is not uncommon and no preventive action can be taken based on the test. General advice should be given to avoid child nurseries where children have coughs, colds and influenza and may harbour CMV infection that is easily transmitted. Syphilis is uncommon, but if detected it is eminently treatable to avoid infection of the fetus and its sequelae. Checking the husband/partner and contact tracing are important. Rubella infection causes major congenital malformations in 25–50% if the mother is infected in the first trimester of pregnancy. If the mother is not immune, she should be immunized postpartum. HIV/AIDS screening is not universal, but it is advisable to make it a routine screening. If found positive, antiretroviral therapy, elective caesarean delivery and avoidance of breast-feeding have reduced the incidence of vertical transmission from 45% to less than 2%.

2. Group B streptococcus:
   C is correct. Group B streptococcus is a gram-positive bacterium and is a commensal organism found in the nose, oropharynx, nasopharynx, anal canal and vagina. Group B streptococcal colonization of the genitourinary tract is associated with higher incidence of pre-term labour and pre-labour rupture of membranes. Screening is not routine in all countries. In the UK screening is not performed, but should there be a high-risk history, suitable precautions are taken, especially intrapartum penicillin therapy if the mother had streptococcal colonization in the vaginal or rectal swab or growth in urine culture.

3. Gestational diabetes:
   E is correct. Gestational diabetes predisposes to macrosomic babies, and those who had higher-birth-weight babies in the previous pregnancy are more prone to gestational diabetes. The cut-off value of when to consider the baby to be macrosomic, i.e. >4 or 4.5 kg, varies with the population studied. Maternal body mass index (BMI) >35 has a known association with gestational diabetes mellitus in pregnancy. Gestational diabetes in previous pregnancy identifies those who are likely to develop early-onset type 2 diabetes in their life, and they also indicate a higher chance of getting gestational diabetes in subsequent pregnan-

cies. Older mothers >35 years of age are more prone to gestational diabetes and not younger mothers.

4. Extra folic acid supplementation:
   E is correct. Folic acid is well known to reduce the overall incidence of congenital malformations. Folic acid facilitates cell division and is an important vitamin in any growth or reparative process. Extra folic acid supplementation (5 mg per day) reduces neural tube defects, and hence it is important to take prior to and in early pregnancy in mothers who had a previous child with neural tube defects. Mothers who have epilepsy, especially those who are on anti-epileptic medication, have a higher chance of having children with neural tube defects, and they should be advised on higher-dose folic acid supplementation. This also applies to mothers with diabetes and those with a high body mass index (BMI), e.g. >35. Down's syndrome is a chromosomal problem, commonly trisomy 21, and the incidence cannot be reduced by taking extra folic acid.

5. Regarding advice in pregnancy:
   D is correct. Moderate exercise for recreation, including swimming, is harmless and is encouraged. Strenuous exercise and competitive sports with active movements are contraindicated. Anti-D Ig is not routinely administered after complete spontaneous miscarriage under 12 weeks' gestation in the absence of surgical evacuation. There is controversy about minimal alcohol consumption and its effects on the fetus. Moderate alcohol consumption may be harmful to the fetus, and severe alcohol consumption is associated with fetal alcohol syndrome, which is associated with microcephaly and mental retardation. Smoking is harmful to the pregnancy and is well known to be associated with intrauterine growth restriction. Paracetamol appears to be safe in pregnancy, though no drug is proven to be completely safe. Non-steroidal anti-inflammatory drugs taken in significant amounts in the third trimester may cause oligohydramnios and premature closure of the ductus arteriosus.

Chapter 8

1. Antepartum haemorrhage at 36 weeks:
   C is correct. Although placental abruption (separation of normally situated placenta) and placenta praevia (low-lying placenta) are major causes of maternal and perinatal morbidity and mortality, the incidence of each of these conditions is less than 1%. The commonest reason is idiopathic. Clinical examination, both general and abdominal, and a speculum examination (to exclude cervical or vaginal lesion and to visualize

whether blood is emerging via the cervical os) and an ultrasound examination (to check the placental position and to visualize the fetal lie and presentation and liquor volume) are vital to identify the other causes and to come to the diagnosis by exclusion of 'idiopathic'.

2. Hypertension in pregnancy:

   D is correct. Normal physiological change is for a decrease in blood pressure (BP) from the first trimester onwards with a later gentle rise to pre-pregnancy levels in the third trimester. More emphasis is now paid to the systolic reading, especially >160 mmHg, as there is a greater tendency for cerebral haemorrhage, and there is a strong recommendation to immediately treat and bring the systolic BP <150 mmHg and preferably <140 mmHg. Hypertension after 20 weeks is gestational in the absence of proteinuria, and the diagnosis would be pre-eclampsia in the additional presence of significant proteinuria. Several factors may contribute to a rise in BP, although it is known that there is a fall in peripheral resistance due to vasodilatory hormones, including oestrogen and progesterone. In pre-eclampsia the vasoconstrictor thromboxane and vasodilatory prostacyclin, mainly liberated by the platelets and endothelial cells of blood vessels, play a major role. HELLP syndrome stands for haemolysis, elevated liver enzymes and low platelets, and it signifies a serious form of the pre-eclamptic process which has affected several systems. It has a poor prognosis, and careful management and early delivery are advised.

3. In twin pregnancy, what is the most appropriate statement?

   B is correct. The prevalence of identical twins appears to be uniformly similar in many countries. Twin peak sign or lambda sign at the attachment of the membranes to the uterus signifies additional chorionic layers in between the amniotic membranes and the diagnosis of dizygotic twins. All complications of pregnancy are increased in twins, and miscarriage is not an exception. Pre-term delivery in twins is twice that of singleton pregnancy, and the average gestational age of delivery of the fetuses are much less than singletons. Twin-to-twin transfusion can appear as early as 18 weeks, and many centres would scan at this stage and decide on the date of the next scan. Earlier diagnosis and treatment by laser transection of anastomotic vessels are associated with better outcome.

4. The causes of an unstable lie include all of the following **except**:

   D is correct. Placenta praevia occupies the lower segment and prevents the head or breech from settling down in the pelvis. Polyhydramnios allows the fetus to 'float' around instead of binding the fetus to a longitudinal lie by the uterine muscular tone and normal amount of amniotic fluid volume. Subseptate uterus limits the space of the uterine cavity, and some fetuses may present with transverse or oblique lie. Primiparity is generally associated with good uterine and abdominal muscle tone and should favour a stable longitudinal lie. In twin pregnancy the first twin usually presents in the longitudinal lie, but the second twin can be in an abnormal lie, and the incidence is made greater if it is associated with polyhydramnios.

5. In prolonged pregnancy, which one of the following statements is correct?

   C is correct. The term *postmaturity syndrome* refers to the condition of the infant and has characteristic features. These are all indicators of intrauterine malnutrition and may therefore occur at any stage of the pregnancy if there is placental dysfunction. Postmaturity is often associated with oligohydramnios, an increased incidence of meconium in the amniotic fluid and an increased risk of intrauterine aspiration of meconium-stained fluid into the fetal lungs. It is found in 2% of pregnancies at 41 weeks and up to 5% of pregnancies at 42 weeks. Prolonged pregnancy is associated with increased perinatal morbidity and mortality. The guidelines from most recognized professional bodies suggest induction by 41 weeks and 3 days to avoid morbidity and mortality based on the evidence from randomized controlled studies.

Chapter 9

1. Anaemia in pregnancy:

   E is correct. Pregnancy causes an increase in both plasma volume and red cell mass. This requires an increase in iron and folate, which is not always met by maternal diet. In addition there are fetal requirements for both these nutrients. The increased requirement for iron is greater than that for folate. Whilst sickle cell disease and thalassaemia can cause anaemia in pregnancy, this is much less common than iron deficiency.

2. Causes of gestational diabetes:

   E is correct. Pregnancy induces a diabetogenic state. This is predominantly because of increased resistance to the actions of insulin due to the placental production of the anti-insulin hormones (oestrogen, human placental lactogen, glucagon and cortisol), though the increased production of maternal glucocorticoids and thyroid hormones during pregnancy also contribute to this. In response, the maternal pancreas must increase its production of insulin to combat this. In some women this is not achieved, and gestational diabetes is the result. Progesterone is the only one listed that does not oppose insulin action.

3. Acute venous thromboembolism in pregnancy:
D is correct. Venous thromboembolism is a leading cause of maternal mortality in the developed world. It is 10 times more likely to occur in pregnancy compared to when a woman is not pregnant. Deep vein thrombosis occurs more frequently in the left leg due to compression of the left common iliac vein. D-Dimer measurements are of limited use in pregnancy, as false-positive results are common. Heparin is the first-line treatment; warfarin use in pregnancy is associated with an embryopathy and with fetal bleeding problems.

4. Zika virus in pregnancy
E is correct. Most people (80%) infected with Zika virus have no symptoms.
Pregnant women are no more susceptible to infection than non-pregnant women.
The majority of cases of Zika virus are acquired from infected mosquito bites; however, a few cases of sexual transmission and some through blood transfusions have been reported. Testing of asymptomatic pregnant women is not recommended. Following a systematic review of the literature up to 30 May 2016, the World Health Organization (WHO) concluded that Zika virus infection during pregnancy is a cause of congenital brain abnormalities.

5. Epilepsy and pregnancy:
C is correct. The effect of pregnancy on epilepsy is variable. Usually the seizure frequency is unchanged, but a minority of women will have increased seizures. Different anti-epileptics confer different risks to the fetus; however, sodium valproate has the greatest risks and should be avoided in women of reproductive age. In women with epilepsy there is a higher risk of congenital abnormalities (3% compared with 1–2% in the general population); this risk is increased further if a woman is taking anti-epileptic drugs (4–9%). The main abnormalities are neural tube defects and heart abnormalities.

As there is an increased risk of neural tube defects, a higher (5 mg) dose of folic acid is recommended. Children of women with epilepsy have a 4–5% chance of developing the condition themselves; this increases to up to 20% if their father is also affected. Breast-feeding is safe for women on most anti-epileptic medications.

Chapter 10

1. Abnormalities detected by ultrasound at 20 weeks:
A is correct. Only 25% of cardiac anomalies are detected. About 60–90% of the central nervous system (CNS) malformations are picked up. More than 90% of skeletal malformations are identified. Depending on the specific gastrointestinal anomaly, 60–90% are diagnosed. In most series about 85% of urogenital anomalies are detected.

2. First-trimester screening test for Down's syndrome:
D is correct. There is an over 99% chance (149/150) that the baby does *not* have the diagnosis. As a result the positive predictive value of the screening test is low at 1/150. As the disease is very unlikely, the negative predictive value of this type of screening test is very high. The background incidence is 1:1500, but the test has placed the chance to be 1:150 (10 times higher). At this stage of pregnancy chorionic villus sampling is an option for this woman, but this procedure has a 0.5–1% chance of leading to a procedure-related miscarriage.

3. Assessment of fetal growth in pregnancy:
C is the only answer which is not correct. Progressive abdominal circumference measurement provides the best measure of fetal growth. If the abdominal and head circumferences are on the same centile in a fetus that is small or large, it is more likely that the extreme of size is constitutional/genetic; if they are divergent (e.g. with head larger than abdomen in a small fetus or head smaller than abdomen in a large fetus), then it is more likely that there is pathological fetal growth. Serial symphysial–fundal height measurements detect as few as 20% of small- or large-for-dates fetuses. Fetal abnormality is associated with growth pathology, and that can have been missed at the 20-week detailed scan; thus it is important to exclude fetal anomaly in cases of intrauterine growth restriction (IUGR). In cases where the fetus is growth restricted, the umbilical artery (UA) Doppler recording will indicate its severity and inform management decisions.

4. Tests in high-risk pregnancies which improve fetal outcome:
B is correct. The only antenatal fetal function test that has shown to improve fetal outcome is the umbilical artery Doppler measurements.

5. Most common chromosomal abnormalities:
B is correct. The commonest abnormality is that associated with trisomy 21 or Down's syndrome. In this condition, in at least 92% of cases the chromosomal abnormality is that each cell has three rather than two number 21 chromosomes (about 8% of cases are translocations). The next most common are abnormalities of the sex chromosomes (Klinefelter's syndrome with one extra sex chromosome in the form of two X chromosomes and one Y chromosome, Triple-X syndrome with an extra sex chromosome in the form of three X chromosomes and Turner's syndrome with only one sex chromosome [an X chromosome] followed by trisomies 13 and 18 [Patau and Edwards syndromes, respectively]).

Chapter 11

1. Diagnosis of labour:
   D is correct. 'Show', which is the discharge of the blood-stained mucus plug or rupture of membranes, may be associated with the onset of labour but can take place independently without progressing to labour. Some mothers have 'show' or rupture of membranes and will take days before going into labour. The painful contractions should be associated with cervical effacement and dilatation or both on two consecutive vaginal examinations to diagnose labour. Painful contractions may persist for several hours without cervical changes, and the pain may subside only to restart in a few days' time. Backache and abdominal pain are not sufficient indicators to diagnose labour.

2. Slow labour progress in first stages of labour:
   C is correct. A fetal weight of 4 kg or even more may have no association with abnormal labour progress. Incoordinate uterine contractions are just the description of how the contraction patterns appear, i.e. two or three together and then one and again two or three together at varying intervals. Incoordinate contractions do not mean inefficient contractions, as progressive cervical dilatation can take place with incoordinate contractions. Malposition of the head presents a larger diameter to the pelvis and can cause relative disproportion and lead to slow progress of labour. A gynaecoid pelvis is roomy and so should not cause slow progress. The labour is slower in primigravid compared with multigravida but is not abnormally slow in most cases.

3. Initiation of labour:
   E is correct. The onset of labour involves local progesterone withdrawal and an increase in oestrogen and prostaglandin action. The mechanisms that regulate these changes are unresolved but are likely to involve placental production of the peptide hormone corticotrophin-releasing hormone (CRH). Placental development across gestation leads to an exponential increase in the number of syncytio-trophoblast nuclei in which transcription of the CRH gene occurs. This maturational process leads to an exponential increase in the levels of maternal and fetal plasma CRH. The CRH has direct actions on the placenta to increase oestrogen synthesis and reduce progesterone synthesis. In the fetus the CRH directly stimulates the fetal zone of the adrenal gland to produce dehydroepiandrosterone (DHEA), the precursor of placental oestrogen synthesis. CRH also stimulates the synthesis of prostaglandins by the membranes. The fall in progesterone and increase in oestrogens and prostaglandins lead to increases in connexin 43 that promote connectivity of uterine myocytes and change uterine myocyte electrical excitability, which in turn leads to increases in generalized uterine contractions. Infection of the amniotic membranes seems to be an important pathological cause of pre-term labour.

3. Malposition and asynclitism of the fetal head present larger diameters to the pelvis and may cause delay in the second stage of labour. Epidural analgesia abolishes the 'Ferguson's reflex' and reflex release of oxytocin due to distension of the cervix and upper vagina and associated increased uterine activity and hence may cause a prolonged second stage. Maternal exhaustion can be a cause, and this should be avoided by preventing early encouragement for the mother to bear down – one should ideally wait until the head descends to the perineal phase. Fetal distress does not cause delay in the second stage; on the contrary, the delayed second stage may cause fetal distress.

4. Complications of epidural analgesia:
   C is correct. Complications include blood-stained tap and accidental dural tap, and if the medication is injected without realizing, this may lead to total spinal blockade. Extremely rarely, nerve injury may take place. It causes hypotension due to vasodilatation and not hypertension.

5. Electronic fetal monitoring:
   A is correct. Accelerations of the fetal heart rate indicate good fetal health, and the fetus is unlikely to be acidotic. Absence of accelerations may be due to infection, fetal sleep phase, administration of sedatives and analgesics and, rarely, intracranial pathology or previous injury. The presence of variable decelerations is suggestive of cord compression, and late decelerations are suggestive of placental insufficiency and are of concern and need to be observed for additional features of concern such as rising baseline rate and reduction in baseline variability. Absent fetal heart rate variability may suggest that the fetus is already hypoxic or has suffered injury.

6. Management of pre-term labour:
   C is correct. Hyaline membrane disease and respiratory distress syndrome are the major concerns with prematurity in addition to concern about other organ maturation. The severity of hyaline membrane disease is reduced by the administration of corticosteroids (dexamethasone or betamethasone 12 mg 12 or 24 hours apart). In order to have the time to bring about this maturity, the labour has to be delayed for at least 48 hours in the absence of contraindications such as infections, and this is achieved by the use of tocolytics. Tocolytic agents (terbutaline, atosiban and GTN) in themselves have not been proven to confer clinical benefit. Antibiotics are shown to be of value in cases of pre-term labour associated with pre-labour rupture of membranes only.

7. Accepted indication for induction of labour:
   C is correct. There are increased morbidity and mortality in high-risk pregnancies associated with diabetes, prolonged pregnancy, pre-eclampsia and intrauterine growth restriction. There is no evidence to suggest that there is maternal, fetal or neonatal advantage by induction for macrosomia.

8. Complications of induction of labour:
   E is correct. Prematurity is a known complication of induction if the gestation is not checked correctly. In modern practice this is less of a problem with ultrasound estimation of gestational age in the first trimester. Cord prolapse is a possibility and is less due to wider use of prostaglandins instead of depending on artificial rupture of membranes. However, one needs to exclude cord presentation prior to rupture and should be cautious when rupture is carried out with a high head. The use of oxytocin or prostaglandin may hyperstimulate the uterus and cause iatrogenic fetal distress. Uterine rupture is rare with induction but is a possibility in women with previous caesarean section (CS) and in grand multiparous women. Induced labour is usually longer than spontaneous labour and may be associated with more contractions and naturally is likely to be more painful.

Chapter 12

1. Normal delivery:
   B is correct. Provided no adverse clinical factors are present, a normal duration of the second stage of labour is commonly regarded as lasting up to 3 hours in a nulliparous woman who has received epidural analgesia. Engagement is considered to have occurred when the fetal head has descended to or beyond the level of the ischial spines. During the descent phase of the second stage of labour, the mother does not normally experience the sensation of bearing down until the head has reached the pelvic floor and perineal phase. Maternal expulsive effort should combine short pushing spells with periods of panting to allow vaginal and perineal tissues to relax and stretch over the advancing head. As part of the mechanism of normal labour, the fetal head is delivered by extension when 'crowning' of the head occurs.

2. Perineal injury and episiotomy:
   D is correct. Where episiotomy is performed, the recommended technique is a mediolateral incision to reduce the risk of extension involving the external sphincter and anus. Third-degree injury to the perineum is classified into three subcategories according to whether the damage to the external sphincter is <50% (3a), >50%

(3b) or complete (3c). A fourth-degree laceration involves the ano/rectal mucosa as well as the external and internal sphincter complex. Instrumental delivery, especially forceps delivery, and delivery of a deflexed fetal head in the occiput posterior (OP) position may result in over-distension of the perineum, resulting in perineal injury. Obstetric anal sphincter injuries may lead to long-term incontinence of flatus and faeces, especially if the injury was not recognized and adequately repaired.

3. Caesarean section:
   E is correct. Despite incidences of 25–30% or greater for caesarean deliveries in most developed countries, the instrumental vaginal delivery rates have remained around 10% for several years. Women who have had one uncomplicated previous lower segment caesarean section for a non-recurrent indication may attempt a vaginal delivery in a subsequent labour, provided no other adverse clinical factors are present. The risk of scar dehiscence or rupture is much greater with a previous classical caesarean section and may occur before the onset of labour. Provided the operator has been adequately trained, most occipitoposterior and transverse positions of the fetal head can be managed safely by forceps or vacuum delivery. Although some babies with a mentoanterior face presentation may deliver vaginally, most obstetricians will perform a caesarean delivery because of the risks associated with this malpresentation.

4. Operative vaginal delivery:
   D is correct. McRobert's manoeuvre is successful in the majority of cases of shoulder dystocia. Only a minority of macrosomic infants will experience shoulder dystocia, and the majority of cases will occur in normal labours with infants weighing less than 4000 g. In almost all reports comparing forceps and vacuum delivery, more infants are successfully delivered with forceps than the vacuum extractor. Significantly more severe perineal lacerations are associated with forceps delivery than vacuum extraction. The prerequisites for vacuum delivery are the same as for the forceps, namely, there should be full dilatation of the cervix and a known position and attitude of the fetal head.

5. Postpartum haemorrhage:
   A is correct. A number of important obstetric factors predispose to atonic uterus, making it the most common cause of postpartum haemorrhage (PPH). Nevertheless, uterine hypotonia may occur following normal delivery. There is little doubt that active management of the third stage of labour reduces postpartum bleeding and should be recommended as preferred management of the third stage. Administration of tranexamic acid within 3 hours of PPH will reduce mortality from PPH by 30%. If the placenta has been expelled and the

haemorrhage continues despite the administration of intravenous oxytocin, ergometrine should be administered intravenously, provided the mother does not have hypertension or a cardiac condition. Recently, uterine tamponade with balloon catheters has become a relatively simple method and is usually effective management for persisting PPH.

Chapter 13

1. Physiological changes in the puerperium:
   B is correct. With the delivery of the fetus and placenta, the hormone-producing fetoplacental unit is detached from the mother. This causes a reduction of these hormones that gradually reduce to non-pregnant levels by 6 weeks. There is an increase in clotting factors in the third stage of labour and immediate puerperium as a defence mechanism to prevent excessive bleeding, which in some women at risk may cause thromboembolism. Prolactin increases with lactation. Platelet counts are stable or increase slightly unless there is increased consumption. Cardiac output remains stable but gradually comes down with diuresis and return of the blood volume to normal.

2. Risk factors for anal sphincter injury:
   C is correct. Occipitoanterior position presents the smallest diameter and has less association with third-degree tears compared with a direct occipitoposterior delivery when a larger diameter is presented. Normal duration of the second stage of labour is not known to increase the incidence of anal sphincter injury. Use of an epidural is associated with a slight increase in anal sphincter injury, probably due to its higher rate of instrumental delivery. Babies that weigh more than 4.5 kg and not less than 4.0 kg are linked to third-degree tears. Multiparous pregnancies are not an independent risk factor for anal sphincter injury.

3. The UK's most common overall cause of maternal death (2006–2008):
   D is correct. Sepsis is a leading cause of maternal morbidity and mortality according to the *Mothers and Babies: Reducing Risk through Audits and Confidential Enquiries across the UK* (MBRRACE-UK) report in 2016. Despite the UK direct death rate from sepsis falling from 0.67 to 0.29 per 100,000 maternities between 2009 and 2014, it remains the second commonest cause of total (combined direct and indirect) deaths in the UK and in London. It was the leading cause of direct maternal deaths in 2016.

4. Regarding postnatal anticoagulation:
   D is correct. Heparin and warfarin are not contraindicated with breast-feeding. Use of warfarin is discour-

aged in the antenatal period due to fear of 'warfarin embryopathy'. Those who were on heparin are converted to warfarin after an interval of 2–3 days due to ease of administration and better effectiveness. Generally 3 months of treatment is advised for those who had thromboembolism for pulmonary embolism (PE) or proximal thrombosis to allow for full resolution of the clots and for the coagulopathy status to have completely abated. Postnatal follow-up is best done by the haematologist, who will be able to control the dosage based on the test results and will also be able to give advice on the long-term follow-up.

5. Examination of the newborn:
   A is correct. Examination of the newborn is to assure normality to the parents by excluding any abnormal signs on general, cardiovascular, respiratory, abdominal and musculoskeletal systems. The best time is within 24 hours of delivery and certainly before the mother and baby are discharged from the hospital. Jaundice is not a normal feature of all babies, particularly in the first 24 hours – it needs to be observed, and infection and other causes should be ruled out. Umbilical hernia in a newborn may be small and should regress by the end of 1–2 years. Follow-up by the paediatrician is needed, and there is no need for immediate referral or surgical repair unless there is a large defect. High-pitched cry is not normal – possible sepsis and meningeal irritation should be checked for, and additional tests may be needed if the baby develops symptoms of vomiting, fever or fits.

Chapter 14

1. Psychiatric disorders of childbirth:
   E is correct. Psychiatric disorders are common in pregnancy, as pregnancy often precipitates the condition – probably at least 1:10 pregnancies are affected in some way. If the mother is on psychiatric medication, the risks and benefits should be analyzed; stopping the drug may cause relapse of the psychiatric condition, and certain drugs can be more teratogenic. Psychiatric disorder is the third commonest single cause of indirect maternal deaths. Elevated severe mood disorders (affective) are linked to increased risk of suicide.

2. Depressive illness in pregnancy:
   D is correct. Depressive illness is likely to recur in 50% of mothers when medication is stopped. Anxiety is a prominent feature in depression. Counselling and cognitive behavioural therapy work well for mild to moderate depression associated with anxiety compared with medication. Selective serotonin reuptake inhibitors (SSRIs) are the commonest antidepressant

drug that is used and is continued in pregnancy. Most women will need to continue antidepressant therapy during pregnancy.

3. Postpartum psychosis in pregnancy:
E is correct. The illness is characterized by the following:
- Sudden onset in the early days following delivery, deteriorating on a daily basis.
- Half will present within the first postpartum week, the majority within 2 weeks and almost all within 3 months of delivery.
- Psychosis, delusions, fear and perplexity, confusion and agitation and sometimes hallucinations.
- Agitation and severe disturbance.
Approximately 50% of women with a previous bipolar illness or postpartum psychosis will become ill.

4. Selective serotonin reuptake inhibitors (SSRIs):
A is correct. SSRIs are associated with congenital malformation, especially ventricular septal defects. There is increased pregnancy loss and intrauterine growth restriction. There is also an increased incidence of hypothermia, hypoglycaemia and pulmonary hypertension.

5. Eating disorders in pregnancy and the puerperium:
C is correct. Some association with anorexia and low birth weight or prematurity have been found, but these findings haven't been reproduced in all studies. The relationship between mother and her unborn is often affected. Mothers who have ambivalent or regretful emotions about being pregnant are more likely to have difficulty establishing a warm relationship with their baby. It is highly likely that postnatally the eating disorder behaviours will escalate further. It is probable that mothers with active eating disorders may be concealing the extent of their illness.

Chapter 15

1. Chaperone during vaginal examination:
D is correct. A chaperone should always be present, even if the doctor is female. If the patient does not want a chaperone, you should record that the offer was made and declined. If a chaperone is present, you should record that fact and make a note of the chaperone's identity. If for justifiable practical reasons you cannot offer a chaperone, you should explain to the patient and, if possible, offer to delay the examination to a later date.

2. Pelvic examination:
D is correct. If a patient indicates during an examination that they have withdrawn their consent you must cease the examination immediately. Although it may be possible to discuss a further attempt at examination, for example, with another instrument, it should be clear that the patient has consented to this and, given the position the patient is in, there could be some question over whether the patient is truly giving consent freely. A better alternative would be to abandon the examination at that time. Alternatives might include scheduling the examination for another appointment and/or discussing alternative methods.

3. Pap smear:
B is correct. The appearance is typical of a cervical ectropion, which is the presence of columnar epithelium on the ectocervix, and is normal, especially in reproductive women on the contraceptive pill. There is no indication to offer sexually transmitted infection (STI) testing in a woman of this age who is asymptomatic unless there is a history of contact. Although ectropions can be treated with cryotherapy, this is not indicated if the patient is asymptomatic. She should come for her next smear at the normal screening interval (e.g. every 3 years at her age in the UK).

4. Bimanual pelvic examination:
C is correct. Uterine retroversion is a normal anatomical variant found in 10% of women. It may be associated with pathology in the pouch of Douglas, but this is less likely if the uterus is mobile. Nodularity in the pouch of Douglas is typical of endometriosis. Although in a thin woman the ovary may be palpable in the adnexal region, this should normally be less than 5 cm in size (to include physiological cysts). Pain on cervical movement (cervical excitation) is associated with peritoneal irritations from blood or inflammation.

5. Sims' speculum:
C is correct. Examination of the cervix, insertion of an intrauterine device and taking swabs are performed by most doctors using a bivalve (e.g. Cuscoe's) speculum. Pelvic floor tone is normally assessed by digital examination. Movement of the anterior vaginal wall can only be seen using the Sims' speculum inserted along the posterior vaginal wall. A bivalve speculum can mask this, as it gets in the way of visualizing the anterior and posterior walls.

Chapter 16

1. Treatment of 7-cm solitary leiomyoma in the posterior uterine wall:
A is correct. Most fibroids are asymptomatic and do not require treatment. In symptomatic women the choice of approach may be dictated by factors such as the patient's desire for future fertility, the importance of uterine preservation, symptom severity and tumour characteristics. Although all the treatments are effective, none

would be indicated in the absence of symptoms. There is a small risk of malignant change (approximately 1:1000), but this would not normally be considered an indication for treatment unless the fibroid began to enlarge rapidly or cause pain. In the normal course of events the fibroid will regress after menopause. Fertility is highly unlikely to be an issue here, so uterine artery embolization (UAE) would not be indicated. Gonadotropin-releasing hormone (GnRh) treatment would be limited by its effect on bone density.

2. Treatment of regular heavy periods:
C is correct. When there is regular heavy bleeding with no underlying structural lesion, heavy menstrual bleeding (HMB) is usually the result of a primary endometrial disorder where the mechanisms regulating local endometrial 'haemostasis' are disturbed. The levonorgestrel-releasing intrauterine system is widely recommended as the first choice for medical therapy of HMB in those women who do not have contraindications to its use and do not desire pregnancy.

3. Oligo-amenorrhoea and a negative pregnancy test:
D is correct. The diagnostic criteria for polycystic ovarian syndrome (PCOS) are any two of the following; three are sufficient to confirm the diagnosis:
   • Oligo-ovulation or anovulation
   • Hyperandrogenism (biochemical or clinical)
   • Polycystic ovaries on ultrasound examination
     Prolactin levels are increased (usually mildly) in 15% of cases of PCOS also.

4. Precocious puberty:
A is correct. In girls precocious puberty is defined as the development of the physical signs of puberty before the age of 8 years. It usually progresses from premature thelarche to menarche because breast tissue responds faster to oestrogen than the endometrium. The majority of cases do not have a pathological basis as long as normal consonance (sequence of thelarche, adrenarche, growth spurt and menarche) is maintained. In girls older than 4 years old specific causes are less likely to be found, with the majority being idiopathic (80%).

5. Hormone replacement therapy (HRT):
E is correct. As she has had a hysterectomy, she would require oestrogen-only treatment and obviously cannot develop endometrial cancer. Although studies in older women on combined HRT showed an increase in cardiovascular disease, this was not seen in younger women or with oestrogen-only treatment. HRT is associated with a reduced risk of carcinoma of the colon and osteoporosis. Oestrogen-only treatment is associated with an increase in breast cancer (long term), venous thrombosis and cholelithiasis.

Chapter 17

1. Premature ovarian failure:
A is correct. These are the characteristic clinical and hormone profiles of disorders of ovulation: hypergonadotropic hypogonadism, due to ovarian failure; hypogonadal hypogonadism resulting from failure of pulsatile gonadotropin secretion from the pituitary; normogonadotropic anovulation, most commonly caused by polycystic ovary syndrome; and suppression of follicle-stimulating hormone (FSH) and luteinizing hormone (LH) by exogenous oestradiol in the pill.

2. Causes of oligospermia:
B is correct. Spermatogenesis and sperm function may be affected by a wide range of toxins and therapeutic agents. Various toxins and drugs may act on the seminiferous tubules and the epididymis to inhibit spermatogenesis. Chemotherapeutic agents, particularly alkylating agents, depress sperm function; and sulfasalazine which is frequently used to treat Crohn's disease, reduces sperm motility and density; and anabolic steroids used for bodybuilding may produce profound hypospermatogenesis. Mesalazine is not associated with abnormal sperm parameters.

3. In vitro fertilization:
E is correct. The chance of a live birth after a single cycle of treatment at age 40 is approximately 12%. Embryos reach the blastocyst stage 5 days after fertilization. In vitro fertilization (IVF) involves stimulation of multiple ovarian follicle development using recombinant or urinary-derived gonadotropins, with concurrent use of a gonadotropin-releasing hormone (GnRH) agonist or antagonist to prevent a premature luteinizing hormone (LH) surge and ovulation before oocytes are harvested.

4. In vitro fertilization (IVF) ovarian hyperstimulation syndrome (OHSS):
A is correct. OHSS results in marked ovarian enlargement with fluid shift from the intravascular compartment into the third space, leading to ascites, pleural effusion, sodium retention and oliguria. Patients may become hypovolaemic and hypotensive and may develop renal failure as well as thromboembolic phenomena and adult respiratory distress syndrome. The pathophysiology of this condition appears to be associated with an *increase* in capillary vascular permeability.

5. Pre-implantation genetic screening (PGS):
B is correct. The purpose of PGS is to screen for aneuploidy in embryos, although both parents have no

identified genetic abnormality. PGS has been used in cases of recurrent pregnancy loss, advanced maternal age, repeated unsuccessful in vitro fertilization (IVF) cycles or severe male factor infertility. The aim is to use PGS to select the best embryo for transfer. The use of PGS for aneuploidy screening in all cases of IVF has been advocated, but the contribution to improve success rates when used indiscriminately remains to be proven.

Chapter 18

1. Miscarriage:
   E is correct. Fifty per cent of spontaneous miscarriages are associated with chromosome abnormality, particularly at her advanced maternal age. This was her first pregnancy, so the causes of recurrent miscarriage are less likely to apply. Cervical incompetence normally presents with painless cervical dilation later in pregnancy.
2. Chromosomal abnormalities:
   B is correct. Chromosomal abnormalities are a common cause of early miscarriage. In any form of miscarriage up to 57% of products of conception will have an abnormal karyotype. The most common chromosomal defects are autosomal trisomies, which account for half the abnormalities, while polyploidy and monosomy X account for a further 20% each. Although chromosome abnormalities are common in sporadic miscarriage, parental chromosomal abnormalities are present in only 2–5% of partners presenting with recurrent pregnancy loss. These are most commonly balance reciprocal or robertsonian translocations or mosaicisms.
3. Bleeding in early pregnancy:
   C is correct. Haemodynamic shock associated with bleeding in early pregnancy is usually due either to ruptured ectopic pregnancy or incomplete miscarriage. In this case the low pulse rate suggests vagal stimulation from products of conception distending the cervix, and the absence of abdominal signs of peritonism is against ruptured ectopic. The immediate priority would be to look for products of conception and remove tissue from the cervix. This will confirm a diagnosis of miscarriage, and delay in doing this will cause ongoing blood loss, as the uterus will not be able to contract properly, even with the administration of ergometrine.
4. Uterine abnormalities and miscarriage:
   D is correct. The exact contribution that congenital abnormalities of the uterine cavity, such as a bicornuate uterus or subseptate uterus, make to miscarriage remains controversial. The reported incidence of uterine

anomalies in women with recurrent miscarriage varies from less than 2% to up to 38%. The impact of the abnormality depends on the nature of the anomaly, and the prevalence appears to be higher in women with second-trimester miscarriage. The fetal survival rate is best where the uterus is septate and worst where the uterus is unicornuate. Following damage to the endometrium and inner uterine walls, the surfaces may become adherent, thus partly obliterating the uterine cavity (Asherman's syndrome). The presence of these synechiae may lead to recurrent miscarriage.

5. Ectopic pregnancy:
   B is correct. Medical and conservative management of ectopic pregnancy is not appropriate for someone with significant pain or haemodynamic instability. Once the diagnosis is confirmed, the options for treatment are:
   * *Salpingectomy* – If the tube is badly damaged, or the contralateral tube appears healthy, the correct treatment is removal of the affected tube.
   * *Salpingotomy* – Where the ectopic pregnancy is contained within the tube, it may be possible to conserve the tube by removing the pregnancy and reconstituting the tube. This is particularly important where the contralateral tube has been lost. The disadvantage is the persistence of trophoblastic tissue requiring further surgery or medical treatment in up to 6% of cases.

   Subsequent intrauterine pregnancy rates are similar after both types of treatment, although the risk of recurrent ectopic pregnancy is greater after salpingotomy.
6. Anti-D immunoglobulin administration:
   D is correct. Non-sensitized rhesus (Rh)–negative women should receive anti-D immunoglobulin for all miscarriages and ectopic pregnancies managed surgically Anti-D immunoglobulin does not need to be given for women who have had only medical or expectant management for miscarriage or ectopic pregnancy, who have a threatened miscarriage or who have a pregnancy of unknown location.

Chapter 19

1. Testing for sexually transmitted infection (STI):
   E is correct. The most common STI organism in the developed world is *Chlamydia trachomatis*. This is best defined by polymerase chain reaction (PCR) testing of urine. It is most unlikely to be found in low vaginal or upper vaginal swabs. Vaginal swabs are useful for screening for bacterial vaginosis such as *Gardnerella* infection, *Candida* infection and group B streptococcus (GBS) screening. Antibody screening is less accurate than PCR for *Chlamydia*.

2. Contraceptive efficacy:
   F is correct. The Implanon contraceptive rod has the lowest failure rate whether assessed overall or just with perfect use, although the periods in the 3–6 months after insertion are often very irregular and unpredictable. Of the other methods given A, B and D have similar failure rates, but the failure rate of C is slightly higher.

3. Choice of the appropriate contraceptive to prescribe:
   D is correct. This woman is likely to have the clinical features of polycystic ovarian syndrome (PCOS) and thus should not be given a pill containing a progestogen derived from testosterone (A, B and C) but should be given the one containing the anti-androgen cyproterone acetate. The failure rate of the low-dose progestogen pill is too high to be validly considered in view of her reproductive desires, particularly in women who are overweight.

4. Intrauterine contraceptive device (IUCD) complications:
   B is correct. If the woman or clinician notices that the strings of the device are missing, it must be assumed that one of the following has occurred: pregnancy, the device has been expelled, the device has turned in the uterine cavity and drawn up the strings or the device has perforated the uterus and lies either partly or completely in the peritoneal cavity. Intrauterine infection is not a cause of missing strings.

5. Risks of the combined oral contraceptive pill (COCP):
   B is correct. The risk of venous thrombosis is increased from 5/100,000 to 15/100,000 women per year (RR = 3) and is further increased in smokers and women with a previous history of venous thrombosis. Risk increases with age. This compares to a risk of venous thrombosis in pregnancy and the puerperium of 60/100,000 women. Several studies have suggested that so-called third- and fourth-generation combined pills containing desogestrel, gestodene or drospirenone are associated with a twofold greater risk of venous thrombosis than those containing other progestogens, although the risk of venous thrombosis was lower in these studies than had previously been reported.

Chapter 20

1. Vulvar cancer:
   B is correct. Vulvar cancer has two distinct histological patterns with two different risk factors. The more common basaloid/warty types occur mainly in younger women and are associated with usual vulvar intraepithelial neoplasia (VIN) and human papilloma virus (HPV) infection sharing similar risk factors as cervical cancer. The keratinizing types occur in older women and are associated with lichen sclerosis. VIN is categorized into usual VIN (classic VIN or Bowen's disease) and differentiated VIN based on the distinctive pathological features.

2. Primary prevention of cervical cancer:
   D is correct. Since we now know that the main cause for cervical cancer is human papilloma virus (HPV) infection, preventing HPV infections would be the best primary preventive measure. Prophylactic HPV vaccines have been developed. Bivalent and quadrivalent vaccines have been in the market for about a decade. The bivalent vaccine targets the two high-risk subtypes, HPV 16 and 18, while the quadrivalent vaccine covers HPV 16 and 18 as well as two low-risk subtypes, HPV 6 and 11, which cause genital warts. The prevention of HPV 16 and 18 infections could theoretically prevent more than 70% of cases of cervical cancer, and indeed evidence from Australia after a decade of use has shown a 77% reduction in high-risk HPV serotypes in women aged 18–24 and a 30–50% reaction in high-grade squamous intraepithelial lesion (HSIL) with a 90% reduction in genital warts. These vaccines are most effective when given before any exposure to the virus, i.e. before sexual debut. They may still have some efficacy once sexually active. Cytological screening has been shown to be an effective secondary prevention measure.

3. Predisposing factor for endometrial cancer:
   C is correct. Specific factors are associated with an increased risk of corpus carcinoma, such as nulliparity, late menopause, diabetes and hypertension. It can also be hereditary. Women with hereditary non-polyposis colorectal cancer (HNPCC) syndrome have increased risk of endometrial cancer and ovarian cancer, as well as colorectal cancer. However, the most important risk factors associated with a hyper-oestrogenic state are:
   • Obesity
   • Exogenous oestrogens
   • Endogenous oestrogens
   • Oestrogen-producing ovarian tumours
   • Tamoxifen in breast cancer
   • Endometrial hyperplasia

Chapter 21

1. Uterosacral ligaments:
   C is correct. The uterosacral ligaments are responsible for providing level 1 support to the upper vagina and the cervix and the uterus.

2. Cystocele:
   C is correct. Typically patients complain of 'something coming down' per vaginam. At times there may be

incomplete emptying of the bladder, and this will be associated with double micturition, the desire to repeat micturition immediately after apparent completion of voiding. The patient may give a history of having to manually replace the prolapse into the vagina to void. Urgency is a symptom of overactive bladder, and a cystocele per se should not cause constipation, bleeding or deep dyspareunia.

3. Stress urinary incontinence:
   A is correct. Stress incontinence should be managed initially by pelvic floor physiotherapy. Surgical treatment is indicated where there is a failure to respond to conservative management.

4. Uterovaginal prolapse:
   E is correct. Surgical repair may have to be repeated if vaginal delivery occurs later.

5. Acute retention of urine:
   E is correct. Radiotherapy is more often associated with urinary frequency or incontinence from fistula formation.

Appendix A

1. Routine preoperative investigations:
   C is correct. Preoperative blood investigations include full blood count, urea and electrolytes for screening for renal disease in patients with hypertension or diabetes and in women on diuretics and liver function test for patients with alcohol abuse or liver disease; group and save prior to procedures with risk of bleeding, and cross-match if heavy bleeding is suspected or antibodies are present. A routine coagulation screen is not necessary unless the patient has a known bleeding disorder or has been on medication that causes anticoagulation.

2. World Health Organization (WHO) surgical checklists:
   D is correct. The WHO surgical safety checklist provides a set of checks to be done at three stages of a surgical procedure (sign in, time out and sign out). A routine part of the postoperative sign out is an acknowledgement of correct swab and instrument counts. Administrative staff are not usually involved in the preoperative huddle. The WHO Surgical Safety Checklist was developed to reduce errors and adverse events, as well as increase teamwork and communication in surgery. The use of this checklist has been associated with significant reductions in both morbidity and mortality, as well as postoperative complications.

3. Contraindications prior to surgery:
   C is correct. The combined oral contraceptive pill should be stopped 4–6 weeks prior to major surgery to minimize the risk of venous thromboembolism (VTE). None of the others carry a major perioperative risk of thromboembolism.

4. Intraoperative/postoperative complications:
   E is correct. Compartment syndrome in the legs may occur due to the lithotomy position when the pressure in the muscle of an osteofascial compartment is increased, causing ischaemia followed by reperfusion, capillary leakage from the ischaemic tissue and further increase in tissue oedema resulting in neuromuscular compromise and rhabdomyolysis. Leg holders, pneumatic compression stockings, high body mass index and prolonged surgical time are risk factors. Femoral neuropathy occurs secondary to excessive hip flexion, abduction and external hip rotation, which contribute to nerve compression.

5. Risk factors for urinary tract injuries:
   C is correct. Risk factors for bladder injury include endometriosis, infection, bladder overdistension and adhesions. Lateral rather than suprapubic trocar insertion will reduce the risk of bladder injury.

6. Postoperative care:
   C is correct. Epidural analgesia, dehydration and bleeding are common causes of postoperative hypotension.

7. Postoperative complications:
   E is correct. Common organisms in surgical site infections (SSIs) of abdominal incisions are *Staphylococcus aureus*, coagulase-negative staphylococci, *Enterococcus* spp. and *Escherichia coli*. Postoperative pelvic abscesses are commonly associated with anaerobes. Risk factors include diabetes, smoking, systemic steroid medication, radiotherapy, poor nutrition, obesity, prolonged hospitalization and blood transfusion. Surgical factors associated with SSIs include prolonged operating time, excessive blood loss, hypothermia, hair removal by shaving and surgical drains.

8. Enhanced recovery pathways:
   E is correct. Enhanced recovery pathways have been associated with reduced pain and nursing requirements and improved patient satisfaction and quality of life. Enhanced recovery focuses on optimizing patient education and perioperative expectations, decreasing the perioperative fasting period, maintaining haemodynamic stability and normothermia, increasing mobilization, providing effective pain relief, nausea and vomiting prophylaxis and decreasing use of catheters and drains. These pathways should be individualized as indicated. Intraoperative elements of enhanced recovery involve both the anaesthetists and surgeons. On the day of the surgical procedure, the period of starvation is reduced to 2 hours for clear fluids prior to anaesthetic to avoid dehydration.

Appendix B

1. Using social media:
   D is correct. There are potential benefits and risks for doctors and health care professionals if they are engaging with social media. Whilst there are advantages of networking professionally and socially and the public accessing health-related information from professionals, challenges exist in maintaining confidentiality and professional and personal boundaries. It is therefore important that all doctors be aware of and adhere to the General Medical Council's guidance on the use of social media.

2. General Data Protection Regulation (GDPR) data protection:
   B is correct. GDPR was introduced on 25 May 2018 to update personal data rules. It is a mandatory regulation in EU law on data protection and privacy for all individuals within the European Union and European Economic Area (EEA). It also addresses the export of personal data outside the EEA and EU. Therefore even companies and organizations registered outside the EEA and EU but operating within Europe must comply with this regulation. The two key terms in GDPR involve personal and sensitive data. Essentially GDPR offers new rights for people to access the information companies/organizations hold about them, and there are obligations for organizations for better management of data or to risk a new regimen of fines.

3. Research and clinical audit:
   B is correct. One complete cycle of a clinical audit demonstrates improvement in patient care and that includes procedures used for diagnosis, treatment, associated use of resources and resulting outcome for the patient, whereas the primary aim of research is to drive generalizable new knowledge. For clinical research, application is made for approval from a research ethics committee, whereas no such approval is required for a clinical audit. It is important that the first cycle of a clinical audit is followed by further audit cycles in order to demonstrate continuing improvement process. This may require several cycles of clinical audits to demonstrate significant improvement in patient outcomes. There are clearly laid out principles around research funding. Several organizations provide funding for research.

4. Clinical guidelines:
   A is correct. Clinical guidelines are developed by a large number of organizations such as World Health Organization (WHO), National Institute for Health and Care Excellence (NICE), Scottish Intercollegiate Guidelines Network (SIGN) and royal colleges, to cite a few. Although guidelines are evidence based and derived from level 1 evidence, not all organizations follow a similar methodology. The guideline developers usually consult previously published guidelines from other organizations, but they do not necessarily follow their methodology. Guidelines production is a very intense, time-consuming process taking between 18 and 24 months. Guidelines recommendations are based on clinical effectiveness. Guidelines published by NICE take account of cost-effectiveness of the recommendation as well.

5. Research:
   E is correct. Descriptive studies test an aetiological hypothesis – such as excessive smoking increases the risk of cancer of the lung. Case control studies compare people with disease and those without it, whereas cohort studies compare people exposed to the suspected causative agent and those not exposed to it. It is unethical for patients to be randomized without ethics committee approval. Furthermore, patients should give valid, informed consent before they can be entered into a clinical trial. If patients do not wish to be randomized to a clinical trial, they should be treated with standard treatment for that condition. Clinicians should not be aware of whether their patients are being treated with an active drug or a dummy preparation and should be treated in a similar way. All side effects should be reported accurately. However, if any patient experiences an undesirable side effect, he or she should be withdrawn from the trial immediately, irrespective of his or her allocation in the trial. Thereafter he or she should be treated following the best practice guidelines. Finally, pregnant women or those who desire to become pregnant should not be exposed to new drugs or new interventions, as data may not be available on the safety of these drugs on embryonic development.

6. Evidence-based health care:
   A is correct. The risk management strategy should be in place in each organization in order to not only improve care of women but also to minimize risk to patients and to the organization. A clinical risk management strategy involves collection of data on all aspects of patient care and that involves elements of process, treatment and outcome. Therefore the focus should not only be on serious outcomes such as maternal and neonatal mortality. By reducing risk to women and to their babies, care can be improved. The focus should be to minimize risk and to learn from errors. This can only be done by learning from near-misses and by implementation of guidelines. Successful implementation of guidelines is always supported by regular clinical audits to ensure that level of adherence to guidelines is above 90%. When clinical

incidents are reported, they should be investigated in a positive and constructive way involving all members of a care team. Lessons should be learned and an action plan be implemented to reduce the risk of recurrence of similar incidences in the future. When patients do complain against staff, it is important to investigate their complaints in an open and transparent way to ensure that issues identified by the patient have been investigated fully. Lessons should be learned and organizations should respond to the issues identified in the patient's complaints.

Appendix C

1. Informed consent:
   D is correct. As the operating surgeon, it is your responsibility to obtain informed consent. You can never be sure exactly what was discussed by other individuals; therefore you must discuss the other treatment options available to this patient and the potential complications which could occur if the planned surgery was performed and the further treatment which might then be necessary. She may well decide against the planned surgery when given all of this information, especially if complications of the surgery, although most unlikely and even at a risk of less than 1%, would distress her considerably. Provision of the college statement on the risks of surgery would be incomplete information and, even if provided, would not cover the requirements of informed consent unless time was given for these matters to be discussed in detail.

2. Legal requirements regarding retention of medical records:
   B is correct. For a problem unrelated to pregnancy, medical records must be retained for at least 7 years and can then be destroyed. For a pregnancy-related record, these need to be retained for 7 years after the child has reached 'maturity' at the age of 18 years. Both the maternal medical record and that of the child must therefore be retained for 25 years. As this case does not involve a pregnancy, the correct response is B.

3. Levels of evidence:
   E is correct. By far the best level of evidence is provided by randomized controlled clinical trials. The remaining options are less valuable in defining the adequacy and accuracy of the evidence given, with these progressively declining in efficacy from level D to level A.

4. Requirements of an adequate medical record:
   E is correct. All of these matters need to be documented in detail. The adequacy of care can only be assessed and the possible cause of any long-term problem in the baby defined with all of this information.

5. Appropriate care of a 15-year-old girl requesting contraception:
   D is correct. If he is less than 3 years older than her and is not a relative, a teacher or other responsible person, then sex would be legal. If he is older, is a close relative, a teacher or youth leader, etc., any sexual relationship would be illegal and is potentially reportable to the police if the actual relationship is confirmed. It is not illegal to give her the pill, provided she understands the implications. Advising the parents or department of health is not necessary to give her the pill. Use of condoms would remove the doctor from the problem, but less-than-adequate contraception would be provided since her partner has indicated he is not prepared to use such methods.

Further reading

Papers marked * indicate those the editors consider landmark studies in the development of obstetrics and gynaecology over the last 40 years. These are mainly clinical trials or meta-analyses that have influenced contemporary practice. They are also beloved of the setters of short-answer questions in postgraduate examinations. Although highly cited, many of these studies have been the source of much debate and do not necessarily represent the 'final word' in evidence-based practice. We are sure that readers of this book will have suggestions of their own as to other studies that should be included (or indeed should be excluded from this list).

Chapter 2

Johnson MH. *Essential Reproduction*. 6th ed. Chichester: John Wiley; 2008.

Moore K. *The Developing Human: Clinically Oriented Embryology*. London: WB Saunders; 1988.

Philipp EE, Setchell M, eds. *Scientific Foundations of Obstetrics and Gynaecology*. London: Heinemann; 1991.

Chapter 3

Broughton Pipkin F. Maternal physiology. In: Chamberlain GV, Steer P, eds. *Turnbull's Obstetrics*. 3rd ed. Edinburgh: Churchill Livingstone; 2001.

Broughton Pipkin F. Maternal physiology. In: Edmonds DK, ed. *Dewhurst's Textbook of Obstetrics and Gynaecology*. 8th ed. Oxford: Blackwell; 2007.

Cartwright JE, Duncan WC, Critchley HO, et al. Remodelling at the maternal–fetal interface: relevance to human pregnancy disorders. *Reproduction*. 2010;140:803–813.

James D, Steer P, Weiner C, et al. *High Risk Pregnancy: Management Options*. London: Elsevier Saunders; 2011.

Chapter 4

De Swiet M, Chamberlain GVP. *Basic Science in Obstetrics and Gynaecology*. Edinburgh: Churchill Livingstone; 1992.

Erikson PS, Secher NJ, Weis-Bentson M. Normal growth of the fetal biparietal diameter and the abdominal diameter in a longitudinal study. *Acta Obstet Gynaecol Scand*. 1985;64:65–70.

Gardosi J, Chang A, Kalyan B, et al. Customised antenatal growth charts. *Lancet*. 1992;339:283–287.

Thorburn GD, Harding R. *Textbook of Fetal Physiology*. Oxford: Oxford University Press; 1994.

Chapter 5

Centre for Maternal and Child Enquiries (CMACE). *Perinatal Mortality 2008 United Kingdom*. London: CMACE; 2010. Available: http://www.publichealth.hscni.net/sites/default/files/Perinatal%20Mortality%202008.pdf.

Centre for Maternal and Child Enquiries (CMACE). Saving mothers' lives: reviewing maternal deaths to make motherhood safer: 2006–08. The eighth report on confidential enquiries into maternal deaths in the United Kingdom. *BJOG*. 2011;118(suppl 1):1–203.

Gardosi J, Kady SM, McGeown P, et al. Classification of stillbirth by relevant condition at death (ReCoDe): population based cohort study. *BMJ*. 2005;331:1113–1117.

World Health Organization. *Beyond the Numbers: Reviewing Maternal Deaths and Complications to Make Pregnancy Safer*. Geneva: WHO Press; 2004. Available: http://apps.who.int/iris/handle/10665/42984.

World Health Organization. *Neonatal and Perinatal Mortality: Country, Regional and Global Estimates*. Geneva: WHO Press; 2006. Available: http://apps.who.int/iris/handle/10665/43444.

World Health Organization. *Neonatal and Perinatal Mortality: Country, Regional and Global Estimates 2004 /Elisabeth Åhman and Jelka Zupan*. Geneva: WHO Press; 2007. Available: http://apps.who.int/iris/bitstream/handle/10665/43800/9789241596145_eng.pdf?sequence=1.

World Health Organization. *Trends in Maternal Mortality: 1990 to 2008. Estimates Developed by WHO, UNICEF, UNFPA and The World Bank. 2010*. Geneva: WHO Press; 2010. Available: https://www.who.int/reproductivehealth/publications/monitoring/9789241500265/en/.

Chapter 6

Chandraharan E, Arulkumaran S. Female pelvis and details of operative delivery; shoulder dystocia and episiotomy. In: Arulkumaran S, Penna LK, Rao Basker, eds. *Management of Labour*. India: Orient Longman; 2005.

Chapter 7

Australian Institute of Health and Welfare, Australian Government, Canberra. Australian Red Cross Blood Service. *Transfusion*. Available: www.transfusion.com.au

Laws PJ, Li Z, Sullivan EA. *Australia's Mothers and Babies 2008. Perinatal Statistics Series No. 24. Cat. No. PER 50*. Canberra: AIHW. National Health and Medical Research Council Immunization Handbook; 2010. Available: http://www.health.gov.au/internet/immunise/publishing.nsf/Content/Handbook-home.

National Organisation for Fetal Alcohol Syndrome and Related Disorders (NOFASARD). Available: http://www.nofasard.org.au/.

Antenatal Care for uncomplicated pregnancies National Institute for Health and Care Excellence (NICE) Clinical Guideline CG62 Updated Feb 2019. Availlable: https://www.nice.org.uk/guidance/cg62.

Qureshi H, Massey E, Kirwan D, et al. BCSH guideline for the use of anti-D immunoglobulin for the prevention of haemolytic disease of the fetus and newborn. *Transfus Med.* 2014;24:8–20.

Royal Australian and New Zealand College of Obstetrics and Gynaecology. Statement C-Obs 6 Guidelines for the use of Rh (D) Immunoglobulin (anti-D) in Obstetrics in Australia. Available: https://www.ranzcog.edu.au/Statements-Guidelines/Obstetrics/RhD-Immunoglobulin-(Anti-D)-in-Obstetrics-in. Austr.

Chapter 8

*CLASP collaborative group. CLASP: a randomised trial of low-dose aspirin for the prevention and treatment of pre-eclampsia among 9364 pregnant women. *Lancet.* 1994;343:619–629.

*Hannah ME, Hannah WJ, Hellman J, et al. Induction of labour as compared with serial antenatal monitoring in post-term pregnancy. *N Engl J Med.* 1992;326:1587–1592.

*Hannah ME, Hannah WJ, Hewson SA, et al. Planned caesarean section versus planned vaginal birth for breech presentation at term: a randomised multicentre trial (Term Breech Trial). *Lancet.* 2000;356:1375–1383.

*Hilder L, Costeloe K, Thilaganathan B. Prolonged pregnancy: evaluating gestation-specific risks of fetal and infant mortality. *BJOG.* 1998;105:169–173.

*Magpie Trial Follow-Up Study Collaborative Group. The Magpie Trial: a randomised trial comparing magnesium sulphate with placebo for pre-eclampsia. Outcome for children at 18 months. *BJOG.* 2007;114:289–299.

National Institute for Health and Clinical Excellence. *The Management of Hypertensive Disorders in Pregnancy. July 2013*; 2010. Available: https://www.nice.org.uk/guidance/qs35/chapter/quality-statement-3-antenatal-blood-pressure-targets.

Royal College of Obstetricians and Gynaecologists Green-top Guideline No. 63. *Antepartum Haemorrhage*; 2011. Available: https://www.rcog.org.uk/globalassets/documents/guidelines/gtg_63.pdf.

Royal College of Obstetricians and Gynaecologists Green-top Guideline No. 20b. *The Management of Breech Presentation*; 2017. Available: https://obgyn.onlinelibrary.wiley.com/doi/epdf/10.1111/1471-0528.14465.

Royal College of Obstetricians and Gynaecologists Green-top Guideline No. 27. *Placenta Praevia, Placenta Accreta. Diagnosis and Management. 27 A*; 2018. https://www.rcog.org.uk/en/guidelines-research-services/guidelines/gtg27a/.

Royal College of Obstetricians and Gynaecologists Green-top Guidelines No. 51. *Management of Monochorionic Twin Pregnancy*; 2016. Available: https://obgyn.onlinelibrary.wiley.com/doi/pdf/10.1111/14711-0528.14188.

Smith GC, Pell JP, Dobbie R. Birth order, gestational age, and risk of delivery related perinatal death in twins: retrospective cohort study. *BMJ.* 2002;325:1004.

Chapter 9

*Crowther CA, Hiller JE, Moss RJ, et al. Effect of treatment of gestational diabetes mellitus on pregnancy outcomes (ACHOIS). *N Engl J Med.* 2005;352:2477–2486.

*HAPO Study Cooperative Research Group. Hyperglycaemia and adverse pregnancy outcomes. *N Engl J Med.* 2008;358:1991–2002.

Royal College of Obstetricians and Gynaecologists Green-top Guideline No. 37b *The Acute Management of Thrombosis and Embolism During Pregnancy and the Puerperium*; 2007, reviewed 2010. Available: https://www.rcog.org.uk/globalassets/documents-guidelines/gtg_37b.pdf.

Royal College of Obstetricians and Gynaecologists & BASH - Management of Genital Herpes in Pregnancy. 2014. Available: https://www.rcog.org.uk/globalassets/documents/guidelines/management-genital-herpes.pdf.

Royal College of Obstetricians and Gynaecologists Green-top Guideline No. 13. *Chickenpox in Pregnancy*; 2015. Available: https://www.rcog.org.uk/en/guidelines-research-services/guidelines/gtg13/.

Royal College of Obstetricians and Gynaecologists Green-top Guideline No. 72. *Care of Women With Obesity in Pregnancy*; 2018. Available at: https://obgyn.onlinelibrary.wiley.com/doi/full/10.1111/1471-0528.15386.

Chapter 10

Baschat AA. Pathophysiology of fetal growth restriction: implications for diagnosis and surveillance. *Obstet Gynecol Surv.* 2004;59:617–627.

Bottomley C, Bourne T. Dating and growth in the first trimester. *Best Pract Res Clin Obstet Gynaecol.* 2009;23:439–452.

Cosmi E, Ambrosini G, D'Antona D, et al. Doppler, cardiotocography, and biophysical profile changes in growth-restricted fetuses. *Obstet Gynecol.* 2005;106:1240–1245.

Devoe LD. Antenatal fetal assessment: contraction stress test, non-stress test, vibroacoustic stimulation, amniotic fluid volume, biophysical profile, and modified biophysical profile – an overview. *Semin Perinatol.* 2008;32:247–252.

Johnstone FD. *Clinical Obstetrics and Gynaecology.* London: Baillière Tindall; 1992.

Langford KS. Infectious disease and pregnancy. *Curr Obstet Gynaecol.* 2002;12:125–130.

*Malone FD, Canick J, Ball R, et al. First-trimester or second-trimester screening, or both, for Down's syndrome (FASTER). *N Engl J Med.* 2003;353:2001–2011.

Inducing Labour National Institute for Health and Care Excellence Clinical Guideline CG70 July 2008. Available at https://www.nice.org.uk/guidance/cg70.

Reed GB, Claireaux AE, Bain AD. *Diseases of the Fetus and Newborn.* London: Chapman and Hall; 1989.

Royal College of Obstetricians and Gynaecologists Green-top Guidelines No. 31. *The Investigation and Management of the Small-for-Gestational-Age Fetus*; 2013. Available: https://www.rcog.org.uk/globalassets/documents/guidelines/gtg_31.pdf.

Spencer K, Spencer CE, Power M, et al. Screening for chromosomal abnormalities in the first trimester using ultrasound and maternal serum biochemistry in a one-stop clinic: a review of three years prospective experience. *BJOG.* 2003;110:281–286.

*The GRIT study group. A randomised trial of timed delivery for the compromised preterm fetus: short term outcomes and Bayesian interpretation. *BJOG.* 2003;110:27–32.

Timor-Tritsch IE, Fuchs KM, Monteagudo A, et al. Performing a fetal anatomy scan at the time of first-trimester screening. *Obstet Gynecol.* 2009;113:402–407.

*Van Bulck B, et al. Infant wellbeing at 2 years of age in the Growth Restriction Intervention Trial. *Lancet.* 2004;364:513–520.

Chapter 11

Backett TF, Arulkumaran S. *Intrapartum Care for the MRCOG and Beyond*. London: RCOG Press; 2001. https://www.cambridge.org/core/books/intrapartum-care-for-the-mrcog-and-beyond/1D5FBAAFF75E23DD10341DE35F0521EC.

*Doyle LW, Crowther CA, Middleton P, et al. Magnesium sulphate for women at risk of preterm birth for neuroprotection of the fetus. *Cochrane Database Syst Rev*. 2009;(Issue 1):Art No: CD004661.

Fonseca EB, Celik E, Parra M, et al. Progesterone and the risk of preterm birth among women with a short cervix. *N Engl J Med*. 2007;357:462–469.

*Kenyon SL, Taylor DJ, Tarnow-Mordi W; ORACLE Collaborative Group. Broad-spectrum antibiotics for preterm, prelabour rupture of fetal membranes: the ORACLE I randomised trial. *Lancet*. 2001;357:979–988.

*Kenyon SL, Taylor DJ, Tarnow-Mordi W, ORACLE Collaborative Group. Broad-spectrum antibiotics for spontaneous preterm labour: the ORACLE II randomised trial. *Lancet*. 2001;357:989–994.

*MacDonald D, Grant A, Sheridan-Pereira M, et al. The Dublin randomised controlled trial of intrapartum fetal heart rate monitoring. *Am J Obstet Gynecol*. 1985;152:524–539.

Mahmood T, Owen P, Arulkumaran S, Dhillon C, eds. *Models of Care in Maternity Services*. London: RCOG Press; 2010. Available: https://www.cambridge.org/core/books/models-of-care-in-maternity-services/C903136D3328C459994BC0098F67363D.

Intrapartum care for healthy women and babies NICE Clinical Guideline CG190 Feb 2017. Available: https://www.nice.org.uk/guidance/cg190.

*O'Driscoll K, Stronge JM, Minogue M, et al. Active management of labour. *BMJ*. 1973;3:135–137.

Royal College of Obstetricians and Gynaecologists Green-top Guideline No. 50. *Umbilical Cord Prolapse*; 2014. Available: https://www.rcog.org.uk/en/guidelines-research-services/guidelines/gtg50/.

Royal College of Obstetricians and Gynaecologists Green-top Guideline No. 7. *Antenatal Corticosteroids to Reduce Neonatal Morbidity. Cross referenced to NICE guidelines on Preterm labour and birth. ND 25) of Nov 2015*; 2010. Available: http://www.rcog.org.uk/files/rcog-corp/GTG 7.pdf https://www.nice.org.uk/guidance/ng25?unlid=9291036072016213201257.

Royal College of Obstetricians and Gynaecologists Green-top Guideline No. 1b. *Tocolysis for Women in Preterm Labour. Cross Referenced to NICE Guidelines on Preterm Labour and Birth. ND 25) of Nov 2015*; 2011. Available: https://www.rcog.org.uk/en/guidelines-research-services/guidelines/gtg1b/.

Royal College of Obstetricians and Gynaecologists Green-top Guideline No. 42. *Shoulder Dystocia*; 2012. Available: http://www.rcog.org.uk/files/rcog-corp/GTG 42_Shoulder dystocia 2nd edition 2012.pdf https://www.rcog.org.uk/globalassets/documents/guidelines/gtg_42.pdf.

Chapter 12

*Landon MB, Hauth JC, Leveno KJ, et al. Maternal and perinatal outcomes associated with a trial of labour after prior caesarean delivery. *N Engl J Med*. 2004;351:2581–2589.

Robson S, Higgs P. Third- and fourth- degree injuries. *Aust N Z J Obstet Gynaecol*. 2011;13(2):20–22.

Royal College of Obstetricians and Gynaecologists Green-top Guideline No. 52. *Prevention and Management of Postpartum Haemorrhage*; 2016. Available: https://www.rcog.org.uk/en/guidelines-research services/guidelines/gtg52/.

Royal College of Obstetricians and Gynaecologists Green-top Guidelines No. 26. *Operative vaginal delivery*; 2011. Available: https://www.rcog.org.uk/en/guidelines-research-services/guidelines/gtg26/.

Chapter 13

Benn C. Milk of humankind: best. *Aust N Z J Obstet Gynaecol*. 2011;13(2):40–41.

Coker A, Oliver R. *Definitions and Classifications in a Textbook of Postpartum Hemorrhage*. Sapiens Publishing; London 2006:11–16.

Kumarasamy R. Infection in the peuperium. *Aust N Z J Obstet Gynaecol*. 2011;13(2):17.

Royal College of Obstetricians and Gynaecologists Green-top Guideline No. 37b. *Thromboembolic Disease in Pregnancy and the Puerperium: Acute Management*; 2015. Available: https://www.rcog.org.uk/en/guidelines-research-services/guidelines/gtg37b/.

Royal College of Obstetricians and Gynaecologists Green-top Guideline No. 29. *The Management of Third and Fourth Degree Perineal Tears*; 2015. Available: https://www.rcog.org.uk/global assets/documents/guidelines/gtg-29.pdf.

Royal College of Obstetricians and Gynaecologists Green-top Guideline No. 47. *Blood Transfusion in Obstetrics*; 2015. Available: https://www.rcog.org.uk/en/guidelines-research-services/guidelines/gtg47/.

Royal College of Obstetricians and Gynaecologists Green-top Guideline No. 56. *Maternal Collapse in Pregnancy and the Peurperium*; 2011. Available: https://www.rcog.org.uk/globalassets/documents/guidelines/gtg_56.pdf.

Thakkar. *Guidelines on neonatal examination. CGCHealth005-1*. Milton Keynes, UK: Milton Keynes NHS Trust; 2004.

Chapter 14

Antenatal and Postnatal Mental Health – Quality standard. QS 115. 2016. Available: https://www.nice.org.uk/guidance/qs115.

British Association of Psychopharmacology Consensus Guidance on Use of Psychotropic Medication in Perinatal Period 2017. Available: https://www.bap.org.uk/pdfs/BAP_Guidelines-Perinatal.pdf.

Howard L, Piot P, Stein A. No health without perinatal mental health. Lancet 2014;15;384(9956):1723–4. Available: www.thelancet.com/journals/lancet/article/PIIS0140-6736(14)62040-7/fulltext.

Maternal Mental Health – Womens Voices RCOG Publications. 2017. Available: https://www.rcog.org.uk/globalassets/documents/patients/information/maternalmental-healthwomensvoices.pdf. MBRRACE-UK:Saving Libes, Improving Mothers Care (2-14-2016). Available at: https://www.npeu.ox.ac.uk/mbrrace-uk/reports.

Mental Health in Pregnancy and the Postnatal Period – Fingertips Tool PHE. 2017. Available: https://fingertips.phe.org.uk/profile-group/mental-health/profile/perinatal-mental-health.

Chapter 15

Critchley HOD, Munro MG, Broder M, et al. A five-year international review process concerning terminologies, definitions and related issues around abnormal uterine bleeding. *Semin Reprod Med*. 2011;29:377–382.

Chapter 16

*Garry R, Fountain J, Mason S, et al. The eVALuate study: two parallel randomised trials, one comparing laparoscopic with abdominal hysterectomy, the other comparing laparoscopic with vaginal hysterectomy. *BMJ*. 2004;328:129.

*Hulley S, Grady D, Bush T, et al. Randomised trial of estrogen plus progestin for secondary prevention of coronary heart disease in postmenopausal women (HERS). *J Am Med Ass*. 1998;280:605–613.

Royal College of Obstetricians and Gynaecologists Green-top Guideline No. 48. *Management of Premenstrual Syndrome*; 2017. Available: https://obgyn.onlinelibrary.wiley.com/doi/epdf/10.1111/1471-0528.14260.

NICE Guideline No 23 Menopause: diagnosis and managment No 2015. Available: https://www.nice.org.uk/guidance/ng23.

Royal College of Obstetricians and Gynaecologists Green-top Guideline No. 41. *The Initial Management of Chronic Pelvic Pain*; 2012. Available: https://www.rcog.org.uk/globalassets/documents/guidelines/gtg_41.pdf.

RANZCOG College Statement C-Gyn 9. Management of the Menopause; 2011. Available: https://www.ranzcog.edu.au/RANZCOG_SITE/media/RANZCOG-MEDIA/Women%27s%20Health/Statement%20and%20guidelines/Clinical%20-%20Gynaecology/Management-of-the-Menopause-(C-Gyn-9)-Review-November-2014_1.pdf?ext=.pdf.

Sampson JA. Perforating hemorrhagic (chocolate) cysts of the ovary. Their importance and especially their relation to pelvic adenomas of the endometrial type ('adenomyoma' of the uterus, rectovaginal septum, sigmoid, etc.). *Arch Surg*. 1921;3:245–323.

*The Women's Health Initiative steering committee. Effects of conjugated equine estrogen in postmenopausal women with hysterectomy: the WHI randomised controlled trial. *J Am Med Ass*. 2004;291:1701–1712.

*Writing group for the Women's Health Initiative (WHI) randomised controlled trial. Risks and benefits of estrogen plus progestin in healthy postmenopausal women: principle results the WHI randomised controlled trial. *J Am Med Ass*. 2002;288:321–333.

Chapter 17

Bhattacharya S, Porter M, Amalraj E, et al. The epidemiology of infertility in the north east of scotland. *Hum Reprod*. 2009;24(12):3096–3107.

Brosens J, Gordon A. *Tubal Infertility*. Philadelphia: J B Lippincott; 1990.

Insler V, Lunenfeld B. *Infertility, Male and Female*. Edinburgh: Churchill Livingstone; 1986.

Lashen H. Investigations for infertility. *Curr Obstet Gynaecol*. 2001;11:239–244.

Ledger WL. In vitro fertilization. *Curr Obstet Gynaecol*. 2002;12:269–275.

Fertility Problems: assessment and treatment NICE Clinical Guideline CG156 Sept 2017. Available: https://www.nice.org.uk/guidance/cg156.

Royal College of Obstetricians and Gynaecologists Green-top Guidelines No. 24. *The Investigation and Management of Endomtreiosis. Cross Referenced to Guideline on the Management of Women With Endometriosis by ESHRE. Sept 2013*; 2006. Available: https://www.eshre.eu/Guidelines-and-Legal/Guidelines/Endometriosis-guideline.aspx.

Taylor A. The subfertile couple. *Curr Obstet Gynaecol*. 2001;11:115–125.

Wakley G. Sexual dysfunction. *Curr Obstet Gynaecol*. 2002;12:35–40.

Chapter 18

Abortion Act. London: HMSO; 1967.

Ankum A. Diagnosing suspected ectopic pregnancy. *BMJ*. 2000;321:1235–1236.

*Clark P, Walker ID, Langhorne P, et al. Scottish pregnancy intervention (SPIN) study: a multicentre, randomised controlled trial of low molecular weight heparin and low dose aspirin in women with recurrent miscarriage. *Blood*. 2010;115:4162–4167.

Demetroulis C, Saridogan E, Kunde D, et al. A prospective RCT comparing medical and surgical treatment for early pregnancy failure. *Hum Reprod*. 2001;16:365–369.

Department of Health, Department for Education and Employment, Home Office. *The Removal, Retention and Use of Human Organs and Tissue Post-Mortem Examination. Advice from the Chief Medical Officer*. London: Stationery Office; 2001.

Eliakim R, Abulafia O, Sherer DM. Hyperemesis: a current review. *Am J Perinatol*. 2000;17(4):207–218.

Graziosi GC, Moi BW, Ankum WM, et al. Management of early pregnancy loss – a systematic review. *Int J Gynaecol Obstet*. 2001;86:337–346.

National Institute for Health and Clinical Excellence. *NICE Clinical Guideline 154 Ectopic Pregnancy and Miscarriage: Diagnosis and Initial Management*; 2012. guidance. Available: https://www.nice.org.uk/guidance/cg154.

Regan L, Rai R. Epidemiology and the medical causes of miscarriage. *Best Pract Res Clin Obstet Gynaecol*. 2000;14(5):839–854.

Royal College of Obstetricians and Gynaecologists Green-top Guideline No. 38. *Management of Gestational Trophoblastic Disease*; 2010. Available: https://www.rcog.org.uk/en/guidelines-research-services/guidelines/gtg38/.

Royal College of Obstetricians and Gynaecologists Green-top Guideline No. 17. *The Investigation and Treatment of Couples with Recurrent First-trimester and Second-trimester Miscarriage*; 2011. Available: https://www.rcog.org.uk/globalassets/documents/guidelines/gtg_17.pdf.

Speroff L, Glass RH, Kase NG. Ectopic pregnancy. In: Speroff L, Glass RH, Kase NG, eds. *Clinical Gynecologic Endocrinology and Infertility*. 32. Baltimore: Williams and Wilkins; 1994:947–964.

*Trinder J, Brocklehurst P, Porter R, et al. Management of miscarriage: expectant, medical or surgical? Results of randomised controlled trial (MIST). *BMJ*. 2006;332:1235–1240.

Zhang J, Gilles JM, Barnhart K, et al. A comparison of medical management with misoprostol and surgical management for early pregnancy failure. *N Engl J Med*. 2005;353:761–769.

Chapter 19

Adaikan PG, Chong YS, Chew SSL, et al. Male sexual dysfunction. *Curr Obstet Gynaecol*. 2000;10:23–28.

Barton SE. Classification, general principles of vulval infections. *Curr Obstet Gynaecol*. 2000;10:2–6.

Berek JS. *Berek and Novak's Gynecology*. 14th ed. Philadelphia: Lippincott, Williams & Wilkins; 2007.

Breen KJ, Cordner SM, Thomson CJH, et al. *Good Medical Practice: Professionalism, Ethics and Law*. Melbourne: Cambridge University Press; 2010.

Bignell CJ. Chlamydial infections in obstetrics and gynaecology. *Curr Obstet Gynaecol*. 1997;7:104–109.

Denman M. Gynaecological aspects of female sexual dysfunction. *Curr Obstet Gynaecol*. 1999;9:88–92.

Department of Health. *Handbook of Contraceptive Practice*. London: HMSO; 1990.

Hampton N. Choice of contraception. *Curr Obstet Gynaecol.* 2001;11:50–53.

Hamoda H, Bignell C. Pelvic Infections. *Curr Obstet Gynaecol.* 2002;12:185–190.

Johnstone FD. *Clinical Obstetrics and Gynaecology.* London: Baillière Tindall; 1992.

Ledger WJ, Witkin SS. *Vulvovaginal Infections.* London: Manson Publishing; 2007.

Loudon N. *Handbook of Family Planning.* 2nd ed. Edinburgh: Churchill Livingstone; 1991.

Masters T, Everett S. Intrauterine and barrier contraception. *Curr Obstet Gynaecol.* 2002;12:28–34.

Robinson C, Kubba AA. Medical problems and oral contraceptives. *Curr Obstet Gynaecol.* 1997;7:173–179.

Royal Australian and New Zealand College of Obstetrics and Gynaecology College Statement C-Gyn 11. *Emergency Contraception;* 2012. Available: http://www.ranzcog.edu.au/component/docman/doc_view/1001-c-gyn-11-emergency-contraception.html?Itemid=341.

Sterilisation Familiy Planning Association (accessed 14th July 2019). Available: https://www.sexwise.fpa.org.uk/contraception/sterilisation.

Royal College of Obstetricians and Gynaecologists. *Evidence-Based Guideline 7: The Care of Women Requesting Induced Abortion.* London: RCOG Press; 2011. Available: https://www.rcog.org.uk/globalassets/documents/guidelines/abortion-guideline_web_1.pdf.

Spagne VA, Prior RB. *Sexually Transmitted Diseases.* New York: Marcel Dekker; 1985.

Stewart P, Fletcher J. Therapeutic termination of pregnancy. *Curr Obstet Gynaecol.* 2002;12:22–27.

Szarciwski A, Guillebaud J. *Contraception.* Oxford: Oxford University Press; 1994.

Walters WAW. *Clinical Obstetrics and Gynaecology.* London: Baillière Tindall; 1991.

Chapter 20

Australian Government Department of Health. *National Cervical Screening Program.* (2017). Available: http://www.cancerscreening.gov.au/cervical.

Berek JS, Neville F, Hacker NF. *Berek and Hacker's Gynecologic Oncology.* 5th ed. Philadelphia: Lippincott, William & Wilkins; 2009.

Brown V, Sridhar T, Symonds RP. Principles of chemotherapy and radiotherapy. *Obstet Gynaecol Reprod Med.* 2011;21(12):339–345.

*Buys SS, Partridge E, Black A, et al. Effect of screening on ovarian cancer mortality: the prostate, lung, colorectal and ovarian cancer screening randomised controlled trial. *J Am Med Ass.* 2011;305:2295–2303.

Freeman S, Hampson F, Addley H, et al. Imaging of the female pelvis. *Obstet Gynaecol Reprod Med.* 2009;19(10):271–281.

Hannemann MH, Alexander HM, Cope NJ, et al. Endometrial hyperplasia: a clinician's review. *Obstet Gynaecol Reprod Med.* 2010;20(4):116–120.

Holland C. Endometrial cancer. *Obstet Gynaecol Reprod Med.* 2010;20(12):347–352.

Iyengar S, Acheson N. Premalignant vulval conditions. *Obstet Gynaecol Reprod Med.* 2008;18(3):60–63.

Kyrgiou M, Shafi MI. Colposcopy and cervical intra-epithelial neoplasia. *Obstet Gynaecol Reprod Med.* 2010;20(5):38–46.

Kyrgiou M, Shafi MI. Invasive cancer of the cervix. *Obstet Gynaecol Reprod Med.* 2010;20(5):47–54.

Palmer J, Gillespie A. Palliative care in gynaecological oncology. *Obstet Gynaecol Reprod Med.* 2012;22(5):123–128.

Peevor R, Fiander AN. Human papillomavirus (including vaccination). *Obstet Gynaecol Reprod Med.* 2010;20(10):295–299.

Robinson Z, Edey K, Murdoch J. Invasive vulval cancer. *Obstet Gynaecol Reprod Med.* 2011;21(5):129–136.

Shafi MI, Earl H, Tan LT. *Gynaecological Oncology.* Cambridge: Cambridge University Press; 2010.

Symonds IM. Screening for gynaecological conditions. *Obstet Gynaecol Reprod Med.* 2012. Available: https://doi.org/10.1016/j.ogrm.2012.11.005.

Taylor SE, Kirwan JM. Ovarian cancer: current management and future directions. *Obstet Gynaecol Reprod Med.* 2012;22(2):33–37.

Chapter 21

*Altman D, Väyrynen T, Engh ME et al; Nordic Transvaginal Mesh Group. Anterior colporrhaphy versus transvaginal mesh for pelvic-organ prolapse. *N Engl J Med.* 2011;364:1826–1836.

DeLancey JO. Anatomic aspects of vaginal eversion after hysterectomy. *Am J Obstet Gynecol.* 1992;166:1717.

National Institutes for Health and Clinical Excellence. Clinical Guideline 40. *Urinary Incontinence. The Management of Urinary Incontinence in Women;* 2006. Available: http://www.nice.org.uk/nicemedia/pdf/CG40NICEguideline.pdf.

*Ward K, Hilton P, United Kingdom and Ireland Tension-free Vaginal Tape Trial Group. Prospective multicentre randomised trial of tension-free vaginal tape and colposuspension as primary treatment for stress incontinence. *BMJ.* 2002; 325:67–70.

Appendix A

Croissant K, Shafi MI. Preoperative and postoperative care in gynaecology. *Obstet Gynaecol Reprod Med.* 2009;(3):68–74.

National Institute for Clinical Excellence (NICE). Clinical Guidline 46. *Venous Thromboembolism: Reducing the Risk of Venous Thromboembolism (Deep Vein Thrombosis and Pulmonary Embolism) in Inpatients Undergoing Surgery;* 2010. Available: https://www.ncbi.nlm.nih.gov/pmc/articles/PMC1871784/.

Royal College of Obstetricians and Gynaecologists Clinical Governance Advice No. 6. *Obtaining Valid Consent;* 2008. Available: http://www.rcog.org.uk/files/rcog-corp/CGA6-15072010.pdf.

Scottish Intercollegiate Guidelines Network (SIGN). *Postoperative Management in Adults. A Practical Guide to Postoperative Care for Clinical Staff.* Edinburgh: SIGN; 2004.

Sharp HT. Prevention and management of complications from gynecologic surgery. *Obstet Gynecol Clin N Am.* 2010;37(3): 461–467.

Appendix B

General Medical Council. Confidentiality: Supplementary Guidance. Available: www.gmc-uk.org.

General Medical Council. Research: The Role and Responsibilities of Doctors. Available: www.gmc-uk.org.

McSherry R, Pearce P, eds. *Clinical Governance: A Guide to Implementation for Healthcare Professionals.* 2nd ed. Oxford: Blackwell; 2007.

Royal College of Obstetricians & Gynaecologists Clinical Governance Advice No. 5. *Understanding Audit;* 2003. Available: https://www.rcog.org.uk/en/guidelines-research-services/guidelines/clinical-governance-advice-5/.

Royal College of Obstetricians and Gynaecologists. *Guideline Compendium: A Compendium of College Guidelines Available.* London: RCOG Press; 2006.

Royal College of Obstetricians and Gynaecologists Clinical Governance Advice No. 2. *Improving Patient Safety: Risk Management for Maternity and Gynaecology*; 2009. Available: https://www.rcog.org.uk/globalassets/documents/guidelines/clinical-governance-advice/cga2improvingpatien.

Scottish Intercollegiate Guidelines Network. SIGN 50. *A Guideline Developer's Handbook*. Scottish Intercollegiate Guidelines Network; 2011:23–27. Available: https://www.sign.ac.uk/assets/sign50_2011.pdf.

Appendix C

Breen KJ, Cordner SM, Thomson CJH, et al. *Good Medical Practice: Professionalism, Ethics and Law*. Melbourne: Cambridge University Press; 2010.

Chamberlain GVP, ed. *How to Avoid Medico-legal Problems in Obstetrics and Gynaecology*. 2nd ed. London: RCOG; 1992.

Clements RV. *Safe Practice in Obstetrics and Gynaecology. A Medico-legal Handbook*. Edinburgh: Churchill Livingstone; 1994.

Further websites

Since the publication of the last edition, the availability of online resources has expanded exponentially. Many of these are open source, and the issue is no longer whether there is information the reader can access online, but which information is reliable and detailed enough for the student who wants to study an area in greater detail yet concise enough not to overwhelm them.

We have included a number of online resources within the relevant sections, but it should be noted that both the Royal College of Obstetrics and Gynaecology (RCOG) in the UK and the Royal Australian and New Zealand College of Obstetrics and Gynaecology (RANZCOG) and the National Institute for Health and Care Excellence publish statements and guidelines about clinical practice. These not only provide a summary of what is considered best practice in each country but often themselves contain further links to other material and reference original evidence. They have the added advantage of being more regularly updated than most textbooks. It should be noted that as documents are updated the URL may change. If you are unable to access the relevant webpage using the URLs listed in the chapters, you can copy the URL into your search engine for the relevant contents webpage given here and search by name for the information.

The National Institute for Clinical Excellence guidelines

http://www.nice.org.uk/guidance/index.jsp?action=byTopic&o=7252.

The Royal College of Obstetrics and Gynaecology (RCOG)

Green-top guidelines

http://www.rcog.org.uk/guidelines?filter0%5B%5D=10.

Clinical governance advice

http://www.rcog.org.uk/guidelines?filter0%5B%5D=6.

Joint guidelines

http://www.rcog.org.uk/guidelines?filter0%5B%5D=11.

National evidence-based guidelines

http://www.rcog.org.uk/guidelines?filter0%5B%5D=12.

Royal Australian and New Zealand College of Obstetrics and Gynaecology (RANZCOG) statements on women's health

Obstetrics

https://www.ranzcog.edu.au/statements-Guidelines/Obstetrics.

Gynaecology

https://www.ranzcog.edu.au/Statements-Guidelines/Gynaecology.

General

https://www.ranzcog.edu.au/Statements-Guidelines/General.

Other websites

The National Electronic Library for Health has links to guidelines for both the UK and United States on: http://www.evidence.nhs.uk.

The most recent version of the Confidential Enquiry into Maternal Deaths in the United Kingdom: http://onlinelibrary.wiley.com/doi/10.1111/bjo.2011.118.issue-s1/issuetoc.

The most recent report on maternal deaths in Australia from the Australian Institute of Health and Welfare: http://www.aihw.gov.au/WorkArea/DownloadAsset.aspx?id=10737421514.

Index

Note: Page numbers followed by "f" indicate figures, "t" indicate tables and "b" indicate boxes.